Basic and Advanced Bayesian Structural Equation Modeling

WILEY SERIES IN PROBABILITY AND STATISTICS

Established by WALTER A. SHEWHART and SAMUEL S. WILKS

A complete list of the titles in this series appears at the end of this volume.

Basic and Advanced Bayesian Structural Equation Modeling

With Applications in the Medical and Behavioral Sciences

Xin-Yuan Song and Sik-Yum Lee

Department of Statistics, The Chinese University of Hong Kong

WILEY

A John Wiley & Sons, Ltd., Publication

This edition first published 2012

Registered office
John Wiley & Sons Ltd, The Atrium, Southern Gate, Chichester, West Sussex, PO19 8SQ, United Kingdom

For details of our global editorial offices, for customer services and for information about how to apply for permission to reuse the copyright material in this book please see our website at www.wiley.com.

Library of Congress Cataloging-in-Publication Data

Lee, Sik-Yum.
Basic and Advanced Bayesian Structural Equation Modeling: With Applications in the Medical and Behavioral Sciences / Sik-Yum Lee and Xin-Yuan Song.
p. cm.
Includes bibliographical references and index.
ISBN 978-0-470-66952-5 (hardback)
1. Structural equation modeling. 2. Bayesian statistical decision theory. I. Song, Xin-Yuan. II. Title.
QA278.3.L439 2012
519.5′3–dc23

2012012199

MIX
Paper from responsible sources
FSC® C013604
FSC www.fsc.org

A catalogue record for this book is available from the British Library.

ISBN: 978-0-470-66952-5

Typeset in 10/12pt Times by Aptara Inc., New Delhi, India

For our family members:

Yulin and Haotian Wu;
Mable, Anna, and Timothy Lee

Contents

About the authors

Xin-Yuan Song is an associate professor at the Department of Statistics of the Chinese University of Hong Kong. She earned her PhD in Statistics at the Chinese University of Hong Kong. She serves as an associate editor for *Psychometrika*, and as a member of the editorial board of *Frontiers in Quantitative Psychology and Measurement* and the *Open Journal of Statistics*. Her research interests are in structural equation models, latent variable models, Bayesian methods, survival analysis, and statistical computing. She has published over 80 papers in prestigious international journals.

Sik-Yum Lee is an emeritus professor of statistics at the Chinese University of Hong Kong. He earned his PhD in biostatistics at the University of California, Los Angeles. He received a distinguished service award from the International Chinese Statistical Association, is a former president of the Hong Kong Statistical Society, and is an elected member of the International Statistical Institute and a Fellow of the American Statistical Association. He had served as an associate editor for *Psychometrika* and *Computational Statistics & Data Analysis*, and as a member of the editorial board of the *British Journal of Mathematical and Statistical Psychology*, *Structural Equation Modeling*, and the *Chinese Journal of Medicine*. His research interests are in structural equation models, latent variable models, Bayesian methods, and statistical diagnostics. He is editor of the *Handbook on Structural Equation Models* and author of *Structural Equation Modeling: A Bayesian Approach*, and over 160 papers.

Preface

Latent variables that cannot be directly measured by a single observed variable are frequently encountered in substantive research. In establishing a model to reflect reality, it is often necessary to assess various interrelationships among observed and latent variables. Structural equation models (SEMs) are well recognized as the most useful statistical model to serve this purpose. In past years, even the standard SEMs were widely applied to behavioral, educational, medical, and social sciences through commercial software, such as AMOS, EQS, LISREL, and M*plus*. These programs basically use the classical covariance structure analysis approach. In this approach, the hypothesized covariance structure of the observed variables is fitted to the sample covariance matrix. Although this works well for many simple situations, its performance is not satisfactory in dealing with complex situations that involve complicated data and/or model structures.

Nowadays, the Bayesian approach is becoming more popular in the field of SEMs. Indeed, we find that when coupled with data augmentation and Markov chain Monte Carlo (MCMC) methods, this approach is very effective in dealing with complex SEMs and/or data structures. The Bayesian approach treats the unknown parameter vector $\boldsymbol{\theta}$ in the model as random and analyzes the posterior distribution of $\boldsymbol{\theta}$, which is essentially the conditional distribution of $\boldsymbol{\theta}$ given the observed data set. The basic strategy is to augment the crucial unknown quantities such as the latent variables to achieve a complete data set in the posterior analysis. MCMC methods are then implemented to obtain various statistical results. The book *Structural Equation Modeling: A Bayesian Approach*, written by one of us (Sik-Yum Lee) and published by Wiley in 2007, demonstrated several advantages of the Bayesian approach over the classical covariance structure analysis approach. In particular, the Bayesian approach can be applied to deal efficiently with nonlinear SEMs, SEMs with mixed discrete and continuous data, multilevel SEMs, finite mixture SEMs, SEMs with ignorable and/or nonignorable missing data, and SEMs with variables coming from an exponential family.

The recent growth of SEMs has been very rapid. Many important new results beyond the scope of *Structural Equation Modeling* have been achieved. As SEMs have wide applications in various fields, many new developments are published not only in journals in social and psychological methods, but also in biostatistics and statistical computing, among others. In order to introduce these useful developments to researchers in different fields, it is desirable to have a textbook or reference book that includes those new contributions. This is the main motivation for writing this book.

Similar to *Structural Equation Modeling*, the theme of this book is the Bayesian analysis of SEMs. Chapter 1 provides an introduction. Chapter 2 presents the basic concepts of standard SEMs and provides a detailed discussion on how to apply these models in practice. Materials in this chapter should be useful for applied researchers. Note that we regard the nonlinear SEM as a standard SEM because some statistical results for analyzing this model can be easily obtained through the Bayesian approach. Bayesian estimation and model comparison are discussed in Chapters 3 and 4, respectively. Chapter 5 discusses some practical SEMs, including models with mixed continuous and ordered categorical data, models with variables coming from an exponential family, and models with missing data. SEMs for analyzing heterogeneous data are presented in Chapters 6 and 7. Specifically, multilevel SEMs and multisample SEMs are discussed in Chapter 6, while finite mixture SEMs are discussed in Chapter 7. Although some of the topics in Chapters 3–7 have been covered by *Structural Equation Modeling*, we include them in this book for completeness. To the best of our knowledge, materials presented in Chapters 8–13 do not appear in other textbooks. Chapters 8 and 9 respectively discuss second-order growth curve SEMs and a dynamic two-level multilevel SEM for analyzing various kinds of longitudinal data. A Bayesian semiparametric SEM, in which the explanatory latent variables are modeled through a general truncated Dirichlet process, is introduced in Chapter 10. The purposes for introducing this model are to capture the true distribution of explanatory latent variables and to handle nonnormal data. Chapter 11 deals with SEMs with unordered categorical variables. The main aim is to provide SEM methodologies for analyzing genotype variables, which play an important role in developing useful models in medical research. Chapter 12 introduces an SEM with a general nonparametric structural equation. This model is particularly useful when researchers have no idea about the functional relationships among outcome and explanatory latent variables. In the statistical analysis of this model, the Bayesian P-splines approach is used to formulate the nonparametric structural equation. As we show in Chapter 13, the Bayesian P-splines approach is also effective in developing transformation SEMs for dealing with extremely nonnormal data. Here, the observed nonnormal random vector is transformed through the Bayesian P-splines into a random vector whose distribution is close to normal. Chapter 14 concludes the book with a discussion. In this book, concepts of the models and the Bayesian methodologies are illustrated through analyses of real data sets in various fields using the software WinBUGS, R, and/or our tailor-made C codes. Chapters 2–4 provide the basic concepts of SEMs and the Bayesian approach. The materials in the subsequent chapters are basically self-contained. To understand the material in this book, all that is required are some fundamental concepts of statistics, such as the concept of conditional distributions.

We are very grateful to organizations and individuals for their generous support in various respects. The Research Grant Council of the Hong Kong Special Administration Region has provided financial support such as GRF446609 and GRF404711 for our research and for writing this book. The World Value Study Group, World Values Survey, 1981–1984 and 1990–1993, the World Health Organization WHOQOL group, Drs. D. E. Morisky, J. A. Stein, J. C. N. Chan, Y. I. Hser, T. Kwok, H. S. Ip, M. Power and Y. T. Hao have been kind enough to let us have their data sets. The Department of Epidemiology and Public Health of the Imperial College, School of Medicine at St. Mary's Hospital (London, UK) provided their WinBUGS software. Many of our graduate students and research collaborators, in particular J. H. Cai, J. H. Pan, Z. H. Lu, P. F. Liu, J. Chen, D. Pan, H. J. He, K. H. Lam, X. N. Feng,

B. Lu, and Y. M. Xia, made very valuable comments which led to improvements to the book. We are grateful to all the wonderful people on the John Wiley editorial staff, particularly Richard Leigh, Richard Davies, Heather Kay, Prachi Sinha Sahay, and Baljinder Kaur for their continued assistance, encouragement and support of our work. Finally, we owe deepest thanks for our family members for their constant support and love over many years.

This book features an accompanying website:
`www.wiley.com/go/medical_behavioral_sciences`

1

Introduction

1.1 Observed and latent variables

Observed variables are those that can be directly measured, such as systolic blood pressure, diastolic blood pressure, waist–hip ratio, body mass index, and heart rate. Measurements from observed variables provide data as the basic source of information for statistical analysis. In medical, social, and psychological research, it is common to encounter latent constructs that cannot be directly measured by a single observed variable. Simple examples are intelligence, health condition, obesity, and blood pressure. To assess the nature of a latent construct, a combination of several observed variables is needed. For example, systolic blood pressure and diastolic blood pressure should be combined to evaluate blood pressure; and waist–hip ratio and body mass index should be combined to evaluate obesity. In statistical inference, a latent construct is analyzed through a latent variable which is appropriately defined by a combination of several observed variables.

For practical research in social and biomedical sciences, it is often necessary to examine the relationships among the variables of interest. For example, in a study that focuses on kidney disease of type 2 diabetic patients (see Appendix 1.1), we have data from the following observed key variables: plasma creatine (PCr), urinary albumin creatinine ratio (ACR), systolic blood pressure (SBP), diastolic blood pressure (DBP), body mass index (BMI), waist–hip ratio (WHR), glycated hemoglobin (HbAlc), and fasting plasma glucose (FPG). From the basic medical knowledge about kidney disease, we know that the severity of this disease is reflected by both PCr and ACR. In order to understand the effects of the explanatory (independent) variables such as SBP and BMI on kidney disease, one possible approach is to apply the well-known regression model by treating PCr and ACR as outcome (dependent) variables and regressing them on the observed explanatory (independent) variables as follows:

$$\text{PCr} = \alpha_1 \text{SBP} + \alpha_2 \text{DBP} + \alpha_3 \text{BMI} + \alpha_4 \text{WHR} + \alpha_5 \text{HbA1c} + \alpha_6 \text{FPG} + \epsilon_1, \quad (1.1)$$

$$\text{ACR} = \beta_1 \text{SBP} + \beta_2 \text{DBP} + \beta_3 \text{BMI} + \beta_4 \text{WHR} + \beta_5 \text{HbA1c} + \beta_6 \text{FPG} + \epsilon_2. \quad (1.2)$$

Basic and Advanced Bayesian Structural Equation Modeling: With Applications in the Medical and Behavioral Sciences,
First Edition. Xin-Yuan Song and Sik-Yum Lee.

From the estimates of the αs and βs, we can assess the effects of the explanatory variables on PCr and ACR. For example, based on the estimates of α_1 and β_1, we can evaluate the effects of SBP on PCr and ACR, respectively. However, this result cannot provide a clear and direct answer to the question about the effect of SBP on kidney disease. Similarly, the effects of other observed explanatory variables on kidney disease cannot be directly assessed from results obtained from regression analysis of equations (1.1) and (1.2). The deficiency of the regression model when applied to this study is due to the fact that kidney disease is a latent variable (construct) rather than an observed variable. A better approach is to appropriately combine PCr and ACR into a latent variable 'kidney disease (KD)' and regress this latent variable on the explanatory variables. Moreover, one may be interested in the effect of blood pressure rather than in the separate effects of SBP and DBP. Although the estimates of α_1 and α_2 can be used to examine the respective effects of SBP and DBP on PCr, they cannot provide a direct and clear assessment on the effect of blood pressure on PCr. Hence, it is desirable to group SBP and DBP together to form a latent variable that can be interpreted as 'blood pressure (BP)', and then use BP as an explanatory variable. Based on similar reasoning, {BMI, WHR} and {HbA1c, FPG} are appropriately grouped together to form latent variables that can be interpreted as 'obesity (OB)' and 'glycemic control (GC)', respectively. To study the effects of blood pressure, obesity, and glycemic control on kidney disease, we consider the following simple regression equation with latent variables:

$$\mathrm{KD} = \gamma_1 \mathrm{BP} + \gamma_2 \mathrm{OB} + \gamma_3 \mathrm{GC} + \delta. \tag{1.3}$$

This simple regression equation can be generalized to the multiple regression equation with product terms. For example, the following regression model can be used to assess the additional interactive effects among blood pressure, obesity, and glycemic control on kidney disease:

$$\begin{aligned} \mathrm{KD} = {} & \gamma_1 \mathrm{BP} + \gamma_2 \mathrm{OB} + \gamma_3 \mathrm{GC} + \gamma_4 (\mathrm{BP} \times \mathrm{OB}) + \gamma_5 (\mathrm{BP} \times \mathrm{GC}) \\ & + \gamma_6 (\mathrm{OB} \times \mathrm{GC}) + \delta. \end{aligned} \tag{1.4}$$

Note that studying these interactive effects by using the regression equations with the observed variables (see (1.1) and (1.2)) is extremely tedious.

It is obvious from the above simple example that incorporating latent variables in developing models for practical research is advantageous. First, it can reduce the number of variables in the key regression equation. Comparing equation (1.3) with (1.1) and (1.2), the number of explanatory variables is reduced from six to three. Second, as highly correlated observed variables are grouped into latent variables, the problem induced by multicollinearity is alleviated. For example, the multicollinearity induced by the highly correlated variables SBP and DBP in analyzing regression equation (1.1) or (1.2) does not exist in regression equation (1.3). Third, it gives better assessments on the interrelationships of latent constructs. For instance, direct and interactive effects among the latent constructs blood pressure, obesity, and glycemic control can be assessed through the regression model (1.4). Hence, it is important to have a statistical method that simultaneously groups highly correlated observed variables into latent variables and assesses interrelationships among latent variables through a regression model of latent variables. This strong demand is the motivation for the development of structural equation models.

1.2 Structural equation model

The structural equation model (SEM) is a powerful multivariate tool for studying interrelationships among observed and latent variables. This statistical method is very popular in behavioral, educational, psychological, and social research. Recently, it has also received a great deal of attention in biomedical research; see, for example, Bentler and Stein (1992) and Pugesek *et al.* (2003).

The basic SEM, for example, the widely used LISREL model (Jöreskogand Sörbom, 1996), consists of two components. The first component is a confirmatory factor analysis (CFA) model which groups the highly correlated observed variables into latent variables and takes the measurement error into account. This component can be regarded as a regression model which regresses the observed variables on a smaller number of latent variables. As the covariance matrix of the latent variables is allowed to be nondiagonal, the correlations/covariances of the latent variables can be evaluated. However, various effects of the explanatory latent variables on the key outcome latent variables of interest cannot be assessed by the CFA model of the first component. Hence, a second component is needed. This component is again a regression type model, in which the outcome latent variables are regressed on the explanatory latent variables. As a result, the SEM is conceptually formulated by the familiar regression type model. However, as latent variables in the model are random, the standard technique in regression analysis cannot be applied to analyze SEMs.

It is often important in substantive research to develop an appropriate model to evaluate a series of simultaneous hypotheses on the impacts of some explanatory observed and latent variables on the key outcome variables. Based on its particular formulation, the SEM is very useful for achieving the above objective. Furthermore, it is easy to appreciate the key idea of the SEM, and to apply it to substantive research; one only needs to understand the basic concepts of latent variables and the familiar regression model. As a result, this model has been extensively applied to behavioral, educational, psychological, and social research. Due to the strong demand, more than a dozen user-friendly SEM software packages have been developed; typical examples are AMOS, EQS6, LISREL, and Mplus. Recently, the SEM has become a popular statistical tool for biomedical and environmental research. For instance, it has been applied to the analysis of the effects of *in utero* methylmercury exposure on neurodevelopment (Sánchez *et al.*, 2005), to the study of ecological and evolutionary biology (Pugesek *et al.*, 2003), and to the evaluation of the interrelationships among latent domains in quality of life (e.g. Lee *et al.*, 2005).

1.3 Objectives of the book

Like most other statistical methods, the methodological developments of standard SEMs depend on crucial assumptions. More specifically, the most basic assumptions are as follows: (i) The regression model in the second component is based on a simple linear regression equation in which higher-order product terms (such as quadratic terms or interaction terms) cannot be assessed. (ii) The observed random variables are assumed to be continuous, and independently and identically normally distributed. As these assumptions may not be valid in substantive research, they induce limitations in applying SEMs to the analysis of real data in relation to complex situations. Motivated by the need to overcome these limitations, the growth of SEMs has been very rapid in recent years. New models and statistical methods have been developed to relax various aspects of the crucial assumptions for better analyses of complex data structure in practical research. These include, but are not limited to: nonlinear SEMs with covariates (e.g. Schumacker and Marcoulides, 1998; Lee and Song, 2003a); SEMs with mixed continuous, ordered and/or unordered categorical variables (e.g. Shi and Lee, 2000; Moustaki, 2003; Song and Lee, 2004; Song *et al.*, 2007); multilevel SEMs (e.g. Lee and Shi, 2001; Rabe-Hesketh *et al.*, 2004; Song and Lee, 2004; Lee and Song, 2005); mixture SEMs (e.g. Dolan and van der Maas, 1998; Zhu and Lee, 2001; Lee and Song, 2003b); SEMs with missing data (e.g. Jamshidian and Bentler, 1999; Lee and Tang, 2006; Song and Lee, 2006); SEMs with variables from exponential family distributions (e.g. Wedel and Kamakura, 2001; Song and Lee, 2007); longitudinal SEMs (Dunson, 2003; Song *et al.*, 2008); semiparametric SEMs (Lee *et al.*, 2008; Song *et al.*, 2009; Yang and Dunson, 2010; Song and Lu, 2010); and transformation SEMs (van Montfort *et al.*, 2009; Song and Lu, 2012). As the existing software packages in SEMs are developed on the basis of the covariance structure approach, and their primary goal is to analyze the standard SEM under usual assumptions, they cannot be effectively and efficiently applied to the analysis of the more complex models and/or data structures mentioned above. Blindly applying these software packages to complex situations has a very high chance of producing questionable results and drawing misleading conclusions.

In substantive research, data obtained for evaluating hypotheses of complex diseases are usually very complicated. In analyzing these complicated data, more subtle models and rigorous statistically methods are important for providing correct conclusions. In view of this, there is an urgent need to introduce into applied research statistically sound methods that have recently been developed. This is the main objective in writing this book. As we write, there has only been a limited amount of work on SEM. Bollen (1989) was devoted to standard SEMs and focused on the covariance structure approach. Compared to Bollen (1989), this book introduces more advanced SEMs and emphasizes the Bayesian approach which is more flexible than the covariance structure approach in handling complex data and models. Lee (2007) provides a Bayesian approach for analyzing the standard and more subtle SEMs. Compared to Lee (2007), the first four chapters of this book provide less technical discussions and explanations of the basic ideas in addition to the more involved, theoretical developments of the statistical methods, so that they can be understood without much difficulty by applied researchers. Another objective of this book is to introduce important models that have recently been developed and were not covered by Lee (2007), including innovative growth curve models and longitudinal SEMs for analyzing longitudinal data and for studying the dynamic changes of characteristics with respect to time; semiparametric SEMs for relaxing the normality assumption and for assessing the true distributions of explanatory latent variables; SEMs with a nonparametric structural equation for capturing the true general relationships among latent variables, and transformation SEMs for analyzing highly nonnormal data. We believe that these advanced SEMs are very useful in substantive research.

1.4 The Bayesian approach

A traditional method in analyzing SEMs is the covariance structure approach which focuses on fitting the covariance structure under the proposed model to the sample covariance matrix computed from the observed data. For simple SEMs, when the underlying distribution of the observed data is normal, this approach works fine with reasonably large sample sizes. However, some serious difficulties may be encountered in many complex situations in which deriving the covariance structure or obtaining an appropriate sample covariance matrix for statistical inferences is difficult.

Thanks to recent advances in statistical computing, such as the development of various efficient Markov chain Monte Carlo (MCMC) algorithms, the Bayesian approach has been extensively applied to analyze many complex statistical models. Inspired by its wide applications in statistics, we will use the Bayesian approach to analyze the advanced SEMs that are useful for medical and social-psychological research. Moreover, in formulating and fitting the model, we emphasize the raw individual random observations rather than the sample covariance matrix. The Bayesian approach coupled with the formulation based on raw individual observations has several advantages. First, the development of statistical methods is based on the first moment properties of the raw individual observations which are simpler than the second moment properties of the sample covariance matrix. Hence, it has the potential to be applied to more complex situations. Second, it produces a direct estimation of latent variables, which cannot be obtained with classical methods. Third, it directly models observed variables with their latent variables through the familiar regression equations; hence, it gives a more direct interpretation and can utilize the common techniques in regression such as outlier and residual analyses in conducting statistical analysis. Fourth, in addition to the information that is available in the observed data, the Bayesian approach allows the use of genuine prior information for producing better results. Fifth, the Bayesian approach provides more easily assessable statistics for goodness of fit and model comparison, and also other useful statistics such as the mean and percentiles of the posterior distribution. Sixth, it can give more reliable results for small samples (see Dunson, 2000; Lee and Song, 2004). For methodological researchers in SEMs, technical details that are necessary in developing the theory and the MCMC methods are given in the appendices to the chapters. Applied researchers who are not interested in the methodological developments can skip those appendices. For convenience, we will introduce the freely available software WinBUGS (Spiegelhalter, *et al.*, 2003) through analyses of simulated and real data sets. This software is able to produce reliable Bayesian statistics including the Bayesian estimates and their standard error estimates for a wide range of statistical models (Congdon, 2003) and for SEMs (Lee, 2007).

1.5 Real data sets and notation

We will use several real data sets for the purpose of motivating the models and illustrating the proposed Bayesian methodologies. These data sets are respectively related to the studies about: (i) job and life satisfaction, work attitude, and other related social-political issues; (ii) effects of some phenotype and genotype explanatory latent variables on kidney disease for type 2 diabetic patients; (iii) quality of life for residents of several countries, and for stroke patients; (iv) the development of and findings from an AIDS preventative intervention for Filipina commercial sex workers; (v) the longitudinal characteristics of cocaine and polydrug use; (vi) the functional relationships between bone mineral density (BMD) and its observed and latent determinants for old men; and (vii) academic achievement and its influential factors for American youth. Some information on these data sets is given in Appendix 1.1.

In the discussion of various models and their associated statistical methods, we will encounter different types of observations in relation to observable continuous and discrete variables or covariates; unobservable measurements in relation to missing data or continuous measurements underlying the discrete data; latent variables; as well as different types of

Table 1.1 Typical notation.

Symbol	Meaning
ω	Latent vector in the measurement equation
η	Outcome (dependent) latent vector in the structural equation
ξ	Explanatory (independent) latent vector in the structural equation
ϵ, δ	Random vectors of measurement errors
$\mathbf{\Lambda}$	Factor loading matrix in the measurement equation
$\mathbf{B}, \mathbf{\Pi}, \mathbf{\Gamma}, \mathbf{\Lambda}_\omega$	Matrices of regression coefficients in the structural equation
$\mathbf{\Phi}$	Covariance matrix of explanatory latent variables
$\mathbf{\Psi}_\epsilon, \mathbf{\Psi}_\delta$	Diagonal covariance matrices of measurement errors, with diagonal elements $\psi_{\epsilon k}$ and $\psi_{\delta k}$, respectively
$\alpha_{0\epsilon k}, \beta_{0\epsilon k}, \alpha_{0\delta k}, \beta_{0\delta k}$	Hyperparameters in the gamma distributions of $\psi_{\epsilon k}$ and $\psi_{\delta k}$
$\mathbf{R}_0, \rho_0$	Hyperparameters in the Wishart distribution related to the prior distribution of $\mathbf{\Phi}$
$\mathbf{\Lambda}_{0k}, \mathbf{H}_{0yk}$	Hyperparameters in the multivariate normal distribution related to the prior distribution of the kth row of $\mathbf{\Lambda}$ in the measurement equation
$\mathbf{\Lambda}_{0\omega k}, \mathbf{H}_{0\omega k}$	Hyperparameters in the multivariate normal distribution related to the prior distribution of the kth row of $\mathbf{\Gamma}$ in the structural equation
$\mathbf{I}_q$	A $q \times q$ identity matrix; sometimes we just use $\mathbf{I}$ to denote an identity matrix if its dimension is clear.

parameters, such as thresholds, structural parameters in the model, and hyperparameters in the prior distributions. Hence, we have a shortage of symbols. If the context is clear, some Greek letters may serve different purposes. For example, α has been used to denote an unknown threshold in defining an ordered categorical variable, and to denote a hyperparameter in some prior distributions. Nevertheless, some general notation is given in Table 1.1.

Appendix 1.1 Information on real data sets

Inter-university Consortium for Political and Social Research (ICPSR) data

The ICPSR data set was collected in the World Values Survey 1981–1984 and 1990–1993 project (World Values Study Group, ICPSR Version). The whole data set consists of answers to a questionnaire survey about work attitude, job and family life, religious belief, interest in politics, attitude towards competition, etc. The items that have been used in the illustrative examples in this book are given below.

Thinking about your reasons for doing voluntary work, please use the following five-point scale to indicate how important each of the reasons below have been in your own case (1 is unimportant and 5 is very important).

V 62 Religious beliefs 1 2 3 4 5

During the past few weeks, did you ever feel . . . (Yes: 1; No: 2)

V 89 Bored 1 2

V 91 Depressed or very unhappy 1 2

V 93 Upset because somebody criticized you 1 2

V 96 All things considered, how satisfied are you with your life as a whole these days?
1 2 3 4 5 6 7 8 9 10
Dissatisfied Satisfied

Here are some aspects of a job that people say are important. Please look at them and tell me which ones you personally think are important in a job. (Mentioned: 1; Not Mentioned: 2)

V 99 Good Pay 1 2

V 100 Pleasant people to work with 1 2

V 102 Good job security 1 2

V 103 Good chances for promotion 1 2

V 111 A responsible job 1 2

V 115 How much pride, if any, do you take in the work that you do?
1 A great deal 2 Some 3 Little 4 None

V 116 Overall, how satisfied or dissatisfied are you with your job?
1 2 3 4 5 6 7 8 9 10
Dissatisfied Satisfied

V 117 How free are you to make decisions in your job?
1 2 3 4 5 6 7 8 9 10
Not at all A great deal

V 129 When jobs are scarce, people should be forced to retire early,
1 Agree, 2 Neither, 3 Disagree

V 132 How satisfied are you with the financial situation of your household?
1 2 3 4 5 6 7 8 9 10
Dissatisfied Satisfied

V 176 How important is God in your life? 10 means very important and 1 means not at all important.

1 2 3 4 5 6 7 8 9 10

V 179 How often do you pray to God outside of religious services? Would you say . . .

1 Often 2 Sometimes
3 Hardly ever 4 Only in times of crisis 5 Never

V 180 Overall, how satisfied or dissatisfied are you with your home life?

1 2 3 4 5 6 7 8 9 10
Dissatisfied Satisfied

V 241 How interested would you say you are in politics?

1 Very interested 2 Somewhat interested
3 Not very interested 4 Not at all interested

Now I'd like you to tell me your views on various issues. How would you place your views on this scale? 1 means you agree completely with the statement on the left, 10 means you agree completely with the statement on the right, or you can choose any number in between.

V 252

1 2 3 4 5 6 7 8 9 10

Individual should take more responsibility for providing for themselves.

The state should take more responsibility to ensure that everyone is provided for.

V 253

1 2 3 4 5 6 7 8 9 10

People who are unemployed should have to take any job available or lose their unemployment benefits.

People who are unemployed should have the right to refuse a job they do not want.

V 254

1 2 3 4 5 6 7 8 9 10

Competition is good. It stimulates people to work hard and develop new ideas.

Competition is harmful. It brings out the worst in people.

V 255

1 2 3 4 5 6 7 8 9 10

In the long run, hard work usually brings a better life.

Hard work doesn't generally bring success – it's more a matter of luck and connections.

Please tell me for each of the following statements whether you think it can always be justified, never be justified, or something in between.

V 296 Claiming government benefits which you are not entitled to

1 2 3 4 5 6 7 8 9 10
Never Always

V 297 Avoiding a fare on public transport

1 2 3 4 5 6 7 8 9 10

Never Always

V 298 Cheating on tax if you have the chance

1 2 3 4 5 6 7 8 9 10

Never Always

V 314 Failing to report damage you've done accidentally to a parked vehicle

1 2 3 4 5 6 7 8 9 10

Never Always

I am going to read out some statements about the government and the economy. For each one, could you tell me how much you agree or disagree?

V 336 Our government should be made much more open to the public

1 2 3 4 5 6

Agree Completely Disagree Completely

V 337 We are more likely to have a healthy economy if the government allows more freedom for individuals to do as they wish

1 2 3 4 5 6

Agree Completely Disagree Completely

V 339 Political reform in this country is moving too rapidly

1 2 3 4 5 6

Agree Completely Disagree Completely

Type 2 diabetic patients data

The data set was collected from an applied genomics program conducted by the Institute of Diabetes, the Chinese University of Hong Kong. It aims to examine the clinical and molecular epidemiology of type 2 diabetes in Hong Kong Chinese, with particular emphasis on diabetic nephropathy. A consecutive cohort of 1188 type 2 diabetic patients was enrolled into the Hong Kong Diabetes Registry. All patients underwent a structured 4-hour clinical and biochemical assessment including renal function measured by plasma creatine (PCr) and urinary albumin creatinine ratio (ACR); continuous phenotype variables such as systolic blood pressure (SBP), diastolic blood pressure (DBP), body mass index (BMI), waist–hip ratio (WHR), glycated hemoglobin (HbA1c), fasting plasma glucose (FPG), non-high-density lipoprotein cholesterol (non-HDL-C), lower-density lipoprotein cholesterol (LDL-C), plasma triglyceride (TG); and multinomial genotype variables such as beta-3 adrenergic receptor (ADRβ3), beta-2 adrenergic receptor SNP1 (ADRβ21), beta-2 adrenergic receptor SNP2 (ADRβ22), angiotensin converting enzyme (DCP1 intro 16 del/ins (DCP1)), and angiotensin II receptor type 1 AgtR1 A1166C (AGTR1).

WHOQOL-BREF quality of life assessment data

The WHOQOL-100 assessment was developed by the WHOQOL group in 15 international field centers for the assessment of quality of life (QOL). The WHOQOL-BREF instrument is a short version of WHOQOL-100 consisting of 24 ordinal categorical items selected from the 100 items. This instrument was established to evaluate four domains: physical health, mental health, social relationships, and environment. The instrument also includes two ordinal categorical items for overall QOL and health-related QOL, giving a total of

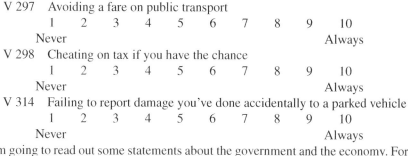

26 items. All of the items are measured on a 5-point scale (1 = 'not at all/very dissatisfied'; 2 = 'a little/dissatisfied'; 3 y 'moderate/neither'; 4 = 'very much/satisfied'; 5 = 'extremely/very satisfied'). The frequencies of the ordinal scores of the items are as follows:

	Ordinal score					
WHOQOL item	1	2	3	4	5	Number of incomplete obs.
Q1 Overall QOL	3	41	90	233	107	1
Q2 Overall health	32	127	104	154	58	0
Q3 Pain and discomfort	21	65	105	156	127	1
Q4 Medical treatment dependence	21	57	73	83	239	2
Q5 Energy and fatigue	15	57	166	111	118	8
Q6 Mobility	16	36	58	120	243	2
Q7 Sleep and rest	28	87	95	182	83	0
Q8 Daily activities	7	73	70	224	100	1
Q9 Work capacity	19	83	88	191	91	3
Q10 Positive feelings	2	30	141	241	59	2
Q11 Spirituality/personal beliefs	13	45	149	203	61	4
Q12 Memory and concentration	4	40	222	184	21	4
Q13 Bodily image and appearance	9	46	175	137	106	2
Q14 Self-esteem	13	72	130	210	50	0
Q15 Negative feelings	4	54	137	239	39	2
Q16 Personal relationships	8	46	68	218	134	1
Q17 Sexual activity	25	55	137	149	76	33
Q18 Social support	2	23	84	228	136	2
Q19 Physical safety and security	2	25	193	191	62	2
Q20 Physical environment	4	29	187	206	43	6
Q21 Financial resources	27	56	231	105	54	2
Q22 Daily life information	5	27	176	194	70	3
Q23 Participation in leisure activity	10	99	156	163	47	0
Q24 Living conditions	9	27	53	235	151	0
Q25 Health accessibility and quality	0	17	75	321	61	1
Q26 Transportation	8	38	61	253	113	2

AIDS preventative intervention data

The data set was collected from female commercial sex workers (CSWs) in 95 establishments (bars, night clubs, karaoke TV and massage parlours) in cities in the Philippines. The whole questionnaire consists of 134 items on areas of demographic knowledge, attitudes, beliefs, behaviors, self-efficacy for condom use, and social desirability. The primary concern is finding an AIDS preventative intervention for Filipina CSWs. Questions are as follows:

(1) How much of a threat do you think AIDS is to the health of people?
no threat at all/very small/moderate/strong/very great

(2) What are the chances that you yourself might get AIDS?
none/very small/moderate/great/very great

(3) How worried are you about getting AIDS?
not worried/slightly/moderate/very/extremely

How great is the risk of getting AIDS or the AIDS virus from sexual intercourse with someone:

(4) Who has the AIDS virus using a condom?
none/very small/moderate/great/very great

(5) Whom you don't know very well without using a condom?
none/very small/moderate/great/very great

(6) Who injects drugs?
none/very small/moderate/great/very great

(7) How often did you perform vaginal sex in the last 7 days?

(8) How often did you perform manual sex in the last 7 days?

(9) How often did you perform oral sex in the last 7 days?

(10) Have you ever used a condom? Yes/No

(11) Did you use a condom the last time you had sex? Yes/No

(12) Have you ever put a condom on a customer? Yes/No

(13) Do you agree or disagree that condoms make sex less enjoyable?
strongly agree/agree/neutral/disagree/strongly disagree

(14) Do you agree or disagree that condoms cause a man to lose his erection?
strongly agree/agree/neutral/disagree/strongly disagree

(15) Do you agree or disagree that condoms cause pain or discomfort?
strongly agree/agree/neutral/disagree/strongly disagree

(16) Are condoms available at your establishment for the workers who work there? Yes/No

(17) How much do you think you know the disease called AIDS?
nothing/a little/somewhat/moderate/a great deal

(18) Have you ever had an AIDS test? Yes/No

Polydrug use and treatment retention data

This is a longitudinal study of polydrug use initiated by California voters and conducted in five California counties in 2004. Proposition 36 directs drug offenders to a community-based drug treatment to reduce drug abuse using proven and effective treatment strategies. One of the objectives of the study is to examine why court-mandated offenders drop out of the drug treatment and to compare the characteristics, treatment experiences, perceptions, and outcomes of treatment completers (see Evans *et al.*, 2009). Data were collected from self-reported and administrative questionnaires about the retention of drug treatment (i.e.

the days of stay in treatment), drug use history, drug-related crime history, and service and test received for 1588 participants at intake, 3-month, and 12-month follow-up interviews. In addition, variables about treatment motivation (Mtsum01, Mtsum02, and Mtsum03) were collected at intake. Variables include:

(1) Drgplm30: Drug problems in past 30 days at intake, which ranges from 0 to 30.

(2) Drgday30: Drug use in past 30 days at intake, which ranges from 0 to 30.

(3) DrgN30: The number of kinds of drugs used in past 30 days at intake, which ranges from 1 to 8.

(4) Incar: The number of incarcerations in lifetime at intake, which ranges from 0 to 216.

(5) ArrN: The number of arrests in lifetime at intake, which ranges from 1 to 115.

(6) Agefirstarrest: The age of first arrest, which ranges from 6 to 57.

(7) Retent: Days of stay in treatment or retention, which ranges from 0 to 365.

(8) M12drg30: Primary drug use in past 30 days at 12-month interview, which ranges from 1 to 5.

(9) Servicem: Services received in past 3 months at TSI 3-month interview.

(10) DrugtestTX: The number of drug tests by TX in past 3 months at TSI 3-month interview, which ranges from 0 to 36.

(11) DrugtestCJ: The number of drug tests by criminal justice in past 3 months at TSI 3-month interview, which ranges from 0 to 12.

(12) Mtm01: Motivation subscale 1 at intake, which ranges from 1 to 5.

(13) Mtm02: Motivation subscale 2 at intake, which ranges from 1 to 5.

(14) Mtm03: Motivation subscale 3 at intake, which ranges from 1 to 5.

Quality of life for stroke survivors data

The setting for this study was the Prince of Wales Hospital (PWH) in Hong Kong which is a regional university hospital with 1500 beds serving a population of 0.7 million people. Patients with acute stroke within 2 days of admission were identified and followed up at 3, 6, and 12 months post stroke. All patients included in the study were ethnic Chinese. As the aim was to study those with a first disabling stroke, patients were excluded if they had moderate or severe premorbid handicap level (Rankin Scale score greater than 2). Outcome measures are obtained from questionnaires, which respectively measure respondents' functional status, depression, health-related quality of life, and handicap situation, including (1) modified Barthel Index (MBI) score, (2) Geriatric Depression Scale (GDS) score, (3) Chinese Mini-Mental State Examination (MMSE) score, (4) World Health Organization Quality of Life measure (abbreviated Hong Kong version) (WHOQOL BREF (HK)) score, and (5) the London Handicap Scale (LHS) score.

Cocaine use data

This data set was obtained from a longitudinal study about cocaine use conducted at the UCLA Center for Advancing Longitudinal Drug Abuse Research. The UCLA Center collected various measures from patients admitted in 1988–1989 to the West Los Angeles Veterans Affairs Medical Center and met the DSM III-R criteria for cocaine dependence. The cocaine-dependent patients were assessed at baseline, 1 year after treatment, 2 years after treatment, and 12 years after treatment in 2002. Measures at each time point include the following:

(1) cocaine use (CC), an ordered categorical variable coded 1 to 5 to denote days of cocaine use per month that are fewer than 2 days, 2–7 days, 8–14 days, 15–25 days, and more than 25 days, respectively;

(2) Beck inventory (BI), an ordered categorical variable coded 1 to 5 to denote scores that are less than 3.0, between 3.0 and 8.0, between 9.0 and 20.0, between 21 and 30, and greater than 30;

(3) depression (DEP), an ordered categorical variable based on the Hopkins Symptom Checklist-58 scores, coded 1 to 5 to denote scores that are less than 1.1, between 1.1 and 1.4, between 1.4 and 1.8, between 1.8 and 2.5, and greater than 2.5;

(4) number of friends (NF), an ordered categorical variable coded 1 to 5 to denote no friend, 1 friend, 2–4 friends, 5–8 friends, and more than 9 friends;

(5) 'have someone to talk to about problem (TP)', $\{0, 1\}$ for $\{\text{No, Yes}\}$;

(6) 'currently employed (EMP)', $\{0, 1\}$ for $\{\text{No, Yes}\}$;

(7) 'alcohol dependence (AD) at baseline', $\{0, 1\}$ for $\{\text{No, Yes}\}$.

Bone mineral density data

This data set was collected from a partial study on osteoporosis prevention and control. The study concerned the influence of serum concentration of sex hormones, their precursors and metabolites on bone mineral density (BMD) in older men. It was part of a multicenter prospective cohort study of risk factors of osteoporotic fractures in older people. A total of 1446 Chinese men aged 65 years and older were recruited using a combination of private solicitation and public advertising from community centers and public housing estates.

The observed variables include: spine BMD, hip BMD, estrone (E1), estrone sulfate (E1-S), estradiol (E2), testosterone (TESTO), 5-androstenediol (5-DIOL), dihydrotestosterone (DHT), androstenedione (4-DIONE), dehydroepiandrosterone (DHEA), DHEA sulfate (DHEA-S), androsterone (ADT), ADT glucuronide (ADT-G), 3α-diol-3G (3G), and 3α-diol-17G (17G). Weight and age were also measured.

National longitudinal surveys of youth (NLSY) data

The four-decade-long NLSY is one of the most comprehensive longitudinal studies of youths conducted in North America. The NLSY data include a nationally representative sample of youths who were 14–21 years old in 1979 and 29–36 years old in 1994.

The data set derived for the illustrative examples in this book includes 1660 observations and the following measures: the Peabody Individual Achievement Tests (PIAT) with continuous scales in the three domains of math, reading recognition, and reading comprehension; the Behavior Problem Index (BPI) with an ordinal scale in the five domains of anti-social, anxious, dependent, headstrong, and hyperactive behavior; home environment in the three domains of cognitive stimulation, emotional support, and household conditions; and friendship in the two domains of the number of boyfriends and the number of girlfriends. The instruments for measuring these constructs were taken from a short form of Home Observation for Measurement of the Environment (HOME) Inventory.

References

Bentler, P. M. and Stein, J. A. (1992) Structural equation models in medical research. *Statistical Methods in Medical Research*, **1**, 159–181.

Bollen, K. A. (1989) *Structural Equations with Latent Variables*. New York: John Wiley & Sons, Inc.

Congdon, P. (2003) *Applied Bayesian Modelling*. Chichester: John Wiley & Sons, Ltd.

Dolan, C. V. and van der Maas, H. L. J. (1998) Fitting multivariage normal finite mixtures subject to structural equation modeling. *Psychometrika*, **63**, 227–253.

Dunson, D. B. (2000) Bayesian latent variable models for clustered mixed outcomes. *Journal of the Royal Statistical Society, Series B*, **62**, 355–366.

Dunson, D. B. (2003) Dynamic latent trait models for multidimensional longitudinal data. *Journal of the American Statistical Association*, **98**, 555–563.

Evans, E., Li, L. and Hser, Y. I. (2009) Client and program factors associated with dropout from court mandated drug treatment. *Evaluation and Program Planning*, **32**, 204–212.

Jöreskog, K. G. and Sörbom, D. (1996) *LISREL 8: Structural Equation Modeling with the SIMPLIS Command Language*. Hove: Scientific Software International.

Jamshidian, M. and Bentler, P. M. (1999) ML estimation of mean and covariance structures with missing data using complete data routines. *Journal of Educational and Behavioral Statistics*, **24**, 21–41.

Lee, S. Y. (2007) *Structural Equation Modeling: A Bayesian Approach*. Chichester: John Wiley & Sons, Ltd.

Lee, S. Y. and Shi, J. Q. (2001) Maximum likelihood estimation of two-level latent variable models with mixed continuous and polytomous data. *Biometrics*, **57**, 787–794.

Lee, S. Y. and Song X. Y. (2003a) Model comparison of nonlinear structural equation models with fixed covariates. *Psychometrika*, **68**, 27–47.

Lee, S. Y. and Song, X. Y. (2003b) Maximum likelihood estimation and model comparison for mixtures of structural equation models with ignorable missing data. *Journal of Classification*, **20**, 221–255.

Lee, S. Y. and Song, X. Y. (2004) Evaluation of the Bayesian and maximum likelihood approaches in analyzing structural equation models with small sample sizes. *Multivariate Behavioral Research*, **39**, 653–686.

Lee, S. Y. and Song, X. Y. (2005) Maximum likelihood analysis of a two-level nonlinear structural equation model with fixed covariates. *Journal of Educational and Behavioral Statistics*, **30**, 1–26.

Lee, S. Y. and Tang, N. S. (2006) Bayesian analysis of nonlinear structural equation models with nonignorable missing data. *Psychometrika*, **71**, 541–564.

Lee, S. Y., Song, X. Y., Skevington, S. and Hao, Y. T. (2005) Application of structural equation models to quality of life. *Structural Equation Modeling – A Multidisciplinary Journal*, **12**, 435–453.

Lee, S. Y., Lu, B. and Song, X. Y. (2008) Semiparametric Bayesian analysis of structural equation models with fixed covariates. *Statistics in Medicine*, **27**, 2341–2360.

Moustaki, I. (2003) A general class of latent variable models for ordinal manifest variables with covariate effects on the manifest and latent variables. *British Journal of Mathematical and Statistical Psychology*, **56**, 337–357.

Pugesek, B. H., Tomer, A. and von Eye, A. (2003) *Structural Equation Modeling: Applications in Ecological and Evolutionary Biology*, Cambridge: Cambridge University Press.

Rabe-Hesketh, S., Skrondal, A. and Pickles, A. (2004) Generalized multilevel structural equation modeling. *Psychometrika*, **69**, 167–190.

Sánchez, B. N., Budtz-Jorgensen, E., Ryan L, M. and Hu, H. (2005) Structural equation models: a review with applications to environmental epidemiology. *Journal of the American Statistical Association*, **100**, 1443–1455.

Schumacker, R. E. and Marcoulides, G. A. (1998) *Interaction and Nonlinear Effects in Structural Equation Modeling*. Mahwah, NJ: Lawrence Erlbaum Associates.

Shi, J. Q. and Lee, S. Y. (2000) Latent variable models with mixed continuous and polytomous data. *Journal of the Royal Statistical Society, Series B*, **62**, 77–87.

Song, X. Y. and Lee, S. Y. (2004) Bayesian analysis of two-level nonlinear structural equation models with continuous and polytomous data. *British Journal of Mathematical and Statistical Psychology*, **57**, 29–52.

Song, X. Y. and Lee, S. Y. (2006) A maximum likelihood approach for multisample nonlinear structural equation models with missing continuous and dichotomous data. *Structural Equation Modeling – A Multidisciplinary Journal*, **13**, 325–351.

Song, X. Y. and Lee, S. Y. (2007) Bayesian analysis of latent variable models with non-ignorable missing outcomes from exponential family. *Statistics in Medicine*, **26**, 681–693.

Song, X. Y. and Lu, Z. H. (2010) Semiparametric latent variable models with Bayesian P-splines. *Journal of Computational and Graphical Statistics*, **19**, 590–608.

Song, X. Y. and Lu, Z. H. (2012) Semiparametric transformation models with Bayesian P-splines. *Statistics and Computing*, to appear.

Song, X. Y., Lee, S. Y., Ng, M. C. Y., So, W. Y. and Chan, J. C. N. (2007) Bayesian analysis of structural equation models with multinomial variables and an application to type 2 diabetic nephropathy. *Statistics in Medicine*, **26**, 2348–2369.

Song, X. Y., Lee, S. Y. and Hser, Y. I. (2008) A two-level structural equation model approach for analyzing multivariate longitudinal responses. *Statistics in Medicine*, **27**, 3017–3041.

Song, X. Y., Xia, Y. M. and Lee, S. Y. (2009) Bayesian semiparametric analysis of structural equation models with mixed continuous and unordered categorical variables. *Statistics in Medicine*, **28**, 2253–2276.

Spiegelhalter, D. J., Thomas, A., Best, N. G. and Lunn, D. (2003) *WinBugs User Manual. Version 1.4*. Cambridge: MRC Biostatistics Unit.

van Montfort, K., Mooijaart, A. and Meijerink, F. (2009) Estimating structural equation models with non-normal variables by using transformations. *Statistica Neerlandica*, **63**, 213–226.

Wedel, M. and Kamakura, W. A. (2001) Factor analysis with (mixed) observed and latent variables in the exponential family. *Psychometrika*, **66**, 515–530.

Yang, M. G. and Dunson, D. B. (2010) Bayesian semiparametric structural equation models with latent variables. *Psychometrika*, **75**, 675–693.

Zhu, H. T. and Lee, S. Y. (2001) A Bayesian analysis of finite mixtures in the LISREL model. *Psychometrika*, **66**, 133–152.

2

Basic concepts and applications of structural equation models

2.1 Introduction

Structural equation models (SEMs) are a flexible class of models that allow complex modeling of correlated multivariate data for assessing interrelationships among observed and latent variables. It is well known in the fields of social and psychological sciences that this class of models subsumes many widely used statistical models, such as regression, factor analysis, canonical correlations, and analysis of variance and covariance. Traditional methods for analyzing SEMs were mainly developed in psychometrics, and have been extensively applied in behavioral, educational, social, and psychological research in the past twenty years. Recently, SEMs have begun to attract a great deal of attention in public health, biological, and medical sciences. Today, due to strong demand in various disciplines, there are more than a dozen SEM software packages, such as AMOS, EQS6, LISREL, and Mplus. Among the various ways to specify SEMs in these software packages, we choose the key idea of the LISREL (Jöreskog and Sörbom, 1996) formulation in defining the basic model through a measurement equation and a structural equation. The main reasons for this choice are as follows: (i) The measurement and structural equations are very similar to the familiar regression models, hence more direct interpretation can be achieved and the common techniques in regression such as outlier and residual analyses can be employed. (ii) It makes a clear distinction between observed and latent variables. (iii) It directly models raw individual observations with latent variables, hence it can be naturally generalized to handle complex situations, and results in a direct estimation of latent variables. (iv) The development of statistical methodologies for subtle SEMs is more natural and comparatively easier.

In practical SEM applications, from the objective of a substantive study researchers usually know which are the outcome latent variables, and which are the explanatory latent variables of interest. In certain cases, a latent variable can be naturally defined by some observed variables;

Basic and Advanced Bayesian Structural Equation Modeling: With Applications in the Medical and Behavioral Sciences, First Edition. Xin-Yuan Song and Sik-Yum Lee.

for example, the latent variable 'blood pressure' is naturally formed by combining systolic and diastolic blood pressures. In other cases, researchers may need to carefully select observed variables in order to measure latent variables of interest to them. Substantive knowledge of the related study is important in making the decision. Hence, in practice, applied researchers of SEMs usually have prior information on which observed variables should be used to define a specific latent variable. This kind of information is useful in formulating the measurement equation which relates latent variables to their corresponding observed variables. From the above discussion, it is clear that the measurement equation in SEMs is a confirmatory tool rather than an exploratory tool. Basically, the measurement equation can be regarded as a confirmatory factor analysis model. The effects of explanatory latent variables on outcome latent variables are assessed through the structural equation in the model. The use of this equation is very similar to the application of the regression model, except that here latent variables are involved. At this stage, we may need to compare several structural equations, and select the most appropriate one. This is done by model comparison via reliable model comparison statistics.

The first objective of this chapter is to introduce the basic concepts of SEMs through models with a linear or a nonlinear structural equation. The second objective is to illustrate how to apply these models to substantive research. Illustrative examples with real medical studies will be presented.

2.2 Linear SEMs

Linear SEMs are formulated with a measurement equation and a structural equation with linear terms of explanatory latent variables. Under the assumption that the observed variables are continuous, and independently and identically normally distributed, the linear SEM is the most basic SEM.

Let $\mathbf{y} = (y_1, \ldots, y_p)^T$ be a $p \times 1$ vector of observed variables that have been selected for the analysis, and let $\boldsymbol{\omega} = (\omega_1, \ldots, \omega_q)^T$ be a $q \times 1$ vector of latent variables that are expected to be formed from the observed variables in $\mathbf{y}$. The link between the observed variables and all the latent variables in $\boldsymbol{\omega}$ is defined by the following measurement equation: for $j = 1, \ldots, p$,

$$y_j = \mu_j + \lambda_{j1}\omega_1 + \ldots + \lambda_{jq}\omega_q + \epsilon_j, \tag{2.1}$$

where μ_j is an intercept, the λ_{jk} are unknown coefficients that relate y_j and ω_k, and ϵ_j is the residual error. In factor analysis terminology, the λ_{jk} are called factor loadings. Now, according to the objective of the underlying substantive research, we have the following partition of $\boldsymbol{\omega} = (\boldsymbol{\eta}^T, \boldsymbol{\xi}^T)^T$, where $\boldsymbol{\eta}$ and $\boldsymbol{\xi}$ are $q_1 \times 1$ and $q_2 (= q - q_1) \times 1$ random vectors which respectively contain the outcome and explanatory latent variables in $\boldsymbol{\omega}$. The effects of $\boldsymbol{\xi} = (\xi_1, \ldots, \xi_{q_2})^T$ on $\boldsymbol{\eta} = (\eta_1, \ldots, \eta_{q_1})^T$ are assessed by the following structural equation: for $j = 1, \ldots, q_1$,

$$\eta_j = \gamma_{j1}\xi_1 + \ldots + \gamma_{jq_2}\xi_{q_2} + \delta_j, \tag{2.2}$$

where the γ_{jk} are unknown coefficients that represent the effects of ξ_k on η_j, and δ_j is the residual error. Equations (2.1) and (2.2) define the most basic linear SEM. These two equations can be rewritten in matrix notation: the measurement equation as

$$\mathbf{y} = \boldsymbol{\mu} + \boldsymbol{\Lambda}\boldsymbol{\omega} + \boldsymbol{\epsilon}, \tag{2.3}$$

and the structural equation as

$$\boldsymbol{\eta} = \boldsymbol{\Gamma}\boldsymbol{\xi} + \boldsymbol{\delta}, \tag{2.4}$$

where $\mathbf{y}$ is a $p \times 1$ random vector of observed variables, $\boldsymbol{\mu}$ is a $p \times 1$ vector of intercepts, $\boldsymbol{\Lambda}$ is a $p \times q$ unknown matrix of factor loadings, $\boldsymbol{\Gamma}$ is a $q_1 \times q_2$ unknown matrix of regression coefficients, and $\boldsymbol{\epsilon}$ and $\boldsymbol{\delta}$ are $p \times 1$ and $q_1 \times 1$ random vectors of measurement (residual) errors, respectively.

2.2.1 Measurement equation

Most applications of SEMs are related to the study of interrelationships among latent variables. In particular, they are useful for examining the effects of explanatory latent variables on outcome latent variables of interest. For such situations, researchers usually have in mind what observed variables should be selected from the whole data set for the analysis, and how these observed variables are grouped to form latent variables. The purpose of the measurement equation in an SEM is to relate the latent variables in $\boldsymbol{\omega}$ to the observed variables in $\mathbf{y}$. It represents the link between observed and latent variables, through the specified factor loading matrix $\boldsymbol{\Lambda}$. The vector of measurement error, $\boldsymbol{\epsilon}$, is used to take the residual errors into account.

The most important issue in formulating the measurement equation is to specify the structure of the factor loading matrix, $\boldsymbol{\Lambda}$, based on the knowledge of the observed variables in the study. Any element of $\boldsymbol{\Lambda}$ can be a free parameter or a fixed parameter with a preassigned value. The positions and the preassigned values of fixed parameters are decided on the basis of the prior knowledge of the observed variables and latent variables, and they are also related to the interpretations of latent variables. We give here a simple example by way of illustration.

Consider a study concerning the effects of blood pressure and obesity on kidney disease of type 2 diabetic patients. From its objective, we are interested in three latent variables, namely one outcome latent variable for kidney disease, and two explanatory latent variables for blood pressure and obesity. Based on the related medical knowledge, plasma creatine (PCr) and urinary albumin creatinine ratio (ACR) are measured to obtain the observed variables to form the latent variable 'kidney disease (KD)'; systolic blood pressure (SBP) and diastolic blood pressure (DBP) are measured to form latent variable 'blood pressure (BP)'; and body mass index (BMI) and waist–hip ratio (WHR) are measured to form the latent variable 'obesity (OB)'. From clear interpretation of BP, and the meaning of the observed variables, BP should only relate to SBP and DBP, but not to other observed variables. This rationale also applies to latent variables KD and OB. Thus, the system of measurement equations is defined as:

$$\begin{aligned}
\text{PCr} &= \mu_1 + \lambda_{11}\text{KD} + \epsilon_1, \\
\text{ACR} &= \mu_2 + \lambda_{21}\text{KD} + \epsilon_2, \\
\text{SBP} &= \mu_3 + \lambda_{32}\text{BP} + \epsilon_3, \\
\text{DBP} &= \mu_4 + \lambda_{42}\text{BP} + \epsilon_4, \\
\text{BMI} &= \mu_5 + \lambda_{53}\text{OB} + \epsilon_5, \\
\text{WHR} &= \mu_6 + \lambda_{63}\text{OB} + \epsilon_6,
\end{aligned} \tag{2.5}$$

or, in matrix notation,

$$\begin{bmatrix} \text{PCr} \\ \text{ACR} \\ \text{SBP} \\ \text{DBP} \\ \text{BMI} \\ \text{WHR} \end{bmatrix} = \begin{bmatrix} \mu_1 \\ \mu_2 \\ \mu_3 \\ \mu_4 \\ \mu_5 \\ \mu_6 \end{bmatrix} + \begin{bmatrix} \lambda_{11} & 0 & 0 \\ \lambda_{21} & 0 & 0 \\ 0 & \lambda_{32} & 0 \\ 0 & \lambda_{42} & 0 \\ 0 & 0 & \lambda_{53} \\ 0 & 0 & \lambda_{63} \end{bmatrix} \begin{bmatrix} \text{KD} \\ \text{BP} \\ \text{OB} \end{bmatrix} + \begin{bmatrix} \epsilon_1 \\ \epsilon_2 \\ \epsilon_3 \\ \epsilon_4 \\ \epsilon_5 \\ \epsilon_6 \end{bmatrix} \tag{2.6}$$

or

$$\mathbf{y} = \boldsymbol{\mu} + \boldsymbol{\Lambda}\boldsymbol{\omega} + \boldsymbol{\epsilon},$$

where $\mathbf{y}$, $\boldsymbol{\mu}$, $\boldsymbol{\Lambda}$, $\boldsymbol{\omega}$, and $\boldsymbol{\epsilon}$ are defined as in (2.3). The interpretations of μ_j and λ_{jk} are the same as the interpretations of the intercept and regression coefficient in a regression model. It is clear from (2.5) or (2.6) that λ_{jk} is the coefficient linking the observed variable y_j with the latent variable ω_k. For instance, PCr and KD are linked via λ_{11}. From the structure of $\boldsymbol{\Lambda}$, we know that KD is only linked with PCr and ACR, BP is only linked to SBP and DBP, and OB is only linked with BMI and WHR. As a result, the interpretation of the latent variables, KD, BP, and OB, is clear. This specific structure of $\boldsymbol{\Lambda}$ is called a non-overlapping structure. In applications of SEMs, factor loading matrices with non-overlapping structures are frequently used. In most situations, it is not necessary, or even not advisable, to use a more general structure for $\boldsymbol{\Lambda}$. For example, if λ_{12} in the above defined factor loading matrix $\boldsymbol{\Lambda}$ (see equation (2.6)) is not zero, then BP is also related to PCr. Hence, BP cannot be interpreted as blood pressure, and the effect of blood pressure on kidney disease cannot be clearly assessed. To achieve a better interpretation, we use $\boldsymbol{\Lambda}$ with a non-overlapping structure in all real applications presented in this book. In other applications with more observed and latent variables, we need to appropriately define a specific loading matrix to formulate their relationships. From the above discussion, we recognize that the measurement equation is a confirmatory tool with a specifically defined loading matrix.

2.2.2 Structural equation and one extension

Recall that the latent variables identified through the measurement equation are made up of a $q_1 \times 1$ vector of outcome latent variables and a $q_2 (= q - q_1) \times 1$ vector of explanatory latent variables. The choices of the outcome and explanatory latent variables, and thus the values of q_1 and q_2, are based on the objective of the substantive study. In the kidney disease study, it is clear from its objective that KD is the outcome latent variable, and BP and OB are the explanatory latent variables; hence, $q_1 = 1$ and $q_2 = 2$. The structural equation (2.2) or (2.4) is essentially a regression type model which regresses $\boldsymbol{\eta}$ on $\boldsymbol{\xi}$. For example, the structural equation of the kidney disease study might be:

$$\text{KD} = \gamma_1 \text{BP} + \gamma_2 \text{OB} + \delta. \tag{2.7}$$

This equation is linear in the variables and linear in the parameters. The interpretations of γ_1 and γ_2 are the same as in a regression model. Hence, they represent the magnitude of the expected changes in KD for a one-unit change in BP and OB, respectively. The outcome latent variables are only partially explained by the explanatory latent variables; the unexplained part is taken into account by the residual error δ.

Sometimes SEMs are called 'causal' models, and they have been used to achieve causality. We wish to emphasize that the structural equation is just a regression model with latent variables. Great care should be taken in using this regression type model to achieve causality. See Bollen (1989) for more discussion on this issue.

A slight extension of structural equation (2.4) that is particularly useful in business and social-psychological research is given by

$$\boldsymbol{\eta} = \boldsymbol{\Pi}\boldsymbol{\eta} + \boldsymbol{\Gamma}\boldsymbol{\xi} + \boldsymbol{\delta}, \tag{2.8}$$

where $\boldsymbol{\Pi}$ is a $q_1 \times q_1$ matrix of unknown coefficients, such that $\mathbf{I} - \boldsymbol{\Pi}$ is nonsingular and the diagonal elements of $\boldsymbol{\Pi}$ are zero; the definitions of $\boldsymbol{\Gamma}$, $\boldsymbol{\xi}$, and $\boldsymbol{\delta}$ are the same as before. Depending on the application, elements in $\boldsymbol{\Pi}$ and $\boldsymbol{\Gamma}$ can be fixed to preassigned values. This structural equation allows some outcome latent variables to depend on the other outcome latent variables through an appropriately defined $\boldsymbol{\Pi}$. For example, we wish to study the effects of BP and OB on KD, as well as a disease A that is represented by an outcome latent variable η_A. Moreover, suppose that it is also of interest to examine the possible effect of KD on disease A. To tackle this problem, the following structural equation can be used:

$$\begin{pmatrix} \mathrm{KD} \\ \eta_A \end{pmatrix} = \begin{pmatrix} 0 & 0 \\ \pi & 0 \end{pmatrix} \begin{pmatrix} \mathrm{KD} \\ \eta_A \end{pmatrix} + \begin{pmatrix} \gamma_1 & \gamma_2 \\ \gamma_3 & \gamma_4 \end{pmatrix} \begin{pmatrix} \mathrm{BP} \\ \mathrm{OB} \end{pmatrix} + \begin{pmatrix} \delta \\ \delta_A \end{pmatrix}. \tag{2.9}$$

Here, $\boldsymbol{\eta} = (\mathrm{KD}, \eta_A)^T$, π is the unknown coefficient that represents the effect of KD on disease A, and $\boldsymbol{\Gamma}$ is the parameter matrix with elements γ_i. The relationship of KD with BP and OB is again given by equation (2.7), while the relationship of disease A with KD, BP, and OB is given by

$$\eta_A = \pi\,\mathrm{KD} + \gamma_3\mathrm{BP} + \gamma_4\mathrm{OB} + \delta_A. \tag{2.10}$$

By allowing elements in $\boldsymbol{\Pi}$ and $\boldsymbol{\Gamma}$ to be fixed at any preassigned values, structural equation (2.8) achieves considerable flexibility in handling rather complex relationships among latent variables. More general structural equations with fixed covariates and nonlinear terms of latent variables will be discussed in Sections 2.3. and 2.4.

2.2.3 Assumptions of linear SEMs

Like most statistical models, the standard linear SEMs involve some assumptions. In practical applications of SEMs, it is important to make sure that these assumptions are valid. Let $\{\mathbf{y}_i, i = 1, \ldots, n\}$ be the observed data set with a sample size n, where $\mathbf{y}_i$ can be modeled via the linear SEM with latent variables $\boldsymbol{\eta}_i$ and $\boldsymbol{\xi}_i$, and measurement errors $\boldsymbol{\epsilon}_i$ and $\boldsymbol{\delta}_i$, as defined by the measurement equation (2.3) and the structural equation (2.8). For $i = 1, \ldots, n$, the assumptions of the model are as follows:

Assumption A1: The random vectors of residual errors $\boldsymbol{\epsilon}_i$ are independently and identically distributed (i.i.d.) according to $N[\mathbf{0}, \boldsymbol{\Psi}_\epsilon]$, where $\boldsymbol{\Psi}_\epsilon$ is a diagonal covariance matrix.

Assumption A2: The random vectors of explanatory latent variables $\boldsymbol{\xi}_i$ are i.i.d. according to $N[\mathbf{0}, \boldsymbol{\Phi}]$, where $\boldsymbol{\Phi}$ is a general covariance matrix.

Assumption A3: The random vectors of residual errors $\boldsymbol{\delta}_i$ are i.i.d. according to $N[\mathbf{0}, \boldsymbol{\Psi}_\delta]$, where $\boldsymbol{\Psi}_\delta$ is a diagonal covariance matrix.

Assumption A4: $\boldsymbol{\delta}_i$ is independent of $\boldsymbol{\xi}_i$, and $\boldsymbol{\epsilon}_i$ is independent of $\boldsymbol{\omega}_i$ and $\boldsymbol{\delta}_i$.

These assumptions introduce three unknown parameter matrices, namely $\mathbf{\Phi}$, $\mathbf{\Psi}_\epsilon$, and $\mathbf{\Psi}_\delta$. As $\boldsymbol{\eta}_i$ is a linear combination of $\boldsymbol{\xi}_i$ and $\boldsymbol{\delta}_i$, the observations of $\boldsymbol{\eta}_i$ are also i.i.d. according to a normal distribution with a covariance matrix that depends on $\mathbf{\Pi}$, $\mathbf{\Gamma}$, $\mathbf{\Phi}$, and $\mathbf{\Psi}_\delta$. As a result, based on Assumptions A2 and A3 and the linear structural equation, the $\boldsymbol{\omega}_i$ are i.i.d. according to a normal distribution. Moreover, these assumptions also implicitly restrict $\mathbf{y}_i$ to be i.i.d. according to a normal distribution.

2.2.4 Model identification

Model identification is an issue relevant to all SEMs. In general, consider an SEM with a measurement equation and a structural equation which are formulated with an unknown parameter vector $\boldsymbol{\theta}$. The traditional definition of identification is based on $\mathbf{\Sigma}(\boldsymbol{\theta})$, the population covariance matrix of the observed variables in $\mathbf{y}$. The model is said to be identified if, for any $\boldsymbol{\theta}_1$ and $\boldsymbol{\theta}_2$, $\mathbf{\Sigma}(\boldsymbol{\theta}_1) = \mathbf{\Sigma}(\boldsymbol{\theta}_2)$ implies $\boldsymbol{\theta}_1 = \boldsymbol{\theta}_2$ (see Bollen, 1989). This definition is difficult to apply to a complex SEM whose $\mathbf{\Sigma}(\boldsymbol{\theta})$ is very complicated or even impossible to derive. For almost all existing SEMs, the parameters involved in the measurement equation are different from those involved in the structural equation, which are respectively defined by distinctive $\boldsymbol{\theta}$ and $\boldsymbol{\theta}^*$ that have no common elements. Hence, we consider a definition of identification on the basis of the fundamental measurement equation $m(\boldsymbol{\theta})$ and structural equation $s(\boldsymbol{\theta}^*)$. We regard the measurement equation as identified if, for any $\boldsymbol{\theta}_1$ and $\boldsymbol{\theta}_2$, $m(\boldsymbol{\theta}_1) = m(\boldsymbol{\theta}_2)$ implies $\boldsymbol{\theta}_1 = \boldsymbol{\theta}_2$. Similarly, we regard the structural equation as identified if, for any $\boldsymbol{\theta}_1^*$ and $\boldsymbol{\theta}_2^*$, $s(\boldsymbol{\theta}_1^*) = s(\boldsymbol{\theta}_2^*)$ implies $\boldsymbol{\theta}_1^* = \boldsymbol{\theta}_2^*$. Moreover, we regard the SEM as identified if both of its measurement equation and structural equation are identified. General necessary and sufficient conditions to guarantee the identifiability of an SEM are difficult to find. Hence, in practical applications of SEMs, we are mainly concerned with the sufficient conditions for achieving an identified model. For most SEMs, such sufficient conditions are usually available, and the issue is approached on a problem-by-problem basis.

Consider linear SEMs. The measurement equation is not identified without imposing some identification condition. This is because, for any nonsingular matrix $\mathbf{M}$, we have

$$\begin{aligned} \mathbf{y} &= \boldsymbol{\mu} + \mathbf{\Lambda}\boldsymbol{\omega} + \boldsymbol{\epsilon} = \boldsymbol{\mu} + \mathbf{\Lambda}\mathbf{M}\mathbf{M}^{-1}\boldsymbol{\omega} + \boldsymbol{\epsilon} \\ &= \boldsymbol{\mu} + \mathbf{\Lambda}^*\boldsymbol{\omega}^* + \boldsymbol{\epsilon}, \end{aligned} \tag{2.11}$$

where $\mathbf{\Lambda}^* = \mathbf{\Lambda}\mathbf{M}$, and $\boldsymbol{\omega}^* = \mathbf{M}^{-1}\boldsymbol{\omega}$, which is a random vector of latent variables with distribution $N[\mathbf{0}, \mathbf{M}^{-1}\mathbf{\Phi}^+(\mathbf{M}^{-1})^T]$, where $\mathbf{\Phi}^+$ is the covariance matrix of $\boldsymbol{\omega}$. To identify the measurement equation, we have to impose restrictions on $\mathbf{\Lambda}$ and/or $\mathbf{\Phi}^+$, such that the only nonsingular matrix $\mathbf{M}$ that satisfies the imposed conditions is the identity matrix. A simple and common method is to use a $\mathbf{\Lambda}$ with the non-overlapping structure. Consider an illustrative example with $p = 10$ observed variables and $q = 3$ latent variables, in which the first four observed variables are related to ω_1, and the next and the last three observed variables are related to ω_2 and ω_3, respectively. A non-overlapping structure of $\mathbf{\Lambda}$ is given by:

$$\mathbf{\Lambda}^T = \begin{bmatrix} 1 & \lambda_{21} & \lambda_{31} & \lambda_{41} & 0 & 0 & 0 & 0 & 0 & 0 \\ 0 & 0 & 0 & 0 & 1 & \lambda_{62} & \lambda_{72} & 0 & 0 & 0 \\ 0 & 0 & 0 & 0 & 0 & 0 & 0 & 1 & \lambda_{93} & \lambda_{10,3} \end{bmatrix},$$

where the 1 and 0 elements are known parameters with fixed values, and the other λ_{jk} are unknown parameters. The fixed value 1 is used to introduce a scale to the corresponding latent variable. In the above $\mathbf{\Lambda}$, λ_{11} is fixed at 1 to introduce a scale to ω_1. The choice of λ_{11} is for convenience only; we can fix λ_{21} at 1 and let λ_{11} be an unknown parameter. Similarly, we can fix λ_{62} (or λ_{72}) and λ_{93} (or $\lambda_{10,3}$) at 1, and let λ_{52} and λ_{83} be unknown parameters. Based on the objective of the underlying confirmatory study about the target latent variables, and the meaning of the observed variables, we can have a clear idea about the positions of the parameters fixed as 0; see Section 2.2.1.

There are other methods to identify the measurement equation. For instance, we may allow λ_{11}, λ_{52}, and/or λ_{83} in the above defined $\mathbf{\Lambda}$ to be unknown parameters, and fix the diagonal elements of $\mathbf{\Phi}^+$ as 1. This method restricts the variances of latent variables to the value 1; hence $\mathbf{\Phi}^+$ is a correlation matrix. As this method is not convenient for identifying an SEM with a structural equation, and induces complication in the Bayesian analysis (see Chapter 3), we use the first identification method to identify the measurement equation throughout this book. After obtaining the estimates of $\mathbf{\Lambda}$ and $\mathbf{\Phi}^+$, say $\hat{\mathbf{\Lambda}}$ and $\hat{\mathbf{\Phi}}^+$, we can get another set of equivalent estimates $\hat{\mathbf{\Lambda}}^*(=\hat{\mathbf{\Lambda}}\mathbf{M})$ and $\hat{\mathbf{\Phi}}^*(=\mathbf{M}^{-1}\hat{\mathbf{\Phi}}^+(\mathbf{M}^{-1})^T)$ that satisfy the same measurement equation via a nonsingular matrix $\mathbf{M}$; see equation (2.11).

For almost all applications of SEMs, the structural equation is identified with the identified measurement equation and latent variables. If necessary, the above simple method (via fixing appropriate parameters) for identifying the measurement equation can be used to identify the structural equation.

2.2.5 Path diagram

A path diagram is a pictorial representation of the measurement and structural equations. It is useful for presenting and discussing the related SEM. In practical applications, it is worthwhile to draw the path diagram related to the hypothesized SEM for effective communication of the basic conceptual ideas behind the real study. We first use the example discussed in Sections 2.2.1 and 2.2.2 to illustrate the relation between a path diagram and the measurement and structural equations. The following conventions (see Jöreskog and Sörbom, 1996) are assumed:

(i) Observed variables such as x- and y-variables are enclosed in rectangles or squares. Latent variables such as ξ- and η-variables are enclosed in ellipses or circles. Residual errors such as δ- and ϵ-variables are included in the path diagram but are not enclosed.

(ii) A one-way arrow between two variables indicates a postulated direct influence of one variable on another. A two-way arrow between two variables indicates that these variables may be correlated.

(iii) The coefficient associated with each arrow indicates the corresponding parameter.

(iv) All direct influences of one variable on another are included in the path diagram. Hence the nonexistence of an arrow between two variables means that these two variables are assumed not directly related.

Sometimes two-way arrows between two correlated variables and/or residual errors are not drawn for clarity. Moreover, the means (intercepts) may not be presented in the diagram.

Following the above conventions, the path diagram for the SEM with measurement equation (2.6) and structural equation (2.7) is presented in Figure 2.1.

In applying SEMs to a complex study with nontrivial relationships among variables, it is worthwhile to first draw the path diagram that can clearly display the conceptual ideas behind

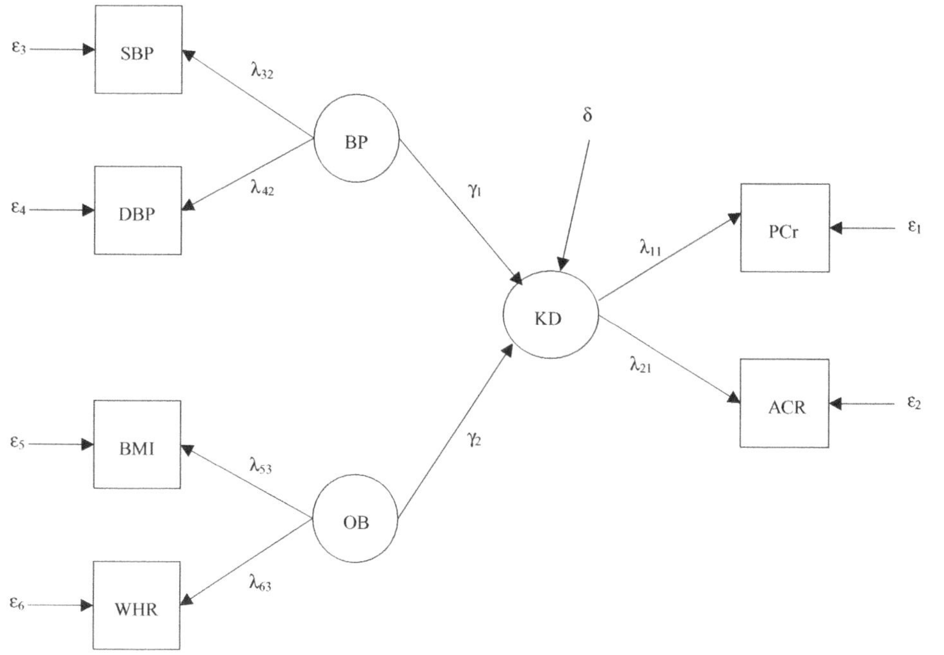

Figure 2.1 Path diagram representing the model defined by (2.6) and (2.7).

the real situation and then formulate the measurement and structural equations of the model on the basis of the path diagram.

2.3 SEMs with fixed covariates

In the basic linear SEMs, $\mathbf{y} = (y_1, \ldots, y_p)^T$ on the left-hand side of the measurement equation (see equation (2.3)) contains only observed variables in the model. These observed variables are related to the latent variables in $\boldsymbol{\omega}$ through the loading matrix $\boldsymbol{\Lambda}$. In order to develop better models, it is often desirable to incorporate explanatory observed variables on the right-hand sides of the measurement and structural equations. In the SEM field these explanatory observed variables are regarded as fixed covariates. Accommodation of fixed covariates into the measurement equation provides additional information about the latent exposure and thus reduces estimation uncertainty for the latent variables. For the structural equation, fixed covariates give more ingredients to account for the outcome latent variables, in addition to the explanatory latent variables. Hence, the residual errors in both equations can be reduced by incorporating fixed covariates.

2.3.1 The model

SEMs with fixed covariates are defined as follows. For an observed $p \times 1$ random vector $\mathbf{y}$, the measurement equation is given by:

$$\mathbf{y} = \mathbf{A}\mathbf{c} + \boldsymbol{\Lambda}\boldsymbol{\omega} + \boldsymbol{\epsilon}, \tag{2.12}$$

where $\mathbf{A}$ is a $p \times r_1$ matrix of unknown coefficients, $\mathbf{c}$ is an $r_1 \times 1$ vector of fixed covariates (with their values observed), and $\mathbf{\Lambda}$, $\boldsymbol{\omega}$, and $\boldsymbol{\epsilon}$ are defined exactly as in Section 2.2. A simple example with one intercept and one fixed covariate c_2 is:

$$\begin{bmatrix} y_1 \\ \vdots \\ y_p \end{bmatrix} = \begin{bmatrix} a_{11} & a_{12} \\ \vdots & \vdots \\ a_{p1} & a_{p2} \end{bmatrix} \begin{bmatrix} 1 \\ c_2 \end{bmatrix} + \begin{bmatrix} \lambda_{11} & \cdots & \lambda_{1q} \\ \vdots & \ddots & \vdots \\ \lambda_{p1} & \cdots & \lambda_{pq} \end{bmatrix} \begin{bmatrix} \omega_1 \\ \vdots \\ \omega_q \end{bmatrix} + \begin{bmatrix} \epsilon_1 \\ \vdots \\ \epsilon_p \end{bmatrix}, \qquad (2.13)$$

or

$$y_j = a_{j1} + a_{j2}c_2 + \lambda_{j1}\omega_1 + \ldots + \lambda_{jq}\omega_q + \epsilon_j, \quad j = 1, \ldots, p.$$

If $c_2 = 0$, and letting $\mu_j = a_{j1}$, equation (2.13) reduces to equation (2.3). The structural equation is defined by:

$$\boldsymbol{\eta} = \mathbf{Bd} + \mathbf{\Pi}\boldsymbol{\eta} + \mathbf{\Gamma}\boldsymbol{\xi} + \boldsymbol{\delta}, \qquad (2.14)$$

where $\mathbf{B}$ is a $q_1 \times r_2$ matrix of unknown coefficients, $\mathbf{d}$ is an $r_2 \times 1$ vector of fixed covariates, and $\mathbf{\Pi}$, $\mathbf{\Gamma}$, and $\boldsymbol{\delta}$ are defined exactly as in Section 2.2. Note that $\mathbf{c}$ and $\mathbf{d}$ may have common elements; and (2.14) reduces to (2.8) if $\mathbf{d} = \mathbf{0}$. A simple example with one outcome latent variable η, two covariates d_1 and d_2, three explanatory latent variables ξ_1, ξ_2, and ξ_3, and $\Pi = 0$ is given by:

$$\eta = b_1 d_1 + b_2 d_2 + \gamma_1\xi_1 + \gamma_2\xi_2 + \gamma_3\xi_3 + \delta,$$

where $\mathbf{B} = (b_1, b_2)$ and $\mathbf{\Gamma} = (\gamma_1, \gamma_2, \gamma_3)$.

The assumptions of SEMs with fixed covariates are the same as Assumptions A1–A4 given in Section 2.2.3. As fixed covariates are observed values, the distributions of $\boldsymbol{\omega}_i$ and $\mathbf{y}_i$ are still normal. Similarly to the basic linear SEMs, SEMs with fixed covariates can be identified by fixing appropriate parameters at given values.

2.3.2 An artificial example

The purpose of this artificial example is to illustrate the flexibility in incorporating fixed covariates in SEMs. After researchers have decided their main objective, it is desirable to use a path diagram to obtain a clear picture of the hypothesized model. For a complicated model with many fixed covariates and latent variables, the path diagram representing the whole model will be rather involved. For clarity, it is worth using one path diagram to represent the measurement equation, and another path diagram to represent the structural equation. Moreover, if the context is clear, the residual errors can be ignored in the path diagrams.

Suppose that the main objective is to study diabetic kidney disease, with emphasis on assessing effects of blood pressure, obesity, lipid control as well as some covariates on that disease. Based on known medical knowledge, data on the observed variables {PCr, ACR, SBP, DBP, BMI, WHR} $= (y_1, \ldots, y_6)$ were collected in order to form the latent variables 'kidney disease (KD)', 'blood pressure (BP)' and 'obesity (OB)'; see also Section 2.2.1. Data from observed variables {non-high-density lipoprotein cholesterol (non-HDL-C), low-density lipoprotein cholesterol (LDL-C), plasma triglyceride (TG)} $= (y_7, y_8, y_9)$ were collected to measure the latent variable 'lipid control (LIP)'. The relationships of the aforementioned observed and latent variables can be assessed through measurement equation (2.3) with an appropriate non-overlapping loading matrix $\mathbf{\Lambda}$. Now, if we know from the real study that smoking and daily alcohol intake may be helpful in relating these observed and latent variables, then 'smoking (c_1)' and 'alcohol (c_2)' can be accommodated in the measurement equation as follows:

$$\begin{bmatrix} y_1 \\ y_2 \\ y_3 \\ y_4 \\ y_5 \\ y_6 \\ y_7 \\ y_8 \\ y_9 \end{bmatrix} = \begin{bmatrix} a_{11} & a_{12} \\ a_{21} & a_{22} \\ a_{31} & a_{32} \\ a_{41} & a_{42} \\ a_{51} & a_{52} \\ a_{61} & a_{62} \\ a_{71} & a_{72} \\ a_{81} & a_{82} \\ a_{91} & a_{92} \end{bmatrix} \begin{bmatrix} c_1 \\ c_2 \end{bmatrix} + \begin{bmatrix} \lambda_{11} & 0 & 0 & 0 \\ \lambda_{21} & 0 & 0 & 0 \\ 0 & \lambda_{32} & 0 & 0 \\ 0 & \lambda_{42} & 0 & 0 \\ 0 & 0 & \lambda_{53} & 0 \\ 0 & 0 & \lambda_{63} & 0 \\ 0 & 0 & 0 & \lambda_{74} \\ 0 & 0 & 0 & \lambda_{84} \\ 0 & 0 & 0 & \lambda_{94} \end{bmatrix} \begin{bmatrix} \text{KD} \\ \text{BP} \\ \text{OB} \\ \text{LIP} \end{bmatrix} + \begin{bmatrix} \epsilon_1 \\ \epsilon_2 \\ \epsilon_3 \\ \epsilon_4 \\ \epsilon_5 \\ \epsilon_6 \\ \epsilon_7 \\ \epsilon_8 \\ \epsilon_9 \end{bmatrix}. \qquad (2.15)$$

To study various explanatory effects on the key outcome latent variable KD, we can incorporate fixed covariates 'age (d_1)' and 'gender (d_2)' into the structural equation as follows:

$$\text{KD} = b_1\text{age} + b_2\text{gender} + \gamma_1\text{BP} + \gamma_2\text{OB} + \gamma_3\text{LIP} + \delta, \qquad (2.16)$$

where b_1 and b_2, γ_1, γ_2, and γ_3 are unknown regression coefficients. The path diagram related to this model is presented in Figure 2.2. Note that the same fixed covariates c_1 and c_2 appear on both the left- and right-hand sides of the path diagram. Moreover, paths related to the residual errors and correlations among latent variables are not presented.

2.4 Nonlinear SEMs

Nonlinear SEMs are formulated with a measurement equation that is basically the same as in linear SEMs, and a structural equation that is nonlinear in the explanatory latent variables. The theoretical motivation for this generalization is natural; it is similar to the extension of simple regression with latent variables to multiple regression with latent variables. From a practical point of view, the development of nonlinear SEMs is motivated by the fact that nonlinear relations among latent variables are important for establishing more meaningful and correct models in some complicated situations; see Schumacker and Marcoulides (1998) and references therein on the importance of interaction and quadratic effects of latent variables in social and psychological research. In biomedical research, the importance of interaction effects has been increasingly recognized. In the study of pathogenesis of complex diseases, it is necessary to consider the gene–gene and gene–environment interactions (Chen *et al.*, 1999). In the case of diabetic kidney disease, there are interactions among glucose, lipid, and hemodynamic pathways in the activation of the renin angiotensin system (Fioretto *et al.*, 1998; Parving *et al.*, 1996).

2.4.1 Basic nonlinear SEMs

Let $\mathbf{y}$, $\boldsymbol{\mu}$, $\boldsymbol{\Lambda}$, $\boldsymbol{\epsilon}$, $\boldsymbol{\omega}$, $\boldsymbol{\eta}$, and $\boldsymbol{\xi}$ denote random vectors and parameters with the same definitions as in Section 2.2. The measurement equation of nonlinear SEMs is defined as

$$\mathbf{y} = \boldsymbol{\mu} + \boldsymbol{\Lambda}\boldsymbol{\omega} + \boldsymbol{\epsilon}, \qquad (2.17)$$

which has exactly the same form as in (2.3). The structural equation is formulated as

$$\boldsymbol{\eta} = \boldsymbol{\Pi}\boldsymbol{\eta} + \boldsymbol{\Gamma}\mathbf{F}(\boldsymbol{\xi}) + \boldsymbol{\delta}, \qquad (2.18)$$

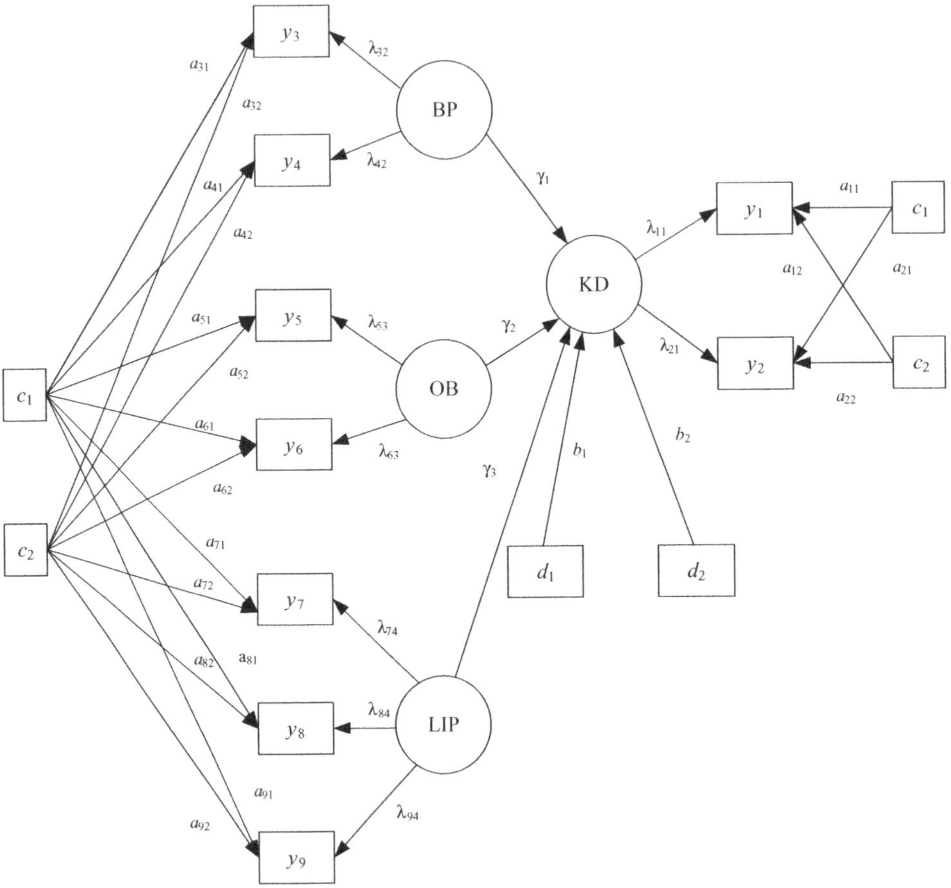

Figure 2.2 Path diagram representing the model defined by (2.15) and (2.16). The residual errors have been omitted.

where $\mathbf{\Pi}$, $\mathbf{\Gamma}$, and $\boldsymbol{\delta}$ are defined the same as before, and $\mathbf{F}(\boldsymbol{\xi}) = (f_1(\boldsymbol{\xi}), \ldots, f_t(\boldsymbol{\xi}))^T$ is a $t \times 1$ vector-valued function with nonzero, known, and linearly independent differentiable functions $f_1, \ldots, f_t$, and $t \geq q_2$.

Let $\{\mathbf{y}_i, i = 1, \ldots, n\}$ be the observed data set with a sample size n, where the $\mathbf{y}_i$ are modeled via a nonlinear SEM with latent variables $\boldsymbol{\eta}_i$ and $\boldsymbol{\xi}_i$, and measurement errors $\boldsymbol{\epsilon}_i$ and $\boldsymbol{\delta}_i$. The assumptions of the model for developing related statistical methods are the same as Assumptions A1–A4 given in Section 2.2.3. Note that, due to the presence of the nonlinear terms of $\boldsymbol{\xi}$ in $\mathbf{F}(\boldsymbol{\xi})$, the distributions of $\boldsymbol{\omega}_i$ and $\mathbf{y}_i$ are no longer normal. In other words, nonlinear SEMs do not assume that $\boldsymbol{\omega}_i$ and $\mathbf{y}_i$ are normal.

Similar to linear SEMs, the measurement equation of nonlinear SEMs can be identified by fixing appropriate parameters (particularly those in $\mathbf{\Lambda}$) at some given values. To achieve an identified structural equation, the choice of $\mathbf{F}(\boldsymbol{\xi})$ in the structural equation is not completely arbitrary. For example, the following obvious cases are not allowed: $\mathbf{F}_1(\boldsymbol{\xi}) = (\xi_1, \xi_2, \xi_1^2, \xi_1^2)^T$ and $\mathbf{F}_2(\boldsymbol{\xi}) = (\xi_1, \xi_2, \xi_1\xi_2, 0)^T$. They should be modified as $\mathbf{F}_1(\boldsymbol{\xi}) = (\xi_1, \xi_2, \xi_1^2)^T$ and

$\mathbf{F}_2(\boldsymbol{\xi}) = (\xi_1, \xi_2, \xi_1\xi_2)^T$, respectively. An example of identified structural equations is:

$$\begin{pmatrix}\eta_1\\ \eta_2\end{pmatrix} = \begin{pmatrix}0 & \pi\\ 0 & 0\end{pmatrix}\begin{pmatrix}\eta_1\\ \eta_2\end{pmatrix} + \begin{pmatrix}\gamma_{11} & \gamma_{12} & 0 & 0 & 0\\ \gamma_{21} & \gamma_{22} & \gamma_{23} & \gamma_{24} & \gamma_{25}\end{pmatrix}\begin{pmatrix}\xi_1\\ \xi_2\\ \xi_1^2\\ \xi_1\xi_2\\ \xi_2^2\end{pmatrix} + \begin{pmatrix}\delta_1\\ \delta_2\end{pmatrix}.$$

The interpretation of the parameter matrices $\boldsymbol{\Lambda}$, $\boldsymbol{\Pi}$, and $\boldsymbol{\Gamma}$ is basically the same as before; that is, they can be interpreted as regression coefficients in regression models. More care is needed to interpret the mean vector of $\mathbf{y}$. Let $\boldsymbol{\Lambda}_k^T$ be the kth row of $\boldsymbol{\Lambda}$. For $k = 1, \ldots, p$, it follows from equation (2.3) that $E(y_k) = \mu_k + \boldsymbol{\Lambda}_k^T E(\boldsymbol{\omega})$. Although $E(\boldsymbol{\xi}) = \mathbf{0}$, it follows from equation (2.18) that $E(\boldsymbol{\eta}) \neq \mathbf{0}$ if $\mathbf{F}(\boldsymbol{\xi})$ is a vector-valued nonlinear function of $\boldsymbol{\xi}$ and $E(\mathbf{F}(\boldsymbol{\xi})) \neq 0$. Hence $E(\boldsymbol{\omega}) \neq \mathbf{0}$ and $E(y_k) \neq \mu_k$. Let $\boldsymbol{\Lambda}_k^T = (\boldsymbol{\Lambda}_{k\eta}^T, \boldsymbol{\Lambda}_{k\xi}^T)$ be a partition of $\boldsymbol{\Lambda}_k^T$ that corresponds to the partition of $\boldsymbol{\omega} = (\boldsymbol{\eta}^T, \boldsymbol{\xi}^T)^T$. Because $E(\boldsymbol{\xi}) = \mathbf{0}$ and $E(\boldsymbol{\eta}) = [(\mathbf{I} - \boldsymbol{\Pi})^{-1}\boldsymbol{\Gamma}]E(\mathbf{F}(\boldsymbol{\xi}))$, it follows from (2.17) that

$$E(y_k) = \mu_k + \boldsymbol{\Lambda}_{k\eta}^T E(\boldsymbol{\eta}) + \boldsymbol{\Lambda}_{k\xi}^T E(\boldsymbol{\xi}) = \mu_k + \boldsymbol{\Lambda}_{k\eta}^T[(\mathbf{I} - \boldsymbol{\Pi})^{-1}\boldsymbol{\Gamma}]E(\mathbf{F}(\boldsymbol{\xi})). \tag{2.19}$$

As $\mathbf{F}(\boldsymbol{\xi})$ is usually not very complicated in most practical applications, $E(\mathbf{F}(\boldsymbol{\xi}))$ is not very complex and thus the computation of $E(y_k)$ is not difficult.

2.4.2 Nonlinear SEMs with fixed covariates

Linear SEMs with fixed covariates can be naturally generalized to nonlinear SEMs with fixed covariates through the following measurement and structural equations:

$$\mathbf{y} = \mathbf{A}\mathbf{c} + \boldsymbol{\Lambda}\boldsymbol{\omega} + \boldsymbol{\epsilon}, \tag{2.20}$$

$$\boldsymbol{\eta} = \mathbf{B}\mathbf{d} + \boldsymbol{\Pi}\boldsymbol{\eta} + \boldsymbol{\Gamma}\mathbf{F}(\boldsymbol{\xi}) + \boldsymbol{\delta}, \tag{2.21}$$

where the definitions of the random vectors and the parameter matrices are the same as in Sections 2.2. and 2.3. In this model, the measurement equation is the same as in (2.12), while the structural equation can be regarded as a natural extension of equations (2.14) and (2.18). As a simple example, we consider a continuation of the artificial example as described in Section 2.3.2. Suppose that we wish to study various interactive effects of the explanatory latent variables BP, OB, and LIP on KD. To achieve our goal, we consider a model with its measurement equation given in (2.15), while the structural equation is formulated as

$$\begin{aligned}\mathrm{KD} = {} & b_1 d_1 + b_2 d_2 + \gamma_1 \mathrm{BP} + \gamma_2 \mathrm{OB} + \gamma_3 \mathrm{LIP} + \gamma_4(\mathrm{BP} \times \mathrm{OB}) + \gamma_5(\mathrm{BP} \times \mathrm{LIP})\\ & + \gamma_6(\mathrm{OB} \times \mathrm{LIP}) + \delta.\end{aligned} \tag{2.22}$$

In this formulation, $\mathbf{B} = (b_1, b_2)$, $\mathbf{d} = (d_1, d_2)^T$, $\boldsymbol{\Gamma} = (\gamma_1, \gamma_2, \gamma_3, \gamma_4, \gamma_5, \gamma_6)$, and $\mathbf{F}(\boldsymbol{\xi}) = (\mathrm{BP}, \mathrm{OB}, \mathrm{LIP}, \mathrm{BP} \times \mathrm{OB}, \mathrm{BP} \times \mathrm{LIP}, \mathrm{OB} \times \mathrm{LIP})^T$.

While the structural equation (2.21) can include nonlinear terms of $\boldsymbol{\xi}$ in predicting $\boldsymbol{\eta}$, it does not accommodate nonlinear terms of $\boldsymbol{\xi}$ and $\mathbf{d}$ simultaneously. A simple extension of the structural equation to cope with the above consideration is

$$\boldsymbol{\eta} = \boldsymbol{\Pi}\boldsymbol{\eta} + \boldsymbol{\Lambda}_\omega \mathbf{G}(\mathbf{d}, \boldsymbol{\xi}) + \boldsymbol{\delta}, \tag{2.23}$$

where $\mathbf{G}(\mathbf{d}, \boldsymbol{\xi}) = (g_1(\mathbf{d}, \boldsymbol{\xi}), \ldots, g_t(\mathbf{d}, \boldsymbol{\xi}))^T$ is a vector-valued function with nonzero, known, and linearly independent differentiable functions. A special case of this general structural equation is the one defined by (2.21) with $\boldsymbol{\Lambda}_\omega = (\mathbf{B}, \boldsymbol{\Gamma})$ and $\mathbf{G}(\mathbf{d}, \boldsymbol{\xi}) = (\mathbf{d}^T, \mathbf{F}(\boldsymbol{\xi})^T)^T$. The assumptions of this nonlinear SEM with nonlinear terms of covariates are the same as Assumptions A1–A4 given in Section 2.2.3. Moreover, identification of the model can be achieved via a method similar to that described in Section 2.2.4. Again, care should be taken to interpret the mean of $\mathbf{y}$. Using the same notation as in Section 2.4.1, we have

$$E(y_k) = \mathbf{A}_k^T \mathbf{c} + \boldsymbol{\Lambda}_{k\eta}^T [(\mathbf{I} - \boldsymbol{\Pi})^{-1} \boldsymbol{\Lambda}_\omega] E[\mathbf{G}(\mathbf{d}, \boldsymbol{\xi})], \tag{2.24}$$

where $\mathbf{A}_k^T$ is the kth row of $\mathbf{A}$. The artificial example presented above is again used to illustrate the key idea of incorporating nonlinear terms of fixed covariates and explanatory latent variables in the structural equation. The measurement equation is again defined by (2.15), while the structural equation can be formulated as

$$\begin{aligned} \mathrm{KD} = {} & b_1 d_1 + b_2 d_2 + \gamma_1 \mathrm{BP} + \gamma_2 \mathrm{OB} + \gamma_3 \mathrm{LIP} + \gamma_4 (\mathrm{BP} \times \mathrm{OB}) + \gamma_5 (\mathrm{BP} \times \mathrm{LIP}) \\ & + \gamma_6 (\mathrm{OB} \times \mathrm{LIP}) + \gamma_7 (d_1 \times \mathrm{BP}) + \gamma_8 (d_1 \times \mathrm{OB}) + \gamma_9 (d_2 \times \mathrm{OB}) \\ & + \gamma_{10} (d_2 \times \mathrm{LIP}) + \delta. \end{aligned} \tag{2.25}$$

Note that more complex product terms of d_1, d_2, BP, OB, and LIP can be assessed via other appropriately defined structural equations. The path diagram corresponding to structural equation (2.25) is presented in Figure 2.3. For clarity, and because the measurement equation is the same as before, Figure 2.3 does not include the observed variables in $\mathbf{y}$, and fixed covariates c_1 and c_2.

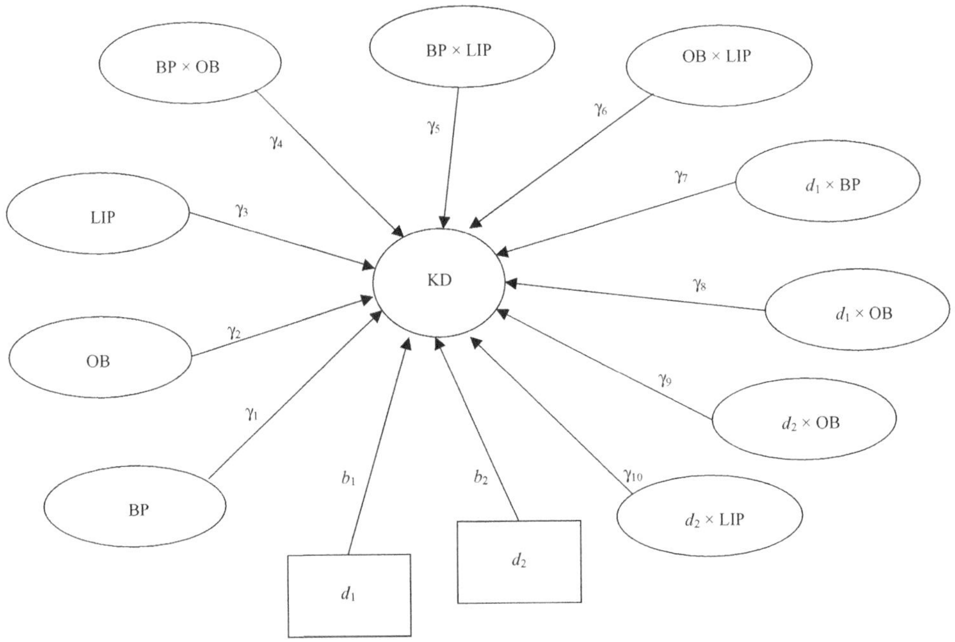

Figure 2.3 Path diagram representing structural equation (2.25). The residual error has been omitted.

In general, as the fixed covariates in $\mathbf{d}$ may come from arbitrary distributions that result in continuous or discrete data, and the functions f_j in $\mathbf{G}(\mathbf{d}, \boldsymbol{\xi})$ are differentiable functions which include any product terms as special cases, the nonlinear SEM defined by (2.20) and (2.23) (or (2.21)) can handle a wide range of situations.

2.4.3 Remarks

Due to the nonnormal distributions associated with the nonlinear terms of latent variables, development of statistical methods for inference based on the traditional approach of covariance structure analysis encounters certain difficulties. Several approaches have been proposed in the past; examples are the product-indicator method (e.g. Jaccard and Wan, 1995), the moment-based method (Wall and Amemiya, 2000), and the latent moderated structural equations (Klein and Moosbrugger, 2000) approaches. Most of these approaches used unnatural or technically involved techniques to handle the nonnormality problem. Hence, nonlinear SEMs have been regarded as complicated models. In the next chapter, we will discuss the application of the Bayesian approach to the analysis of SEMs. Using the Bayesian approach, the development of statistical methods for analyzing nonlinear SEMs is essentially the same as for linear SEMs. Hence, we regard nonlinear SEMs as standard models rather than complicated models.

2.5 Discussion and conclusions

Real analyses of most complicated studies (e.g. complex diseases) usually involve a large number of observed and latent variables of interest. Although the emphasis is on assessing the effects of explanatory latent variables on the key outcome latent variables, some particular explanatory latent variables may be significantly related to other explanatory latent variables and/or fixed covariates. For instance, in the artificial example discussed in Section 2.3.2, although KD is the key outcome latent variable, the explanatory latent variables BP and OB, as well as the fixed covariates, age (d_1) and gender (d_2), are also expected to have effects on the latent variable LIP. To provide a more concrete illustration, suppose that we are interested in assessing the SEM with the corresponding path diagram presented in Figure 2.4. Compared to the SEM presented in Figure 2.2, we also have: (i) two additional observed genetic variables GV1 and GV2 which correspond to a latent variable LGV, (ii) a path from LGV to LIP, (iii) a path from OB to LIP, and (iv) a path from age (d_1) to LIP.

The measurement equation is defined by:

$$\begin{bmatrix} y_1 \\ y_2 \\ y_3 \\ y_4 \\ y_5 \\ y_6 \\ y_7 \\ y_8 \\ y_9 \\ \mathrm{GV}_1 \\ \mathrm{GV}_2 \end{bmatrix} = \begin{bmatrix} a_{11} & a_{12} \\ a_{21} & a_{22} \\ a_{31} & a_{32} \\ a_{41} & a_{42} \\ a_{51} & a_{52} \\ a_{61} & a_{62} \\ a_{71} & a_{72} \\ a_{81} & a_{82} \\ a_{91} & a_{92} \\ 0 & 0 \\ 0 & 0 \end{bmatrix} \begin{bmatrix} c_1 \\ c_2 \end{bmatrix} + \begin{bmatrix} \lambda_{11} & 0 & 0 & 0 & 0 \\ \lambda_{21} & 0 & 0 & 0 & 0 \\ 0 & \lambda_{32} & 0 & 0 & 0 \\ 0 & \lambda_{42} & 0 & 0 & 0 \\ 0 & 0 & \lambda_{53} & 0 & 0 \\ 0 & 0 & \lambda_{63} & 0 & 0 \\ 0 & 0 & 0 & \lambda_{74} & 0 \\ 0 & 0 & 0 & \lambda_{84} & 0 \\ 0 & 0 & 0 & \lambda_{94} & 0 \\ 0 & 0 & 0 & 0 & \lambda_{10,5} \\ 0 & 0 & 0 & 0 & \lambda_{11,5} \end{bmatrix} \begin{bmatrix} \mathrm{KD} \\ \mathrm{BP} \\ \mathrm{OB} \\ \mathrm{LIP} \\ \mathrm{LGV} \end{bmatrix} + \begin{bmatrix} \epsilon_1 \\ \epsilon_2 \\ \epsilon_3 \\ \epsilon_4 \\ \epsilon_5 \\ \epsilon_6 \\ \epsilon_7 \\ \epsilon_8 \\ \epsilon_9 \\ \epsilon_{10} \\ \epsilon_{11} \end{bmatrix}. \tag{2.26}$$

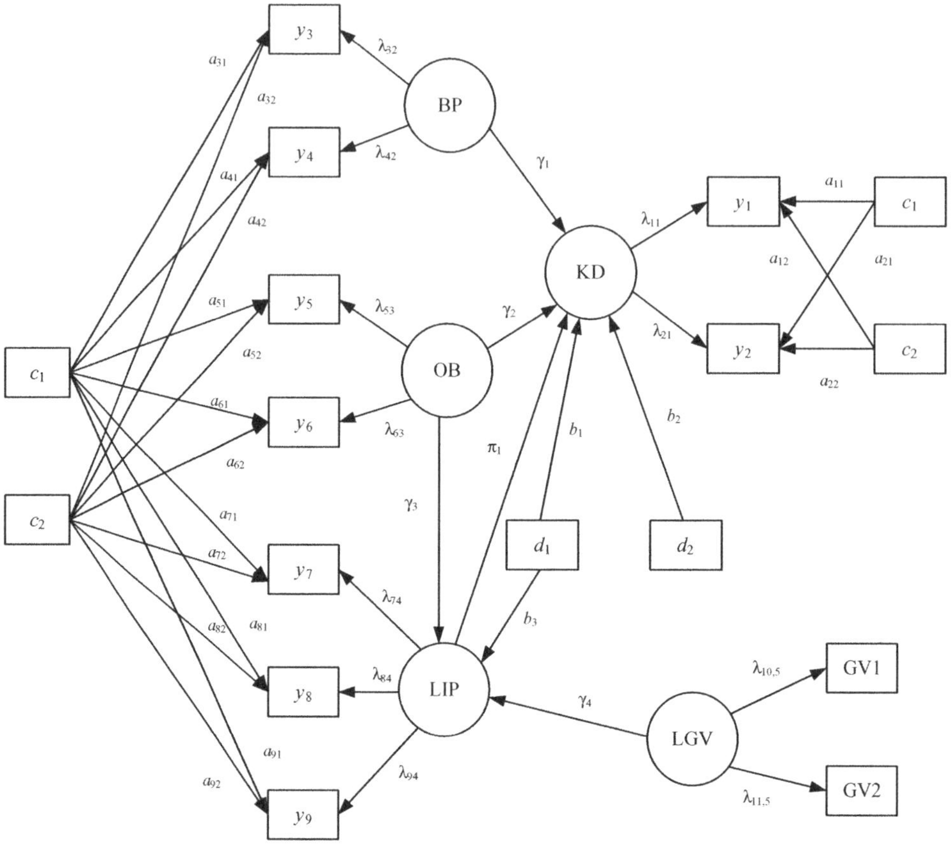

Figure 2.4 Path diagram representing the model defined by (2.26) and (2.27). The residual errors have been omitted.

To formulate the structural equation associated with this path diagram, LIP is treated as an outcome latent variable. More specifically, the structural equation is defined as:

$$\begin{pmatrix} \text{KD} \\ \text{LIP} \end{pmatrix} = \begin{pmatrix} b_1 & b_2 \\ b_3 & 0 \end{pmatrix} \begin{pmatrix} d_1 \\ d_2 \end{pmatrix} + \begin{pmatrix} 0 & \pi_1 \\ 0 & 0 \end{pmatrix} \begin{pmatrix} \text{KD} \\ \text{LIP} \end{pmatrix} + \begin{pmatrix} \gamma_1 & \gamma_2 & 0 \\ 0 & \gamma_3 & \gamma_4 \end{pmatrix} \begin{pmatrix} \text{BP} \\ \text{OB} \\ \text{LGV} \end{pmatrix} + \begin{pmatrix} \delta_1 \\ \delta_2 \end{pmatrix}. \tag{2.27}$$

Hence, through an appropriate formulation of the structural equation, SEMs provide considerable flexibility in assessing various kinds of relationships among latent variables and covariates. Here, as OB has a direct effect on LIP, which itself also has a direct effect on KD, OB has an indirect effect ($\pi_1 \times \gamma_3$) on KD. Hence, the total effect of OB on KD is $\gamma_2 + \pi_1\gamma_3$. Given the flexibility in formulating different structural equations, the above modeling concerning LIP can be considered for explanatory latent variables BP and OB.

In general, latent variables involved in the study of complex situations commonly have interrelationships with other observed and latent variables similar to those discussed above.

There is a temptation to develop a comprehensive SEM that takes into account all the interrelationships of the observed and latent variables. From a practical point of view, the following issues have to be carefully considered in the development of a comprehensive model:

(i) Due to the large amount of observed variables and latent variables, the size of the comprehensive SEM and the number of its unknown parameters are large. It is important to make sure the sample size of the available data set is large enough to yield accurate statistical results.

(ii) The data structures associated with complex situations are usually complicated. Researchers may encounter mixed types of continuous, ordered and unordered categorical data with missing entries, and hierarchical or heterogeneous structures. Although Bayesian methods (to be introduced in next chapter) are efficient and can be applied to handle such complex data, if the size of the proposed SEM and the number of parameters are large, we may encounter difficulties in achieving convergence of the related computing algorithm and thus in obtaining statistical results.

(iii) Researchers need to make sure that the hypothesized model can be analyzed under the proposed SEM framework. In this chapter, the most general SEM is the nonlinear SEM with fixed covariates defined by equations (2.20) and (2.23). This model has limitations. Note that the vector-valued function $\mathbf{G}(\mathbf{d}, \boldsymbol{\xi})$ for assessing nonlinear terms of $\mathbf{d}$ and $\boldsymbol{\xi}$ does not involve any outcome latent variables in $\boldsymbol{\eta}$. Hence, once a latent variable is treated as an outcome latent variable, nonlinear terms of this latent variable and interactive effects between this latent variable and other explanatory latent variables (or fixed covariates) cannot be used to predict the other outcome latent variables. For instance, consider the previous artificial example related to the SEM with structural equation (2.27). In this model, as LIP is treated as an outcome variable, it is an element in $\boldsymbol{\eta}$. Hence, it cannot be accommodated in $\mathbf{G}(\mathbf{d}, \boldsymbol{\xi})$, and nonlinear effects of LIP on the key outcome variable KD cannot be assessed.

Ideally, establishing a comprehensive model that simultaneously takes into account all the interrelationships among all observed variables, latent variables, as well as fixed covariates is desirable. In practice, however, if the comprehensive model involves a large number of variables and unknown parameters, and the underlying data structure is complex, one may encounter serious difficulties in developing such a comprehensive model. In these situations, it is advantageous to separate the comprehensive model into submodels, and then conduct the SEM analysis for each submodel. Of course, among the submodels, the one that involves the key outcome variables of main interest is the most important.

For example, in the analysis of the above artificial example, the comprehensive SEM that treats LIP as an outcome latent variable and accommodates its nonlinear effects in the structural equation associated with the path diagram in Figure 2.4 can be separated into two submodels. One is the SEM represented by measurement equation (2.15), and structural equation (2.25) with main focus on the outcome latent variable KD. In this submodel, LIP is only treated as an explanatory latent variable (no paths from d_1, BP, and OB to LIP; see Figure 2.3). Hence, its nonlinear effects BP $\times$ LIP, OB $\times$ LIP, and $d_2 \times$ LIP on KD can be assessed. To further assess the relationships among LIP and the other covariates and/or latent variables, the following submodel is used. The measurement equation is defined by

$$\begin{bmatrix} y_5 \\ y_6 \\ y_7 \\ y_8 \\ y_9 \\ \mathrm{GV}_1 \\ \mathrm{GV}_2 \end{bmatrix} = \begin{bmatrix} a_{51} & a_{52} \\ a_{61} & a_{62} \\ a_{71} & a_{72} \\ a_{81} & a_{82} \\ a_{91} & a_{92} \\ 0 & 0 \\ 0 & 0 \end{bmatrix} \begin{bmatrix} c_1 \\ c_2 \end{bmatrix} + \begin{bmatrix} \lambda_{53} & 0 & 0 \\ \lambda_{63} & 0 & 0 \\ 0 & \lambda_{74} & 0 \\ 0 & \lambda_{84} & 0 \\ 0 & \lambda_{94} & 0 \\ 0 & 0 & \lambda_{10,5} \\ 0 & 0 & \lambda_{11,5} \end{bmatrix} \begin{bmatrix} \mathrm{OB} \\ \mathrm{LIP} \\ \mathrm{LGV} \end{bmatrix} + \begin{bmatrix} \epsilon_5 \\ \epsilon_6 \\ \epsilon_7 \\ \epsilon_8 \\ \epsilon_9 \\ \epsilon_{10} \\ \epsilon_{11} \end{bmatrix}. \quad (2.28)$$

The structural equation is given by

$$\mathrm{LIP} = b_3 d_1 + \gamma_4 \mathrm{OB} + \gamma_5 \mathrm{LGV} + \delta. \quad (2.29)$$

A path diagram representing the submodel defined by (2.28) and (2.29) is given in Figure 2.5. Here, LIP is treated as an outcome latent variable. Based on the estimates of the path coefficients γ_3 in the submodel associated with Figure 2.3, and γ_4 in the submodel defined by equations (2.28) and (2.29) (see also Figure 2.5), we can get some idea about the indirect effect of OB on KD via $\hat{\gamma}_3 \times \hat{\gamma}_4$. However, as $\hat{\gamma}_3$ and $\hat{\gamma}_4$ are not simultaneously estimable through a single model, the estimate of this indirect effect is not optimal and should be interpreted with care. It should also be noted that there are two sets of estimates for the common parameters in these two submodels. One set of estimates is obtained through the analysis of the submodel defined by (2.15) and (2.25), while the other set of estimates is obtained through analysis of

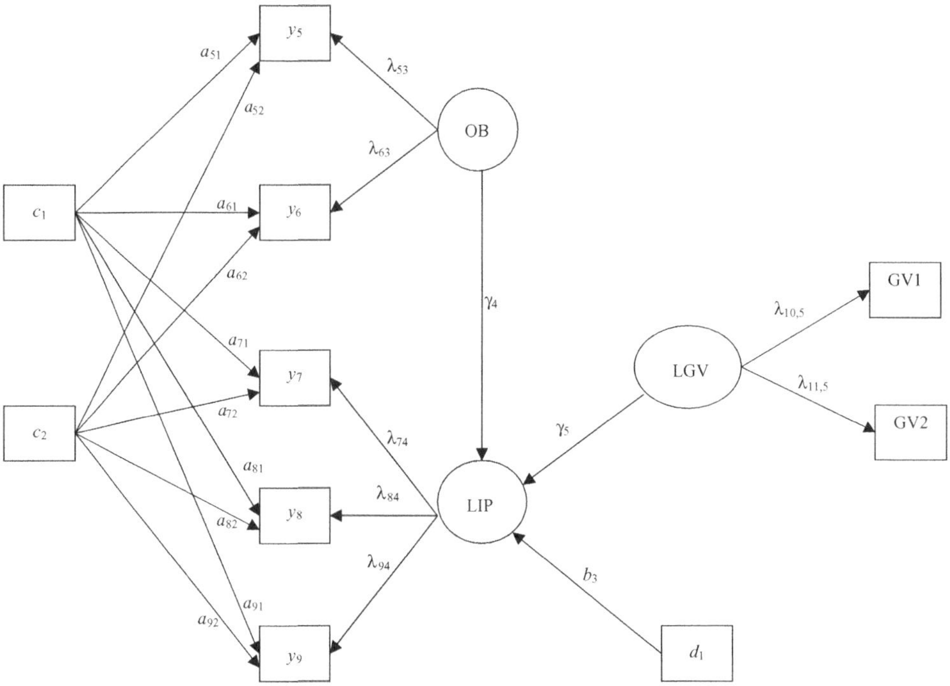

Figure 2.5 Path diagram representing the submodel defined by (2.28) and (2.29). The residual errors have been omitted.

the submodel defined by (2.28) and (2.29). However, the differences between these two sets of estimates are very small; and in practice, they would not result in different interpretations of the results. Hence, this issue is not important. The tradeoff of these disadvantages in using submodels is the possibility of assessing various nonlinear effects in relation to LIP through the submodel associated with Figure 2.3. In practice, the choice between the different approaches in applying SEMs heavily depends on the objective of the real study. For instance, if assessing the nonlinear effect of LIP on KD is more important, it may be worthwhile to use submodels in the analysis.

In the analysis of SEMs, sound statistical methods that seriously take into consideration the structures of the hypothesized model and data should be used. Parameter estimates should be obtained via valid statistical procedures. It is necessary to develop rigorous goodness of fit and model comparison statistics for assessing the goodness of fit of the hypothesized model to the sample data and for comparing competing models. In the next chapter, we will introduce the Bayesian approach with optimal statistical properties for estimation, goodness of fit analysis, and model comparison.

In this chapter, we have discussed the basic SEMs, namely the linear SEMs and nonlinear SEMs with fixed covariates, and their applications to the analysis of practical data. While these SEMs are helpful for analyzing real data sets related to biomedical research, they have limitations which are mainly induced by their underlying assumptions. There is a need to develop more subtle generalizations of these models to overcome the limitations. Based on the requirements of substantive research, certain generalizations will be discussed in subsequent chapters. Given the developments of the basic models and their generalizations, SEMs provide efficient tools with great flexibility for analyzing multivariate data in behavioral, educational, medical, social, and psychological sciences.

References

Bollen, K. A. (1989) *Structural Equations with Latent Variables*. New York: John Wiley & Sons, Inc.

Chen, C. C., Lu, R. B., Chen, Y. C., Wang, M. F., Chang, Y. C., Li, T. K. and Yin, S. J. (1999) Interaction between the functional polymorphisms of the alcohol-metabolism genes in protection against alcoholism. *American Journal of Human Genetics*, **65**, 795–807.

Fioretto, P., Steffes, M. W., Sutherland, D. E. R., Goetz, F. C. and Mauer, M. (1998) Reversal of lesions of diabetic nephropathy after pancreas transplantation. *New England Journal of Medicine*, **339**, 69–75.

Jaccard, J. and Wan, C. K. (1995) Measurement error in the analysis of interaction effects between continuous predictors using multiple regression: Multiple indicator and structural equation approaches. *Psychological Bulletin*, **117**, 348–357.

Jöreskog, K. G. and Sörbom, D. (1996) *LISREL 8: Structural Equation Modeling with the SIMPLIS Command Language*. Hove: Scientific Software International.

Klein, A. and Moosbrugger, H. (2000) Maximum likelihood estimation of latent interaction effects with the LMS method. *Psychometrika*, **65**, 457–474.

Parving, H. H., Tarnow, L. and Rossing, P. (1996) Genetics of diabetic nephropathy. *Journal of the American Society of Nephrology*, **7**, 2509–2517.

Schumacker, R. E. and Marcoulides, G. A. (1998) *Interaction and Nonlinear Effects in Structural Equation Modeling*. Mahwah, NJ: Lawrence Erlbaum Associates.

Wall, M. M. and Amemiya, Y. (2000) Estimation for polynomial structural equation modeling. *Journal of the American Statistical Association*, **95**, 929–940.

3

Bayesian methods for estimating structural equation models

3.1 Introduction

In Chapter 2 we presented some basic SEMs and discussed how these models can be used in practice. In substantive applications of these basic SEMs or their generalizations (to be discussed in subsequent chapters) for coping with complex situations, it is important to introduce sound statistical methods that give accurate statistical results. The traditional approach for analyzing SEMs is that of covariance structure analysis. In this approach, the statistical theory as well as the computational algorithms are developed on the basis of the sample covariance matrix **S** and its asymptotic distribution. Under some standard assumptions, for example that the random observations are i.i.d. normal, this approach works fine. As a result, almost all classical commercial SEM software was developed on the basis of this approach with the sample covariance matrix **S**. Unfortunately, under slightly more complex situations that are common in substantive research, the covariance structure analysis approach based on **S** is not effective and may encounter theoretical and computational problems. For instance, in the presence of nonlinear terms of explanatory latent variables, outcome latent variables and the related observed variables in $\mathbf{y}_i$ are not normally distributed. Hence, **S** is not suitable for modeling nonlinear relationships; and the application of the covariance structure analysis approach via some unnatural methods, for example the product-indicator method, produces inferior results. See Lee (2007) for further discussion of the disadvantages of using the covariance structure analysis approach to analyze subtle SEMs and data structures that are common in substantive research. In this chapter, we will introduce an attractive Bayesian approach which can be effectively applied to analyze not only the standard SEMs but also useful generalizations of SEMs that have been developed in recent years.

The basic nice feature of a Bayesian approach is its flexibility in utilizing useful prior information to achieve better results. In many practical problems, statisticians may have good

Basic and Advanced Bayesian Structural Equation Modeling: With Applications in the Medical and Behavioral Sciences,
First Edition. Xin-Yuan Song and Sik-Yum Lee.

prior information from some sources, for example the knowledge of the experts, and analyses of similar data and/or past data. For situations without accurate prior information, some types of noninformative prior distributions can be used in a Bayesian approach. In these cases, the accuracy of Bayesian estimates is close to that of maximum likelihood (ML) estimates.

It is well known that the statistical properties of the ML approach are asymptotic. Hence, they are valid for situations with large sample sizes. In the context of some basic SEMs, several studies (e.g. Boomsma, 1982; Chou *et al.*, 1991; Hu *et al.*, 1992; Hoogland and Boomsma, 1998) showed that the statistical properties of the ML approach are not robust to small sample sizes. In contrast, as pointed out by many important articles in Bayesian analyses of SEMs (see Scheines *et al.*, 1999; Ansari and Jedidi, 2000; Dunson, 2000; Lee and Song, 2004), the sampling-based Bayesian methods depend less on asymptotic theory, and hence have the potential to produce reliable results even with small samples.

Recently, Bayesian methods have been developed with various Markov chain Monte Carlo (MCMC) algorithms. Usually, a sufficiently large number of observations are simulated from the joint posterior distribution through these MCMC algorithms. Means as well as quantiles of this joint posterior distribution can be estimated from the simulated observations. These quantities are useful for making statistical inferences. For example, the Bayesian estimates of the unknown parameters and the latent variables can be obtained from the corresponding sample means of observations simulated from the posterior distribution. Moreover, from these estimates, the estimated residuals which are useful for assessing the goodness of fit of the proposed model and for detecting outliers can be obtained. Finally, various model comparison statistics that are closely related to the Bayesian approach, such as the Bayes factor, give more flexible and natural tools for model comparison than the classical likelihood ratio test (see Kass and Raftery, 1995; Lee, 2007). We will give a detailed discussion on model comparison in Chapter 4.

Basic statistical inferences of SEMs include estimation of the unknown parameters and latent variables, assessment of the goodness of fit of the proposed model, and model comparison. The objective of this chapter is to provide an introduction to the Bayesian approach to conducting statistical inferences of SEMs. It is not our intention to provide full coverage of the general Bayesian theory. Readers may refer to other excellent books such as Box and Tiao (1973), and Gelman *et al.* (2003) for more details. Section 3.2 of this chapter presents the basic ideas of the Bayesian approach to estimation, including the prior distribution. Posterior analyses through applications of some MCMC methods are considered in Section 3.3. An application of the MCMC methods is presented in Section 3.4. Section 3.5 describes how to use the WinBUGS software to obtain Bayesian estimation and to conduct simulation studies. Some technical details are given in the appendices.

3.2 Basic concepts of the Bayesian estimation and prior distributions

The Bayesian approach is recognized in the statistics literature as an attractive approach in analyzing a wide variety of models (Berger, 1985; Congdon, 2003). To introduce this approach for SEMs, let M be an arbitrary SEM with a vector of unknown parameters $\boldsymbol{\theta}$, and let $\mathbf{Y} = (\mathbf{y}_1, \ldots, \mathbf{y}_n)$ be the observed data set of raw observations with a sample size n. In a non-Bayesian approach, $\boldsymbol{\theta}$ is not considered as random. In a Bayesian approach, $\boldsymbol{\theta}$ is considered to be random with a distribution (called a prior distribution) and an associated (prior) density function, say, $p(\boldsymbol{\theta}|M)$. We give here a simple example to show the rationale for regarding an unknown parameter as random. Suppose that we wish to estimate the mean of systolic blood pressure, say μ. It is not necessary to assume that μ is fixed with a certain value; instead, μ is allowed to vary randomly, for example with a higher (or lower) probability at some values. Hence, it is more reasonable to treat μ as random with a prior distribution and a prior density $p(\mu)$. See Berger (1985) and the references therein for theoretical and practical rationales for treating $\boldsymbol{\theta}$ as random.

For simplicity, we use $p(\boldsymbol{\theta})$ to denote $p(\boldsymbol{\theta}|M)$. Bayesian estimation is based on the observed data $\mathbf{Y}$ and the prior distribution of $\boldsymbol{\theta}$. Let $p(\mathbf{Y}, \boldsymbol{\theta}|M)$ be the probability density function of the joint distribution of $\mathbf{Y}$ and $\boldsymbol{\theta}$ under M. The behavior of $\boldsymbol{\theta}$ under the given data $\mathbf{Y}$ is fully described by the conditional distribution of $\boldsymbol{\theta}$ given $\mathbf{Y}$. This conditional distribution is called the posterior distribution of $\boldsymbol{\theta}$. Let $p(\boldsymbol{\theta}|\mathbf{Y}, M)$ be the density function of the posterior distribution, which is called the posterior density function. The posterior distribution of $\boldsymbol{\theta}$ or its density plays the most important role in the Bayesian analysis of the model. Based on a well-known identity in probability, we have $p(\mathbf{Y}, \boldsymbol{\theta}|M) = p(\mathbf{Y}|\boldsymbol{\theta}, M)p(\boldsymbol{\theta}) = p(\boldsymbol{\theta}|\mathbf{Y}, M)p(\mathbf{Y}|M)$. As $p(\mathbf{Y}|M)$ does not depend on $\boldsymbol{\theta}$, and can be regarded as a constant with fixed $\mathbf{Y}$, we have

$$\begin{aligned} p(\boldsymbol{\theta}|\mathbf{Y}, M) &\propto p(\mathbf{Y}|\boldsymbol{\theta}, M)p(\boldsymbol{\theta}), \quad \text{or} \\ \log p(\boldsymbol{\theta}|\mathbf{Y}, M) &= \log p(\mathbf{Y}|\boldsymbol{\theta}, M) + \log p(\boldsymbol{\theta}) + \text{constant}. \end{aligned} \tag{3.1}$$

Note that $p(\mathbf{Y}|\boldsymbol{\theta}, M)$ can be regarded as the likelihood function because it is the probability density of $\mathbf{y}_1, \ldots, \mathbf{y}_n$ conditional on the parameter vector $\boldsymbol{\theta}$. It follows from (3.1) that the posterior density function incorporates the sample information through the likelihood function $p(\mathbf{Y}|\boldsymbol{\theta}, M)$, and the prior information through the prior density function $p(\boldsymbol{\theta})$. Note also that $p(\mathbf{Y}|\boldsymbol{\theta}, M)$ depends on the sample size, whereas $p(\boldsymbol{\theta})$ does not. When the sample size becomes arbitrarily large, $\log p(\mathbf{Y}|\boldsymbol{\theta}, M)$ could be very large and hence $\log p(\mathbf{Y}|\boldsymbol{\theta}, M)$ dominates $\log p(\boldsymbol{\theta})$. In this situation, the prior distribution of $\boldsymbol{\theta}$ plays a less important role, and the logarithm of posterior density function $\log p(\boldsymbol{\theta}|\mathbf{Y}, M)$ is close to the log-likelihood function $\log p(\mathbf{Y}|\boldsymbol{\theta}, M)$. Hence, Bayesian and ML approaches are asymptotically equivalent, and the Bayesian estimates have the same optimal properties as the ML estimates. When the sample sizes are small or moderate, the prior distribution of $\boldsymbol{\theta}$ plays a more substantial role in Bayesian estimation. Hence, in substantive research problems where the sample sizes are small or moderate, prior information on the parameter vector $\boldsymbol{\theta}$ incorporated into the Bayesian analysis is useful for achieving better results (see below for the utilization of useful prior information in the analysis). For many problems in biomedical and behavioral sciences, researchers may have good prior information from the subject experts, from analyses of similar or past data, or from some other sources. As more accurate results can be obtained by incorporating appropriate prior information in the analysis through the prior distribution of $\boldsymbol{\theta}$, the selection of $p(\boldsymbol{\theta})$ is an important issue in Bayesian analysis. In the following sections and chapters, the symbol M will be suppressed if the context is clear; for example, $p(\boldsymbol{\theta}|\mathbf{Y})$ will denote the posterior density of $\boldsymbol{\theta}$ under M, and $[\boldsymbol{\theta}|\mathbf{Y}]$ will denote the posterior distribution of $\boldsymbol{\theta}$ under M.

3.2.1 Prior distributions

The prior distribution of $\boldsymbol{\theta}$ represents the distribution of possible parameter values, from which the parameter $\boldsymbol{\theta}$ has been drawn. Basically, there are two kinds of prior distributions, noninformative and informative. Noninformative prior distributions are associated with situations when the prior distributions have no population basis. They are used when we have little prior information, and hence the prior distributions play a minimal role in the posterior distribution of $\boldsymbol{\theta}$. The associated prior densities are chosen to be vague, diffuse, flat, or noninformative, for example a density that is proportional to a constant or has a huge variance. In this case, the Bayesian estimation is unaffected by information external to the observed data. For an informative prior distribution, we may have useful prior knowledge about this distribution, either from closely related data or from subjective knowledge of experts. An informative prior distribution usually has its own parameters, which are called hyperparameters.

A commonly used informative prior distribution in the general Bayesian approach for statistical problems is the conjugate prior distribution. We consider the univariate binomial model in order to motivate this kind of prior distribution. Considered as a function of θ, the likelihood of an observation y is of the form

$$p(y|\theta) = \binom{n}{y}\theta^y(1-\theta)^{n-y}.$$

If the prior density of θ is of the same form, it can be seen from (3.1) that the posterior density will also be of this form. More specifically, consider the following prior density of θ:

$$p(\theta) \propto \theta^{\alpha-1}(1-\theta)^{\beta-1}, \tag{3.2}$$

which is a beta distribution with hyperparameters α and β. Then,

$$\begin{aligned} p(\theta|y) &\propto p(y|\theta)p(\theta) \\ &\propto \theta^y(1-\theta)^{n-y}\theta^{\alpha-1}(1-\theta)^{\beta-1} \\ &= \theta^{y+\alpha-1}(1-\theta)^{n-y+\beta-1}, \end{aligned} \tag{3.3}$$

which is a beta distribution with parameters $y+\alpha$ and $n-y+\beta$. We see that $p(\theta)$ and $p(\theta|y)$ are of the same form. The property that the posterior distribution follows the same parametric form as the prior distribution is called conjugacy, and the prior distribution is called a conjugate prior distribution (Gelman *et al.*, 2003). One advantage of this kind of prior distribution is that it provides a manageable posterior distribution for developing the MCMC algorithm for statistical inference.

If the hyperparameters in the conjugate prior distributions are unknown, then they may be treated as unknown parameters and thus have their own prior distributions in a full Bayesian analysis. These hyperprior distributions again have their own hyperparameters. As a result, the problem will become very tedious. Hence, in developing the Bayesian methods for analyzing SEMs, we usually assign fixed known values to the hyperparameters in the conjugate prior distributions.

3.2.2 Conjugate prior distributions in Bayesian analyses of SEMs

In the field of SEMs, almost all previous work in Bayesian analysis has used conjugate prior distributions with the given hyperparameter values; see Lee (2007) and the references therein. It has been shown that these distributions work well for many SEMs. Therefore, in this book, we will use the conjugate prior distributions in our Bayesian analyses. In general, it has been shown that for a univariate normal distribution, the conjugate prior distributions of the unknown mean and variance are normal and inverted gamma, respectively (see Gelman *et al.*, 2003; Lee, 2007). This fact motivates the selection of conjugate prior distributions for the parameters in SEMs, which are basically the regression coefficients related to the mean vector of a multivariate normal distribution, and variance and covariance matrix related to the residual errors and latent vector, respectively.

Without loss of generality, we illustrate the selection of prior distributions in the context of a nonlinear SEM with fixed covariates in the structural equation. More specifically, we first consider the following measurement equation and structural equation for the model:

$$\mathbf{y}_i = \boldsymbol{\mu} + \boldsymbol{\Lambda}\boldsymbol{\omega}_i + \boldsymbol{\epsilon}_i, \tag{3.4}$$

$$\boldsymbol{\eta}_i = \mathbf{B}\mathbf{d}_i + \boldsymbol{\Pi}\boldsymbol{\eta}_i + \boldsymbol{\Gamma}\mathbf{F}(\boldsymbol{\xi}_i) + \boldsymbol{\delta}_i, \tag{3.5}$$

where $\mathbf{y}_i$ is a $p \times 1$ vector of observed variables, $\boldsymbol{\mu}$ is a vector of intercepts, $\boldsymbol{\omega}_i = (\boldsymbol{\eta}_i^T, \boldsymbol{\xi}_i^T)^T$ is a vector of latent variables which is partitioned into a $q_1 \times 1$ vector of outcome latent variables $\boldsymbol{\eta}_i$ and a $q_2 \times 1$ vector of explanatory latent variables $\boldsymbol{\xi}_i$, $\boldsymbol{\epsilon}_i$ and $\boldsymbol{\delta}_i$ are residual errors, $\mathbf{d}_i$ is an $r \times 1$ vector of fixed covariates, $\boldsymbol{\Lambda}$, $\mathbf{B}$, $\boldsymbol{\Pi}$, and $\boldsymbol{\Gamma}$ are parameter matrices of unknown regression coefficients, and $\mathbf{F}(\cdot)$ is a given vector of differentiable functions of $\boldsymbol{\xi}_i$. Similarly to the model described in Chapter 2, the distributions of $\boldsymbol{\xi}_i$, $\boldsymbol{\epsilon}_i$, and $\boldsymbol{\delta}_i$ are $N[\mathbf{0}, \boldsymbol{\Phi}]$, $N[\mathbf{0}, \boldsymbol{\Psi}_\epsilon]$, and $N[\mathbf{0}, \boldsymbol{\Psi}_\delta]$, respectively; and the assumptions as given in Chapter 2 are satisfied. In this model, the unknown parameters are $\boldsymbol{\mu}$, $\boldsymbol{\Lambda}$, $\mathbf{B}$, $\boldsymbol{\Pi}$, and $\boldsymbol{\Gamma}$ which are related to the mean vectors of $\mathbf{y}_i$ and $\boldsymbol{\eta}_i$; and $\boldsymbol{\Phi}$, $\boldsymbol{\Psi}_\epsilon$, and $\boldsymbol{\Psi}_\delta$ which are the covariance matrices. Now consider the prior distributions of the parameters $\boldsymbol{\mu}$, $\boldsymbol{\Lambda}$, and $\boldsymbol{\Psi}_\epsilon$ that are involved in the measurement equation. Let $\boldsymbol{\Lambda}_k^T$ be the kth row of $\boldsymbol{\Lambda}$, and $\psi_{\epsilon k}$ be the kth diagonal element of $\boldsymbol{\Psi}_\epsilon$. It can be shown (see Lee, 2007) that the conjugate type prior distributions of $\boldsymbol{\mu}$ and $(\boldsymbol{\Lambda}_k, \psi_{\epsilon k})$ are

$$\psi_{\epsilon k} \stackrel{D}{=} \mathrm{IG}[\alpha_{0\epsilon k}, \beta_{0\epsilon k}] \text{ or equivalently } \psi_{\epsilon k}^{-1} \stackrel{D}{=} \mathrm{Gamma}[\alpha_{0\epsilon k}, \beta_{0\epsilon k}],$$

$$\boldsymbol{\mu} \stackrel{D}{=} N[\boldsymbol{\mu}_0, \boldsymbol{\Sigma}_0], \text{ and } [\boldsymbol{\Lambda}_k|\psi_{\epsilon k}] \stackrel{D}{=} N\left[\boldsymbol{\Lambda}_{0k}, \psi_{\epsilon k}\mathbf{H}_{0yk}\right], \tag{3.6}$$

where IG$[\cdot, \cdot]$ denotes the inverted gamma distribution, $\alpha_{0\epsilon k}$, $\beta_{0\epsilon k}$, and elements in $\boldsymbol{\mu}_0$, $\boldsymbol{\Lambda}_{0k}$, $\boldsymbol{\Sigma}_0$, and $\mathbf{H}_{0yk}$ are hyperparameters, and $\boldsymbol{\Sigma}_0$ and $\mathbf{H}_{0yk}$ are positive definite matrices. For simplicity of notation, we rewrite the structural equation (3.5) as

$$\boldsymbol{\eta}_i = \boldsymbol{\Lambda}_\omega \mathbf{G}(\boldsymbol{\omega}_i) + \boldsymbol{\delta}_i, \tag{3.7}$$

where $\boldsymbol{\Lambda}_\omega = (\mathbf{B}, \boldsymbol{\Pi}, \boldsymbol{\Gamma})$ and $\mathbf{G}(\boldsymbol{\omega}_i) = (\mathbf{d}_i^T, \boldsymbol{\eta}_i^T, \mathbf{F}(\boldsymbol{\xi}_i)^T)^T$. Let $\boldsymbol{\Lambda}_{\omega k}^T$ be the kth row of $\boldsymbol{\Lambda}_\omega$, and $\psi_{\delta k}$ be the kth diagonal element of $\boldsymbol{\Psi}_\delta$. Based on reasoning similar to that used earlier, the conjugate type prior distributions of $\boldsymbol{\Phi}$ and $(\boldsymbol{\Lambda}_{\omega k}, \psi_{\delta k})$ are:

$$\boldsymbol{\Phi} \stackrel{D}{=} \mathrm{IW}_{q_2}\left[\mathbf{R}_0^{-1}, \rho_0\right], \text{ or equivalently } \boldsymbol{\Phi}^{-1} \stackrel{D}{=} W_{q_2}[\mathbf{R}_0, \rho_0],$$

$$\psi_{\delta k} \stackrel{D}{=} \mathrm{IG}[\alpha_{0\delta k}, \beta_{0\delta k}] \text{ or equivalently } \psi_{\delta k}^{-1} \stackrel{D}{=} \mathrm{Gamma}[\alpha_{0\delta k}, \beta_{0\delta k}],$$

$$[\boldsymbol{\Lambda}_{\omega k}|\psi_{\delta k}] \stackrel{D}{=} N[\boldsymbol{\Lambda}_{0\omega k}, \psi_{\delta k}\mathbf{H}_{0\omega k}], \tag{3.8}$$

where $W_{q_2}[\mathbf{R}_0, \rho_0]$ is a q_2-dimensional Wishart distribution with hyperparameters ρ_0 and a positive definite matrix $\mathbf{R}_0$, $\mathrm{IW}_{q_2}[\mathbf{R}_0^{-1}, \rho_0]$ is a q_2-dimensional inverted Wishart distribution with hyperparameters ρ_0 and a positive definite matrix $\mathbf{R}_0^{-1}$, $\alpha_{0\delta k}$, $\beta_{0\delta k}$, and elements in $\boldsymbol{\Lambda}_{0\omega k}$ and $\mathbf{H}_{0\omega k}$ are hyperparameters, and $\mathbf{H}_{0\omega k}$ is a positive definite matrix. Note that the prior distribution of $\boldsymbol{\Phi}^{-1}$ (or $\boldsymbol{\Phi}$) is a multivariate extension of the prior distribution of $\psi_{\delta k}^{-1}$ (or $\psi_{\delta k}$).

For clarity, the gamma, inverted gamma, Wishart, and inverted Wishart distributions as well as their characteristics are given in Appendix 3.1.

In specifying conjugate prior distributions, we assign values to their hyperparameters. These preassigned values (prior inputs) represent the available prior knowledge. In general, if we are confident of having good prior information about a parameter, then it is advantageous to select the corresponding prior distribution with a small variance; otherwise the prior distribution with a larger variance should be selected. We use the prior distributions given in (3.6) to illustrate this. If we have confidence that the true $\mathbf{\Lambda}_k$ is not too far away from the preassigned hyperparameter value $\mathbf{\Lambda}_{0k}$, then $\mathbf{H}_{0yk}$ should be taken as a matrix with small variances (such as $0.5\mathbf{I}$). The choice of $\alpha_{0\epsilon k}$ and $\beta_{0\epsilon k}$ is based on the same general rationale and the nature of $\psi_{\epsilon k}$ in the model. First, we note that the distribution of ϵ_k is $N[0, \psi_{\epsilon k}]$. Hence, if we think that the variation of ϵ_k is small (i.e. $\mathbf{\Lambda}_k^T \boldsymbol{\omega}_i$ is a good predictor of y_{ik}), then the prior distribution of $\psi_{\epsilon k}$ should have a small mean as well as a small variance. Otherwise, the prior distribution of $\psi_{\epsilon k}$ should have a large mean and/or a large variance. This gives some idea in choosing the hyperparameters $\alpha_{0\epsilon k}$ and $\beta_{0\epsilon k}$ in the inverted gamma distribution. Note that for the inverted gamma distribution, the mean is equal to $\beta_{0\epsilon k}/(\alpha_{0\epsilon k} - 1)$, and the variance is equal to $\beta_{0\epsilon k}^2/\{(\alpha_{0\epsilon k} - 1)^2(\alpha_{0\epsilon k} - 2)\}$. Hence, we may take $\alpha_{0\epsilon k} = 9$ and $\beta_{0\epsilon k} = 4$ for a situation where we have confidence that $\mathbf{\Lambda}_k^T \boldsymbol{\omega}_i$ is a good predictor of y_{ik} in the measurement equation. Under this choice, the mean of $\psi_{\epsilon k}$ is $4/8 = 0.5$, and the variance of $\psi_{\epsilon k}$ is $4^2/\{(9-1)^2(9-2)\} = 1/28$. For a situation with little confidence, we may take $\alpha_{0k} = 6$ and $\beta_{0\epsilon k} = 10$, so that the mean of $\psi_{\epsilon k}$ is 2.0 and the variance is 1.0. The above ideas for choosing preassigned hyperparameter values can similarly be used in specifying $\mathbf{\Lambda}_{0\omega k}$, $\alpha_{0\delta k}$, and $\beta_{0\delta k}$ in the conjugate prior distributions of $\mathbf{\Lambda}_{\omega k}$ and $\psi_{\delta k}$; see (3.8). We now consider the choice of $\mathbf{R}_0$ and ρ_0 in the prior distribution of $\mathbf{\Phi}$. It follows from Muirhead (1982, p.97) that the mean of $\mathbf{\Phi}$ is $\mathbf{R}_0^{-1}/(\rho_0 - q_2 - 1)$. Hence, if we have confidence that $\mathbf{\Phi}$ is not too far away from a known matrix $\mathbf{\Phi}_0$, we can choose $\mathbf{R}_0^{-1}$ and ρ_0 such that $\mathbf{R}_0^{-1} = (\rho_0 - q_2 - 1)\mathbf{\Phi}_0$. Other values of $\mathbf{R}_0^{-1}$ and ρ_0 may be considered for situations without good prior information.

We now discuss some methods for obtaining $\mathbf{\Lambda}_{0k}$, $\mathbf{\Lambda}_{0\omega k}$, and $\mathbf{\Phi}_0$. As mentioned before, these hyperparameter values may be obtained from subjective knowledge of experts in the field, and/or analysis of past or closely related data. If this kind of information is not available and the sample size is small, we may consider using the following noninformative prior distributions:

$$
\begin{aligned}
p(\mathbf{\Lambda}, \mathbf{\Psi}_\epsilon) &\propto p(\psi_{\epsilon 1}, \ldots, \psi_{\epsilon p}) \propto \prod_{k=1}^{p} \psi_{\epsilon k}^{-1}, \\
p(\mathbf{\Lambda}_\omega, \mathbf{\Psi}_\delta) &\propto p(\psi_{\delta 1}, \ldots, \psi_{\delta q_1}) \propto \prod_{k=1}^{q_1} \psi_{\delta k}^{-1}, \\
p(\mathbf{\Phi}) &\propto |\mathbf{\Phi}|^{-(q_2+1)/2}.
\end{aligned} \tag{3.9}
$$

In (3.9), the prior distributions of the unknown parameters in $\mathbf{\Lambda}$ and $\mathbf{\Lambda}_\omega$ are implicitly taken to be proportional to a constant. Note that no hyperparameters are involved in these noninformative prior distributions. Bayesian analysis on the basis of the above noninformative prior distributions is basically close to the Bayesian analysis with conjugate prior distributions given by (3.6) and (3.8) with very large variances. If the sample size is large, one possible method for obtaining $\mathbf{\Lambda}_{0k}$, $\mathbf{\Lambda}_{0\omega k}$, and $\mathbf{\Phi}_0$ is to use a portion of the data, say one-third or less, to conduct an auxiliary Bayesian estimation with noninformative priors to produce initial Bayesian estimates. The remaining data are then used to conduct the actual Bayesian analysis with the initial Bayesian estimates as hyperparameter values in relation to $\mathbf{\Lambda}_{0k}$, $\mathbf{\Lambda}_{0\omega k}$, and $\mathbf{\Phi}_0$. For situations with moderate sample sizes, Bayesian analysis may be done by applying data-dependent prior inputs that are obtained from an initial estimation with the whole data set. Although the above methods are reasonable, we emphasize that we are not routinely recommending them for every practical application. In general, the issue of choosing prior inputs should be carefully approached on a problem-by-problem basis. Moreover, under situations without useful prior information, a sensitivity analysis should be conducted to see whether the results are robust to prior inputs. This can be done by perturbing the given hyperparameter values or considering some *ad hoc* prior inputs.

3.3 Posterior analysis using Markov chain Monte Carlo methods

The Bayesian estimate of $\boldsymbol{\theta}$ is usually defined as the mean or the mode of the posterior distribution $[\boldsymbol{\theta}|\mathbf{Y}]$. In this book, we are mainly interested in estimating the unknown parameters via the mean of the posterior distribution. Theoretically, it could be obtained via integration. For most situations, the integration does not have a closed form. However, if we can simulate a sufficiently large number of observations from $[\boldsymbol{\theta}|\mathbf{Y}]$ (or $p(\boldsymbol{\theta}|\mathbf{Y})$), we can approximate the mean and other useful statistics through the simulated observations. Hence, to solve the problem, it suffices to develop efficient and dependable methods for drawing observations from the posterior distribution. For most nonstandard SEMs, the posterior distribution $[\boldsymbol{\theta}|\mathbf{Y}]$ is complicated. It is difficult to derive this distribution and simulate observations from it. A major breakthrough for posterior simulation is the idea of data augmentation proposed by Tanner and Wong (1987). The strategy is to treat latent quantities as hypothetical missing data and to augment the observed data with them so that the posterior distribution based on the complete data set is relatively easy to analyze. This strategy has been widely adopted in analyzing many statistical models (e.g. Rubin, 1991; Albert and Chib, 1993; Dunson, 2000). It is particularly useful for SEMs which involve latent variables (see Lee, 2007). The feature that makes SEMs different from the common regression model and the simultaneous equation model is the existence of random latent variables. In many situations, the presence of latent variables causes major difficulties in the analysis of the model. However, if the random latent variables are given, SEMs will become familiar regression models that can be handled without much difficulty.

Hence, the above mentioned strategy based on data augmentation provides a useful approach to cope with the problem that is induced by latent variables. By augmenting the observed variables in complicated SEMs with the latent variables that are treated as hypothetical missing data, we can obtain the Bayesian solution based on the complete data set. More specifically, instead of working on the intractable posterior density $p(\boldsymbol{\theta}|\mathbf{Y})$, we will work on $p(\boldsymbol{\theta}, \boldsymbol{\Omega}|\mathbf{Y})$, where $\boldsymbol{\Omega}$ is the set of latent variables in the model. For most cases, $p(\boldsymbol{\theta}, \boldsymbol{\Omega}|\mathbf{Y})$ is still not in closed form and it is difficult to deal with it directly. However, on the basis of the complete data set $(\boldsymbol{\Omega}, \mathbf{Y})$, the conditional distribution $p(\boldsymbol{\theta}|\boldsymbol{\Omega}, \mathbf{Y})$ is usually standard, and the conditional distribution $p(\boldsymbol{\Omega}|\boldsymbol{\theta}, \mathbf{Y})$ can also be derived from the definition of the model without much difficulty. As a result, we can apply some MCMC methods to simulate observations from $p(\boldsymbol{\theta}, \boldsymbol{\Omega}|\mathbf{Y})$ by drawing observations iteratively from their full conditional densities $p(\boldsymbol{\theta}|\boldsymbol{\Omega}, \mathbf{Y})$ and $p(\boldsymbol{\Omega}|\boldsymbol{\theta}, \mathbf{Y})$. Following the terminology in MCMC methods, we may call $p(\boldsymbol{\theta}|\boldsymbol{\Omega}, \mathbf{Y})$ and $p(\boldsymbol{\Omega}|\boldsymbol{\theta}, \mathbf{Y})$ conditional distributions if the context is clear. Note that as $\boldsymbol{\Omega}$ is given in $p(\boldsymbol{\theta}|\boldsymbol{\Omega}, \mathbf{Y})$, the derivation of this conditional distribution is possible. A useful algorithm for this purpose is the following Gibbs sampler (Geman and Geman, 1984).

In the model M, suppose the parameter vector $\boldsymbol{\theta}$ and the latent matrix $\boldsymbol{\Omega}$ are respectively decomposed into the following components: $\boldsymbol{\theta} = (\boldsymbol{\theta}_1, \ldots, \boldsymbol{\theta}_a)$ and $\boldsymbol{\Omega} = (\boldsymbol{\Omega}_1, \ldots, \boldsymbol{\Omega}_b)$. The Gibbs sampler is an MCMC algorithm which performs an alternating conditional sampling at each of its iteration. It cycles through the components of $\boldsymbol{\theta}$ and $\boldsymbol{\Omega}$, drawing each component conditional on the values of all the other components. More specifically, at the jth iteration with current values $\boldsymbol{\theta}^{(j)} = (\boldsymbol{\theta}_1^{(j)}, \ldots, \boldsymbol{\theta}_a^{(j)})$ and $\boldsymbol{\Omega}^{(j)} = (\boldsymbol{\Omega}_1^{(j)}, \ldots, \boldsymbol{\Omega}_b^{(j)})$, it simulates in turn

$$\begin{aligned}
&\boldsymbol{\theta}_1^{(j+1)} \text{ from } p\big(\boldsymbol{\theta}_1|\boldsymbol{\theta}_2^{(j)}, \ldots, \boldsymbol{\theta}_a^{(j)}, \boldsymbol{\Omega}^{(j)}, \mathbf{Y}\big),\\
&\boldsymbol{\theta}_2^{(j+1)} \text{ from } p\big(\boldsymbol{\theta}_2|\boldsymbol{\theta}_1^{(j+1)}, \ldots, \boldsymbol{\theta}_a^{(j)}, \boldsymbol{\Omega}^{(j)}, \mathbf{Y}\big),\\
&\quad\vdots \qquad\qquad \vdots\\
&\boldsymbol{\theta}_a^{(j+1)} \text{ from } p\big(\boldsymbol{\theta}_a|\boldsymbol{\theta}_1^{(j+1)}, \ldots, \boldsymbol{\theta}_{a-1}^{(j+1)}, \boldsymbol{\Omega}^{(j)}, \mathbf{Y}\big),\\
&\boldsymbol{\Omega}_1^{(j+1)} \text{ from } p\big(\boldsymbol{\Omega}_1|\boldsymbol{\theta}^{(j+1)}, \boldsymbol{\Omega}_2^{(j)}, \ldots, \boldsymbol{\Omega}_b^{(j)}, \mathbf{Y}\big),\\
&\boldsymbol{\Omega}_2^{(j+1)} \text{ from } p\big(\boldsymbol{\Omega}_2|\boldsymbol{\theta}^{(j+1)}, \boldsymbol{\Omega}_1^{(j+1)}, \ldots, \boldsymbol{\Omega}_b^{(j)}, \mathbf{Y}\big),\\
&\quad\vdots \qquad\qquad \vdots\\
&\boldsymbol{\Omega}_b^{(j+1)} \text{ from } p\big(\boldsymbol{\Omega}_b|\boldsymbol{\theta}^{(j+1)}, \boldsymbol{\Omega}_1^{(j+1)}, \ldots, \boldsymbol{\Omega}_{b-1}^{(j+1)}, \mathbf{Y}\big).
\end{aligned} \tag{3.10}$$

There are $a+b$ steps in the jth iteration of the Gibbs sampler. At each step, each component in $\boldsymbol{\theta}$ and $\boldsymbol{\Omega}$ is updated conditionally on the latest values of the other components. We may simulate the components in $\boldsymbol{\Omega}$ first, then the components in $\boldsymbol{\theta}$; or vice versa. For basic linear SEMs, the full conditional distribution in (3.10) is usually normal, gamma, or inverted Wishart. Simulating observations from these is straightforward and fast. For nonstandard conditional distributions, the Metropolis–Hastings (MH) algorithm (Metropolis *et al.*, 1953; Hastings, 1970) may be used for efficient simulation. A brief description of the MH algorithm is given in Appendix 3.2.

It has been shown (Geman and Geman, 1984) that under mild regularity conditions, the joint distribution of $(\boldsymbol{\theta}^{(j)}, \boldsymbol{\Omega}^{(j)})$ converges to the desired posterior distribution $[\boldsymbol{\theta}, \boldsymbol{\Omega}|\mathbf{Y}]$ after a sufficiently large number of iterations, say J. It should be noted that if the iterations have not proceeded long enough, the simulated observations may not be representative of the posterior distribution. Moreover, even if the algorithm has reached approximate convergence, observations obtained in the early iterations should be discarded because they still do not belong to the desired posterior distribution. The required number of iterations for achieving convergence of the Gibbs sampler, that is, the burn-in iterations J, can be determined by plots of the simulated sequences of the individual parameters. At convergence, parallel sequences generated with different starting values should mix well together. Examples of sequences from which convergence looks reasonable, and sequences that have not reached convergence are presented in Figure 3.1. A minor problem with iterative simulation draws is their within-sequence correlation. In general, statistical inference from correlated observations is less

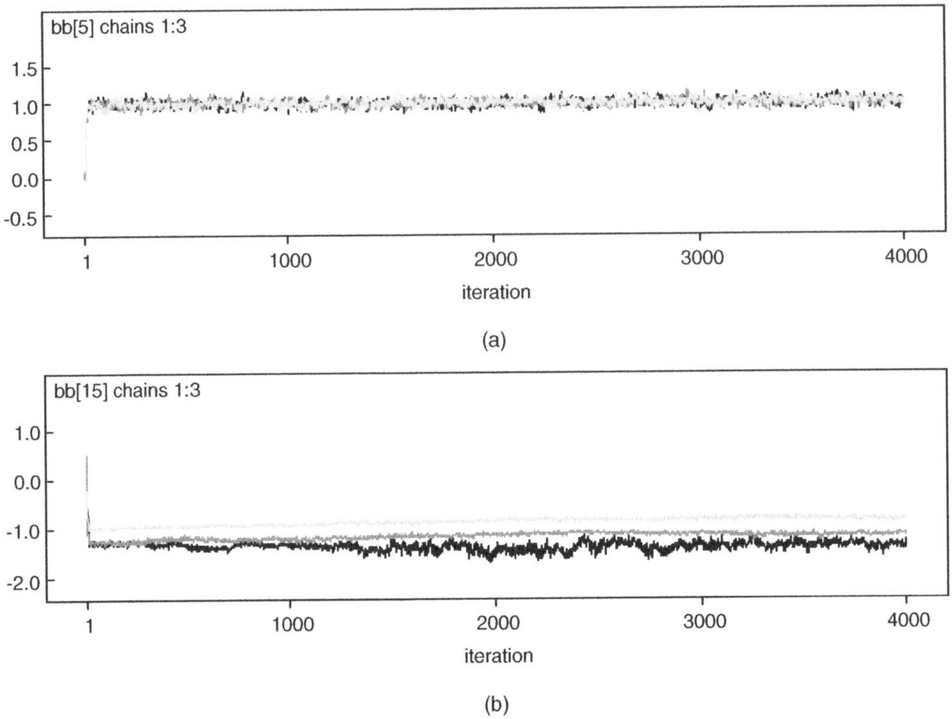

Figure 3.1 Sample traces of chains from which: (a) convergence looks reasonable; (b) convergence is not reached.

precise than that from the same number of independent observations. To obtain a less correlated sample, observations may be collected in cycles with indices $J + s, J + 2s, \ldots, J + Ts$ for some spacing s (Gelfand and Smith, 1990). However, in most practical applications a small s will be sufficient for many statistical analyses such as getting estimates of the parameters (see Albert and Chib, 1993). In the numerical illustrations of the remaining chapters, we will use $s = 1$.

Statistical inference of the model can then be conducted on the basis of a simulated sample of observations from $p(\boldsymbol{\theta}, \boldsymbol{\Omega}|\mathbf{Y})$, namely, $\{(\boldsymbol{\theta}^{(t)}, \boldsymbol{\Omega}^{(t)}) : t = 1, \ldots, T^*\}$. The Bayesian estimate of $\boldsymbol{\theta}$ as well as the numerical standard error estimate can be obtained from

$$\hat{\boldsymbol{\theta}} = T^{*-1} \sum_{t=1}^{T^*} \boldsymbol{\theta}^{(t)}, \tag{3.11}$$

$$\widehat{\mathrm{Var}}(\boldsymbol{\theta}|\mathbf{Y}) = (T^* - 1)^{-1} \sum_{t=1}^{T^*} (\boldsymbol{\theta}^{(t)} - \hat{\boldsymbol{\theta}})(\boldsymbol{\theta}^{(t)} - \hat{\boldsymbol{\theta}})^T. \tag{3.12}$$

It has been shown (Geyer, 1992) that $\hat{\boldsymbol{\theta}}$ tends to $E(\boldsymbol{\theta}|\mathbf{Y})$ as T^* tends to infinity. Other statistical inference on $\boldsymbol{\theta}$ can be carried out based on the simulated sample, $\{\boldsymbol{\theta}^{(t)} : t = 1, \ldots, T^*\}$. For instance, the 2.5% and 97.5% quantiles of the sampled distribution of an individual parameter can give a 95% posterior credible interval and convey skewness in its marginal posterior density. The total number of draws, T^*, that is required for accurate statistical analysis depends on the complexity of the posterior distribution. For most simple SEMs, 3000 draws after convergence are sufficient. Different choices of sufficiently large T^* would produce close estimates, although they may not be exactly equal.

As the posterior distribution of $\boldsymbol{\theta}$ given $\mathbf{Y}$ describes the distributional behaviors of $\boldsymbol{\theta}$ with the given data, the dispersion of $\boldsymbol{\theta}$ can be assessed through $\text{Var}(\boldsymbol{\theta}|\mathbf{Y})$, with an estimate given by (3.12), based on the sample covariance matrix of the simulated observations. Let θ_k be the kth element of $\boldsymbol{\theta}$. The positive square root of the kth diagonal element in $\widehat{\text{Var}}(\boldsymbol{\theta}|\mathbf{Y})$ can be taken as the estimate of the standard deviation of θ_k. Although this estimate is commonly taken as the standard error estimate and provides some information about the variation of $\hat{\theta}_k$, it may not be appropriate to construct a 'z-score' for hypothesis testing. In general Bayesian analysis, the issue of hypothesis testing is formulated as a model comparison problem, and is handled by some model comparison statistics such as the Bayes factor. See Chapter 4 for a more detailed discussion.

For any individual $\mathbf{y}_i$, let $\boldsymbol{\omega}_i$ be the vector of latent variables, and $E(\boldsymbol{\omega}_i|\mathbf{y}_i)$ be the posterior mean. A Bayesian estimate $\hat{\boldsymbol{\omega}}_i$ can be obtained through $\{\boldsymbol{\Omega}^{(t)}, t = 1, \ldots, T^*\}$ as follows:

$$\hat{\boldsymbol{\omega}}_i = T^{*-1} \sum_{t=1}^{T^*} \boldsymbol{\omega}_i^{(t)}, \tag{3.13}$$

where $\boldsymbol{\omega}_i^{(t)}$ is the ith column of $\boldsymbol{\Omega}^{(t)}$. This gives a direct Bayesian estimate that is not expressed in terms of the structural parameter estimates. Hence, in contrast to the classical methods in estimating latent variables, no sampling errors of the estimates are involved in the Bayesian method. It can be shown (Geyer, 1992) that $\hat{\boldsymbol{\omega}}_i$ is a consistent estimate of $E(\boldsymbol{\omega}_i|\mathbf{y}_i)$. These estimates $\hat{\boldsymbol{\omega}}_i$ can be used for outlier and residual analyses, and the assessment of goodness of fit of the measurement equation or the structural equation, particularly in the analysis of complicated SEMs. See examples in Lee (2007) or other chapters in this book. It should be noted that as the data information for estimating $\hat{\boldsymbol{\omega}}_i$ is only given by the single observation $\mathbf{y}_i$, $\hat{\boldsymbol{\omega}}_i$ is not an accurate estimate of the true latent variable $\boldsymbol{\omega}_{i0}$; see the simulation study reported in Lee and Shi (2000) on the estimation of factor scores in a factor analysis model. However, the empirical distribution of the Bayesian estimates $\{\hat{\boldsymbol{\omega}}_1, \ldots, \hat{\boldsymbol{\omega}}_n\}$ is close to the distribution of the true factor scores $\{\boldsymbol{\omega}_{10}, \ldots, \boldsymbol{\omega}_{n0}\}$; see Shi and Lee (1998).

3.4 Application of Markov chain Monte Carlo methods

In this section, we illustrate the implementation of MCMC methods through their application to some SEMs described in Chapter 2. First, we consider the following linear SEM with fixed covariates. Its measurement equation for a $p \times 1$ observed random vector $\mathbf{y}_i$ measured on an individual i is given by

$$\mathbf{y}_i = \mathbf{A}\mathbf{c}_i + \boldsymbol{\Lambda}\boldsymbol{\omega}_i + \boldsymbol{\epsilon}_i, \quad i = 1, \ldots, n, \tag{3.14}$$

in which $\mathbf{A}$ and $\boldsymbol{\Lambda}$ are unknown parameter matrices, $\mathbf{c}_i$ is an $r_1 \times 1$ vector of fixed covariates, $\boldsymbol{\omega}_i$ is a $q \times 1$ latent random vector, and $\boldsymbol{\epsilon}_i$ is a random vector of residual errors with distribution $N[\mathbf{0}, \boldsymbol{\Psi}_\epsilon]$, where $\boldsymbol{\Psi}_\epsilon$ is diagonal and $\boldsymbol{\epsilon}_i$ is independent of $\boldsymbol{\omega}_i$. The structural equation is defined as

$$\boldsymbol{\eta}_i = \mathbf{B}\mathbf{d}_i + \boldsymbol{\Pi}\boldsymbol{\eta}_i + \boldsymbol{\Gamma}\boldsymbol{\xi}_i + \boldsymbol{\delta}_i, \tag{3.15}$$

where $\mathbf{d}_i$ is an $r_2 \times 1$ vector of fixed covariates; $\boldsymbol{\omega}_i = (\boldsymbol{\eta}_i^T, \boldsymbol{\xi}_i^T)^T$, $\boldsymbol{\eta}_i$ and $\boldsymbol{\xi}_i$ being $q_1 \times 1$ and $q_2 \times 1$ latent vectors, respectively; $\mathbf{B}$, $\boldsymbol{\Pi}$, and $\boldsymbol{\Gamma}$ are unknown parameter matrices; and $\boldsymbol{\xi}_i$ and $\boldsymbol{\delta}_i$ are independently distributed as $N[\mathbf{0}, \boldsymbol{\Phi}]$ and $N[\mathbf{0}, \boldsymbol{\Psi}_\delta]$, respectively, where $\boldsymbol{\Psi}_\delta$ is a diagonal covariance matrix. To simplify notation, equation (3.15) is rewritten as

$$\boldsymbol{\eta}_i = \boldsymbol{\Lambda}_\omega \mathbf{v}_i + \boldsymbol{\delta}_i, \tag{3.16}$$

where $\boldsymbol{\Lambda}_\omega = (\mathbf{B}, \boldsymbol{\Pi}, \boldsymbol{\Gamma})$ and $\mathbf{v}_i = (\mathbf{d}_i^T, \boldsymbol{\eta}_i^T, \boldsymbol{\xi}_i^T)^T$. See Section 2.3.1 for a more detailed discussion of this model, such as the required assumptions and identification conditions.

Let $\mathbf{Y} = (\mathbf{y}_1, \ldots, \mathbf{y}_n)$, $\mathbf{C} = (\mathbf{c}_1, \ldots, \mathbf{c}_n)$, and $\mathbf{D} = (\mathbf{d}_1, \ldots, \mathbf{d}_n)$ be the data matrices; and let $\boldsymbol{\Omega} = (\boldsymbol{\omega}_1, \ldots, \boldsymbol{\omega}_n)$ be the matrix of latent vectors, and $\boldsymbol{\theta}$ be the structural parameter vector that contains all the unknown parameters in $\{\mathbf{A}, \boldsymbol{\Lambda}, \mathbf{B}, \boldsymbol{\Pi}, \boldsymbol{\Gamma}, \boldsymbol{\Phi}, \boldsymbol{\Psi}_\epsilon, \boldsymbol{\Psi}_\delta\} = \{\mathbf{A}, \boldsymbol{\Lambda}, \boldsymbol{\Lambda}_\omega, \boldsymbol{\Phi}, \boldsymbol{\Psi}_\epsilon, \boldsymbol{\Psi}_\delta\}$. Our main objective is to use MCMC methods to obtain the Bayesian estimates of $\boldsymbol{\theta}$ and $\boldsymbol{\Omega}$. To this end, a sequence of random observations from the joint posterior distribution $[\boldsymbol{\theta}, \boldsymbol{\Omega}|\mathbf{Y}]$ will be generated via the Gibbs sampler which is implemented as follows: At the jth iteration with current value $\boldsymbol{\theta}^{(j)}$:

A. Generate a random variate $\boldsymbol{\Omega}^{(j+1)}$ from the conditional distribution $[\boldsymbol{\Omega}|\mathbf{Y}, \boldsymbol{\theta}^{(j)}]$.
B. Generate a random variate $\boldsymbol{\theta}^{(j+1)}$ from the conditional distribution $[\boldsymbol{\theta}|\mathbf{Y}, \boldsymbol{\Omega}^{(j+1)}]$, and return to step A if necessary.

Here $\boldsymbol{\theta}$ has six components that correspond to unknown parameters in $\mathbf{A}$, $\boldsymbol{\Lambda}$, $\boldsymbol{\Lambda}_\omega$, $\boldsymbol{\Phi}$, $\boldsymbol{\Psi}_\epsilon$, and $\boldsymbol{\Psi}_\delta$, while $\boldsymbol{\Omega}$ has only one component. Conjugate prior distributions for parameters in various components of $\boldsymbol{\theta}$ can be similarly obtained as before; see equations (3.6) and (3.8). For readers who are interested in developing their own computer programs, full conditional distributions for implementing step A and B of the Gibbs sampler are presented in Appendix 3.3. These full conditional distributions are the familiar normal, gamma, and inverted Wishart distributions. Simulating observations from them is fast and straightforward. For applied researchers, we will discuss the use of the freely available WinBUGS software (Spiegelhalter *et al.*, 2003) to obtain the Bayesian results in Section 3.5.

As we discussed at the beginning of Section 3.3, the main difference between SEMs and the familiar regression model is the presence of latent variables in SEMs. Since latent variables are random rather than observed, classical techniques in regression cannot be applied in estimating parameters in SEMs. The idea of data augmentation is used to solve the problem. We augment $\boldsymbol{\Omega}$, the matrix containing all latent variables, with the observed data $\mathbf{Y}$ and work on the joint posterior distribution $[\boldsymbol{\theta}, \boldsymbol{\Omega}|\mathbf{Y}]$. In step B of the Gibbs sampler, we need to simulate $\boldsymbol{\theta}$ from $[\boldsymbol{\theta}|\mathbf{Y}, \boldsymbol{\Omega}]$, the conditional distribution of $\boldsymbol{\theta}$ given $\mathbf{Y}$ and $\boldsymbol{\Omega}$. It is important to note that once $\boldsymbol{\Omega}$ is given rather than random, the SEM becomes the familiar regression model. Consequently, the conditional distribution $[\boldsymbol{\theta}|\mathbf{Y}, \boldsymbol{\Omega}]$ can be derived and the implementation of Gibbs sampler is possible.

The above strategy based on data augmentation is very useful for developing Bayesian methods in the analysis of various complex SEMs with complicated data structures; see detailed discussions in subsequent chapters. Here, we present an application of this strategy to the analysis of nonlinear SEMs for illustration.

Consider a generalization of linear SEMs with fixed covariates to nonlinear SEMs with fixed covariates by extending the structural equation (3.15) to a nonlinear structural equation as follows:

$$\eta_i = \mathbf{Bd}_i + \mathbf{\Pi}\eta_i + \mathbf{\Gamma F}(\xi_i) + \delta_i, \qquad (3.17)$$

where $\mathbf{F}(\xi_i)$ is a vector-valued nonlinear function of ξ_i, and the definitions of other random vectors and parameter matrices are the same as before. The distributions of the nonlinear terms of ξ_i in $\mathbf{F}(\xi_i)$ are not normal and hence induce serious difficulties in the use of traditional methods such as the covariance structure analysis approach, and of existing commercial structural equation modeling software. In contrast, the nonlinear terms of ξ_i can be easily handled using the Bayesian approach with data augmentation. First note that the Gibbs sampler is similarly implemented with steps A and Bb as before, although $[\mathbf{\Omega}|\boldsymbol{\theta}, \mathbf{Y}]$ and $[\boldsymbol{\theta}|\mathbf{Y}, \mathbf{\Omega}]$ are slightly different. The nonlinear terms of ξ_i induce no difficulties in deriving these conditional distributions. In fact, $[\mathbf{\Omega}|\boldsymbol{\theta}, \mathbf{Y}]$ can be derived on the basis of the distribution of the latent variables and the definition of the model. For $[\boldsymbol{\theta}|\mathbf{Y}, \mathbf{\Omega}]$, as $\mathbf{\Omega}$ is given, the nonlinear SEM again becomes the familiar regression model. The conditional distributions for the implementation of the MCMC methods in nonlinear SEMs are presented in Appendix 3.4. We note that the differences between the conditional distributions corresponding to linear and nonlinear SEMs are minor. Hence, we regard nonlinear SEMs as basic SEMs.

3.5 Bayesian estimation via WinBUGS

The freely available WinBUGS (**W**indows version of **B**ayesian inference **U**sing **G**ibbs **S**ampling) software is useful for producing reliable Bayesian statistics for a wide range of statistical models. WinBUGS relies on the use of MCMC techniques, such as the Gibbs sampler (Geman and Geman, 1984) and the MH algorithm (Metropolis *et al.*, 1953; Hastings, 1970). It has been shown that under broad conditions, this software can provide simulated samples from the joint posterior distribution of the unknown quantities, such as parameters and latent variables in the model. As discussed in previous sections, Bayesian estimates of the unknown parameters and latent variables in the model can be obtained from these samples for conducting statistical inferences.

The advanced version of the program is WinBUGS 1.4, developed by the Medical Research Council (MRC) Biostatistics Unit (Cambridge, UK) and the Department of Epidemiology and Public Health of the Imperial College School of Medicine at St. Mary's Hospital (London). It can be downloaded from the website: http://www.mrc-bsu.cam.ac.uk/bugs/. The WinBUGS manual (Spiegelhalter *et al.*, 2003), which is available online, gives brief instructions on WinBUGS; see also Lawson *et al.* (2003, Chapter 4) for supplementary descriptions.

We illustrate the use of WinBUGS through the analysis of an artificial example that is based on the following nonlinear SEM with a linear covariate (see Lee *et al.*, 2007; Lee, 2007). For easy application of the program, we use the following scalar representation of the model. Let $y_{ij} \stackrel{D}{=} N[\mu^*_{ij}, \psi_j]$, where

$$\begin{aligned}
&\mu^*_{i1} = \mu_1 + \eta_i, \quad \mu^*_{ij} = \mu_j + \lambda_{j1}\eta_i, \quad j = 2, 3,\\
&\mu^*_{i4} = \mu_4 + \xi_{i1}, \quad \mu^*_{ij} = \mu_j + \lambda_{j2}\xi_{i1}, \quad j = 5, 6, 7, \quad \text{and}\\
&\mu^*_{i8} = \mu_8 + \xi_{i2}, \quad \mu^*_{ij} = \mu_j + \lambda_{j3}\xi_{i2}, \quad j = 9, 10, \qquad (3.18)
\end{aligned}$$

where the μ_j are intercepts, and the ηs and ξs are the latent variables. The structural equation is reformulated by defining the conditional distribution of η_i given ξ_{i1} and ξ_{i2} as $N[\nu_i, \psi_\delta]$, where

$$\nu_i = b_1 d_i + \gamma_1 \xi_{i1} + \gamma_2 \xi_{i2} + \gamma_3 \xi_{i1} \xi_{i2} + \gamma_4 \xi_{i1}^2 + \gamma_5 \xi_{i2}^2, \tag{3.19}$$

in which d_i is a fixed covariate coming from a t distribution with 5 degrees of freedom. The true population values of the unknown parameters in the model were taken to be:

$$\begin{aligned}
&\mu_1 = \ldots = \mu_{10} = 0.0, \lambda_{21} = \lambda_{52} = \lambda_{93} = 0.9, \lambda_{31} = \lambda_{62} = \lambda_{10,3} = 0.7,\\
&\lambda_{72} = 0.5, \psi_{\epsilon 1} = \psi_{\epsilon 2} = \psi_{\epsilon 3} = 0.3, \psi_{\epsilon 4} = \ldots = \psi_{\epsilon 7} = 0.5, \psi_{\epsilon 8} = \psi_{\epsilon 9} = \psi_{\epsilon 10} = 0.4,\\
&b_1 = 0.5, \gamma_1 = \gamma_2 = 0.4, \gamma_3 = 0.3, \gamma_4 = 0.2, \gamma_5 = 0.5, \text{ and}\\
&\phi_{11} = \phi_{22} = 1.0, \phi_{12} = 0.3, \psi_\delta = 0.36.
\end{aligned} \tag{3.20}$$

Based on the model formulation and these true parameter values, a random sample of continuous observations $\{\mathbf{y}_i, i = 1, \ldots, 500\}$ was generated, which gave the observed data set $\mathbf{Y}$. The following hyperparameter values were taken for the conjugate prior distributions in equations (3.6) and (3.8):

$$\begin{aligned}
&\boldsymbol{\mu}_0 = (0.0, \cdots, 0.0)^T, \boldsymbol{\Sigma}_0 = \mathbf{I}_{10}, \alpha_{0\epsilon k} = \alpha_{0\delta} = 9, \beta_{0\epsilon k} = \beta_{0\delta} = 4,\\
&\text{elements in } \boldsymbol{\Lambda}_{0k} \text{ and } \boldsymbol{\Lambda}_{0\omega k} \text{ are taken to be the true values,}\\
&\mathbf{H}_{0yk} = \mathbf{I}_{10}, \mathbf{H}_{0\omega k} = \mathbf{I}_6, \rho_0 = 4, \mathbf{R}_0 = \boldsymbol{\Phi}_0^{-1},
\end{aligned} \tag{3.21}$$

where $\boldsymbol{\Phi}_0$ is the matrix with true values of ϕ_{11}, ϕ_{22}, and ϕ_{12}. These hyperparameter values represent accurate prior inputs. The WinBUGS code and data are respectively given in the following website:

www.wiley.com/go/medical_behavioral_sciences

We observed that the WinBUGS program converged in less than 4000 iterations. Plots of some simulated sequences of observations for monitoring convergence are presented in Figure 3.2. Based on equations (3.11) and (3.12), Bayesian estimates of the parameters and their standard error estimates as obtained from 6000 iterations after the 4000 burn-in iterations are presented in Table 3.1. We observe that the Bayesian estimates (EST) are close to the true values, and that the standard error estimates (SE) are reasonable. WinBUGS also produces estimates of the latent variables $\{\hat{\boldsymbol{\omega}}_i = (\hat{\eta}_i, \hat{\xi}_{i1}, \hat{\xi}_{i2})^T, i = 1, \ldots, n\}$. Histograms that correspond to the sets of latent variable estimates $\hat{\xi}_{i1}$ and $\hat{\xi}_{i2}$ are displayed in Figure 3.3. We observe from these histograms that the corresponding empirical distributions are close to the normal distributions. The elements in the sample covariance matrix of $\{\hat{\boldsymbol{\xi}}_i, i = 1, \ldots, n\}$ are $s_{11} = 0.902$, $s_{12} = 0.311$, and $s_{22} = 0.910$, and hence this sample covariance matrix is close to the true covariance matrix of $\boldsymbol{\xi}_i$; see (3.20). The residuals can be estimated via $\hat{\boldsymbol{\theta}}$ and $\hat{\boldsymbol{\omega}}_i = (\hat{\eta}_i, \hat{\xi}_{i1}, \hat{\xi}_{i2})^T$ for $i = 1, \ldots, n$ as follows:

$$\begin{aligned}
&\hat{\epsilon}_{i1} = y_{i1} - \hat{\mu}_1 - \hat{\eta}_i, \quad \hat{\epsilon}_{ij} = y_{ij} - \hat{\mu}_j - \hat{\lambda}_{j1}\hat{\eta}_i, \quad j = 2, 3,\\
&\hat{\epsilon}_{i4} = y_{i4} - \hat{\mu}_4 - \hat{\xi}_{i1}, \quad \hat{\epsilon}_{ij} = y_{ij} - \hat{\mu}_j - \hat{\lambda}_{j2}\hat{\xi}_{i1}, \quad j = 5, 6, 7,\\
&\hat{\epsilon}_{i8} = y_{i8} - \hat{\mu}_8 - \hat{\xi}_{i2}, \quad \hat{\epsilon}_{ij} = y_{ij} - \hat{\mu}_j - \hat{\lambda}_{j3}\hat{\xi}_{i2}, \quad j = 9, 10,\\
&\hat{\delta}_i = \hat{\eta}_i - \hat{b}_1 d_i - \hat{\gamma}_1\hat{\xi}_{i1} - \hat{\gamma}_2\hat{\xi}_{i2} - \hat{\gamma}_3\hat{\xi}_{i1}\hat{\xi}_{i2} - \hat{\gamma}_4\hat{\xi}_{i1}^2 - \hat{\gamma}_5\hat{\xi}_{i2}^2.
\end{aligned}$$

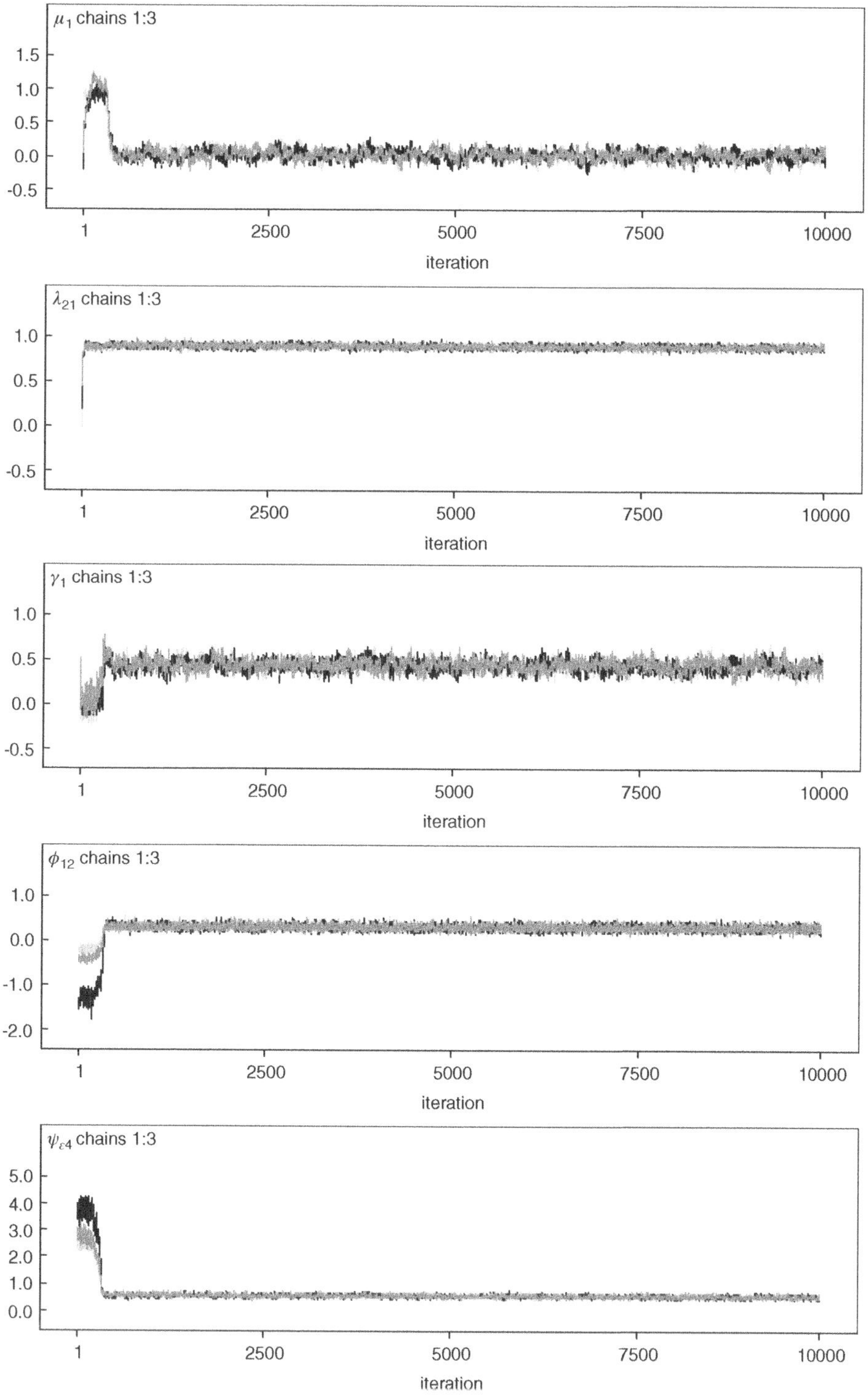

Figure 3.2 From top to bottom, plots represent three chains of observations corresponding to μ_1, λ_{21}, γ_1, ϕ_{12} and $\psi_{\epsilon 4}$, generated by different initial values.

Table 3.1 Bayesian estimates obtained from WinBUGS for the artificial example.

Par	True value	EST	SE	Par	True value	EST	SE
μ_1	0.0	0.022	0.069	$\psi_{\epsilon 1}$	0.3	0.324	0.032
μ_2	0.0	0.065	0.062	$\psi_{\epsilon 2}$	0.3	0.285	0.027
μ_3	0.0	0.040	0.052	$\psi_{\epsilon 3}$	0.3	0.284	0.022
μ_4	0.0	0.003	0.058	$\psi_{\epsilon 4}$	0.5	0.558	0.050
μ_5	0.0	0.036	0.056	$\psi_{\epsilon 5}$	0.5	0.480	0.045
μ_6	0.0	0.002	0.047	$\psi_{\epsilon 6}$	0.5	0.554	0.041
μ_7	0.0	0.004	0.042	$\psi_{\epsilon 7}$	0.5	0.509	0.035
μ_8	0.0	0.092	0.053	$\psi_{\epsilon 8}$	0.4	0.382	0.035
μ_9	0.0	0.032	0.050	$\psi_{\epsilon 9}$	0.4	0.430	0.035
μ_{10}	0.0	−0.000	0.044	$\psi_{\epsilon 10}$	0.4	0.371	0.029
λ_{21}	0.9	0.889	0.022	b_1	0.5	0.525	0.075
λ_{31}	0.7	0.700	0.019	γ_1	0.4	0.438	0.059
λ_{52}	0.9	0.987	0.053	γ_2	0.4	0.461	0.034
λ_{62}	0.7	0.711	0.046	γ_3	0.3	0.304	0.045
λ_{72}	0.5	0.556	0.040	γ_4	0.2	0.184	0.060
λ_{93}	0.9	0.900	0.042	γ_5	0.5	0.580	0.050
$\lambda_{10,3}$	0.7	0.766	0.038	ϕ_{11}	1.0	1.045	0.120
				ϕ_{12}	0.3	0.302	0.057
				ϕ_{22}	1.0	1.023	0.089
				ψ_δ	0.36	0.376	0.045

Some estimated residual plots, $\hat{\epsilon}_{i2}$, $\hat{\epsilon}_{i3}$, $\hat{\epsilon}_{i8}$, and $\hat{\delta}_i$, against case number are presented in Figure 3.4. The plots of estimated residuals $\hat{\delta}_i$ versus $\hat{\xi}_{i1}$ and $\hat{\xi}_{i2}$ are presented in Figure 3.5, and those of $\hat{\epsilon}_{i2}$ versus $\hat{\xi}_{i1}$, $\hat{\xi}_{i2}$, and $\hat{\eta}_i$ are presented in Figure 3.6. Other residual plots are similar. The interpretation of these residual plots is similar to that in regression models. We observe that the plots lie within two parallel horizontal lines that are centered at zero, and no linear or quadratic trends are detected. This roughly indicates that the proposed measurement equation and structural equation are adequate. Moreover, based on $\hat{\boldsymbol{\theta}}$ and $\hat{\boldsymbol{\Omega}}$, we can compute the estimate of the proportion of the variance of $\mathbf{y}$ that can be explained by the measurement equation, using exactly the same method as in analyzing a regression model. Similarly, the proportion of the variance of η that can be explained by the structural equation can also be estimated.

WinBUGS is rather flexible in the analysis of SEMs. In this example, it is applied to analyze nonlinear SEMs with covariates. In the program setup (see the above mentioned website), it only requires a single program statement for the structural equation given by (3.19). In fact, even with more complicated quadratic or interaction terms of the explanatory latent variables and fixed covariates, one program statement is sufficient. Hence, nonlinear SEMs with covariates can be easily analyzed via WinBUGS. This is why we regard nonlinear SEMs as basic SEMs.

WinBUGS is an interactive program, and it is not convenient to use it directly to do a simulation study. However, WinBUGS can be run in batch mode using scripts, and the R package R2WinBUGS (Sturtz *et al.*, 2005) uses this feature and provides tools to directly call

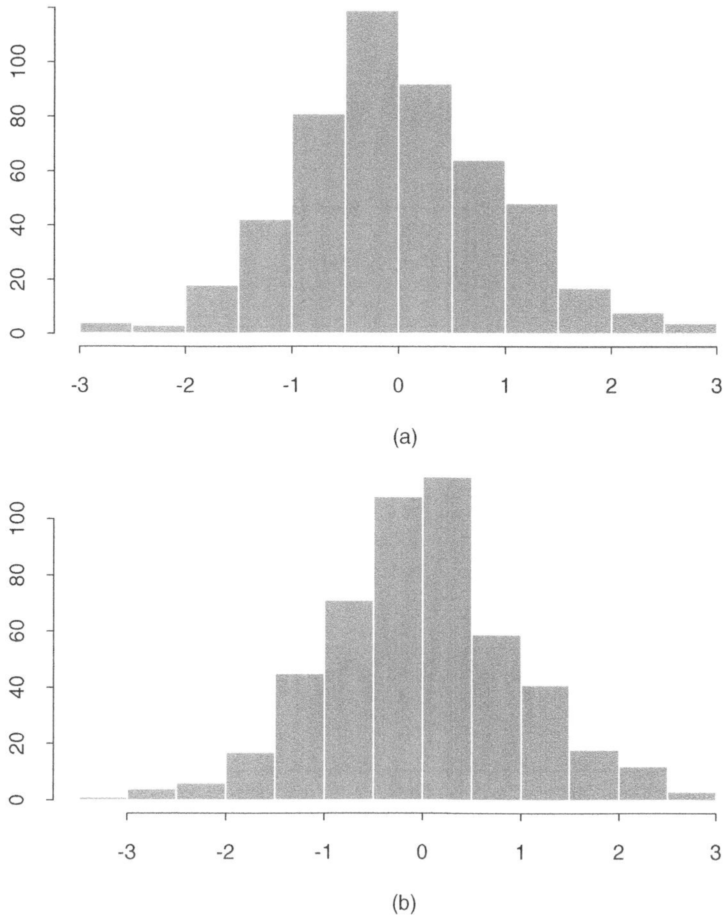

Figure 3.3 Histograms of the latent variables (a) $\hat{\xi}_{i1}$ and (b) $\hat{\xi}_{i2}$.

WinBUGS after the manipulation in R. Furthermore, it is possible to work on the results after importing them back into R. The implementation of R2WinBUGS is mainly based on the R function 'bugs($\cdots$)', which takes data and initial values as input. It automatically writes a WinBUGS script, calls the model, and saves the simulation for easy access in R.

To illustrate the applications of WinBUGS together with R2WinBUGS, we present a simulation study based on the settings of the artificial example described above; see equations (3.18)–(3.20). The sample size was again taken to be 500, and the conjugate prior distributions with hyperparameter values as given in (3.21) were used. Based on 100 replications, the simulation results reported in Table 3.2 were obtained. In the simulation study, we use R to generate the data sets, and input these data sets into WinBUGS to obtain the Bayesian estimates from the WinBUGS outputs. We then use R to store and analyze the Bayesian estimates and the associated results. The WinBUGS and R codes for the simulation study are presented in Appendices 3.5 and 3.6, respectively.

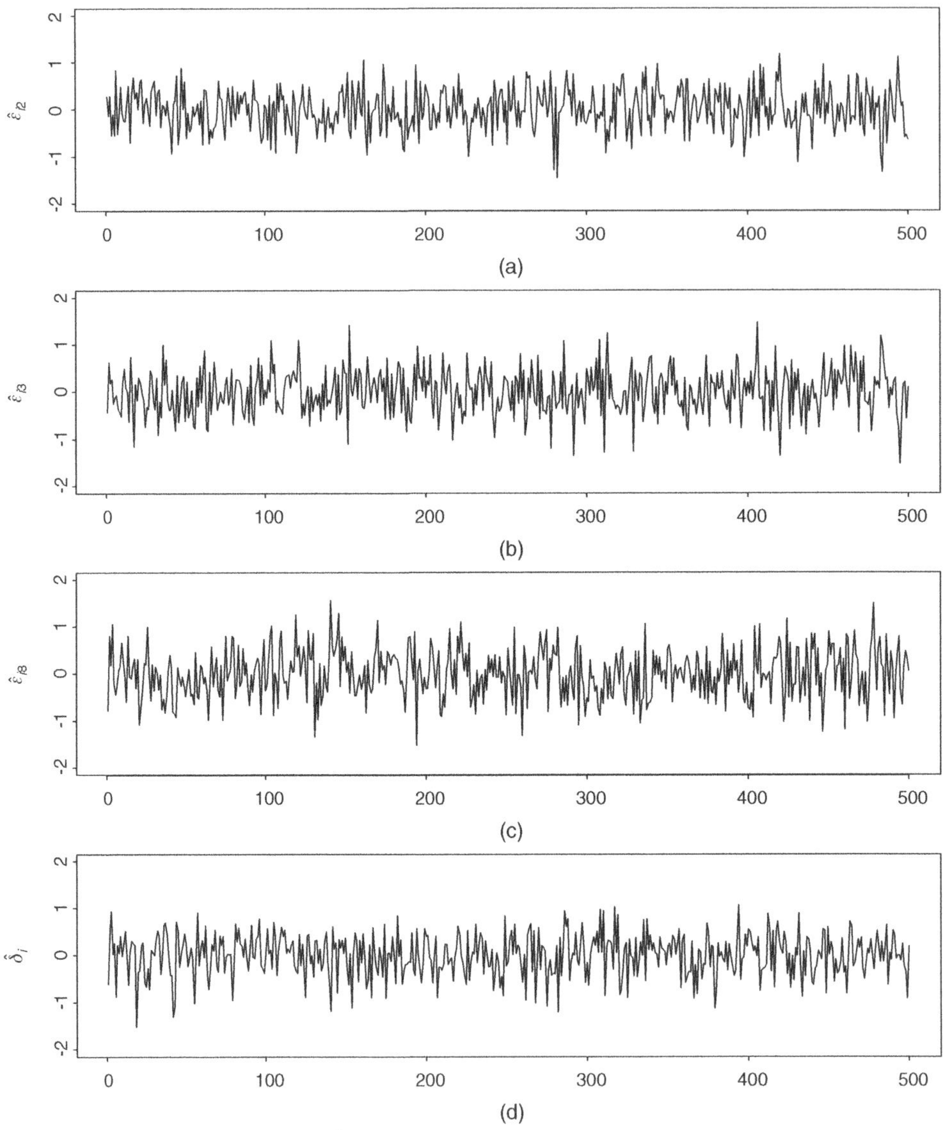

Figure 3.4 Estimated residual plots: (a) $\hat{\epsilon}_{i2}$, (b) $\hat{\epsilon}_{i3}$, (c) $\hat{\epsilon}_{i8}$, and (d) $\hat{\delta}_i$.

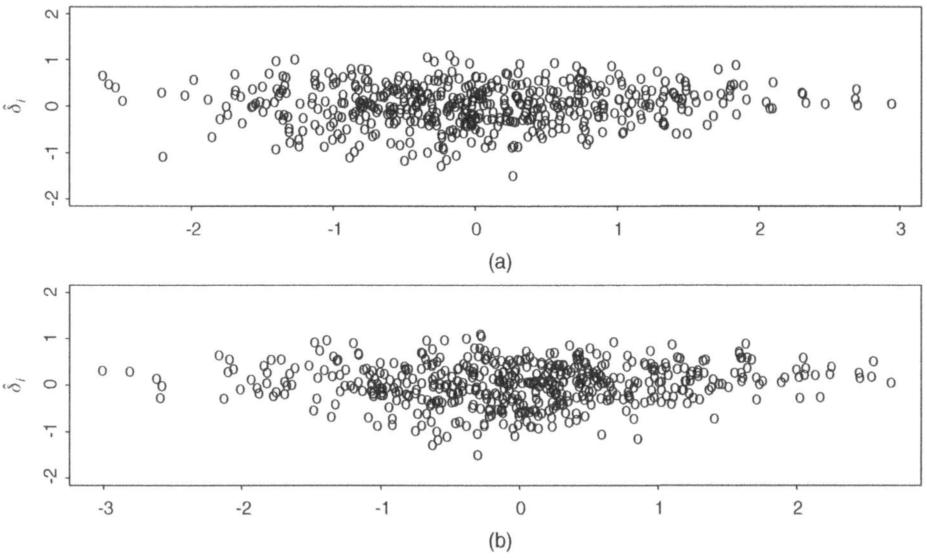

Figure 3.5 Plots of estimated residuals $\hat{\delta}_i$ versus (a) $\hat{\xi}_{i1}$, (b) $\hat{\xi}_{i2}$.

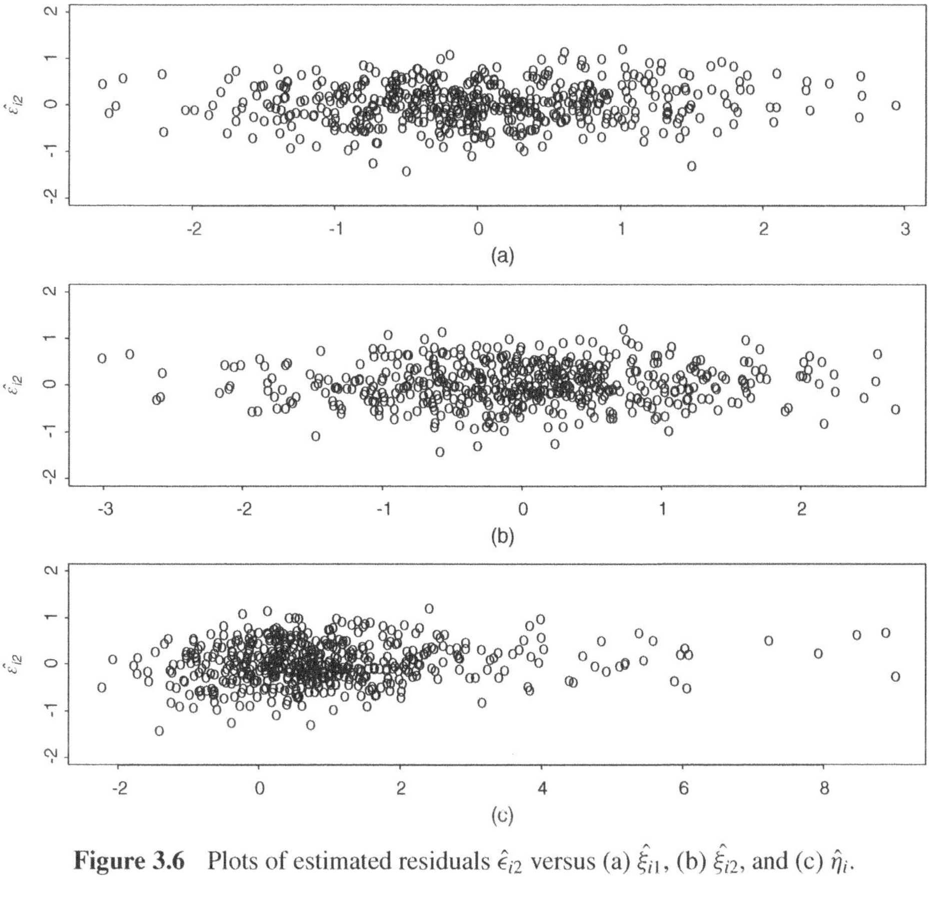

Figure 3.6 Plots of estimated residuals $\hat{\epsilon}_{i2}$ versus (a) $\hat{\xi}_{i1}$, (b) $\hat{\xi}_{i2}$, and (c) $\hat{\eta}_i$.

Table 3.2 Bayesian estimates obtained from WinBUGS for the artificial example, based on 100 replications.

Par	AB	RMS	Par	AB	RMS
μ_1	0.009	0.068	$\psi_{\epsilon 1}$	0.008	0.027
μ_2	0.001	0.064	$\psi_{\epsilon 2}$	0.010	0.028
μ_3	0.003	0.050	$\psi_{\epsilon 3}$	0.004	0.021
μ_4	0.008	0.058	$\psi_{\epsilon 4}$	0.012	0.046
μ_5	0.000	0.055	$\psi_{\epsilon 5}$	0.000	0.047
μ_6	0.005	0.046	$\psi_{\epsilon 6}$	0.002	0.038
μ_7	0.005	0.041	$\psi_{\epsilon 7}$	0.009	0.036
μ_8	0.002	0.051	$\psi_{\epsilon 8}$	0.012	0.037
μ_9	0.001	0.048	$\psi_{\epsilon 9}$	0.001	0.032
μ_{10}	0.001	0.037	$\psi_{\epsilon 10}$	0.006	0.031
λ_{21}	0.006	0.021	b_1	0.001	0.030
λ_{31}	0.001	0.022	γ_1	0.019	0.056
λ_{52}	0.021	0.063	γ_2	0.000	0.066
λ_{62}	0.016	0.047	γ_3	0.003	0.071
λ_{72}	0.015	0.043	γ_4	0.021	0.048
λ_{93}	0.004	0.046	γ_5	0.018	0.062
$\lambda_{10,3}$	0.003	0.037	ϕ_{11}	0.046	0.107
			ϕ_{21}	0.017	0.053
			ϕ_{22}	0.088	0.040
			ψ_δ	0.013	0.040

Note: 'AB' and 'RMS' denote the averages of the absolute bias and the root mean square values, respectively.

Appendix 3.1 The gamma, inverted gamma, Wishart, and inverted Wishart distributions and their characteristics

Let θ and $\mathbf{W}$ denote an unknown parameter and unknown covariance matrix, respectively; and let $p(\cdot)$, $E(\cdot)$, and $\mathrm{Var}(\cdot)$ denote the density function, expectation, and variance, respectively.

1. *Gamma distribution:* $\theta \overset{D}{=} \mathrm{Gamma}[\alpha, \beta]$

$$p(\theta) = \frac{\beta^\alpha}{\Gamma(\alpha)} \theta^{\alpha-1} e^{-\beta\theta},$$

$$E(\theta) = \alpha/\beta, \mathrm{Var}(\theta) = \alpha/\beta^2.$$

2. *Inverted gamma distribution:* $\theta \overset{D}{=} \mathrm{IG}[\alpha, \beta]$

$$p(\theta) = \frac{\beta^\alpha}{\Gamma(\alpha)} \theta^{-(\alpha+1)} e^{-\beta/\theta},$$

$$E(\theta) = \frac{\beta}{\alpha - 1}, \mathrm{Var}(\theta) = \frac{\beta^2}{(\alpha-1)^2(\alpha-2)}.$$

3. *Relation between gamma and inverted gamma distributions*

$$\text{If } \theta \overset{D}{=} \mathrm{IG}[\alpha, \beta], \quad \text{then} \quad \theta^{-1} \overset{D}{=} \mathrm{Gamma}[\alpha, \beta].$$

4. *Wishart distribution:* $\mathbf{W} \overset{D}{=} W_q[\mathbf{R}_0, \rho_0]$

$$p(\mathbf{W}) = \left[2^{\rho_0 q/2} \pi^{q(q-1)/4} \prod_{i=1}^{q} \Gamma\left(\frac{\rho_0 + 1 - i}{2} \right) \right]^{-1}$$

$$\times |\mathbf{R}_0|^{-\rho_0/2} \times |\mathbf{W}|^{(\rho_0-q-1)/2} \times \exp\left\{ -\frac{1}{2} \mathrm{tr}\left(\mathbf{R}_0^{-1}\mathbf{W}\right) \right\},$$

$$E(\mathbf{W}) = \rho_0 \mathbf{R}_0.$$

5. *Inverted Wishart distribution:* $\mathbf{W} \overset{D}{=} \mathrm{IW}_q[\mathbf{R}_0^{-1}, \rho_0]$

$$p(\mathbf{W}) = \left[2^{\rho_0 q/2} \pi^{q(q-1)/4} \prod_{i=1}^{q} \Gamma\left(\frac{\rho_0 + 1 - i}{2} \right) \right]^{-1}$$

$$\times |\mathbf{R}_0|^{-\rho_0/2} \times |\mathbf{W}|^{-(\rho_0+q+1)/2} \times \exp\left\{ -\frac{1}{2} \mathrm{tr}\left(\mathbf{R}_0^{-1}\mathbf{W}^{-1}\right) \right\},$$

$$E(\mathbf{W}) = \frac{\mathbf{R}_0^{-1}}{\rho_0 - q - 1}.$$

6. *Relation between Wishart and inverted Wishart distributions*

$$\text{If } \mathbf{W} \overset{D}{=} \mathrm{IW}\left[\mathbf{R}_0^{-1}, \rho_0\right], \quad \text{then} \quad \mathbf{W}^{-1} \overset{D}{=} W[\mathbf{R}_0, \rho_0].$$

Appendix 3.2 The Metropolis–Hastings algorithm

Suppose we wish to simulate observations, say $\{X_j, j = 1, 2, \ldots\}$, from a conditional distribution with target density $p(\cdot)$. At the jth iteration of the Metropolis–Hastings algorithm with a current value X_j, the next value X_{j+1} is chosen by first sampling a candidate point Y from a proposal distribution $q(\cdot|X_j)$ which is easy to sample. This candidate point Y is accepted as X_{j+1} with probability

$$\min\left(1, \frac{p(Y)q(X_j|Y)}{p(X_j)q(Y|X_j)}\right).$$

If the candidate point Y is rejected, then $X_{j+1} = X_j$ and the chain does not move.

The proposal distribution $q(\cdot|\cdot)$ can have any form and the stationary distribution of the Markov chain will be the target distribution with density $p(\cdot)$. In most analyses of SEMs considered in this book, we will take $q(\cdot|X)$ to be a normal distribution with mean X and a fixed covariance matrix.

Appendix 3.3 Conditional distributions $[\boldsymbol{\Omega}|\mathbf{Y},\boldsymbol{\theta}]$ and $[\boldsymbol{\theta}|\mathbf{Y},\boldsymbol{\Omega}]$

Conditional Distribution $[\boldsymbol{\Omega}|\mathbf{Y},\boldsymbol{\theta}]$

We first note that for $i = 1, \ldots, n$, the $\boldsymbol{\omega}_i$ are conditionally independent given $\boldsymbol{\theta}$, and the $\mathbf{y}_i$ are also conditionally independent given $(\boldsymbol{\omega}_i, \boldsymbol{\theta})$. Hence,

$$p(\boldsymbol{\Omega}|\mathbf{Y},\boldsymbol{\theta}) \propto \prod_{i=1}^{n} p(\boldsymbol{\omega}_i|\boldsymbol{\theta})\, p(\mathbf{y}_i|\boldsymbol{\omega}_i,\boldsymbol{\theta}). \tag{3.A1}$$

This implies that the conditional distributions of $\boldsymbol{\omega}_i$ given $(\mathbf{y}_i, \boldsymbol{\theta})$ are mutually independent for different i, and $p(\boldsymbol{\omega}_i|\mathbf{y}_i,\boldsymbol{\theta}) \propto p(\boldsymbol{\omega}_i|\boldsymbol{\theta})p(\mathbf{y}_i|\boldsymbol{\omega}_i,\boldsymbol{\theta})$. Let $\boldsymbol{\Pi}_0 = \mathbf{I} - \boldsymbol{\Pi}$ and the covariance matrix of $\boldsymbol{\omega}_i$ be

$$\boldsymbol{\Sigma}_\omega = \begin{bmatrix} \boldsymbol{\Pi}_0^{-1}(\boldsymbol{\Gamma\Phi\Gamma}^T + \boldsymbol{\Psi}_\delta)\boldsymbol{\Pi}_0^{-T} & \boldsymbol{\Pi}_0^{-1}\boldsymbol{\Gamma\Phi} \\ \boldsymbol{\Phi\Gamma}^T\boldsymbol{\Pi}_0^{-T} & \boldsymbol{\Phi} \end{bmatrix}.$$

It can be shown that

$$[\boldsymbol{\omega}_i|\boldsymbol{\theta}] \overset{D}{=} N\left[\begin{pmatrix} \boldsymbol{\Pi}_0^{-1}\mathbf{B}\mathbf{d}_i \\ \mathbf{0} \end{pmatrix}, \boldsymbol{\Sigma}_\omega\right],$$

and$[\mathbf{y}_i|\boldsymbol{\omega}_i,\boldsymbol{\theta}] \overset{D}{=} N[\mathbf{A}\mathbf{c}_i + \boldsymbol{\Lambda\omega}_i, \boldsymbol{\Psi}_\epsilon]$. Thus,

$$[\boldsymbol{\omega}_i|\mathbf{y}_i,\boldsymbol{\theta}] \overset{D}{=} N\left[\boldsymbol{\Sigma}^{*-1}\boldsymbol{\Lambda}^T\boldsymbol{\Psi}_\epsilon^{-1}(\mathbf{y}_i - \mathbf{A}\mathbf{c}_i) + \boldsymbol{\Sigma}^{*^{-1}}\boldsymbol{\Sigma}_\omega^{-1}\begin{pmatrix} \boldsymbol{\Pi}_0^{-1}\mathbf{B}\mathbf{d}_i \\ \mathbf{0} \end{pmatrix}, \boldsymbol{\Sigma}^{*-1}\right] \tag{3.A2}$$

where $\boldsymbol{\Sigma}^* = \boldsymbol{\Sigma}_\omega^{-1} + \boldsymbol{\Lambda}^T\boldsymbol{\Psi}_\epsilon^{-1}\boldsymbol{\Lambda}$. We see that the conditional distribution $[\boldsymbol{\omega}_i|\mathbf{y}_i,\boldsymbol{\theta}]$ is a normal distribution.

Conditional Distribution $[\boldsymbol{\theta}|\mathbf{Y},\boldsymbol{\Omega}]$

The conditional distribution of $\boldsymbol{\theta}$ given $(\mathbf{Y},\boldsymbol{\Omega})$ is proportional to $p(\boldsymbol{\theta})p(\mathbf{Y},\boldsymbol{\Omega}|\boldsymbol{\theta})$. We note that as $\boldsymbol{\Omega}$ is given, the equations defined in (3.14) and (3.15) are linear models with fixed covariates. Let $\boldsymbol{\theta}_y$ be the unknown parameters in $\mathbf{A}$, $\boldsymbol{\Lambda}$, and $\boldsymbol{\Psi}_\epsilon$ associated with the measurement equation, and $\boldsymbol{\theta}_\omega$ be the unknown parameters in $\mathbf{B}$, $\boldsymbol{\Pi}$, $\boldsymbol{\Gamma}$, $\boldsymbol{\Phi}$, and $\boldsymbol{\Psi}_\delta$ associated with the structural equation. It is assumed that the prior distribution of $\boldsymbol{\theta}_y$ is independent of the prior distribution of $\boldsymbol{\theta}_\omega$, that is, $p(\boldsymbol{\theta}) = p(\boldsymbol{\theta}_y)p(\boldsymbol{\theta}_\omega)$. Moreover, as $p(\mathbf{Y}|\boldsymbol{\Omega},\boldsymbol{\theta}) = p(\mathbf{Y}|\boldsymbol{\Omega},\boldsymbol{\theta}_y)$ and $p(\boldsymbol{\Omega}|\boldsymbol{\theta}) = p(\boldsymbol{\Omega}|\boldsymbol{\theta}_\omega)$, it can be shown that the marginal conditional densities of $\boldsymbol{\theta}_y$ and $\boldsymbol{\theta}_\omega$ given $(\mathbf{Y},\boldsymbol{\Omega})$ are proportional to $p(\mathbf{Y}|\boldsymbol{\Omega},\boldsymbol{\theta}_y)p(\boldsymbol{\theta}_y)$ and $p(\boldsymbol{\Omega}|\boldsymbol{\theta}_\omega)p(\boldsymbol{\theta}_\omega)$, respectively. Hence, these conditional densities can be treated separately.

Consider first the marginal conditional distribution of $\boldsymbol{\theta}_y$. Let $\boldsymbol{\Lambda}_y = (\mathbf{A},\boldsymbol{\Lambda})$ with general elements λ_{ykj}, $j = 1, \ldots, r_1 + q$, $k = 1, \ldots, p$, and $\mathbf{u}_i = (\mathbf{c}_i^T, \boldsymbol{\omega}_i^T)^T$. It follows that $\mathbf{y}_i = \boldsymbol{\Lambda}_y\mathbf{u}_i + \boldsymbol{\epsilon}_i$. This simple transformation reformulates the model with fixed covariate $\mathbf{c}_i$ as the original factor analysis model. The positions of the fixed elements in $\boldsymbol{\Lambda}_y$ are identified via an index matrix $\mathbf{L}_y$ with the following elements:

$$l_{ykj} = \begin{cases} 0, & \text{if } \lambda_{ykj} \text{ is fixed,} \\ 1, & \text{if } \lambda_{ykj} \text{ is free;} \end{cases} \quad \text{for } j = 1, \ldots, r_1 + q \text{ and } k = 1, \ldots, p.$$

Let $\psi_{\epsilon k}$ be the kth diagonal element of $\boldsymbol{\Psi}_\epsilon$, and $\boldsymbol{\Lambda}_{yk}^T$ be the row vector that contains the unknown parameters in the kth row of $\boldsymbol{\Lambda}_y$. The following commonly used conjugate type prior distributions are used. For any $k \neq h$, we assume that the prior distribution of $(\psi_{\epsilon k}, \boldsymbol{\Lambda}_{yk})$ is independent of $(\psi_{\epsilon h}, \mathbf{\Lambda}_{yh})$, and

$$\psi_{\epsilon k}^{-1} \stackrel{D}{=} \text{Gamma}[\alpha_{0\epsilon k}, \beta_{0\epsilon k}], \text{ and } [\mathbf{\Lambda}_{yk}|\psi_{\epsilon k}] \stackrel{D}{=} N[\mathbf{\Lambda}_{0yk}, \psi_{\epsilon k}\mathbf{H}_{0yk}], \quad k = 1, \ldots, p, \quad (3.\text{A}3)$$

where $\alpha_{0\epsilon k}, \beta_{0\epsilon k}, \mathbf{\Lambda}_{0yk}^T = (\mathbf{A}_{0k}^T, \mathbf{\Lambda}_{0k}^T)$, and the positive definite matrix $\mathbf{H}_{0yk}$ are hyperparameters whose values are assumed to be given from the prior information of previous studies or other sources.

Let $\mathbf{U} = (\mathbf{u}_1, \ldots, \mathbf{u}_n)$ and $\mathbf{U}_k$ be the submatrix of $\mathbf{U}$ such that all the rows corresponding to $l_{ykj} = 0$ are deleted; and let $\mathbf{Y}_k^{*T} = (y_{1k}^*, \ldots, y_{nk}^*)$ with

$$y_{ik}^* = y_{ik} - \sum_{j=1}^{r_1+q} \lambda_{ykj} u_{ij}(1 - l_{ykj}),$$

where u_{ij} is the jth element of $\mathbf{u}_i$. Then, for $k = 1, \ldots, p$, it can be shown (see Lee, 2007, Appendix 4.3) that

$$\left[\psi_{\epsilon k}^{-1}|\mathbf{Y}, \mathbf{\Omega}\right] \stackrel{D}{=} \text{Gamma}[n/2 + \alpha_{0\epsilon k}, \beta_{\epsilon k}], \quad \left[\mathbf{\Lambda}_{yk}|\mathbf{Y}, \mathbf{\Omega}, \psi_{\epsilon k}^{-1}\right] \stackrel{D}{=} N[\mathbf{a}_{yk}, \psi_{\epsilon k}\mathbf{A}_{yk}], \quad (3.\text{A}4)$$

where $\mathbf{A}_{yk} = (\mathbf{H}_{0yk}^{-1} + \mathbf{U}_k\mathbf{U}_k^T)^{-1}$, $\mathbf{a}_{yk} = \mathbf{A}_{yk}(\mathbf{H}_{0yk}^{-1}\mathbf{\Lambda}_{0yk} + \mathbf{U}_k\mathbf{Y}_k^*)$, and

$$\beta_{\epsilon k} = \beta_{0\epsilon k} + \frac{1}{2}\left(\mathbf{Y}_k^{*T}\mathbf{Y}_k^* - \mathbf{a}_{yk}^T\mathbf{A}_{yk}^{-1}\mathbf{a}_{yk} + \mathbf{\Lambda}_{0yk}^T\mathbf{H}_{0yk}^{-1}\mathbf{\Lambda}_{0yk}\right).$$

Since $[\mathbf{\Lambda}_{yk}, \psi_{\epsilon k}^{-1}|\mathbf{Y}, \mathbf{\Omega}]$ equals $[\psi_{\epsilon k}^{-1}|\mathbf{Y}, \mathbf{\Omega}][\mathbf{\Lambda}_{yk}|\mathbf{Y}, \mathbf{\Omega}, \psi_{\epsilon k}^{-1}]$, it can be obtained via (3.A4). This gives the conditional distribution in relation to $\boldsymbol{\theta}_y$.

Now consider the conditional distribution of $\boldsymbol{\theta}_\omega$, which is proportional to $p(\mathbf{\Omega}|\boldsymbol{\theta}_\omega)p(\boldsymbol{\theta}_\omega)$. Let $\mathbf{\Omega}_1 = (\boldsymbol{\eta}_1, \ldots, \boldsymbol{\eta}_n)$ and $\mathbf{\Omega}_2 = (\boldsymbol{\xi}_1, \ldots, \boldsymbol{\xi}_n)$. Since the distribution of $\boldsymbol{\xi}_i$ only involves $\mathbf{\Phi}$, $p(\mathbf{\Omega}_2|\boldsymbol{\theta}_\omega) = p(\mathbf{\Omega}_2|\mathbf{\Phi})$. Under the assumption that the prior distribution of $\mathbf{\Phi}$ is independent of the prior distributions of $\mathbf{B}$, $\mathbf{\Pi}$, $\mathbf{\Gamma}$, and $\mathbf{\Psi}_\delta$, we have

$$p(\mathbf{\Omega}|\boldsymbol{\theta}_\omega)p(\boldsymbol{\theta}_\omega) = [p(\mathbf{\Omega}_1|\mathbf{\Omega}_2, \mathbf{B}, \mathbf{\Pi}, \mathbf{\Gamma}, \mathbf{\Psi}_\delta)p(\mathbf{B}, \mathbf{\Pi}, \mathbf{\Gamma}, \mathbf{\Psi}_\delta)][p(\mathbf{\Omega}_2|\mathbf{\Phi})p(\mathbf{\Phi})].$$

Hence, the marginal conditional densities of $(\mathbf{B}, \mathbf{\Pi}, \mathbf{\Gamma}, \mathbf{\Psi}_\delta)$ and $\mathbf{\Phi}$ can be treated separately.

Consider a conjugate type prior distribution for $\mathbf{\Phi}$ with $\mathbf{\Phi} \stackrel{D}{=} \text{IW}_{q_2}[\mathbf{R}_0^{-1}, \rho_0]$ or $\mathbf{\Phi}^{-1} \stackrel{D}{=} W_{q_2}[\mathbf{R}_0, \rho_0]$, with hyperparameters ρ_0 and $\mathbf{R}_0^{-1}$ or $\mathbf{R}_0$.

To derive $p(\mathbf{\Phi}|\mathbf{\Omega}_2)$, we first note that it is proportional to $p(\mathbf{\Phi})p(\mathbf{\Omega}_2|\mathbf{\Phi})$. As $\boldsymbol{\xi}_i$ are independent, we have

$$p(\mathbf{\Phi}|\mathbf{\Omega}_2) \propto p(\mathbf{\Phi}) \prod_{i=1}^n p(\boldsymbol{\xi}_i|\boldsymbol{\theta}).$$

Moreover, since the distribution of $\boldsymbol{\xi}_i$ given $\mathbf{\Phi}$ is $N(\mathbf{0}, \mathbf{\Phi})$, we have

$$\begin{aligned} p(\mathbf{\Phi}|\mathbf{\Omega}_2) &\propto \left[|\mathbf{\Phi}|^{-(\rho_0+q_2+1)/2} \exp\left\{-\frac{1}{2}\text{tr}[\mathbf{R}_0^{-1}\mathbf{\Phi}^{-1}]\right\}\right]\left[|\mathbf{\Phi}|^{-n/2} \exp\left\{-\frac{1}{2}\sum_{i=1}^n \boldsymbol{\xi}_i^T\mathbf{\Phi}^{-1}\boldsymbol{\xi}_i\right\}\right] \\ &= |\mathbf{\Phi}|^{-(n+\rho_0+q_2+1)/2} \exp\left\{-\frac{1}{2}\,\text{tr}\left[\mathbf{\Phi}^{-1}\left(\mathbf{\Omega}_2\mathbf{\Omega}_2^T + \mathbf{R}_0^{-1}\right)\right]\right\}. \end{aligned} \quad (3.\text{A}5)$$

Since the right-hand side of (3.A5) is proportional to the density function of an inverted Wishart distribution (Zellner, 1971), it follows that the conditional distribution of $\mathbf{\Phi}$ given $\mathbf{\Omega}_2$

is given by

$$[\boldsymbol{\Phi}|\boldsymbol{\Omega}_2] \stackrel{D}{=} \mathrm{IW}_{q_2}\big[\big(\boldsymbol{\Omega}_2\boldsymbol{\Omega}_2^T + \mathbf{R}_0^{-1}\big), n + \rho_0\big] \tag{3.A6}$$

Recall that $\boldsymbol{\eta}_i = \boldsymbol{\Lambda}_\omega \mathbf{v}_i + \boldsymbol{\delta}_i$, where $\boldsymbol{\Lambda}_\omega = (\mathbf{B}, \boldsymbol{\Pi}, \boldsymbol{\Gamma})$ with general elements $\lambda_{\omega kj}$ for $k = 1, \ldots, q_1$, and let $\mathbf{v}_i = (\mathbf{d}_i^T, \boldsymbol{\eta}_i^T, \boldsymbol{\xi}_i^T)^T = (\mathbf{d}_i^T, \boldsymbol{\omega}_i^T)^T$ be an $(r_2 + q_1 + q_2) \times 1$ vector. The model $\boldsymbol{\eta}_i = \boldsymbol{\Lambda}_\omega \mathbf{v}_i + \boldsymbol{\delta}_i$ is similar to $\mathbf{y}_i = \boldsymbol{\Lambda}_y \mathbf{u}_i + \boldsymbol{\epsilon}_i$ considered before. Hence, the derivations for the conditional distributions corresponding to $\boldsymbol{\theta}_\omega$ are similar to those corresponding to $\boldsymbol{\theta}_y$. Let $\mathbf{V} = (\mathbf{v}_1, \ldots, \mathbf{v}_n)$, $\mathbf{L}_\omega$ be the index matrix with general elements $l_{\omega kj}$ defined similarly to $\mathbf{L}_y$ to indicate the fixed known parameters in $\boldsymbol{\Lambda}_\omega$; $\psi_{\delta k}$ be the kth diagonal element of $\boldsymbol{\Psi}_\delta$; and $\boldsymbol{\Lambda}_{\omega k}^T$ be the row vector that contains the unknown parameters in the kth row of $\boldsymbol{\Lambda}_\omega$. The prior distributions of $\boldsymbol{\Lambda}_{\omega k}$ and $\psi_{\delta k}^{-1}$ are similarly selected as the following conjugate type distributions:

$$\psi_{\delta k}^{-1} \stackrel{D}{=} \mathrm{Gamma}[\alpha_{0\delta k}, \beta_{0\delta k}], \text{ and } [\boldsymbol{\Lambda}_{\omega k}|\psi_{\delta k}] \stackrel{D}{=} N[\boldsymbol{\Lambda}_{0\omega k}, \psi_{\delta k}\mathbf{H}_{0\omega k}], \quad k = 1, \ldots, q_1, \tag{3.A7}$$

where $\alpha_{0\delta k}$, $\beta_{0\delta k}$, $\boldsymbol{\Lambda}_{0\omega k}$, and $\mathbf{H}_{0\omega k}$ are given hyperparameters. Moreover, it is assumed that, for $h \neq k$, $(\psi_{\delta k}, \boldsymbol{\Lambda}_{\omega k})$ and $(\psi_{\delta h}, \boldsymbol{\Lambda}_{\omega h})$ are independent. Let $\mathbf{V}_k$ be the submatrix of $\mathbf{V}$ such that all the rows corresponding to $l_{\omega kj} = 0$ are deleted; and let $\boldsymbol{\Xi}_k^T = (\eta_{1k}^*, \ldots, \eta_{nk}^*)$ where

$$\eta_{ik}^* = \eta_{ik} - \sum_{j=1}^{r_2+q} \lambda_{\omega kj} v_{ij}(1 - l_{\omega kj}).$$

Then, it can be shown that

$$[\psi_{\delta k}^{-1}|\boldsymbol{\Omega}] \stackrel{D}{=} \mathrm{Gamma}[n/2 + \alpha_{0\delta k}, \beta_{\delta k}] \quad \text{and} \quad [\boldsymbol{\Lambda}_{\omega k}|\boldsymbol{\Omega}, \psi_{\delta k}^{-1}] \stackrel{D}{=} N[\mathbf{a}_{\omega k}, \psi_{\delta k}\mathbf{A}_{\omega k}], \tag{3.A8}$$

where $\mathbf{A}_{\omega k} = (\mathbf{H}_{0\omega k}^{-1} + \mathbf{V}_k\mathbf{V}_k^T)^{-1}$, $\mathbf{a}_{\omega k} = \mathbf{A}_{\omega k}(\mathbf{H}_{0\omega k}^{-1}\boldsymbol{\Lambda}_{0\omega k} + \mathbf{V}_k\boldsymbol{\Xi}_k)$, and

$$\beta_{\delta k} = \beta_{0\delta k} + \frac{1}{2}\big(\boldsymbol{\Xi}_k^T\boldsymbol{\Xi}_k - \mathbf{a}_{\omega k}^T\mathbf{A}_{\omega k}^{-1}\mathbf{a}_{\omega k} + \boldsymbol{\Lambda}_{0\omega k}^T\mathbf{H}_{0\omega k}^{-1}\boldsymbol{\Lambda}_{0\omega k}\big).$$

The conditional distribution $[\boldsymbol{\theta}_\omega|\boldsymbol{\Omega}] = [\mathbf{B}, \boldsymbol{\Pi}, \boldsymbol{\Gamma}, \boldsymbol{\Psi}_\delta|\boldsymbol{\Omega}]$ can be obtained through (3.A8).

In this appendix, we use $\boldsymbol{\Lambda}_{yk}^T$ and $\boldsymbol{\Lambda}_{\omega k}^T$ to denote the row vectors that contain the unknown parameters in the kth rows of $\boldsymbol{\Lambda}_y$ and $\boldsymbol{\Lambda}_\omega$, respectively. However, in the subsequent chapters we sometimes assume for simplicity that all the elements in the kth rows of $\boldsymbol{\Lambda}_y$ and $\boldsymbol{\Lambda}_\omega$ are unknown parameters. Under these assumptions, $\boldsymbol{\Lambda}_{yk}^T$ and $\boldsymbol{\Lambda}_{\omega k}^T$ simply denote the kth rows of $\boldsymbol{\Lambda}_y$ and $\boldsymbol{\Lambda}_\omega$, respectively.

Appendix 3.4 Conditional distributions $[\mathbf{\Omega}|\mathbf{Y}, \boldsymbol{\theta}]$ and $[\boldsymbol{\theta}|\mathbf{Y}, \mathbf{\Omega}]$ in nonlinear SEMs with covariates

Conditional Distribution $[\mathbf{\Omega}|\mathbf{Y}, \boldsymbol{\theta}]$

First note that the measurement equation of a nonlinear SEM with covariates is the same as given in equation (3.14), while the structural equation is defined as in equation (3.17). Again to simplify notation, equation (3.17) is rewritten as

$$\boldsymbol{\eta}_i = \mathbf{\Lambda}_\omega \mathbf{G}(\boldsymbol{\omega}_i) + \boldsymbol{\delta}_i, \tag{3.A9}$$

where $\mathbf{\Lambda}_\omega = (\mathbf{B}, \mathbf{\Pi}, \mathbf{\Gamma})$ and $\mathbf{G}(\boldsymbol{\omega}_i) = (\mathbf{d}_i^T, \boldsymbol{\eta}_i^T, \mathbf{F}(\boldsymbol{\xi}_i)^T)^T$. Similar reasoning can be used to derive the conditional distribution $[\mathbf{\Omega}|\mathbf{Y}, \boldsymbol{\theta}]$. It can be shown on the basis of the definition and assumptions that

$$p(\mathbf{\Omega}|\mathbf{Y}, \boldsymbol{\theta}) = \prod_{i=1}^{n} p(\boldsymbol{\omega}_i|\mathbf{y}_i, \boldsymbol{\theta}) \propto \prod_{i=1}^{n} p(\mathbf{y}_i|\boldsymbol{\omega}_i, \boldsymbol{\theta}) p(\boldsymbol{\eta}_i|\boldsymbol{\xi}_i, \boldsymbol{\theta}) p(\boldsymbol{\xi}_i|\boldsymbol{\theta}). \tag{3.A10}$$

As the $\boldsymbol{\omega}_i$ are mutually independent, and $\mathbf{y}_i$ are also mutually independent given $\boldsymbol{\omega}_i$, $p(\boldsymbol{\omega}_i|\mathbf{y}_i, \boldsymbol{\theta})$ is proportional to

$$\exp\left\{ -\frac{1}{2}\boldsymbol{\xi}_i^T \mathbf{\Phi}^{-1}\boldsymbol{\xi}_i - \frac{1}{2}(\mathbf{y}_i - \mathbf{A}\mathbf{c}_i - \mathbf{\Lambda}\boldsymbol{\omega}_i)^T \mathbf{\Psi}_\epsilon^{-1}(\mathbf{y}_i - \mathbf{A}\mathbf{c}_i - \mathbf{\Lambda}\boldsymbol{\omega}_i) \right.$$
$$\left. -\frac{1}{2}(\boldsymbol{\eta}_i - \mathbf{\Lambda}_\omega \mathbf{G}(\boldsymbol{\omega}_i))^T \mathbf{\Psi}_\delta^{-1}(\boldsymbol{\eta}_i - \mathbf{\Lambda}_\omega \mathbf{G}(\boldsymbol{\omega}_i)) \right\}. \tag{3.A11}$$

This distribution is nonstandard and complex. Hence, the MH algorithm is used to generate observations from the target density $p(\boldsymbol{\omega}_i|\mathbf{y}_i, \boldsymbol{\theta})$ as given in (3.A11). In this algorithm, we choose $N[\mathbf{0}, \sigma^2\mathbf{\Sigma}_\omega]$ as the proposal distribution, where $\mathbf{\Sigma}_\omega^{-1} = \mathbf{\Sigma}_\delta^{-1} + \mathbf{\Lambda}^T\mathbf{\Psi}_\epsilon^{-1}\mathbf{\Lambda}$ and $\mathbf{\Sigma}_\delta^{-1}$ is given by

$$\mathbf{\Sigma}_\delta^{-1} = \begin{bmatrix} \mathbf{\Pi}_0^T \mathbf{\Psi}_\delta^{-1} \mathbf{\Pi}_0 & -\mathbf{\Pi}_0^T \mathbf{\Psi}_\delta^{-1} \mathbf{\Gamma}\mathbf{\Delta} \\ -\mathbf{\Delta}^T \mathbf{\Gamma}^T \mathbf{\Psi}_\delta^{-1} \mathbf{\Pi}_0 & \mathbf{\Phi}^{-1} + \mathbf{\Delta}^T \mathbf{\Gamma}^T \mathbf{\Psi}_\delta^{-1} \mathbf{\Gamma}\mathbf{\Delta} \end{bmatrix}$$

in which $\mathbf{\Pi}_0 = \mathbf{I} - \mathbf{\Pi}$ and $\mathbf{\Delta} = [\partial \mathbf{F}(\boldsymbol{\xi}_i)/\partial \boldsymbol{\xi}_i]^T|_{\boldsymbol{\xi}_i=\mathbf{0}}$. Let $p(\cdot|\boldsymbol{\omega}, \sigma^2\mathbf{\Sigma}_\omega)$ be the proposal density corresponding to $N[\boldsymbol{\omega}, \sigma^2\mathbf{\Sigma}_\omega]$. The MH algorithm for our problem is implemented as follows: At the rth iteration with the current value $\boldsymbol{\omega}_i^{(r)}$, a new candidate $\boldsymbol{\omega}_i$ is generated from $p(\cdot|\boldsymbol{\omega}_i^{(r)}, \sigma^2\mathbf{\Sigma}_\omega)$, and this new candidate is accepted with probability

$$\min\left\{1, \frac{p(\boldsymbol{\omega}_i|\mathbf{y}_i, \boldsymbol{\theta})}{p(\boldsymbol{\omega}_i^{(r)}|\mathbf{y}_i, \boldsymbol{\theta})}\right\}.$$

The variance σ^2 is chosen such that the acceptance rate is approximately 0.25 or more (see Gelman *et al.*, 1996).

Conditional Distribution $[\boldsymbol{\theta}|\mathbf{Y}, \boldsymbol{\Omega}]$

When $\boldsymbol{\Omega}$ is given, the structural equation (see (3.17)) is just a multiple regression equation, which is slightly different from the linear regression equation (see (3.15)) associated with the linear SEMs. Hence, the components of the conditional distribution $[\boldsymbol{\theta}|\boldsymbol{\Omega}, \mathbf{Y}]$ involved in the Gibbs sampler in analyzing nonlinear SEMs are very similar to those in analyzing linear SEMs. To obtain $[\boldsymbol{\theta}|\mathbf{Y}, \boldsymbol{\Omega}]$ for nonlinear SEMs, we only need to replace $\boldsymbol{\xi}_i$ by $\mathbf{F}(\boldsymbol{\xi}_i)$ in the corresponding conditional distributions that are derived for linear SEMs and are presented in Appendix 3.3.

Appendix 3.5 WinBUGS code

```
model {
    for (i in 1:N) {
        for (j in 1:10) { y[i,j]~dnorm(mu[i,j], psi[j]) }
        mu[i,1]<-u[1]+eta[i]
        mu[i,2]<-u[2]+lam[1]*eta[i]
        mu[i,3]<-u[3]+lam[2]*eta[i]
        mu[i,4]<-u[4]+xi[i,1]
        mu[i,5]<-u[5]+lam[3]*xi[i,1]
        mu[i,6]<-u[6]+lam[4]*xi[i,1]
        mu[i,7]<-u[7]+lam[5]*xi[i,1]
        mu[i,8]<-u[8]+xi[i,2]
        mu[i,9]<-u[9]+lam[6]*xi[i,2]
        mu[i,10]<-u[10]+lam[7]*xi[i,2]

        #structural equation
        eta[i] ~dnorm(nu[i], psd)

        nu[i]<-b*d[i]+gam[1]*xi[i,1]+gam[2]*xi[i,2]+gam[3]*xi[i,1]*xi[i,2]
               +gam[4]*xi[i,1]*xi[i,1]+gam[5]*xi[i,2]*xi[i,2]

        xi[i,1:2] ~dmnorm(zero[1:2], phi[1:2,1:2])
    }   #end of i

    #prior distribution
    lam[1] ~dnorm(0.9,psi[2])       lam[2] ~dnorm(0.7,psi[3])
    lam[3] ~dnorm(0.9,psi[5])       lam[4] ~dnorm(0.7,psi[6])
    lam[5] ~dnorm(0.5,psi[7])       lam[6] ~dnorm(0.9,psi[9])
    lam[7] ~dnorm(0.7,psi[10])

    b ~dnorm(0.5, psd)              gam[1] ~dnorm(0.4,psd)
    gam[2] ~dnorm(0.4,psd)          gam[3] ~dnorm(0.3,psd)
    gam[4] ~dnorm(0.2,psd)          gam[5] ~dnorm(0.5,psd)

    for (j in 1:10) {
        psi[j] dgamma(9,4)        sgm[j]<-1/psi[j]
        u[j] ~dnorm(0,1)
    }

    psd dgamma(9,4)     sgd<-1/psd

    phi[1:2,1:2] dwish(R[1:2,1:2], 4)
    phx[1:2,1:2]<-inverse(phi[1:2,1:2])
} #end of model
```

Appendix 3.6 R2WinBUGS code

```
library(mvtnorm)   #Load mvtnorm package
library(R2WinBUGS) #Load R2WinBUGS package

N=500                          #Sample size
BD=numeric(N)                  #Fixed covariate in structural equation
XI=matrix(NA, nrow=N, ncol=2)  #Explanatory latent variables
Eta=numeric(N)                 #Outcome latent variables
Y=matrix(NA, nrow=N, ncol=8)   #Observed variables

#The covariance matrix of xi
phi=matrix(c(1, 0.3, 0.3, 1), nrow=2)

#Estimates and standard error estimates
Eu=matrix(NA, nrow=100, ncol=10);    SEu=matrix(NA, nrow=100, ncol=10)
Elam=matrix(NA, nrow=100, ncol=7);   SElam=matrix(NA, nrow=100, ncol=7)
Eb=numeric(100);                     SEb=numeric(100)
Egam=matrix(NA, nrow=100, ncol=5);   SEgam=matrix(NA, nrow=100, ncol=5)
Esgm=matrix(NA, nrow=100, ncol=10);  SEsgm=matrix(NA, nrow=100, ncol=10)
Esgd=numeric(100);                   SEsgd=numeric(100)
Ephx=matrix(NA, nrow=100, ncol=3);   SEphx=matrix(NA, nrow=100, ncol=3)

R=matrix(c(1.0, 0.3, 0.3, 1.0), nrow=2)

parameters=c(''u'', ''lam'', ''b'', ''gam'', ''sgm'', ''sgd'', ''phx'')

init1=list(u=rep(0,10), lam=rep(0,7), b=0, gam=rep(0,5), psi=rep(1,10),
           psd=1, phi=matrix(c(1, 0, 0, 1), nrow=2))

init2=list(u=rep(1,10), lam=rep(1,7), b=1, gam=rep(1,5), psi=rep(2,10),
           psd=2, phi=matrix(c(2, 0, 0, 2), nrow=2))

inits=list(init1, init2)

eps=numeric(10)

for (t in 1:100) {
    #Generate Data
    for (i in 1:N) {
        BD[i]=rt(1, 5)

        XI[i,]=rmvnorm(1, c(0,0), phi)

        delta=rnorm(1, 0, sqrt(0.36))
        Eta[i]=0.5*BD[i]+0.4*XI[i,1]+0.4*XI[i,2]+0.3*XI[i,1]*XI[i,2]
               +0.2*XI[i,1]*XI[i,1]+0.5*XI[i,2]*XI[i,2]+delta

        eps[1:3]=rnorm(3, 0, sqrt(0.3))
        eps[4:7]=rnorm(4, 0, sqrt(0.5))
        eps[8:10]=rnorm(3, 0, sqrt(0.4))
        Y[i,1]=Eta[i]+eps[1]
        Y[i,2]=0.9*Eta[i]+eps[2]
        Y[i,3]=0.7*Eta[i]+eps[3]
        Y[i,4]=XI[i,1]+eps[4]
```

```
        Y[i,5]=0.9*XI[i,1]+eps[5]
        Y[i,6]=0.7*XI[i,1]+eps[6]
        Y[i,7]=0.5*XI[i,1]+eps[7]
        Y[i,8]=XI[i,2]+eps[8]
        Y[i,9]=0.9*XI[i,2]+eps[9]
        Y[i,10]=0.7*XI[i,2]+eps[10]
    }

    #Run WinBUGS
    data=list(N=500, zero=c(0,0), d=BD, R=R, y=Y)

    model<-bugs(data,inits,parameters,
                model.file=''C:/Simulation/model.txt'',
                n.chains=2,n.iter=10000,n.burnin=4000,n.thin=1,
                bugs.directory=''C:/Program Files/WinBUGS14/'',
                working.directory=''C:/Simulation/'')

    #Save Estimates
    Eu[t,]=model$mean$u;                    SEu[t,]=model$sd$u
    Elam[t,]=model$mean$lam;                SElam[t,]=model$sd$lam
    Eb[t]=model$mean$b;                     SEb[t]=model$sd$b
    Egam[t,]=model$mean$gam;                SEgam[t,]=model$sd$gam
    Esgm[t,]=model$mean$sgm;                SEsgm[t,]=model$sd$sgm
    Esgd[t]=model$mean$sgd;                 SEsgd[t]=model$sd$sgd
    Ephx[t,1]=model$mean$phx[1,1];          SEphx[t,1]=model$sd$phx[1,1]
    Ephx[t,2]=model$mean$phx[1,2];          SEphx[t,2]=model$sd$phx[1,2]
    Ephx[t,3]=model$mean$phx[2,2];          SEphx[t,3]=model$sd$phx[2,2]
}
```

References

Albert, J. H. and Chib, S. (1993) Bayesian analysis of binary and polychotomous response data. *Journal of the American Statistical Association*, **88**, 669–679.

Ansari, A. and Jedidi, K. (2000) Bayesian factor analysis for multilevel binary observations. *Psychometrika*, **65**, 475–496.

Berger, J. O. (1985) *Statistical Decision Theory and Bayesian Analysis*. New York: Springer-Verlag.

Boomsma, A. (1982) The robustness of LISREL against small sample sizes in factor analysis models. In K. G. Jöreskog and H. Wold (eds), *Systems under Indirect Observation: Causality, Structure, Prediction*, pp. 149–173. Amsterdam: North-Holland.

Box, G. E. P. and Tiao, G. C. (1973) *Bayesian Inference in Statistical Analysis*. Reading, MA: Addison-Wesley.

Chou, C. P., Bentler, P. M. and Satorra, A. (1991) Scaled test statistics and robust standard errors for non-normal data in covariance structure analysis: A Monte Carlo study. *British Journal of Mathematical and Statistical Psychology*, **44**, 347–357.

Congdon, P. (2003) *Applied Bayesian Modelling*. Chichester: John Wiley & Sons, Ltd.

Dunson, D. B. (2000) Bayesian latent variable models for clustered mixed outcomes. *Journal of the Royal Statistical Society, Series B*, **62**, 355–366.

Gelfand, A. E. and Smith, A. F. M. (1990) Sampling-based approaches to calculating marginal densities. *Journal of the American Statistical Association*, **85**, 398–409.

Gelman, A., Carlin, J. B., Stern, H. S. and Rubin, D. B. (2003) *Bayesian Data Analysis*, (2nd edn). London: Chapman & Hall /CRC.

Gelman, A., Roberts, G. O. and Gilks, W. R. (1996) Efficient Metropolis jumping rules. In J. M. Bernardo, J. O. Berger, A. P. Dawid and A. F. M. Smith (eds), *Bayesian Statistics 5*, pp. 599–607. Oxford: Oxford University Press.

Geman, S. and Geman, D. (1984) Stochastic relaxation, Gibbs distributions, and the Bayesian restoration of images. *IEEE Transactions on Pattern Analysis and Machine Intelligence*, **6**, 721–741.

Geyer, C. J. (1992) Practical Markov chain Monte Carlo. *Statistical Science*, **7**, 473–483.

Hastings, W. K. (1970) Monte Carlo sampling methods using Markov chains and their applications. *Biometrika*, **57**, 97–109.

Hoogland, J. J. and Boomsma, A. (1998) Robustness studies in covariance structure modeling: An overview and a meta-analysis. *Sociological Methods & Research*, **26**, 329–367.

Hu, L., Bentler, P. M. and Kano, Y. (1992) Can test statistics in covariance structure analysis be trusted? *Psychological Bulletin*, **112**, 351–362.

Kass, R. E. and Raftery, A. E. (1995) Bayes factors. *Journal of the American Statistical Association*, **90**, 773–795.

Lawson, A. B., Browne, W. J. and Vidal Rodeiro, C. L. (2003) *Disease Mapping with WinBUGS and MLWIN*. Chichester: John Wiley & Sons, Ltd.

Lee, S. Y. (2007) *Structural Equation Modeling: A Bayesian Approach*. Chichester: John Wiley & Sons, Ltd.

Lee, S. Y. and Shi, J. Q. (2000) Joint Bayesian analysis of factor scores and structural parameters in the factor analysis model. *Annals of the Institute of Statistical Mathematics*, **52**, 722–736.

Lee, S. Y. and Song, X. Y. (2004) Evaluation of the Bayesian and maximum likelihood approaches in analyzing structural equation models with small sample sizes. *Multivariate Behavioral Research*, **39**, 653–686.

Lee, S. Y., Song, X. Y. and Tang, N. S. (2007) Bayesian methods for analyzing structural equation models with covariates, interaction and quadratic latent variables. *Structural Equation Modeling: A Multidisciplinary Journal*, **14**, 404–434.

Metropolis, N., Rosenbluth, A. W., Rosenbluth, M. N., Teller, A. H. and Teller, E. (1953) Equation of state calculations by fast computing machines. *Journal of Chemical Physics*, **21**, 1087–1092.

Muirhead, R. J. (1982) *Aspects of Multivariate Statistical Theory*. New York: John Wiley & Sons, Inc.

Rubin, D. B. (1991) EM and beyond. *Psychometrika*, **56**, 241–254.

Scheines, R., Hoijtink, H. and Boomsma, A. (1999) Bayesian estimation and testing of structural equation models. *Psychometrika*, **64**, 37–52.

Shi, J. Q. and Lee, S. Y. (1998) Bayesian sampling-based approach for factor analysis models with continuous and polytomous data. *British Journal of Mathematical and Statistical Psychology*, **51**, 233–252.

Spiegelhalter, D. J., Thomas, A., Best, N. G. and Lunn, D. (2003) *WinBUGS User Manual. Version 1.4*. Cambridge: MRC Biostatistics Unit.

Sturtz, S., Ligges, U. and Gelman, A. (2005) R2WinBUGS: A package for running WinBUGS from R. *Journal of Statistical Software*, **12**, 1–16.

Tanner, M. A. and Wong, W. H. (1987) The calculation of posterior distributions by data augmentation (with discussion). *Journal of the American Statistical Association*, **82**, 528–550.

Zellner, A. (1971) *An Introduction to Bayesian Inference in Econometrics*. New York: John Wiley & Sons, Inc.

4

Bayesian model comparison and model checking

4.1 Introduction

In Chapter 3, we introduced the Bayesian approach for estimating parameters in SEMs. We showed that this approach, when coupled with MCMC methods, provides an efficient and flexible tool for fitting SEMs. As one of the main goals of SEMs is the evaluation of simultaneous hypotheses about the interrelationships among the observed variables, latent variables, and fixed covariates, the testing of various hypotheses about the model is certainly an important topic of interest. In the field of structural equation modeling, the classical approach to hypothesis testing is to use significance tests based on p-values determined by asymptotic distributions of the test statistics. In general, as pointed out in the statistics literature (e.g. Berger and Delampady, 1987; Berger and Sellke, 1987; Kass and Raftery, 1995), there are serious problems associated with such an approach. See Lee (2007, Chapter 5) for a discussion of these problems in relation to SEMs.

The main objectives of this chapter are (i) to introduce various Bayesian statistics for hypothesis testing and model comparison, and (ii) to provide some statistical methods for assessment of the goodness of fit of the posited model and for model diagnosis. In our Bayesian approach, we will consider the issue of hypothesis testing as model comparison, mainly because a hypothesis can be represented via a specific model. Hence, testing the null hypothesis H_0 against its alternative hypothesis H_1 can be regarded as comparing two models corresponding to H_0 and H_1. We use the artificial example presented in Section 3.5 as an illustrative example of the above idea. Suppose that we are interested in testing $H_0 : \gamma_3 = \gamma_4 = \gamma_5 = 0$, against $H_1 : \gamma_3 \neq 0, \gamma_4 \neq 0$, and $\gamma_5 \neq 0$; see equation ((3.19). We can define an SEM, M_0, with a measurement equation defined by (3.18) and a structural equation defined by $\nu_i = b_1 d_i + \gamma_1 \xi_{i1} + \gamma_2 \xi_{i2}$. This gives a model corresponding to H_0. The model M_1 that corresponds to the alternative hypothesis H_1 is defined by equations (3.18) and

Basic and Advanced Bayesian Structural Equation Modeling: With Applications in the Medical and Behavioral Sciences, First Edition. Xin-Yuan Song and Sik-Yum Lee.

(3.19). Similarly, other null and alternative hypotheses can be assessed as a model comparison problem. Hence, in this book, we will use the general term 'model comparison' to represent hypothesis testing and model selection.

A common Bayesian statistic for model comparison in the field of SEMs is the Bayes factor (see Lee, 2007). This statistic has been shown to have many nice statistical properties (see Kass and Raftery, 1995). Computationally, the evaluation of the Bayes factor can be difficult. Recently, various algorithms for computing the Bayes factor have been developed based on of posterior simulation via MCMC methods. Based on a comparative study on a variety of algorithms, DiCiccio *et al.* (1997) concluded that bridge sampling is an attractive method. However, Gelman and Meng (1998) showed that path sampling is a direct extension of bridge sampling and can give even better results. In addition to the Bayes factor, we will introduce several other Bayesian statistics for model comparison, namely the Bayesian information criterion (BIC), Akaike information criterion (AIC), deviance information criterion (DIC), and the L_ν-measure, a criterion-based statistic. The Bayes factor and/or the above mentioned statistics will be applied to cope with the model comparison problem in the context of various complex SEMs and data structures (see subsequent chapters in this book).

We will give sufficient technical details for researchers to implement their own program in computing the aforementioned Bayesian statistics. For applied researchers who do not want to write their own program, WinBUGS provides the DIC values directly for many complex SEMs and data structures. Moreover, by utilizing the program R2WinBUGS, results provided by WinBUGS can be conveniently used to compute other model comparison statistics.

An introduction of the Bayes factor will be presented in Section 4.2. Here, discussions related to path sampling and WinBUGS for computing this statistic will be included; and an application of the methodology to SEMs with fixed covariates will be provided. Some other methods for model comparison are given in Section 4.3. An illustrative example is given in Section 4.4. Methods for model checking and goodness of fit are discussed in Section 4.5.

4.2 Bayes factor

In this section, we introduce an important Bayesian statistic, the Bayes factor (Berger, 1985) for model comparison. This statistic has a solid logical foundation that offers great flexibility. It has been extensively applied to many statistical models (Kass and Raftery, 1995) and SEMs (Lee, 2007).

Suppose that the given data set $\mathbf{Y}$ with a sample size n has arisen under one of the two competing models M_1 and M_0 according to probability density $p(\mathbf{Y}|M_1)$ or $p(\mathbf{Y}|M_0)$. Let $p(M_0)$ be the prior probability of M_0 and $p(M_1) = 1 - p(M_0)$, and let $p(M_k|\mathbf{Y})$ be the posterior probability for $k = 0, 1$. From Bayes' theorem, we have

$$p(M_k|\mathbf{Y}) = \frac{p(\mathbf{Y}|M_k)p(M_k)}{p(\mathbf{Y}|M_1)p(M_1) + p(\mathbf{Y}|M_0)p(M_0)}, \qquad k = 0, 1.$$

Hence,

$$\frac{p(M_1|\mathbf{Y})}{p(M_0|\mathbf{Y})} = \frac{p(\mathbf{Y}|M_1)p(M_1)}{p(\mathbf{Y}|M_0)p(M_0)}. \tag{4.1}$$

The Bayes factor for comparing M_1 and M_0 is defined as

$$B_{10} = \frac{p(\mathbf{Y}|M_1)}{p(\mathbf{Y}|M_0)}. \tag{4.2}$$

From (4.1), we see that posterior odds = Bayes factor × prior odds. In the special case where M_1 and M_0 are equally probable *a priori* so that $p(M_1) = p(M_0) = 0.5$, the Bayes factor is equal to the posterior odds in favor of M_1. In general, it is a summary of evidence provided by the data in favor of M_1 as oppose to M_0, or in favor of M_0 as oppose to M_1. It may reject a null hypothesis associated with M_0, or may equally provide evidence in favor of the null hypothesis or the alternative hypothesis associated with M_1. Unlike the significance test approach, which is based on the likelihood ratio criterion and its asymptotic test statistic, the comparison based on the Bayes factor does not depend on the assumption that either model is 'true'. Moreover, it can be seen from (4.2) that the same data set is used in the comparison; hence, it does not favor the alternative hypothesis (or M_1) in extremely large samples. Finally, it can be applied to compare nonnested models M_0 and M_1.

The criterion (see Kass and Raftery, 1995) that is used for interpreting B_{10} and $2 \log B_{10}$ is given in Table 4.1. Kass and Raftery (1995) pointed out that these categories furnish appropriate guidelines for practical applications of the Bayes factor. Depending on the competing models M_0 and M_1 in fitting a given data set, if B_{10} (or $2 \log B_{10}$) rejects the null hypothesis H_0 that is associated with M_0, we can conclude that the data give evidence to support the alternative hypothesis H_1 that is associated with M_1. Similarly, if the Bayes factor rejects H_1, a definite conclusion of supporting H_0 can be attained.

The interpretation of evidence provided by Table 4.1 depends on the specific context. For two nonnested competing models, say M_1 and M_0, we should select M_0 if $2 \log B_{10}$ is negative. If $2 \log B_{10}$ is in (0, 2), we may take this to mean that M_1 is slightly better than M_0 and hence it may be better to select M_1. The choice of M_1 is more definite if $2 \log B_{10}$ is larger than 6. For two nested competing models (say, M_0 is nested in M_1), $2 \log B_{10}$ is most likely larger than zero. If M_1 is significantly better than M_0, $2 \log B_{10}$ can be much larger than 6. Then the above criterion will suggest a decisive conclusion in favor of selecting M_1. However, if $2 \log B_{10}$ is in (0, 2), then the difference between M_0 and M_1 is 'not worth more than a bare mention'. Under this situation, great care should be taken in drawing conclusions. According to the 'parsimony' guideline in practical applications, it may be desirable to select the simpler model M_0. The criterion given in Table 4.1 is a suggestion, rather than a strict rule. Similar

Table 4.1 Interpretation of Bayes factor.

B_{10}	$2 \log B_{10}$	Evidence against $H_0(M_0)$
<1	<0	Negative (supports $H_0(M_0)$)
1 to 3	0 to 2	Not worth more than a bare mention
3 to 20	2 to 6	Positive (supports $H_1(M_1)$)
20 to 150	6 to 10	Strong
>150	>10	Decisive

Reproduced by permission of *Psychometrika* from Lee, S. Y. and Song, X. Y. (2003a). Model comparison of nonlinear structural equation models with fixed covariates. *Psychometrika*, **68**, 27–47.

to other data analyses, for conclusions drawn from the marginal cases, it is always helpful to conduct another analysis, for example a residual analysis, to cross-validate the results. Generally speaking, model selection should be approached on a problem-by-problem basis. In certain circumstances, the opinions of experts may also be taken into account.

The prior distribution of $\boldsymbol{\theta}$, $p(\boldsymbol{\theta})$, has to be specified in computing a Bayes factor. Compared to Bayesian estimates, the value of the Bayes factor is more sensitive to prior inputs. Hence, the choice of prior inputs is an important issue when applying the Bayes factor to the comparison of M_0 and M_1. As pointed out by Kass and Raftery (1995), using a prior with such a large spread on the parameters under M_1 as to make it 'noninformative' will force the Bayes factor to favor the competing model M_0. This is known as the 'Bartlett's paradox'. To avoid this difficulty, priors on parameters under the model comparison are generally taken to be proper and not having too large a spread. The conjugate families with reasonable spreads are appropriate choices. Prior inputs for the hyperparameters in the conjugate prior distributions may come from analyses of past or similar data, or from the subjective knowledge of experts. To cope with situations without prior information, a simple method suggested by Kass and Raftery (1995) is to set aside part of the data to use as a training sample which is combined with a noninformative prior distribution to produce an informative prior distribution. The Bayes factor is then computed from the remainder of the data. More advanced methods have been suggested (e.g. O'Hagan, 1995; Berger and Pericchi, 1996). To study the sensitivity of the Bayes factor to the choice of prior inputs in terms of the hyperparameter values, a common method (e.g. Kass and Raftery, 1995; Lee and Song, 2003b) is to perturb the prior inputs. For example, if the prior distribution is $N[\mu_0, \sigma_0^2]$, in which the given hyperparameters are μ_0 and σ_0^2, the hyperparameters may be perturbed by changing μ_0 to $\mu_0 \pm c$ and halving or doubling σ_0^2, and the Bayes factor is recomputed accordingly.

4.2.1 Path sampling

From its definition, we observe that Bayes factor involves the density $p(\mathbf{Y}|M_k)$. Let $\boldsymbol{\theta}_k$ be the random parameter vector associated with M_k. From the fact that $p(\boldsymbol{\theta}_k, \mathbf{Y}|M_k) = p(\mathbf{Y}|\boldsymbol{\theta}_k, M_k)p(\boldsymbol{\theta}_k|M_k)$, we have

$$p(\mathbf{Y}|M_k) = \int p(\mathbf{Y}|\boldsymbol{\theta}_k, M_k)p(\boldsymbol{\theta}_k|M_k)d\boldsymbol{\theta}_k, \tag{4.3}$$

where $p(\boldsymbol{\theta}_k|M_k)$ is the prior density of $\boldsymbol{\theta}_k$ and $p(\mathbf{Y}|\boldsymbol{\theta}_k, M_k)$ is the probability density of $\mathbf{Y}$ given $\boldsymbol{\theta}_k$. The dimension of this integral is equal to the dimension of $\boldsymbol{\theta}_k$. This quantity can be interpreted as the marginal likelihood of the data, obtained by integrating the joint density of $(\mathbf{Y}, \boldsymbol{\theta}_k)$ over $\boldsymbol{\theta}_k$. It can also be interpreted as the predictive probability of the data; that is, the probability of observing the data that actually were observed, calculated before any data became available. Sometimes, it is also called an integrated likelihood. Note that, as in the computation of the likelihood ratio statistic but unlike in some other applications of the likelihood, all constants appearing in the definition of the likelihood $p(\mathbf{Y}|\boldsymbol{\theta}_k, M_k)$ must be retained when computing B_{10}. It is very often difficult to obtain B_{10} analytically, and various analytic and numerical approximations have been proposed in the literature. For example, Chib (1995) and Chib and Jeliazkov (2001) developed efficient algorithms for computing the marginal likelihood through MCMC chains produced by the Gibbs sampler and by the MH algorithm, respectively. Based on the results of DiCiccio *et al.* (1997), and the recommendation of Gelman and Meng (1998), we will discuss the application of path sampling to compute the Bayes factor for model comparison. To simplify notation, 'M_k' will be suppressed; hence $p(\mathbf{Y}) = p(\mathbf{Y}|M_k)$, etc.

In general, let $\mathbf{Y}$ be the matrix of observed data, and $\mathbf{\Omega}$ be the matrix of latent variables in the model. For SEMs which involve latent variables, direct application of path sampling (Gelman and Meng, 1998) in computing the Bayes factor is difficult. Similar to Bayesian estimation, we utilize the idea of data augmentation (Tanner and Wong, 1987) to solve the problem. Below we use reasoning similar to that of Gelman and Meng (1998) to briefly show that path sampling can be applied to compute the logarithm of the Bayes factor by augmenting $\mathbf{Y}$ with $\mathbf{\Omega}$. The main result is given by equations (4.8) and (4.9), with the definition of $U(\mathbf{Y}, \mathbf{\Omega}, \boldsymbol{\theta}, t)$ given by (4.7). Readers who are not interested in the technical derivation may jump to these equations. From the equality $p(\mathbf{\Omega}, \boldsymbol{\theta}|\mathbf{Y}) = p(\mathbf{Y}, \mathbf{\Omega}, \boldsymbol{\theta})/p(\mathbf{Y})$, the marginal density $p(\mathbf{Y})$ can be treated as the normalizing constant of $p(\mathbf{\Omega}, \boldsymbol{\theta}|\mathbf{Y})$, with the complete-data probability density $p(\mathbf{Y}, \mathbf{\Omega}, \boldsymbol{\theta})$ taken as the unnormalized density. Now, consider the following class of densities which are denoted by a continuous parameter t in [0, 1]:

$$p(\mathbf{\Omega}, \boldsymbol{\theta}|\mathbf{Y}, t) = \frac{1}{z(t)} p(\mathbf{Y}, \mathbf{\Omega}, \boldsymbol{\theta}|t), \tag{4.4}$$

where

$$z(t) = p(\mathbf{Y}|t) = \int p(\mathbf{Y}, \mathbf{\Omega}, \boldsymbol{\theta}|t) d\mathbf{\Omega} d\boldsymbol{\theta} = \int p(\mathbf{Y}, \mathbf{\Omega}, |\boldsymbol{\theta}, t) p(\boldsymbol{\theta}) d\mathbf{\Omega} d\boldsymbol{\theta}, \tag{4.5}$$

with $p(\boldsymbol{\theta})$ the prior density of $\boldsymbol{\theta}$ which is assumed to be independent of t.

In computing the Bayes factor, we construct a path using the parameter $t \in [0, 1]$ to link two competing models M_1 and M_0 together, so that $z(1) = p(\mathbf{Y}|1) = p(\mathbf{Y}|M_1)$, $z(0) = p(\mathbf{Y}|0) = p(\mathbf{Y}|M_0)$, and $B_{10} = z(1)/z(0)$. Taking logarithms and then differentiating (4.5) with respect to t, and assuming it is legitimate to interchange integration and differentiation; then we have

$$\begin{aligned} \frac{d \log z(t)}{dt} &= \int \frac{1}{z(t)} \frac{d}{dt} p(\mathbf{Y}, \mathbf{\Omega}, \boldsymbol{\theta}|t) d\mathbf{\Omega} d\boldsymbol{\theta} \\ &= \int \frac{d}{dt} \log p(\mathbf{Y}, \mathbf{\Omega}, \boldsymbol{\theta}|t) \cdot p(\mathbf{\Omega}, \boldsymbol{\theta}|\mathbf{Y}, t) d\mathbf{\Omega} d\boldsymbol{\theta} \\ &= E_{\Omega,\theta}\left[\frac{d}{dt} \log p(\mathbf{Y}, \mathbf{\Omega}, \boldsymbol{\theta}|t)\right], \end{aligned} \tag{4.6}$$

where $E_{\Omega,\theta}$ denotes the expectation with respect to the distribution $p(\mathbf{\Omega}, \boldsymbol{\theta}|\mathbf{Y}, t)$. Let

$$U(\mathbf{Y}, \mathbf{\Omega}, \boldsymbol{\theta}, t) = \frac{d}{dt} \log p(\mathbf{Y}, \mathbf{\Omega}, \boldsymbol{\theta}|t) = \frac{d}{dt} \log p(\mathbf{Y}, \mathbf{\Omega}|\boldsymbol{\theta}, t), \tag{4.7}$$

which does not involve the prior density $p(\boldsymbol{\theta})$, we have

$$\log B_{10} = \log \frac{z(1)}{z(0)} = \int_0^1 E_{\Omega,\theta}[U(\mathbf{Y}, \mathbf{\Omega}, \boldsymbol{\theta}, t)] dt.$$

The method given in Ogata (1989) is used to numerically evaluate the integral over t. Specifically, we first order the unique values of fixed grids $\{t_{(s)}\}_{s=1}^S$ in the interval [0, 1] such that

$0 = t_{(0)} < t_{(1)} < \ldots < t_{(S)} < t_{(S+1)} = 1$, and estimate $\log B_{10}$ by

$$\widehat{\log B_{10}} = \frac{1}{2} \sum_{s=0}^{S} \left(t_{(s+1)} - t_{(s)} \right) \left(\bar{U}_{(s+1)} + \bar{U}_{(s)} \right), \tag{4.8}$$

where $\bar{U}_{(s)}$ is the following average of the values of $U(\mathbf{Y}, \mathbf{\Omega}, \boldsymbol{\theta}, t)$ based on simulation draws at $t = t_{(s)}$:

$$\bar{U}_{(s)} = J^{-1} \sum_{j=1}^{J} U\left(\mathbf{Y}, \mathbf{\Omega}^{(j)}, \boldsymbol{\theta}^{(j)}, t_{(s)} \right), \tag{4.9}$$

in which $\{(\mathbf{\Omega}^{(j)}, \boldsymbol{\theta}^{(j)}), j = 1, \ldots, J\}$ are observations drawn from $p(\mathbf{\Omega}, \boldsymbol{\theta}|\mathbf{Y}, t_{(s)})$.

To apply the path sampling procedure, we need to define a link model M_t to link M_0 and M_1, such that when $t = 0, M_t = M_0$; and when $t = 1, M_t = M_1$. Then we obtain $U(\mathbf{Y}, \mathbf{\Omega}, \boldsymbol{\theta}, t)$ by differentiating the logarithm of the complete-data likelihood function under M_t with respect to t, and finally estimate $\log B_{10}$ via (4.7) and (4.8). Note that the form and the derivative of the complete-data likelihood are not difficult. The main computation is in simulating the sample of observations $\{(\mathbf{\Omega}^{(j)}, \boldsymbol{\theta}^{(j)}), j = 1, \ldots, J\}$ from $p(\mathbf{\Omega}, \boldsymbol{\theta}|\mathbf{Y}, t_{(s)})$, for $s = 0, \ldots, S + 1$. This task can be done via some efficient MCMC methods, such as the Gibbs sampler and the MH algorithm as described in the previous chapter; see illustrative examples given in other chapters in this book. For most SEMs, $S = 20$ and $J = 1000$ provide results that are accurate enough for many practical applications. Experiences indicate that $S = 10$ is also acceptable for simple SEMs. However, a smaller J is not recommended.

The path sampling approach has several nice features. Its implementation is simple; the main programming task is simulating observations from $p(\mathbf{\Omega}, \boldsymbol{\theta}|\mathbf{Y}, t_{(s)})$. As pointed out by Gelman and Meng (1998), we can always construct a continuous path to link two competing models. Thus, the method can be applied to the comparison of a wide variety of models. Bayesian estimates of the unknown parameters and latent variables under M_0 and M_1 can be obtained easily via the simulated observations at $t = 0$ and $t = 1$. In contrast to most existing methods in computing the Bayes factor, the path sampling procedure does not directly include the prior density in the computation. Furthermore, the logarithm scale of the Bayes factor is computed, which is generally more stable than the ratio scale. Finally, as path sampling is a generalization of bridge sampling, it has potential to produce more accurate results.

In applying path sampling, it is required to find a path $t \in [0, 1]$ to link the competing models M_0 and M_1. For most cases, finding such a path is fairly straightforward. However, for some complex situations that involve very different M_1 and M_0, it is difficult to find a path that directly links the competing models. Most of the time, this difficulty can be solved by using appropriate auxiliary models, $M_a, M_b, \ldots$, in between M_1 and M_0. For example, suppose that M_a and M_b are appropriate auxiliary models such that M_a can be linked with M_1 and M_b, and M_b can be linked with M_0. Then

$$\frac{p(\mathbf{Y}|M_1)}{p(\mathbf{Y}|M_0)} = \frac{p(\mathbf{Y}|M_1)/p(\mathbf{Y}|M_a)}{p(\mathbf{Y}|M_0)/p(\mathbf{Y}|M_a)} \quad \text{and} \quad \frac{p(\mathbf{Y}|M_0)}{p(\mathbf{Y}|M_a)} = \frac{p(\mathbf{Y}|M_0)/p(\mathbf{Y}|M_b)}{p(\mathbf{Y}|M_a)/p(\mathbf{Y}|M_b)}.$$

Hence, $\log B_{10} = \log B_{1a} + \log B_{ab} - \log B_{0b}$. Each logarithm of the Bayes factor can be computed through path sampling. An illustrative example is given in Section 5.2.4.

4.2.2 A simulation study

The objectives of this simulation study are to reveal the performance of path sampling in computing the Bayes factor, and to evaluate the sensitivity of the results to prior inputs. Random observations were generated from a nonlinear SEM with fixed covariates defined by (2.20) and (2.21). The specific model involves eight observed variables which are related to two fixed covariates $\{c_{i1}, c_{i2}\}$ in the measurement equation, and three latent variables $\{\eta_i, \xi_{i1}, \xi_{i2}\}$ and one fixed covariate d_i in the structural equation. The first fixed covariate c_{i1} is sampled from a multinomial distribution which takes values 1.0, 2.0, and 3.0 with probabilities $\Phi^*(-0.5)$, $\Phi^*(0.5) - \Phi^*(-0.5)$, and $1.0 - \Phi^*(0.5)$, respectively, where $\Phi^*(\cdot)$ is the distribution function of $N[0, 1]$; while the second covariate c_{i2} is sampled from $N[0, 1]$. The true population values in the matrices $\mathbf{A}$, $\mathbf{\Lambda}$, and $\mathbf{\Psi}_\epsilon$ are given as follows:

$$\mathbf{A}^T = \begin{bmatrix} 1.0 & 1.0 & 1.0 & 1.0 & 1.0 & 1.0 & 1.0 & 1.0 \\ 0.7 & 0.7 & 0.7 & 0.7 & 0.7 & 0.7 & 0.7 & 0.7 \end{bmatrix},$$

$$\mathbf{\Lambda}^T = \begin{bmatrix} 1 & 1.5 & 1.5 & 0 & 0 & 0 & 0 & 0 \\ 0 & 0 & 0 & 1 & 1.5 & 0 & 0 & 0 \\ 0 & 0 & 0 & 0 & 0 & 1 & 1.5 & 1.5 \end{bmatrix}, \quad \mathbf{\Psi}_\epsilon = \mathbf{I}_8,$$

where the 1s and 0s in $\mathbf{\Lambda}$ are fixed to identify the model, and $\mathbf{I}_8$ is an 8×8 identity matrix. The true variances and covariance of ξ_{i1} and ξ_{i2} are $\phi_{11} = \phi_{22} = 1.0$, and $\phi_{21} = 0.15$. These two explanatory latent variables are related to the outcome latent variable η_i by

$$\eta_i = 1.0d_i + 0.5\xi_{i1} + 0.5\xi_{i2} + 1.0\xi_{i2}^2 + \delta_i,$$

where d_i is sampled from a Bernoulli distribution that takes 1.0 with probability 0.7 and 0.0 with probability 0.3; and $\mathbf{\Psi}_\delta = \psi_\delta = 1.0$. Based on these specifications, random samples $\{\mathbf{y}_i, i = 1, \ldots, n\}$ with $n = 300$ were generated for the simulation study. A total of 100 replications were taken for each case.

We are interested in comparing models with different structural equations. Hence, models with the same measurement equation and the following structural equations are considered in the model comparison:

$$\begin{aligned}
M_0 &: \eta_i = bd_i + \gamma_1\xi_{i1} + \gamma_2\xi_{i2} + \gamma_{22}\xi_{i2}^2 + \delta_i, \\
M_1 &: \eta_i = bd_i + \gamma_1\xi_{i1} + \gamma_2\xi_{i2} + \delta_i, \\
M_2 &: \eta_i = bd_i + \gamma_1\xi_{i1} + \gamma_2\xi_{i2} + \gamma_{12}\xi_{i1}\xi_{i2} + \delta_i, \\
M_3 &: \eta_i = bd_i + \gamma_1\xi_{i1} + \gamma_2\xi_{i2} + \gamma_{11}\xi_{i1}^2 + \delta_i, \\
M_4 &: \eta_i = bd_i + \gamma_1\xi_{i1} + \gamma_2\xi_{i2} + \gamma_{12}\xi_{i1}\xi_{i2} + \gamma_{11}\xi_{i1}^2 + \delta_i, \\
M_5 &: \eta_i = \gamma_1\xi_{i1} + \gamma_2\xi_{i2} + \gamma_{22}\xi_{i2}^2 + \delta_i, \\
M_6 &: \eta_i = bd_i + \gamma_1\xi_{i1} + \gamma_2\xi_{i2} + \gamma_{12}\xi_{i1}\xi_{i2} + \gamma_{11}\xi_{i1}^2 + \gamma_{22}\xi_{i2}^2 + \delta_i.
\end{aligned}$$

Here, M_0 is the true model, M_1 is a linear model, M_2, M_3, and M_4 are nonnested in M_0, M_5 is nested in M_0, and M_0 is nested in the most general model M_6. To provide a more detailed illustration for the application of path sampling procedure to model comparison of nonlinear SEMs, the implementation of path sampling in estimating $\log B_{02}$ for comparing M_0 and M_2 is given here. Let $\boldsymbol{\theta} = (\tilde{\boldsymbol{\theta}}, \mathbf{\Gamma}_\omega)$ and $\boldsymbol{\theta}_t = (\tilde{\boldsymbol{\theta}}, \mathbf{\Gamma}_{t\omega})$, where $\mathbf{\Gamma}_\omega = (b, \gamma_1, \gamma_2, \gamma_{12}, \gamma_{22})$,

$\boldsymbol{\Gamma}_{t\omega} = (b, \gamma_1, \gamma_2, (1-t)\gamma_{12}, t\gamma_{22})$, and $\tilde{\boldsymbol{\theta}}$ includes other unknown common parameters in M_0 and M_2. The procedure consists of the following steps:

1. Select a link model M_t to link M_0 and M_2. Here, M_t is defined with the same measurement model as in M_0 and M_2, but with the following structural equation:

$$M_t : \eta_i = bd_i + \gamma_1\xi_{i1} + \gamma_2\xi_{i2} + (1-t)\gamma_{12}\xi_{i1}\xi_{i2} + t\gamma_{22}\xi_{i2}^2 + \delta_i.$$

   Clearly, when $t = 1, M_t = M_0$; when $t = 0, M_t = M_2$.

2. On the fixed grid $t = t_{(s)}$, generate observations $\{(\boldsymbol{\Omega}^{(j)}, \boldsymbol{\theta}^{(j)}), j = 1, \ldots, J\}$ from $p(\boldsymbol{\Omega}, \boldsymbol{\theta}|\mathbf{Y}, t_{(s)})$ by using MCMC methods, such as the Gibbs sampler and the MH algorithm, as in the Bayesian estimation.

3. Calculate $U(\mathbf{Y}, \boldsymbol{\Omega}^{(j)}, \boldsymbol{\theta}^{(j)}, t_{(s)})$ by substituting $\{(\boldsymbol{\Omega}^{(j)}, \boldsymbol{\theta}^{(j)}), j = 1, \ldots, J\}$ into the following equation:

$$U(\mathbf{Y}, \boldsymbol{\Omega}, \boldsymbol{\theta}, t_{(s)}) = d\log p(\mathbf{Y}, \boldsymbol{\Omega}|\boldsymbol{\theta}, t)/dt\Big|_{t=t_{(s)}}$$
$$= -\sum_{i=1}^{n}\left(\eta_i - bd_i - \gamma_1\xi_{i1} - \gamma_2\xi_{i2} - (1-t_{(s)})\gamma_{12}\xi_{i1}\xi_{i2} - t_{(s)}\gamma_{22}\xi_{i2}^2\right)\left(\gamma_{12}\xi_{i1}\xi_{i2} - \gamma_{22}\xi_{i2}^2\right)/\psi_\delta.$$

4. Calculate $\bar{U}_{(s)}$; see (4.9).

5. Repeat steps 2–4 until all $\bar{U}_{(s)}, s = 0, \ldots, S+1$ are calculated. Then $\widehat{\log B_{02}}$ is estimated via (4.8).

Conjugate prior distributions (see, for example, equations (3.6) and (3.8)) are used in the Bayesian analysis. In the sensitivity analysis concerned with the prior inputs, we followed the suggestion of Kass and Raftery (1995) to perturb them as follows. Under prior inputs $\alpha_{0\epsilon k} = \alpha_{0\delta k} = 8$, $\beta_{0\epsilon k} = \beta_{0\delta k} = 10$, and $\rho_0 = 20$, we consider the following three types of prior inputs for $\mathbf{A}_{0k}$, $\boldsymbol{\Lambda}_{0k}$, $\boldsymbol{\Lambda}_{0\omega k}$, and $\mathbf{R}_0^{-1}$:

(I) $\mathbf{A}_{0k}$, $\boldsymbol{\Lambda}_{0k}$, and $\boldsymbol{\Lambda}_{0\omega k}$ are selected to be the true parameter matrices, and $\mathbf{R}_0^{-1} = (\rho_0 - q_2 - 1)\boldsymbol{\Phi}_0$, where elements in $\boldsymbol{\Phi}_0$ are the true parameters values.

(II) The hyperparameters specified in (I) are equal to half those given in (I).

(III) The hyperparameters specified in (I) are equal to twice those given in (I).

Moreover, under type (I) prior inputs as given above, we consider the following prior inputs for $\alpha_{0\epsilon k}$, $\alpha_{0\delta k}$, $\beta_{0\epsilon k}$, $\beta_{0\delta k}$, and ρ_0:

(IV) $\alpha_{0\epsilon k} = \alpha_{0\delta k} = 3$, $\beta_{0\epsilon k} = \beta_{0\delta k} = 5$, and $\rho_0 = 12$.

(V) $\alpha_{0\epsilon k} = \alpha_{0\delta k} = 12$, $\beta_{0\epsilon k} = \beta_{0\delta k} = 15$, and $\rho_0 = 30$.

For every case, the covariance matrices $\boldsymbol{\Sigma}_0$, $\mathbf{H}_{0yk}$, and $\mathbf{H}_{0\omega k}$ were taken as the identity matrices with appropriate dimensions. Moreover, we took 20 grids in [0, 1], and collected $J = 1000$ iterations after discarding 500 burn-in iterations at each grid in the computation of the logarithm of the Bayes factor via path sampling. Estimates of $\log B_{0k}, k = 1, \ldots, 6$, under the different prior inputs were computed. The mean and standard deviation of $\widehat{\log B_{0k}}$ were

Table 4.2 Means and standard deviations of the estimated $\log B_{0k}$ in the simulation study.

	Mean (Std)				
	prior I	prior II	prior III	prior IV	prior V
$\log B_{01}$	106.28 (25.06)	107.58 (25.15)	102.96 (24.81)	103.87 (22.71)	104.61 (23.92)
$\log B_{02}$	102.16 (24.91)	103.45 (25.02)	99.17 (24.54)	99.98 (22.67)	100.49 (23.47)
$\log B_{03}$	109.51 (25.63)	111.23 (25.74)	105.96 (25.19)	107.20 (23.81)	108.24 (24.59)
$\log B_{04}$	105.23 (25.31)	106.61 (25.47)	101.83 (24.90)	103.16 (23.78)	103.69 (24.12)
$\log B_{05}$	17.50 (5.44)	18.02 (5.56)	16.65 (5.21)	18.02 (5.34)	17.85 (5.30)
$\log B_{60}$	0.71 (0.54)	0.71 (0.51)	0.69 (0.55)	0.78 (0.67)	0.75 (0.65)

Reproduced by permission of *Psychometrika* from Lee, S. Y. and Song, X. Y. (2003a). Model comparison of nonlinear structural equation models with fixed covariates. *Psychometrika*, **68**, 27–47.

also computed on the basis of 100 replications. Results corresponding to $\widehat{\log B_{0k}}, k = 1, \ldots, 5$, and $\widehat{\log B_{60}}$ are reported in Table 4.2. Moreover, for each $k = 1, \ldots, 6$, we evaluate

$$D(\text{I} - \text{II}) = \max\{|\widehat{\log B_{0k}}(\text{I}) - \widehat{\log B_{0k}}(\text{II})|\}$$

and similarly $D(\text{I} - \text{III})$ and $D(\text{IV} - \text{V})$, where $\widehat{\log B_{0k}}(\text{I})$ is the estimate of $\log B_{0k}$ under prior (I) and so on, and 'max' is the maximum taken over the 100 replications. The results are presented in Table 4.3; for example, the maximum difference of the estimates of $\log B_{01}$ obtained via priors (I) and (II) is 6.55. From the rows of Table 4.2, we observe that the means and standard deviations of $\widehat{\log B_{0k}}$ obtained under different prior inputs are close to each other. This indicates that the estimate of $\log B_{0k}$ is not very sensitive to these prior inputs for a sample size of 300. We also see from Table 4.3 that even for the worst situation with the maximum absolute deviation, the estimated log Bayes factors under different prior inputs give the same conclusion for selecting the model based on the criterion given in Table 4.1.

It is clear from Table 4.2 that M_0 is much better than the linear model M_1, the nonnested models M_2, M_3, and M_4, and the nested model M_5. Thus, the correct model is selected. In comparison with the encompassing model M_6, we found that out of 100 replications under prior (I), 75 of the $\widehat{\log B_{60}}$ were in the interval (0.0, 1.0), 23 of them were in (1.0, 2.0), and

Table 4.3 Maximum absolute differences of $\log B_{0k}$ for several different prior settings.

	$\log B_{01}$	$\log B_{02}$	$\log B_{03}$	$\log B_{04}$	$\log B_{05}$	$\log B_{60}$
$D(\text{I} - \text{II})$	6.55	5.47	8.22	5.24	2.18	0.27
$D(\text{I} - \text{III})$	7.84	9.33	10.23	10.17	3.07	0.31
$D(\text{IV} - \text{V})$	14.03	17.86	13.65	4.87	1.91	0.25

Reproduced by permission of *Psychometrika* from Lee, S. Y. and Song, X. Y. (2003a). Model comparison of nonlinear structural equation models with fixed covariates. *Psychometrika*, **68**, 27–47.

only 2 of them were in (2.0, 3.0). Since M_0 is simpler than M_6, it should be selected if $\widehat{\log B_{60}}$ is in (0.0, 2.0). Thus, the true model is selected in 98 out of the 100 replications. Owing to randomness, only in 2 of 100 replications does the value of $\widehat{\log B_{60}}$ mildly support the encompassing model. Although the encompassing model is not the true model, it should not be regarded as an incorrect model for fitting the data.

WinBUGS does not have an option to compute the Bayes factor. However, as mentioned in Section 3.5, WinBUGS can be run in batch mode using scripts, and the R2WinBUGS (Sturtz *et al.*, 2005) package makes use of this feature and provides tools to call WinBUGS directly after data manipulation in R. Hence, the Bayes factor can be computed via WinBUGS and R2WinBUGS. The WinBUGS code for comparing M_0 and M_2 is given in Appendix 4.1. This WinBUGS code must be stored in a separate file (say, 'model.txt') within an appropriate directory (say, C:\Bayes Factor\) when computing the logarithm of the Bayes factor via path sampling, and $\bar{U}_{(s)}$ at each grid is computed from WinBUGS via the bugs(·) function in R2WinBUGS; the logarithm of the Bayes factor is then computed using the $\bar{U}_{(s)}$, $s = 0, \ldots, S+1$. The related R code for computing $\log B_{02}$, including data generation, is given in Appendix 4.2.

4.3 Other model comparison statistics

4.3.1 Bayesian information criterion and Akaike information criterion

An approximation of $2\log B_{10}$ that does not depend on the prior density is the following Schwarz criterion S^* (Schwarz, 1978):

$$2\log B_{10} \cong 2S^* = 2\{\log p(\mathbf{Y}|\tilde{\boldsymbol{\theta}}_1, M_1) - \log p(\mathbf{Y}|\tilde{\boldsymbol{\theta}}_0, M_0)\} - (d_1 - d_0)\log n, \qquad (4.10)$$

where $\tilde{\boldsymbol{\theta}}_1$ and $\tilde{\boldsymbol{\theta}}_0$ are the maximum likelihood (ML) estimates of $\boldsymbol{\theta}_1$ and $\boldsymbol{\theta}_0$ under M_1 and M_0, respectively; d_1 and d_0 are the dimensions of $\boldsymbol{\theta}_1$ and $\boldsymbol{\theta}_0$, and n is the sample size. Multiplying the quantity in (4.10) by -1 gives the following well-known Bayesian information criterion (BIC) for comparing M_1 and M_0:

$$\text{BIC}_{10} = -2S^* \cong -2\log B_{10} = 2\log B_{01}. \qquad (4.11)$$

The interpretation of BIC_{10} can be based on Table 4.1. Alternatively, for each M_k, $k = 0, 1$, we can define

$$\text{BIC}_k = -2\log p(\mathbf{Y}|\tilde{\boldsymbol{\theta}}_k, M_k) + d_k \log n. \qquad (4.12)$$

Hence $2\log B_{10} \cong \text{BIC}_0 - \text{BIC}_1$. Based on Table 4.1, the model M_k with the smaller BIC_k value is selected.

As n tends to infinity, it has been shown (Schwarz, 1978) that

$$\frac{S^* - \log B_{10}}{\log B_{10}} \to 0,$$

thus S^* may be viewed as an approximation to $\log B_{10}$. This approximation is of order $O(1)$, thus S^* does not give the exact $\log B_{10}$ even for large samples. However, as pointed out by Kass and Raftery (1995), it can be used for scientific reporting as long as the number of degrees of freedom $(d_1 - d_0)$ involved in the comparison is small relative to the sample size n.

The BIC is appealing in that it is relatively simple and can be applied even when the priors $p(\boldsymbol{\theta}_k|M_k)$ $(k = 1, 0)$ are hard to specify precisely. The ML estimates of $\boldsymbol{\theta}_1$ and $\boldsymbol{\theta}_0$ are involved in the computation of BIC. In practice, since the Bayesian estimates and the ML estimates are close to each other, they can be used to compute the BIC. The order of approximation is not changed and the BIC obtained can be interpreted using the criterion given in Table 4.1. See Raftery (1993) for an application of BIC to the standard LISREL model that is based on the normal assumption and a linear structural equation. In this simple case, the computation of the observed-data log-likelihood $\log p(\mathbf{Y}|\tilde{\boldsymbol{\theta}}_k, M_k)$ is in closed form and its computation is straightforward. For complex SEMs, the observed-data log-likelihoods are usually intractable multiple integrals. In such situations, path sampling can be applied to evaluate $p(\mathbf{Y}|\tilde{\boldsymbol{\theta}}_k, M_k)$, by fixing $\boldsymbol{\theta}_k$ at its estimate $\tilde{\boldsymbol{\theta}}_k$ rather than treating it as random. See Song and Lee (2006) for an application of path sampling to evaluate the observed-data log-likelihood function.

The Akaike information criterion (AIC; Akaike, 1973) associated with a competing model M_k is given by

$$\text{AIC}_k = -2\log p(\mathbf{Y}|\tilde{\boldsymbol{\theta}}_k, M_k) + 2d_k, \tag{4.13}$$

which does not involve the sample size n. The interpretation of AIC_k is similar to that of BIC_k. Hence, M_k is selected if its AIC_k is smaller. Comparing (4.12) with (4.13), we see that BIC tends to favor simpler models.

4.3.2 Deviance information criterion

Another model comparison statistic that compromises between the goodness of fit and model complexity is the deviance information criterion (DIC); see Spiegelhalter *et al.* (2002). This statistic is intended as a generalization of the AIC. Under a competing model M_k with a vector of unknown parameter $\boldsymbol{\theta}_k$, the DIC is defined as

$$\text{DIC}_k = \overline{D(\boldsymbol{\theta}_k)} + d_k, \tag{4.14}$$

where $\overline{D(\boldsymbol{\theta}_k)}$ measures the goodness of fit of the model, and is defined as

$$\overline{D(\boldsymbol{\theta}_k)} = E_{\boldsymbol{\theta}_k}\{-2\log p(\mathbf{Y}|\boldsymbol{\theta}_k, M_k)|\mathbf{Y}\}. \tag{4.15}$$

Here, d_k is the effective number of parameters in M_k, and is defined as

$$d_k = E_{\boldsymbol{\theta}_k}\{-2\log p(\mathbf{Y}|\boldsymbol{\theta}_k, M_k)|\mathbf{Y}\} + 2\log p(\mathbf{Y}|\tilde{\boldsymbol{\theta}}_k), \tag{4.16}$$

in which $\tilde{\boldsymbol{\theta}}_k$ is the Bayesian estimate of $\boldsymbol{\theta}_k$. Let $\{\boldsymbol{\theta}_k^{(j)}, j = 1, \ldots, J\}$ be a sample of observations simulated from the posterior distribution. The expectations in (4.15) and (4.16) can be estimated as follows:

$$E_{\boldsymbol{\theta}_k}\{-2\log p(\mathbf{Y}|\boldsymbol{\theta}_k, M_k)|\mathbf{Y}\} = -\frac{2}{J}\sum_{j=1}^{J}\log p\big(\mathbf{Y}|\boldsymbol{\theta}_k^{(j)}, M_k\big). \tag{4.17}$$

In practical applications, the model with the smaller DIC value is selected.

The computational burden of DIC lies in simulating $\{\boldsymbol{\theta}_k^{(j)}, j = 1, \ldots, J\}$ from the posterior distribution, and thus is lighter than that of the Bayes factor. In the analysis of a hypothesized model, WinBUGS (Spiegelhalter, *et al.*, 2003) produces a DIC value which can be used for model comparison. Thus, it is very convenient to apply DIC in practice. As pointed out in the WinBUGS manual (Spiegelhalter *et al.*, 2003), it is important to note the following in practical application of the DIC: (i) DIC assumes the posterior mean to be a good estimate of the parameter. There are circumstances, such as mixture models, in which WinBUGS does not give the DIC values. (ii) If the difference in DIC is small, for example less than 5, and the models make very different inferences, then just reporting the model with the lowest DIC could be misleading. (iii) DIC can be applied to nonnested models. Moreover, similar to the Bayes factor, BIC, and AIC, DIC gives a clear conclusion to support the null hypothesis or the alternative hypothesis. Detailed discussions of the DIC can be found in Spiegelhalter *et al.* (2002) and Celeux *et al.* (2006).

4.3.3 L_ν-measure

The L_ν-measure can be viewed as a criterion-based method for Bayesian model assessment founded on the predictive approach with future values of a replicate experiment. More specifically, this statistic is based on the predictive distribution of the data with a sum of two components. One component involves the means of the posterior predictive distribution, while the other is related to the variances. Hence, it measures the performance of a model by a combination of how close its predictions are to the observed data and the variability of the predictions.

Let $\mathbf{Y}$ be the observed data, and let $p(\mathbf{Y}, \boldsymbol{\theta})$ be the joint density that corresponds to a model M with a parameter vector $\boldsymbol{\theta}$. Considering the predictive approach of using a future response vector for model comparison, we propose a Bayesian model selection statistic through future responses $\mathbf{Y}^{\text{rep}} = (\mathbf{y}_1^{\text{rep}}, \ldots, \mathbf{y}_n^{\text{rep}})$, which have the same sampling density as $p(\mathbf{Y}|\boldsymbol{\theta})$. The basic idea is that good models should give predictions close to what have been observed. Several criteria, such as the Euclidean distance between $\mathbf{Y}$ and $\mathbf{Y}^{\text{rep}}$, can be considered. In this book, we first consider the following statistic: for some $\delta > 0$, let

$$L_1(\mathbf{Y}, \mathbf{B}, \delta) = E[\text{tr}(\mathbf{Y}^{\text{rep}} - \mathbf{B})^T(\mathbf{Y}^{\text{rep}} - \mathbf{B})] + \delta \, \text{tr}(\mathbf{Y} - \mathbf{B})^T(\mathbf{Y} - \mathbf{B}), \tag{4.18}$$

where the expectation is taken with respect to the posterior predictive distribution of $[\mathbf{Y}^{\text{rep}}|\mathbf{Y}]$. Note that this statistic reduces to the Euclidean distance if $\mathbf{B} = \mathbf{Y}$. By setting $\mathbf{B}$ as the minimizer of (4.18), and substituting it into (4.18), it can be shown (Ibrahim *et al.*, 2001) that

$$L_\nu(\mathbf{Y}) = \sum_{i=1}^{n} \text{tr}\{\text{Cov}(\mathbf{y}_i^{\text{rep}}|\mathbf{Y})\} + \nu \sum_{i=1}^{n} \text{tr}[\{E(\mathbf{y}_i^{\text{rep}}|\mathbf{Y}) - \mathbf{y}_i\}\{E(\mathbf{y}_i^{\text{rep}}|\mathbf{Y}) - \mathbf{y}_i\}^T], \tag{4.19}$$

where $\nu = \delta/(\delta + 1)$. This statistic is called the L_ν-measure. Note that this L_ν-measure is a sum of two components. The first component relates to the variability of the predictions, and the second component measures how close its predictions are to the observed data. Clearly, a small value of the L_ν-measure indicates that the corresponding model gives a prediction close to the observed value, and the variability of the prediction is also low. Hence, the model with the smallest L_ν-measure is selected from a collection of competing models.

Obviously $0 \leq \nu \leq 1$, where $\nu = 0$ if $\delta = 0$, and ν tends to 1 as δ tends to infinity. This quantity can be interpreted as a weight term in the second component of $L_\nu(\mathbf{Y})$. Using $\nu = 1$ gives equal weight to the squared bias and the variance component. However, allowing ν to vary provides more flexibility in the tradeoff between bias and variance. In the context of a linear model, Ibrahim *et al.* (2001) provided some theoretical results and argued that $\nu = 0.5$ is a desirable and justifiable choice for model selection.

In applying the L_ν-measure for model assessment and model selection for SEMs, we have to evaluate $\text{Cov}(\mathbf{y}_i^{\text{rep}}|\mathbf{Y})$ and $E(\mathbf{y}_i^{\text{rep}}|\mathbf{Y})$, which involve intractable multiple integrals. Based on the identities

$$E(\mathbf{y}_i^{\text{rep}}|\mathbf{Y}) = E\{E(\mathbf{y}_i^{\text{rep}}|\boldsymbol{\Omega}, \boldsymbol{\theta})|\mathbf{Y}\} \quad \text{and} \quad E\{\mathbf{y}_i^{\text{rep}}(\mathbf{y}_i^{\text{rep}})^T|\mathbf{Y}\} = E[E\{\mathbf{y}_i^{\text{rep}}(\mathbf{y}_i^{\text{rep}})^T|\boldsymbol{\Omega}, \boldsymbol{\theta}\}|\mathbf{Y}],$$

the consistent estimates of $E(\mathbf{y}_i^{\text{rep}}|\mathbf{Y})$ and $\text{Cov}(\mathbf{y}_i^{\text{rep}}|\mathbf{Y})$ can be obtained from the MCMC sample simulated from the full conditional distributions via the Gibbs sampler and/or the MH algorithm.

4.4 Illustration

In this section, we present an example to illustrate the application of the above discussed statistics to model comparison related to nonlinear SEMs. As discussed in Section 2.4.1, the model is defined by

$$\mathbf{y}_i = \boldsymbol{\mu} + \boldsymbol{\Lambda}\boldsymbol{\omega}_i + \boldsymbol{\epsilon}_i, \tag{4.20}$$

$$\boldsymbol{\eta}_i = \boldsymbol{\Pi}\boldsymbol{\eta}_i + \boldsymbol{\Gamma}\mathbf{F}(\boldsymbol{\xi}_i) + \boldsymbol{\delta}_i, \tag{4.21}$$

where the definitions of $\boldsymbol{\mu}$, $\boldsymbol{\Lambda}$, $\boldsymbol{\omega}_i, \ldots$ are the same as in that section.

To compute the L_ν-measure, let $\boldsymbol{\Lambda}_\eta$ and $\boldsymbol{\Lambda}_\xi$ be the submatrices of $\boldsymbol{\Lambda}$ corresponding to $\boldsymbol{\eta}_i$ and $\boldsymbol{\xi}_i$, respectively. It follows that

$$\mathbf{y}_i = \boldsymbol{\mu} + \boldsymbol{\Lambda}_\eta\boldsymbol{\Pi}_0^{-1}\{\boldsymbol{\Gamma}\mathbf{F}(\boldsymbol{\xi}_i) + \boldsymbol{\delta}_i\} + \boldsymbol{\Lambda}_\xi\boldsymbol{\xi}_i + \boldsymbol{\epsilon}_i, \tag{4.22}$$

where $\boldsymbol{\Pi}_0 = \mathbf{I} - \boldsymbol{\Pi}$. As $\mathbf{Y}^{\text{rep}} = (\mathbf{y}_1^{\text{rep}}, \ldots, \mathbf{y}_n^{\text{rep}})$ has the same density as $p(\mathbf{Y}|\boldsymbol{\Omega}, \boldsymbol{\theta})$, we have

$$E(\mathbf{y}_i^{\text{rep}}|\boldsymbol{\Omega}, \boldsymbol{\theta}) = \boldsymbol{\mu} + \boldsymbol{\Lambda}_\eta\boldsymbol{\Pi}_0^{-1}\boldsymbol{\Gamma}\mathbf{F}(\boldsymbol{\xi}_i) + \boldsymbol{\Lambda}_\xi\boldsymbol{\xi}_i, \tag{4.23}$$

$$\text{Cov}(\mathbf{y}_i^{\text{rep}}|\boldsymbol{\Omega}, \boldsymbol{\theta}) = \boldsymbol{\Lambda}_\eta\boldsymbol{\Pi}_0^{-1}\boldsymbol{\Psi}_\delta(\boldsymbol{\Lambda}_\eta\boldsymbol{\Pi}_0^{-1})^T + \boldsymbol{\Psi}_\epsilon. \tag{4.24}$$

To compute the L_ν-measure given in (4.19), we employ the following identities to utilize the simulated observations already available in the estimation:

$$E(\mathbf{y}_i^{\text{rep}}|\mathbf{Y}) = E\{E(\mathbf{y}_i^{\text{rep}}|\boldsymbol{\Omega}, \boldsymbol{\theta})|\mathbf{Y}\},$$
$$\text{Cov}(\mathbf{y}_i^{\text{rep}}|\mathbf{Y}) = E\{\text{Cov}(\mathbf{y}_i^{\text{rep}}|\boldsymbol{\Omega}, \boldsymbol{\theta})|\mathbf{Y}\} + \text{Cov}\{E(\mathbf{y}_i^{\text{rep}}|\boldsymbol{\Omega}, \boldsymbol{\theta})|\mathbf{Y}\}.$$

Let $\{(\boldsymbol{\theta}^{(j)}, \boldsymbol{\Omega}^{(j)}), j = 1, \ldots, J\}$ be simulated observations from $p(\boldsymbol{\theta}, \boldsymbol{\Omega}|\mathbf{Y})$. It follows from (4.20), (4.21), and the above identities that:

$$\widehat{E}(\mathbf{y}_i^{\text{rep}}|\mathbf{Y}) = \frac{1}{J}\sum_{j=1}^J \mathbf{m}_i^{(j)},$$

$$\widehat{\text{Cov}}(\mathbf{y}_i^{\text{rep}}|\mathbf{Y}) = \frac{1}{J}\sum_{j=1}^J [\boldsymbol{\Lambda}_\eta^{(j)}(\boldsymbol{\Pi}_0^{(j)})^{-1}\boldsymbol{\Psi}_\delta^{(j)}(\boldsymbol{\Lambda}_\eta^{(j)}(\boldsymbol{\Pi}_0^{(j)})^{-1})^T + \boldsymbol{\Psi}_\epsilon^{(j)}]$$
$$+\frac{1}{J}\sum_{j=1}^J \mathbf{m}_i^{(j)}\mathbf{m}_i^{(j)T} - \left(\frac{1}{J}\sum_{j=1}^J \mathbf{m}_i^{(j)}\right)\left(\frac{1}{J}\sum_{j=1}^J \mathbf{m}_i^{(j)}\right)^T,$$

where $\mathbf{m}_i^{(j)} = \boldsymbol{\mu}^{(j)} + \boldsymbol{\Lambda}_\eta^{(j)}(\boldsymbol{\Pi}_0^{(j)})^{-1}\{\boldsymbol{\Gamma}^{(j)}\mathbf{F}(\boldsymbol{\xi}_i^{(j)})\} + \boldsymbol{\Lambda}_\xi^{(j)}\boldsymbol{\xi}_i^{(j)}$. Hence, an estimate of the L_ν measure defined by (4.19) can be obtained.

We use the following data set to illustrate model comparison via various statistics. A small portion of the Inter-university Consortium for Political and Social Research (ICPSR) data set collected by the World Values Survey 1981–1984 and 1990–1993 (World Values Study Group, 1994) is considered. Six variables in the original data set obtained from the United Kingdom (variables 180, 96, 62, 176, 116 and 117; see Appendix 1.1) that related to respondents' job, religious belief, and home life were taken as observed variables in $\mathbf{y} = (y_1, \ldots, y_6)^T$. After deleting missing data, the sample size was 197. The variables (y_1, y_2) were related to life, (y_3, y_4) to religious belief, and (y_5, y_6) to job satisfaction. Variable y_3 was measured on a five-point scale, while the rest were measured on a ten-point scale. As this example is for illustration purposes, they were all treated as continuous for brevity.

The competing models are defined with a measurement equation with three latent variables $\{\eta, \xi_1, \xi_2\}$ and the loading matrix

$$\boldsymbol{\Lambda}^T = \begin{bmatrix} 1 & \lambda_{21} & 0 & 0 & 0 & 0 \\ 0 & 0 & 1 & \lambda_{42} & 0 & 0 \\ 0 & 0 & 0 & 0 & 1 & \lambda_{63} \end{bmatrix}.$$

Hence, η, ξ_1, and ξ_2 can be roughly interpreted as 'life', 'religious belief', and 'job satisfaction', respectively. The structural equations of the competing models are as follows: for $i = 1, \ldots, n$,

$$\begin{aligned} M_1 &: \eta_i = \gamma_1\xi_{i1} + \gamma_2\xi_{i2} + \delta_i, \\ M_2 &: \eta_i = \gamma_1\xi_{i1} + \gamma_2\xi_{i2} + \gamma_3\xi_{i1}^2 + \delta_i, \\ M_3 &: \eta_i = \gamma_1\xi_{i1} + \gamma_2\xi_{i2} + \gamma_3\xi_{i2}^2 + \delta_i, \\ M_4 &: \eta_i = \gamma_1\xi_{i1} + \gamma_2\xi_{i2} + \gamma_3\xi_{i1}\xi_{i2} + \delta_i, \\ M_5 &: \eta_i = \gamma_1\xi_{i1} + \gamma_2\xi_{i2} + \gamma_3\xi_{i1}^2 + \gamma_4\xi_{i2}^2 + \gamma_5\xi_{i1}\xi_{i2} + \delta_i. \end{aligned}$$

The following hyperparameters were selected in the analysis: $\alpha_{0\epsilon k} = \alpha_{0\delta} = 10$, $\beta_{0\epsilon k} = \beta_{0\delta} = 8$, $\mathbf{H}_{0yk}$ and $\mathbf{H}_{0\omega k}$ are diagonal matrices with diagonal element 0.25, $\rho_0 = 20$, $\boldsymbol{\Sigma}_0 = \mathbf{I}_6$, $\mathbf{R}_0^{-1} = 2\tilde{\boldsymbol{\Phi}}$, $\boldsymbol{\Lambda}_{0k} = \tilde{\boldsymbol{\Lambda}}_{0k}$, and $\boldsymbol{\Gamma}_{0k} = \tilde{\boldsymbol{\Gamma}}_{0k}$, where $\tilde{\boldsymbol{\Lambda}}_{0k}$, $\tilde{\boldsymbol{\Gamma}}_{0k}$, and $\tilde{\boldsymbol{\Phi}}$ were the Bayesian estimates obtained on the basis of M_1 and noninformative prior distributions. We found that the MCMC algorithm converged within 2000 iterations. Results were obtained from 2000 observations collected after convergence. The following values of the $L_{0.5}$ measure were obtained: $L_{(1)} = 3657.8$, $L_{(2)} = 3652.67$, $L_{(3)} = 3702.8$, $L_{(4)} = 3568.4$, and $L_{(5)} = 3853.5$, where $L_{(k)}$ is the $L_{0.5}$ measure corresponding to M_k. Based on these results, M_4 is selected. The DIC values obtained from WinBUGS were $\text{DIC}_{(1)} = 4093.0$, $\text{DIC}_{(2)} = 4090.5$, $\text{DIC}_{(3)} = 4093.9$, $\text{DIC}_{(4)} = 4081.6$, and $\text{DIC}_{(5)} = 4087.6$. Based on the DIC values, M_4 is again selected. We used the Bayes factor to compare M_4 with the other models, and obtained the following results: $2\log B_{14} = -5.336$, $2\log B_{24} = -8.626$, $2\log B_{34} = -5.748$, and $2\log B_{54} = 0.246$. Again,

M_4 is selected. Hence, we draw the same conclusion that a nonlinear SEM with an interaction is selected for fitting the data set.

4.5 Goodness of fit and model checking methods

4.5.1 Posterior predictive p-value

The model comparison statistics discussed in previous sections can be used to assess the goodness of fit of the hypothesized model by taking M_0 or M_1 to be the saturated model. However, for some complex SEMs, it is rather difficult to define a saturated model. For example, in the analysis of nonlinear SEMs, the distribution of the observed random vector associated with the hypothesized model is not normal. Thus, the model assuming a normal distribution with a general unstructured covariance matrix cannot be regarded as a saturated model. In these situations, model comparison statistics such as the Bayes factor, BIC, AIC, and DIC cannot be applied to assess the goodness of fit of the hypothesized model. A simple and more convenient alternative without involving basic saturated model is the posterior predictive (PP) p-values introduced by Meng (1994) on the basis of the posterior assessment in Rubin (1984). Let $D(\mathbf{Y}|\boldsymbol{\theta}, \boldsymbol{\Omega})$ be a discrepancy measure that is used to capture the discrepancy between the hypothesized model M_0 and the data, and let $\mathbf{Y}^{\text{rep}}$ be the generated hypothetical replicate data. The PP p-value is defined by

$$p_B(\mathbf{Y}) = \Pr\{D(\mathbf{Y}^{\text{rep}}|\boldsymbol{\theta}, \boldsymbol{\Omega}) \geq D(\mathbf{Y}|\boldsymbol{\theta}, \boldsymbol{\Omega})|\mathbf{Y}, M_0\}, \tag{4.25}$$

which is the upper-tail probability of the discrepancy measure under its posterior predictive distribution. See Appendix 4.3 for computation of $p_B(\mathbf{Y})$. PP p-values not far from 0.5 indicate that the realized discrepancies are near the center of the posterior predictive distribution of the discrepancy measure. Hence, a hypothesized model may be considered as plausible when its PP p-value is reasonably close to 0.5.

4.5.2 Residual analysis

Many common model checking methods in data analysis, such as residual analysis, can be incorporated into the Bayesian analysis. An advantage of the sampling-based Bayesian approach for SEMs is that we can obtain the estimates of the latent variables through the posterior simulation so that reliable estimates of the residuals in the measurement equation and the structural equation can be obtained. The graphical interpretation of these residuals is similar to those in other statistical models, for example, regression.

As an illustration of the basic idea, consider the SEMs with fixed covariates as described in Section 2.3. Estimates of the residuals in the measurement equation can be obtained from (2.12) as

$$\hat{\boldsymbol{\epsilon}}_i = \mathbf{y}_i - \hat{\mathbf{A}}\mathbf{c}_i - \hat{\boldsymbol{\Lambda}}\hat{\boldsymbol{\omega}}_i, \quad i = 1, \ldots, n, \tag{4.26}$$

where $\hat{\mathbf{A}}$, $\hat{\boldsymbol{\Lambda}}$, and $\hat{\boldsymbol{\omega}}_i$ are Bayesian estimates obtained from the corresponding simulated observations through MCMC methods. Plots of $\hat{\boldsymbol{\epsilon}}_i$ versus $\hat{\boldsymbol{\omega}}_i$ give useful information for the fit of the measurement equation. For a reasonably good fit, the plots should lie within two parallel horizontal lines that are not widely separated and centered at zero. Estimates of residuals in the structural equation can be obtained from (2.14) as

$$\hat{\boldsymbol{\delta}}_i = (\mathbf{I} - \hat{\boldsymbol{\Pi}})\hat{\boldsymbol{\eta}}_i - \hat{\mathbf{B}}\mathbf{d}_i - \hat{\boldsymbol{\Gamma}}\hat{\boldsymbol{\xi}}_i, \quad i = 1, \ldots, n, \tag{4.27}$$

where $\hat{\boldsymbol{\Pi}}$, $\hat{\mathbf{B}}$, $\hat{\boldsymbol{\Gamma}}$, $\hat{\boldsymbol{\eta}}_i$, and $\hat{\boldsymbol{\xi}}_i$ are Bayesian estimates. The use and interpretation of plots of $\hat{\boldsymbol{\delta}}_i$ and $\hat{\boldsymbol{\epsilon}}_i$ are similar. More concrete examples of residual analysis in the context of real data sets will be presented in subsequent chapters.

The residual estimates $\hat{\boldsymbol{\epsilon}}_i$ can also be used for outlier analysis. A particular observation $\mathbf{y}_i$ whose residual is far from zero may be informally regarded as an outlier. Moreover, the quantile–quantile plots of $\hat{\epsilon}_{ij}$, $j = 1, \ldots, p$, and $\hat{\delta}_{ik}$, $k = 1, \ldots, q_1$, can be used to check the assumption of normality.

Appendix 4.1 WinBUGS code

```
model {
    for (i in 1:N) {
        for (j in 1:8) { y[i,j]~dnorm(mu[i,j], psi[j]) }
        mu[i,1]<-a[1,1]*x[i,1]+a[1,2]*x[i,2]+eta[i]
        mu[i,2]<-a[2,1]*x[i,1]+a[2,2]*x[i,2]+lam[1]*eta[i]
        mu[i,3]<-a[3,1]*x[i,1]+a[3,2]*x[i,2]+lam[2]*eta[i]
        mu[i,4]<-a[4,1]*x[i,1]+a[4,2]*x[i,2]+xi[i,1]
        mu[i,5]<-a[5,1]*x[i,1]+a[5,2]*x[i,2]+lam[3]*xi[i,1]
        mu[i,6]<-a[6,1]*x[i,1]+a[6,2]*x[i,2]+xi[i,2]
        mu[i,7]<-a[7,1]*x[i,1]+a[7,2]*x[i,2]+lam[4]*xi[i,2]
        mu[i,8]<-a[8,1]*x[i,1]+a[8,2]*x[i,2]+lam[5]*xi[i,2]

        #structural equation
        eta[i]~dnorm(nu[i], psd)

        nu[i]<-b*z[i]+gam[1]*xi[i,1]+gam[2]*xi[i,2]
              +t*gam[3]*xi[i,1]*xi[i,2]+(1-t)*gam[4]*xi[i,2]*xi[i,2]

        u[i]<-(eta[i]-nu[i])*psd*(gam[3]*xi[i,1]*xi[i,2]
             -gam[4]*xi[i,2]*xi[i,2])

        xi[i,1:2]~dmnorm(zero[1:2], phi[1:2,1:2])
    }   #end of i

    ubar<-sum(u[])

    #prior distribution
    lam[1]~dnorm(1.5,psi[2])     lam[2]~dnorm(1.5,psi[3])
    lam[3]~dnorm(1.5,psi[5])     lam[4]~dnorm(1.5,psi[7])
    lam[5]~dnorm(1.5,psi[8])

    b~dnorm(1, psd)              gam[1]~dnorm(0.5,psd)
    gam[2]~dnorm(0.5,psd)        gam[3]~dnorm(1.0,psd)
    gam[4]~dnorm(0.0,psd)

    for (j in 1:8) {
        psi[j]~dgamma(8,10)
        a[j,1]~dnorm(1.0,1)      a[j,2]~dnorm(0.7,1)
    }

    psd~dgamma(8,10)    phi[1:2,1:2]~dwish(R[1:2,1:2], 20)
} #end of model
```

Appendix 4.2 R code in Bayes factor example

```
library(mvtnorm)   #Load mvtnorm package
library(R2WinBUGS) #Load R2WinBUGS package

N=300                          #Sample size
AZ=matrix(NA, nrow=N, ncol=2)  #Fixed covariates in measurement equation
BZ=numeric(N)                  #Fixed covariate in structural equation
XI=matrix(NA, nrow=N, ncol=2)  #Explanatory latent variables
Eta=numeric(N)                 #Outcome latent variables
Y=matrix(NA, nrow=N, ncol=8)   #Observed variables

#The covariance matrix of xi
phi=matrix(c(1, 0.15, 0.15, 1), nrow=2)

p=numeric(3); p[1]=pnorm(-0.5); p[2]=pnorm(0.5)-p[1]; p[3]=1-pnorm(0.5)

#Generate the data
for (i in 1:N) {
    AZ[i,1]=sample(1:3, 1, prob=p); AZ[i,2]=rnorm(1,0,1)
    BZ[i]=rbinom(1,1,0.7)

    XI[i,]=rmvnorm(1, c(0,0), phi)

    delta=rnorm(1,0,1)
    Eta[i]=BZ[i]+0.5*XI[i,1]+0.5*XI[i,2]+XI[i,2]*XI[i,2]+delta

    eps=rnorm(8,0,1)
    Y[i,1]=Eta[i]+eps[1]
    Y[i,2]=1.5*Eta[i]+eps[2]
    Y[i,3]=1.5*Eta[i]+eps[3]
    Y[i,4]=XI[i,1]+eps[4]
    Y[i,5]=1.5*XI[i,1]+eps[5]
    Y[i,6]=XI[i,2]+eps[6]
    Y[i,7]=1.5*XI[i,2]+eps[7]
    Y[i,8]=1.5*XI[i,2]+eps[8]

    for (j in 1:8) { Y[i,j]=Y[i,j]+AZ[i,1]+0.7*AZ[i,2] }
}

R=matrix(c(17.0 2.55, 2.55, 17.0), nrow=2)

data=list(N=300, zero=c(0,0), x=AZ, z=BZ, R=R, y=Y, t=NA) #Data

init1=list(lam=rep(0,5), a=matrix(rep(0,16), nrow=8, byrow=T),
           gam=rep(0,4), b=0,    psi=rep(1,8),     psd=1,
           phi=matrix(c(1, 0, 0, 1), nrow=2))

init2=list(lam=rep(1,5), a=matrix(rep(1,16), nrow=8, byrow=T),
           gam=rep(1,4), b=1,    psi=rep(2,8),     psd=2,
           phi=matrix(c(2, 0, 0, 2), nrow=2))

inits=list(init1, init2) #Initial values

parameters=c(''ubar'')
```

```
#Path sampling
for (i in 1:21) {
    data$t<-(i-1)*0.05
    model<-bugs(data,inits,parameters,
                model.file=''C:/Bayes Factor/model.txt'',
                n.chains=2,n.iter=1500,n.burnin=500,n.thin=1,
                bugs.directory=''C:/Program Files/WinBUGS14/'',
                working.directory=''C:/Bayes Factor/'')
    u[i]<-model$mean$ubar
}

#Calculate log Bayes factor
logBF=0
for (i in 1:20) { logBF=logBF+(u[i+1]+u[i])*0.05/2 }
print(logBF)
```

Appendix 4.3 Posterior predictive p-value for model assessment

Based on the posterior predictive assessment as discussed in Rubin (1984), Gelman *et al.* (1996) introduced a Bayesian counterpart of the classical p-value by defining a posterior predictive p-value for model checking. To apply the approach in order to make a goodness of fit assessment of a hypothesized model M_0 with parameter vector $\boldsymbol{\theta}$, observed data $\mathbf{Y}$ and latent data $\boldsymbol{\Omega}$, we consider a discrepancy variable $D(\mathbf{Y}|\boldsymbol{\theta}, \boldsymbol{\Omega})$ for measuring the discrepancy between $\mathbf{Y}$ and the generated hypothetical replicate data $\mathbf{Y}^{\text{rep}}$. Then the PP p-value is defined as

$$\begin{aligned} p_B(\mathbf{Y}) &= \Pr\{D(\mathbf{Y}^{\text{rep}}|\boldsymbol{\theta}, \boldsymbol{\Omega}) \geq D(\mathbf{Y}|\boldsymbol{\theta}, \boldsymbol{\Omega})|\mathbf{Y}, M_0\}, \\ &= \int I\{D(\mathbf{Y}^{\text{rep}}|\boldsymbol{\theta}, \boldsymbol{\Omega}) \geq D(\mathbf{Y}|\boldsymbol{\theta}, \boldsymbol{\Omega})\}p(\mathbf{Y}^{\text{rep}}, \boldsymbol{\theta}, \boldsymbol{\Omega}|\mathbf{Y}, M_0)d\mathbf{Y}^{\text{rep}}d\boldsymbol{\theta}d\boldsymbol{\Omega}, \end{aligned}$$

where $I(\cdot)$ is an indicator function. The probability is taken over the following joint posterior distribution of $(\mathbf{Y}^{\text{rep}}, \boldsymbol{\theta}, \boldsymbol{\Omega})$ given $\mathbf{Y}$ and M_0:

$$p(\mathbf{Y}^{\text{rep}}, \boldsymbol{\theta}, \boldsymbol{\Omega}|\mathbf{Y}, M_0) = p(\mathbf{Y}^{\text{rep}}|\boldsymbol{\theta}, \boldsymbol{\Omega})p(\boldsymbol{\theta}, \boldsymbol{\Omega}|\mathbf{Y}).$$

In almost all our applications to SEMs considered in this book, we take the chi-square discrepancy variable such that $D(\mathbf{Y}^{\text{rep}}|\boldsymbol{\theta}, \boldsymbol{\Omega})$ has a chi-square distribution with d^* degrees of freedom. Thus, the PP p-value is equal to

$$\int p\{\chi^2(d^*) \geq D(\mathbf{Y}|\boldsymbol{\theta}, \boldsymbol{\Omega})\}p(\boldsymbol{\theta}, \boldsymbol{\Omega}|\mathbf{Y})d\boldsymbol{\theta}d\boldsymbol{\Omega}.$$

A Rao-Blackwellized type estimate of this PP p-value is

$$\hat{p}_B(\mathbf{Y}) = J^{-1}\sum_{j=1}^{J} \Pr\{\chi^2(d^*) \geq D(\mathbf{Y}|\boldsymbol{\theta}^{(j)}, \boldsymbol{\Omega}^{(j)})\},$$

where $\{(\boldsymbol{\theta}^{(j)}, \boldsymbol{\Omega}^{(j)}), j = 1, \ldots, J\}$ are observations simulated during the estimation. The computational burden of obtaining this $\hat{p}_B(\mathbf{Y})$ is light.

References

Akaike, H. (1973) Information theory and an extension of the maximum likelihood principle. In B. N. Petrov and F. Csáki (eds), *Second International Symposium on Information Theory*, pp. 267–281. Budapest, Hungary: Akadémiai Kiadó.

Berger, J. O. (1985) *Statistical Decision Theory and Bayesian Analysis*. New York: Springer-Verlag.

Berger, J. O. and Delampady, M. (1987) Testing precise hypotheses. *Statistical Science*, **3**, 317–352.

Berger, J. O. and Pericchi, L. R. (1996) The intrinsic Bayes factor for model selection and prediction. *Journal of the American Statistical Association*, **91**, 109–122.

Berger, J. O. and Sellke, T. (1987) Testing a point null hypothesis: The irreconcilability of P values and evidence. *Journal of the American Statistical Association*, **82**, 112–122.

Celeux, G., Forbes, F., Robert, C. P. and Titterington, D. M. (2006) Deviance information criteria for missing data models. *Bayesian Analysis*, **1**, 651–674.

Chib, S. (1995) Marginal likelihood from the Gibbs output. *Journal of the American Statistical Association*, **90**, 1313–1321.

Chib, S. and Jeliazkov, I. (2001) Marginal likelihood from the Metropolis–Hastings output. *Journal of the American Statistical Association*, **96**, 270–281.

DiCiccio, T. J., Kass, R. E., Raftery, A. and Wasserman, L. (1997) Computing Bayes factors by combining simulation and asymptotic approximations. *Journal of the American Statistical Association*, **92**, 903–915.

Gelman, A. and Meng, X. L. (1998) Simulating normalizing constants: From importance sampling to bridge sampling to path sampling. *Statistical Science*, **13**, 163–185.

Gelman, A., Meng, X. L. and Stern, H. (1996) Posterior predictive assessment of model fitness via realized discrepancies. *Statistica Sinica*, **6**, 733–760.

Ibrahim, J. G., Chen, M. H. and Sinha, D. (2001) Criterion-based methods for Bayesian model assessment. *Statistica Sinica*, **11**, 419–443.

Kass, R. E. and Raftery, A. E. (1995) Bayes factors. *Journal of the American Statistical Association*, **90**, 773–795.

Lee, S. Y. (2007) *Structural Equation Modeling: A Bayesian Approach*. Chichester: John Wiley & Sons, Ltd.

Lee, S. Y. and Song X. Y. (2003a) Model comparison of nonlinear structural equation models with fixed covariates. *Psychometrika*, **68**, 27–47.

Lee, S. Y. and Song, X. Y. (2003b) Bayesian model selection for mixtures of structural equation models with an unknown number of components. *British Journal of Mathematical and Statistical Psychology*, **56**, 145–165.

Meng, X. L. (1994) Posterior predictive *p*-values. *Annals of Statistics*, **22**, 1142–1160.

Ogata, Y. (1989) A Monte Carlo method for high dimensional integration. *Numerische Mathematik*, **55**, 137–157.

O'Hagan, A. (1995) Fractional Bayes factor for model comparison. *Journal of the Royal Statistical Society, Series B*, **57**, 99–138.

Raftery, A. E. (1993) Bayesian model selection in structural equation models. In K. A. Bollen and J. S. Long (eds), *Testing Structural Equation Models*, pp. 163–180. Beverly Hills, CA: Sage.

Rubin, D. B. (1984) Bayesianly justifiable and relevant frequency calculations for the applied statistician. *Annals of Statistics*, **12**, 1151–1172.

Schwarz, G. (1978) Estimating the dimension of a model. *Annals of Statistics*, **6**, 461–464.

Song, X. Y. and Lee, S. Y. (2006) Model comparison of generalized linear mixed models. *Statistics in Medicine*, **25**, 1685–1698.

Spiegelhalter, D. J., Best, N. G., Carlin, B. P. and van der Linde, A. (2002) Bayesian measures of model complexity and fit. *Journal of the Royal Statistical Society, Series B*, **64**, 583–639.

Spiegelhalter, D. J., Thomas, A., Best, N. G. and Lunn, D. (2003) *WinBUGS User Manual. Version 1.4*. Cambridge: MRC Biostatistics Unit.

Sturtz, S., Ligges, U. and Gelman, A. (2005) R2WinBUGS: A package for running WinBUGS from R. *Journal of Statistical Software*, **12**, 1–16.

Tanner, M. A. and Wong, W. H. (1987) The calculation of posterior distributions by data augmentation (with discussion). *Journal of the American statistical Association*, **82**, 528–550.

World Values Study Group (1994) World Values Survey, 1981–1984 and 1990–1993. ICPSR version. Ann Arbor, MI: Institute for Social Research (producer). Ann Arbor, MI: Inter-university Consortium for Political and Social Research (distributor).

5

Practical structural equation models

5.1 Introduction

In Chapter 2, we introduced standard linear and nonlinear SEMs and explained in detail how to apply these models in practice. Bayesian methods for estimating parameters in the model and model comparison are presented in Chapters 3 and 4, respectively. While these developments provide sound statistical methods for solving many practical problems, they depend on certain assumptions. As these assumptions may not be satisfied by many complex data sets coming from substantive research, it is important to deal with those complex data structures.

In subsequent sections, we will introduce some generalizations of the standard SEMs for analyzing complex data sets. These include SEMs with mixed continuous and ordered categorical variables, SEMs with variables coming from an exponential family distribution, and SEMs with missing data. Moreover, we will illustrate how the Bayesian methodologies can be naturally extended to these generalizations, again through data augmentation and MCMC techniques.

5.2 SEMs with continuous and ordered categorical variables

5.2.1 Introduction

Due to questionnaire design and the nature of the problems in social, behavioral, and medical sciences, data often come from ordered categorical variables with observations in discrete form. Examples of such variables are attitude items, Likert items, rating scales and the like. A typical case is when a subject is asked to report the effect of a drug on a scale such as

Basic and Advanced Bayesian Structural Equation Modeling: With Applications in the Medical and Behavioral Sciences, First Edition. Xin-Yuan Song and Sik-Yum Lee.

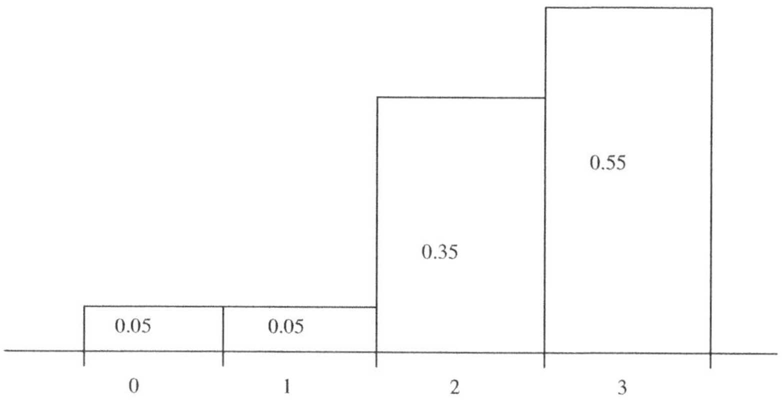

Figure 5.1 Histogram of a hypothetical ordered categorical data set.

'getting worse', 'no change', 'getting better'. One common approach in analyzing ordered categorical data is to treat the assigned integers as continuous data from a normal distribution. This approach may not lead to a serious problem if the histograms of the observations are symmetrical and with the highest frequencies at the center – that is, when most subjects choose the 'no change' category. To claim multivariate normality of the observed variables, we need to have most subjects choosing the middle category in all the corresponding items. However, for interesting items in a questionnaire, most subjects would likely select categories at both ends. Hence, in practice, histograms corresponding to most variables are either skewed or bimodal; and routinely treating them as normal may lead to erroneous conclusions (see Olsson, 1979; Lee *et al.*, 1990).

A better approach for analyzing this kind of discrete data is to treat them as observations that come from a latent continuous normal distribution with a threshold specification. Suppose that, for a given data set, the values 0, 1, 2, 3 occur with proportions 0.05, 0.05, 0.35, 0.55, respectively. The discrete data are highly skewed to the left; see the histogram in Figure 5.1. The threshold approach for analyzing this highly skewed discrete variable is to treat the ordered categorical data as manifestations of an underlying normal variable y. The exact continuous measurements of y are not available, but are related to the observed ordered categorical variable z as follows: for $m = 0, 1, 2, 3$,

$$z = m \quad \text{if}\, \alpha_m \leq y < \alpha_{m+1},$$

where $-\infty = \alpha_0 < \alpha_1 < \alpha_2 < \alpha_3 < \alpha_4 = \infty$, and α_1, α_2, and α_3 are thresholds. Then the ordered categorical observations can be captured by $N[0, 1]$ with appropriate thresholds; see Figure 5.2. As $\alpha_2 - \alpha_1$ can be different from $\alpha_3 - \alpha_2$, unequal-interval scales are allowed. Thus, this threshold approach allows flexible modeling. As it is related to a common normal distribution, it also provides easy interpretation of the parameters.

Analysis of SEMs with mixed continuous and ordered categorical data is not straightforward, because we need to compute the multiple integrals associated with the cell probabilities that are induced by the ordered categorical outcomes. Some multistage methods have been proposed to reduce the computational burden in evaluating these integrals. The basic procedure of these multistage methods is as follows: first, partition the multivariate model into

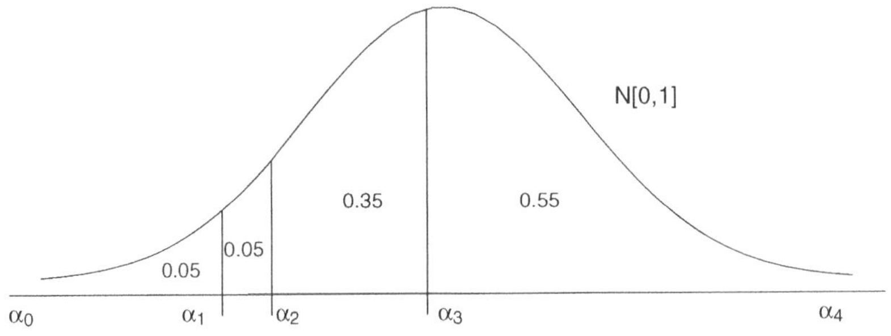

Figure 5.2 The underlying normal distribution with a threshold specification.

several bivariate submodels and estimate the polychoric and polyserial correlations, and the thresholds based on the bivariate submodels; then derive the asymptotic distributions of the estimates and analyze the SEM with a covariance structure analysis approach through a generalized least square (GLS) procedure. However, as pointed out by Shi and Lee (2000), such multistage estimators are not statistically optimal, and it is necessary to invert at each iteration of the GLS minimization a huge matrix whose dimension increases very rapidly with the number of observed variables.

The main objective of this section is to introduce a Bayesian approach for analyzing SEMs with mixed continuous and ordered categorical variables. The basic idea in handling the ordered categorical variables is to treat the underlying latent continuous measurements as hypothetical missing data, and to augment them with the observed data in the posterior analysis. Using this data augmentation strategy, the model that is based on the complete data set becomes one with continuous variables. Again, in estimation, sequences of observations of the structural parameters, latent variables, and thresholds are simulated from the joint posterior distribution via MCMC algorithms. In addition to estimation, we consider model selection via some Bayesian model selection statistics. Finally, an application related to quality of life (QOL) is presented to illustrate the Bayesian methodologies.

5.2.2 The basic model

Consider the following measurement equation for a $p \times 1$ observed random vector $\mathbf{v}_i$:

$$\mathbf{v}_i = \boldsymbol{\mu} + \boldsymbol{\Lambda}\boldsymbol{\omega}_i + \boldsymbol{\epsilon}_i, \quad i = 1, \ldots, n, \tag{5.1}$$

where $\boldsymbol{\mu}$, $\boldsymbol{\Lambda}$, $\boldsymbol{\omega}_i$, and $\boldsymbol{\epsilon}_i$ are defined as in (2.3). Let $\boldsymbol{\eta}_i(q_1 \times 1)$ and $\boldsymbol{\xi}_i(q_2 \times 1)$ be latent subvectors of $\boldsymbol{\omega}_i$, and consider the structural equation

$$\boldsymbol{\eta}_i = \boldsymbol{\Pi}\boldsymbol{\eta}_i + \boldsymbol{\Gamma}\boldsymbol{\xi}_i + \boldsymbol{\delta}_i, \tag{5.2}$$

where $\boldsymbol{\Pi}(q_1 \times q_1)$, $\boldsymbol{\Gamma}(q_1 \times q_2)$, $\boldsymbol{\xi}_i$, and $\boldsymbol{\delta}_i$ are defined as in (2.8). Let $\boldsymbol{\Lambda}_\omega = (\boldsymbol{\Pi}, \boldsymbol{\Gamma})$; then equation (5.2) can be written as $\boldsymbol{\eta}_i = \boldsymbol{\Lambda}_\omega\boldsymbol{\omega}_i + \boldsymbol{\delta}_i$. Let $\mathbf{v} = (\mathbf{x}^T, \mathbf{y}^T)^T$, where $\mathbf{x} = (x_1, \ldots, x_r)^T$ is a subset of variables whose exact continuous measurements are observable, while $\mathbf{y} = (y_1, \ldots, y_s)^T$ is the remaining subset of variables such that the corresponding continuous measurements are unobservable. The information associated with $\mathbf{y}$ is given by an observable ordered categorical vector $\mathbf{z} = (z_1, \ldots, z_s)^T$. Any latent variable in $\boldsymbol{\eta}$ or $\boldsymbol{\xi}$ may be related to observed variables in either $\mathbf{x}$ or $\mathbf{z}$. That is, any latent variable may have continuous and/or ordered categorical observed variables as its indicators. The relationship between $\mathbf{y}$ and $\mathbf{z}$ is defined by a set of thresholds as follows:

$$\mathbf{z} = \begin{bmatrix} z_1 \\ \vdots \\ z_s \end{bmatrix} \quad \text{if} \quad \begin{array}{c} \alpha_{1,z_1} \le y_1 < \alpha_{1,z_1+1}, \\ \vdots \\ \alpha_{s,z_s} \le y_s < \alpha_{s,z_s+1}, \end{array} \tag{5.3}$$

where, for $k = 1, \ldots, s$, z_k is an integer value in $\{0, 1, \ldots, b_k\}$, and $\alpha_{k,0} < \alpha_{k,1} < \ldots < \alpha_{k,b_k} < \alpha_{k,b_k+1}$. In general, we set $\alpha_{k,0} = -\infty$, $\alpha_{k,b_k+1} = \infty$. For the kth variable, there are $b_k + 1$ categories defined by the unknown thresholds $\alpha_{k,j}$. The integer values $\{0, 1, \ldots, b_k\}$ of z_k are used to specify the categories that contain the corresponding elements in y_k. In order to indicate the 'ordered' nature of the categorical values and their thresholds, it is better to choose an ordered set of integers for each z_k. In the Bayesian analysis, these integer values are neither directly used in the posterior simulation nor involved in any actual computation. In this section, the SEM with continuous and ordered categorical variables $\{(\mathbf{x}_i^T, \mathbf{z}_i^T)^T, i = 1, \ldots, n\}$ is analyzed.

The SEM defined by (5.1) and (5.2) is not identified without imposing appropriate identification conditions. There are two kinds of indeterminacies involved in this model. One is the common indeterminacy coming from the covariance structure of the model that can be solved with the common method of fixing appropriate elements in $\mathbf{\Lambda}$, $\mathbf{\Pi}$, and/or $\mathbf{\Gamma}$ at preassigned values. The other indeterminacy is induced by the ordered categorical variables. To tackle this identification problem, we should keep in mind the following two issues. First, obtaining a necessary and sufficient condition for identification is difficult, so we are mainly interested in finding a reasonable and convenient way to identify the model. Second, for an ordered categorical variable, the location and dispersion of its underlying continuous normal variable are unknown. As we have no idea about these latent values, it is desirable to take a unified scale for every ordered categorical variable, and to interpret in a relative sense the statistical results obtained.

Now let z_k be the ordered categorical variable that is defined with a set of thresholds and an underlying continuous variable y_k whose distribution is $N[\mu, \sigma^2]$. The indeterminacy is caused by the fact that the thresholds, μ and σ^2 are not simultaneously estimable. We follow the common practice (see, for example, Shi and Lee, 1998) of imposing identification conditions on the thresholds, which are the less interesting nuisance parameters. More specifically, we propose to fix the thresholds at both ends, $\alpha_{k,1}$ and α_{k,b_k}, at preassigned values. This method implicitly picks measures for the location and dispersion of y_k. For instance, the range from α_{k,b_k} to $\alpha_{k,1}$ provides a standard for measuring the dispersion. This method can be applied to the multivariate case by imposing the above restrictions on the appropriate thresholds for every component in $\mathbf{z}$. If the model is scale invariant, the choice of the preassigned values for the fixed thresholds only changes the scale of the estimated covariance matrix (see Lee *et al.*, 1990). For better interpretation of the statistical results, it is advantageous to assign the values of the fixed thresholds so that the scale of each variable is the same. One common method is to use the observed frequencies and the standard normal distribution, $N[0, 1]$. More specifically, for every k, we may fix $\alpha_{k,1} = \Phi^{*-1}(f_{k,1}^*)$ and $\alpha_{k,b_k} = \Phi^{*-1}(f_{k,b_k}^*)$, where $\Phi^*(\cdot)$ is the distribution function of $N[0, 1]$, $f_{k,1}^*$ is the frequency of the first category, and f_{k,b_k}^* is the cumulative frequency of the category with $z_k < b_k$. For linear SEMs, these restrictions imply that the mean and variance of the underlying continuous variable y_k are 0 and 1, respectively. For nonlinear SEMs, however, fixing $\alpha_{k,1}$ and α_{k,b_k} at preassigned values is only related to the location and dispersion of y_k, and the results should be interpreted with great caution.

5.2.3 Bayesian analysis

We will utilize the useful strategy of data augmentation described in Chapter 3 in the Bayesian estimation of SEMs with continuous and ordered categorical variables. Let $\mathbf{X} = (\mathbf{x}_1, \ldots, \mathbf{x}_n)$ and $\mathbf{Z} = (\mathbf{z}_1, \ldots, \mathbf{z}_n)$ be the observed continuous and ordered categorical data matrices, respectively; and let $\mathbf{Y} = (\mathbf{y}_1, \ldots, \mathbf{y}_n)$ and $\boldsymbol{\Omega} = (\boldsymbol{\omega}_1, \ldots, \boldsymbol{\omega}_n)$ be the matrices of latent continuous measurements and latent variables, respectively. The observed data $[\mathbf{X}, \mathbf{Z}]$ are augmented with the latent data $[\mathbf{Y}, \boldsymbol{\Omega}]$ in the posterior analysis. The joint Bayesian estimates of $\boldsymbol{\Omega}$, unknown thresholds in $\boldsymbol{\alpha} = (\boldsymbol{\alpha}_1, \ldots, \boldsymbol{\alpha}_s)$, and the structural parameter vector $\boldsymbol{\theta}$ that contains all unknown parameters in $\boldsymbol{\mu}$, $\boldsymbol{\Phi}$, $\boldsymbol{\Lambda}$, $\boldsymbol{\Lambda}_\omega$, $\boldsymbol{\Psi}_\epsilon$, and $\boldsymbol{\Psi}_\delta$ will be obtained.

In the Bayesian estimation, we draw samples from the posterior distribution $[\boldsymbol{\alpha}, \boldsymbol{\theta}, \boldsymbol{\Omega}, \mathbf{Y}|\mathbf{X}, \mathbf{Z}]$ through the Gibbs sampler (Geman and Geman, 1984), which iteratively simulates $\boldsymbol{\alpha}$, $\boldsymbol{\theta}$, $\boldsymbol{\Omega}$, and $\mathbf{Y}$ from the full conditional distributions. To implement the Gibbs sampler, we start with initial values $(\boldsymbol{\alpha}^{(0)}, \boldsymbol{\theta}^{(0)}, \boldsymbol{\Omega}^{(0)}, \mathbf{Y}^{(0)})$, then simulate $(\boldsymbol{\alpha}^{(1)}, \boldsymbol{\theta}^{(1)}, \boldsymbol{\Omega}^{(1)}, \mathbf{Y}^{(1)})$ and so on according to the following procedure. At the jth iteration with current values $(\boldsymbol{\alpha}^{(j)}, \boldsymbol{\theta}^{(j)}, \boldsymbol{\Omega}^{(j)}, \mathbf{Y}^{(j)})$:

A. Generate $\boldsymbol{\Omega}^{(j+1)}$ from $p(\boldsymbol{\Omega}|\boldsymbol{\theta}^{(j)}, \boldsymbol{\alpha}^{(j)}, \mathbf{Y}^{(j)}, \mathbf{X}, \mathbf{Z})$.
B. Generate $\boldsymbol{\theta}^{(j+1)}$ from $p(\boldsymbol{\theta}|\boldsymbol{\Omega}^{(j+1)}, \boldsymbol{\alpha}^{(j)}, \mathbf{Y}^{(j)}, \mathbf{X}, \mathbf{Z})$.
C. Generate $(\boldsymbol{\alpha}^{(j+1)}, \mathbf{Y}^{(j+1)})$ from $p(\boldsymbol{\alpha}, \mathbf{Y}|\boldsymbol{\theta}^{(j+1)}, \boldsymbol{\Omega}^{(j+1)}, \mathbf{X}, \mathbf{Z})$.

Convergence of the Gibbs sampler can be monitored by the 'estimated potential scale reduction' (EPSR) values suggested by Gelman (1996), or by plots of simulated sequences of the individual parameters with different starting points. Sequences of the quantities simulated from the joint posterior distribution will be used to calculate the Bayesian estimates and other related statistics. Based on the conjugate prior distributions of the parameters, conditional distributions required in the Gibbs sampler are presented in Appendix 5.1. The efficiency of the Gibbs sampler algorithm heavily depends on how easily one can sample observations from the conditional distributions. It can be seen from Appendix 5.1 that some of the conditional distributions are the familiar normal, gamma, and inverted Wishart distributions. Drawing observations from these standard distributions is straightforward and fast. However, the joint conditional distribution $p(\boldsymbol{\alpha}, \mathbf{Y}|\mathbf{Z}, \boldsymbol{\theta}, \boldsymbol{\Omega})$ is nonstandard and complex. The Metropolis–Hastings (MH) algorithm (Metropolis *et al.*, 1953; Hastings, 1970) for sampling from $p(\boldsymbol{\alpha}, \mathbf{Y}|\mathbf{Z}, \boldsymbol{\theta}, \boldsymbol{\Omega})$ is also given in Appendix 5.1.

It has been shown (Geman and Geman, 1984; Geyer, 1992) that under mild conditions and for a sufficiently large j, the joint distribution of $(\boldsymbol{\alpha}^{(j)}, \boldsymbol{\theta}^{(j)}, \boldsymbol{\Omega}^{(j)}, \mathbf{Y}^{(j)})$ converges at an exponential rate to the desired posterior distribution $[\boldsymbol{\alpha}, \boldsymbol{\theta}, \boldsymbol{\Omega}, \mathbf{Y}|\mathbf{X}, \mathbf{Z}]$. Hence, $[\boldsymbol{\alpha}, \boldsymbol{\theta}, \boldsymbol{\Omega}, \mathbf{Y}|\mathbf{X}, \mathbf{Z}]$ can be approximated by the empirical distribution of a sufficiently large number of simulated observations collected after convergence of the algorithm. After obtaining a sufficiently large sample from the posterior distribution $[\boldsymbol{\alpha}, \boldsymbol{\theta}, \boldsymbol{\Omega}, \mathbf{Y}|\mathbf{X}, \mathbf{Z}]$ with the MCMC algorithm, the Bayesian estimates of $\boldsymbol{\alpha}$, $\boldsymbol{\theta}$, and $\boldsymbol{\Omega}$ can be obtained easily via the corresponding sample means of the simulated observations. Moreover, values of the goodness of fit and model comparison statistics can be obtained via the procedures discussed in Chapter 4.

5.2.4 Application: Bayesian analysis of quality of life data

There is increasing recognition that measures of quality of life (QOL) and health-related QOL have great value for clinical work and the planning and evaluation of health care as well as for medical research. It has been commonly accepted that QOL is a multidimensional concept (Staquet *et al.*, 1998) that is best evaluated by a number of different latent constructs such as physical health status, mental health status, social relationships, and environmental conditions. As these latent constructs often cannot be measured objectively and directly, they are treated as latent variables in QOL analysis. The most popular way to assess a latent construct is to use a survey which incorporates a number of related items that are intended to reflect the underlying latent construct of interest.

An exploratory factor analysis has been used as a method for exploring the structure of a new QOL instrument (WHOQOL Group, 1998; Fayers and Machin, 1998), while a confirmatory factor analysis has been used to confirm the factor structure of the instrument. Recently, SEMs based on continuous observations with a normal distribution have been applied to QOL analysis (Power *et al.*, 1999). Items in a QOL instrument are usually measured on an ordered categorical scale, typically a three- to five-point scale. The discrete ordinal nature of the items also draws much attention in QOL analysis (Fayers and Machin, 1998; Fayers and Hand, 1997). It has been pointed out that nonrigorous treatment of ordinal items as continuous can be subjected to criticism (Glonek and McCullagh, 1995), and thus models such as the item response model and ordinal regression that incorporate the ordinal nature of the items are more appropriate (Olschewski and Schumacker, 1990). The aim of this section is to apply the Bayesian methods for analyzing the following common QOL instrument with ordered categorical items.

The WHOQOL-BREF instrument is a short version of WHOQOL-100 (Power *et al.*, 1999) consisting of 24 ordinal categorical items selected from the 100 items for evaluating four latent constructs. The first seven items (Q3–Q9) are intended to address physical health, the next six items (Q10–Q15) are intended to address psychological health, the three items (Q16–Q18) that follow measure social relationships, and the last eight items (Q19–Q26) measure environment. In addition to the 24 ordered categorical items, this instrument includes two ordered categorical items for the overall QOL (Q1) and overall health (Q2), giving a total of 26 items. All of the items are measured on a five-point scale (1 = 'not at all/very dissatisfied'; 2 = 'a little/dissatisfied'; 3 = 'moderate/neither'; 4 = 'very much/satisfied'; 5 = 'extremely/very satisfied'). The sample size of the whole data set is extremely large. To illustrate the Bayesian methods, we only analyze a synthetic data set given in Lee (2007) with sample size $n = 338$. Appendix 1.1 presents the frequencies of all the ordered categorical items, which shows that many items are skewed to the left. Treating these ordered categorical data as coming from a normal distribution is problematic. Hence, the Bayesian approach that considers the discrete nature of the data is applied to the analysis of this ordered categorical data set.

To illustrate the path sampling procedure, we compare an SEM with four explanatory latent variables to another SEM with three explanatory latent variables (see Lee *et al.*, 2005). Let M_1 be the SEM whose measurement equation is given by

$$\mathbf{y}_i = \mathbf{\Lambda}_1\boldsymbol{\omega}_{1i} + \boldsymbol{\epsilon}_i, \tag{5.4}$$

where $\boldsymbol{\omega}_{1i} = (\eta_i, \xi_{i1}, \xi_{i2}, \xi_{i3}, \xi_{i4})^T$, $\boldsymbol{\epsilon}_i$ is distributed as $N[\mathbf{0}, \mathbf{\Psi}_{\epsilon 1}]$, and

$$\mathbf{\Lambda}_1^T = \begin{bmatrix} 1 & \lambda_{21} & 0 & 0 & \cdots & 0 & 0 & 0 & \cdots & 0 & 0 & 0 & 0 & 0 & 0 & \cdots & 0 \\ 0 & 0 & 1 & \lambda_{42} & \cdots & \lambda_{92} & 0 & 0 & \cdots & 0 & 0 & 0 & 0 & 0 & 0 & \cdots & 0 \\ 0 & 0 & 0 & 0 & \cdots & 0 & 1 & \lambda_{11,3} & \cdots & \lambda_{15,3} & 0 & 0 & 0 & 0 & 0 & \cdots & 0 \\ 0 & 0 & 0 & 0 & \cdots & 0 & 0 & 0 & \cdots & 0 & 1 & \lambda_{17,4} & \lambda_{18,4} & 0 & 0 & \cdots & 0 \\ 0 & 0 & 0 & 0 & \cdots & 0 & 0 & 0 & \cdots & 0 & 0 & 0 & 0 & 1 & \lambda_{20,5} & \cdots & \lambda_{26,5} \end{bmatrix}.$$

The structural equation of M_1 is given by

$$\eta_i = \gamma_1\xi_{i1} + \gamma_2\xi_{i2} + \gamma_3\xi_{i3} + \gamma_4\xi_{i4} + \delta_i, \tag{5.5}$$

where $(\xi_{i1}, \xi_{i2}, \xi_{i3}, \xi_{i4})^T$ and δ_i are independently distributed as $N[\mathbf{0}, \mathbf{\Phi}_1]$ and $N[0, \sigma^2_{\delta 1}]$, respectively. Let M_2 be the SEM whose measurement equation is given by

$$\mathbf{y}_i = \mathbf{\Lambda}_2\boldsymbol{\omega}_{2i} + \boldsymbol{\epsilon}_i, \tag{5.6}$$

where $\boldsymbol{\omega}_{2i} = (\eta_i, \xi_{i1}, \xi_{i2}, \xi_{i3})^T$, and $\boldsymbol{\epsilon}_i$ is distributed according to $N[\mathbf{0}, \mathbf{\Psi}_{\epsilon 2}]$. The first three columns of $\mathbf{\Lambda}_2$ are the same as those in $\mathbf{\Lambda}_1$ except without the rows corresponding to Q19–Q26, while the last column is given by $[0, \ldots, 0, 1, \lambda_{17,4}, \lambda_{18,4}]^T$. The structural equation of M_2 is given by

$$\eta_i = \gamma_1\xi_{i1} + \gamma_2\xi_{i2} + \gamma_3\xi_{i3} + \delta_i, \tag{5.7}$$

where $(\xi_{i1}, \xi_{i2}, \xi_{i3})^T$ and δ_i are independently distributed as $N[\mathbf{0}, \mathbf{\Phi}_2]$ and $N[0, \sigma^2_{\delta 2}]$, respectively. The Bayesian analysis is conducted using the conjugate prior distributions. The hyperparameter values corresponding to the prior distributions of the unknown loadings in $\mathbf{\Lambda}_1$ and $\mathbf{\Lambda}_2$ are all taken to be 0.8; those corresponding to $\{\gamma_1, \gamma_2, \gamma_3, \gamma_4\}$ are $\{0.6, 0.6, 0.4, 0.4\}$; those corresponding to $\mathbf{\Phi}_1$ and $\mathbf{\Phi}_2$ are $\rho_0 = 30$ and $\mathbf{R}_0^{-1} = 8\mathbf{I}$; other hyperparameter values are taken as $\mathbf{H}_{0yk} = 0.25\mathbf{I}$, $\mathbf{H}_{0\omega k} = 0.25\mathbf{I}$, $\alpha_{0\epsilon k} = \alpha_{0\delta k} = 10$, and $\beta_{0\epsilon k} = \beta_{0\delta k} = 8$, where $\mathbf{I}$ denotes the identity matrix of appropriate dimension. In the path sampling procedure in computing the Bayes factor, we take $S = 10$, and $J = 2000$ after a 'burn-in' phase of 1000 iterations.

It is not easy to find a link model M_t that directly links M_1 and M_2. Hence, we first compare M_1 with the following simple model M_0:

$$M_0 : \mathbf{y}_i = \boldsymbol{\epsilon}_i,$$

where $\boldsymbol{\epsilon}_i \overset{D}{=} N[\mathbf{0}, \mathbf{\Psi}_\epsilon]$ and $\mathbf{\Psi}_\epsilon$ is a diagonal matrix. The measurement equation of the link model of M_0 and M_1 is given by $M_t : \mathbf{y}_i = t\mathbf{\Lambda}_1\boldsymbol{\omega}_i + \boldsymbol{\epsilon}_i$, and the structural equation is given by (5.5). We obtain $\widehat{\log B_{10}} = 81.05$. Similarly, we compare M_2 and M_0 via the path sampling procedure, and find that $\widehat{\log B_{20}} = 57.65$. From the above results, we can get an estimate of $\log B_{12}$, that is, $\widehat{\log B_{12}} = \widehat{\log B_{10}} - \widehat{\log B_{20}} = 23.40$. Hence, M_1, the SEM with four explanatory latent variables, is selected. Bayesian estimates of the unknown structural parameters in M_1 are presented in Figure 5.3. The less interesting threshold estimates are not presented. All the factor loading estimates – except $\hat{\lambda}_{17,4}$, which is associated with the indicator 'sexual activity' – are high. This indicates a strong association between each of the latent variables and their corresponding indicators. From the meaning of the items, η, ξ_1, ξ_2, ξ_3 and ξ_4 can be interpreted as the overall QOL, physical health, psychological health, social relationship, and environment, respectively. The correlations $\{\phi_{12}, \phi_{13}, \phi_{14}, \phi_{23}, \phi_{24}, \phi_{34}\}$ among the explanatory latent variables are estimated to be $\{0.46, 0.29, 0.42, 0.48, 0.51, 0.48\}$, indicating that these explanatory latent variables are highly correlated. The estimated structural equation that addresses the relation between QOL and the latent constructs for physical and psychological health, social relationships, and environment is

$$\eta = 0.72\xi_1 + 0.32\xi_2 + 0.17\xi_3 - 0.04\xi_4.$$

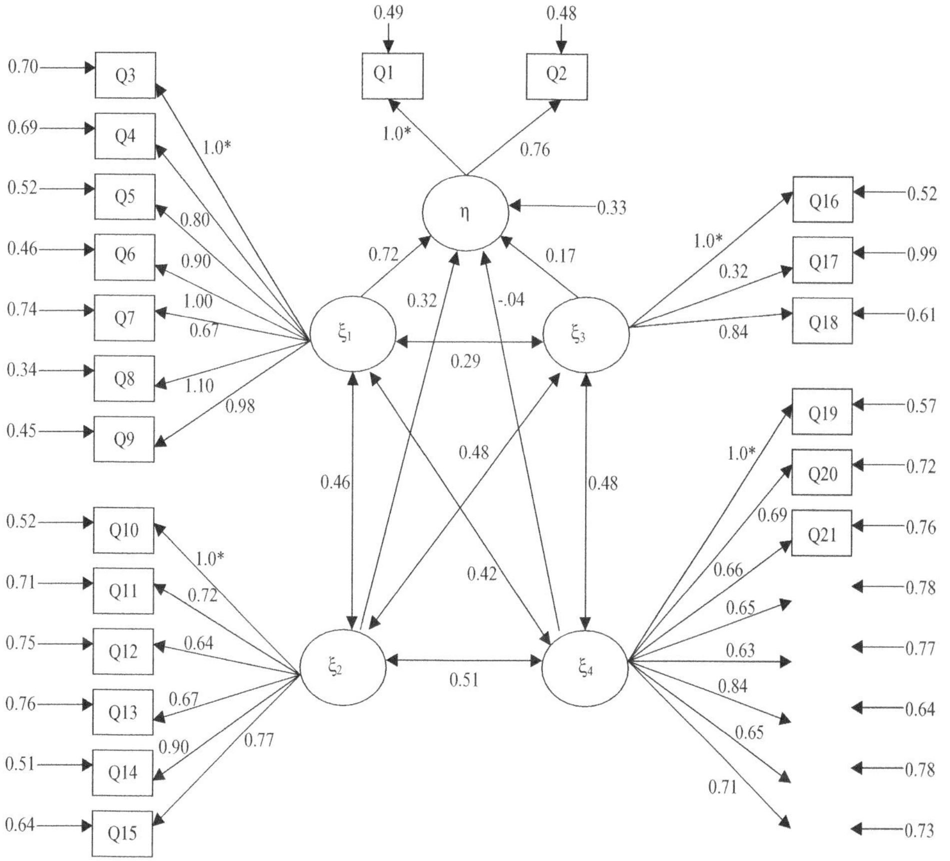

Figure 5.3 Path diagram and Bayesian estimates of parameters in the analysis of the QOL data. Note that Bayesian estimates of ϕ_{11}, ϕ_{22}, ϕ_{33}, and ϕ_{44} are 0.65, 0.71, 0.69, and 0.68, respectively. Source: Lee (2007).

Thus, physical health has the most important effect on QOL, followed by psychological health and social relationships, while the effect of environment is not important.

The WinBUGS software (Spiegelhalter *et al.*, 2003) can produce Bayesian estimates of the structural parameters and latent variables for SEMs with ordered categorical variables. According to our understanding of WinBUGS, it is not straightforward to apply this software to simultaneously estimate the unknown thresholds and structural parameters. Hence, in applying WinBUGS, we first estimate all the thresholds through the method described in Section 5.2.2. Then the thresholds are fixed in the WinBUGS program in producing the Bayesian solutions. Note that this procedure may underestimate the standard errors. Hence, hypothesis testing should be conducted using the DIC, rather than the *z*-score which depends on the standard error estimate. The WinBUGS code and the data relating to the above QOL analysis can respectively be found on the following website:

`www.wiley.com/go/medical_behavioral_sciences`

5.2.5 SEMs with dichotomous variables

In this subsection we will focus on dichotomous variables that are ordered binary and defined with one threshold. Dichotomous variables arise when respondents are asked to answer 'yes' or 'no' when asked about the presence of a symptom, 'feeling better' or 'feeling worse' about the effect of a drug, 'true' or 'false' about a test item, etc. The usual numerical values assigned to these variables are *ad hoc* numbers with an ordering such as '0' and '1', or '1' and '2'. In analyzing dichotomous data, the basic assumption in SEM that the data come from a continuous normal distribution is clearly violated, and rigorous analysis that takes into account the dichotomous nature is necessary. Analysis of SEMs with dichotomous variables is similar to but not exactly the same as the analysis with ordered categorical variables.

In much substantive research, especially in education, it is important to explore and determine a small number of intrinsic latent factors under a number of test items. Item factor analysis is an important model that has been proposed for explaining the underlying factor structures; see Bock and Aitkin (1981), Meng and Schilling (1996), and Lee and Song (2003). Another direction of analysis is motivated by the fact that correlated dichotomous data arise frequently in many medical and biological studies, ranging from measurements of random cross-section subjects to repeated measurements in longitudinal studies. A popular model is the multivariate probit (MP) model in biostatistics and other fields. This model is described in terms of a correlated multivariate normal distribution of the underlying latent variables that are manifested as discrete variables, again through a threshold specification. The emphasis of the MP model is on the mean structure, and the main difficulty in the analysis is in evaluating the multivariate normal orthant probabilities induced by the dichotomous variables; see Gibbons and Wilcox-Gök (1998) and Chib and Greenberg (1998). Analysis of the MP model requires the simulation of observations from a multivariate truncated normal distribution with an arbitrary covariance matrix. Even with the efficient methods in statistical computing, the underlying computational effort is heavy. We will show below that this computational burden can be reduced by adopting an SEM approach.

Consider a common SEM defined by (5.1) and (5.2). Now suppose that the exact measurement of $\mathbf{y}_i = (y_{i1}, \ldots, y_{ip})^T$ is not available and its information is given by an observed dichotomous vector $\mathbf{z}_i = (z_{i1}, \ldots, z_{ip})^T$ such that, for $k = 1, \ldots, p$,

$$z_{ik} = \begin{cases} 1, & \text{if } y_{ik} > 0, \\ 0, & \text{otherwise.} \end{cases} \tag{5.8}$$

The available observed data set is $\{\mathbf{z}_i, i = 1, \ldots, n\}$. Consider the relationship between the measurement equation model given by (5.1) and the dichotomous variables in $\mathbf{z}$. Let $\mathbf{\Lambda}_k^T$, μ_k, and $\psi_{\epsilon k}$ be the kth row of $\mathbf{\Lambda}$, the kth element of $\boldsymbol{\mu}$, and the kth diagonal element of $\mathbf{\Psi}_\epsilon$, respectively. It follows from (5.8) that

$$\Pr(z_{ik}=1|\boldsymbol{\omega}_i, \mu_k, \mathbf{\Lambda}_k, \psi_{\epsilon k}) = \Pr(y_{ik} > 0|\boldsymbol{\omega}_i, \mu_k, \mathbf{\Lambda}_k, \psi_{\epsilon k}) = \Phi^* \left\{ \left(\mathbf{\Lambda}_k^T / \psi_{\epsilon k}^{1/2} \right) \boldsymbol{\omega}_i + \mu_k / \psi_{\epsilon k}^{1/2} \right\},$$

where $\Phi^*(\cdot)$ is the distribution function of $N[0, 1]$. Note that μ_k, $\mathbf{\Lambda}_k$, and $\psi_{\epsilon k}$ cannot be estimated, because $C\mathbf{\Lambda}_k^T/(C\psi_{\epsilon k}^{1/2}) = \mathbf{\Lambda}_k^T/\psi_{\epsilon k}^{1/2}$ and $C\mu_k/(C\psi_{\epsilon k}^{1/2}) = \mu_k/\psi_{\epsilon k}^{1/2}$ for any positive constant C. There are many ways to solve this identification problem. Here, we fix $\psi_{\epsilon k} = 1.0$. Note that the value 1.0 is chosen for convenience, and any other value would give an equivalent solution up to a change of scale. Again the measurement and structural equations are identified by fixing the approximate elements of $\mathbf{\Lambda}$ and $\mathbf{\Lambda}_\omega$ at preassigned values.

Let $u_{ik} = \mathbf{\Lambda}_k^T \boldsymbol{\omega}_i + \epsilon_{ik}$, that is, $u_{ik} + \mu_k = y_{ik}$. Thus, $y_{ik} \geq 0$ if and only if $u_{ik} \geq -\mu_k$, or equivalently $z_{ik} = 1$ if and only if $u_{ik} \geq -\mu_k$. Consequently, $-\mu_k$ is the threshold corresponding to u_{ik}. Because there are at least two thresholds associated with an ordered categorical variable, the relation of the thresholds and μ_k is not as clear. Also, the identification conditions are slightly different. Thus, methods for analyzing these two types of discrete variables are not exactly the same.

Let $\mathbf{Z} = (\mathbf{z}_1, \ldots, \mathbf{z}_n)$ be the observed data set of dichotomous variables, let $\boldsymbol{\theta}$ be the unknown parameter vector, which contains parameters in $\boldsymbol{\mu}$, $\mathbf{\Lambda}$, $\mathbf{\Lambda}_\omega$, $\mathbf{\Phi}$, and $\mathbf{\Psi}_\delta$, let $\mathbf{\Omega} = (\boldsymbol{\omega}_1, \ldots, \boldsymbol{\omega}_n)$ be the matrix of latent variables in the model, and $\mathbf{Y} = (\mathbf{y}_1, \ldots, \mathbf{y}_n)$ be the matrix of latent continuous measurements underlying the matrix of observed dichotomous data $\mathbf{Z}$. In the Bayesian analysis, the observed data $\mathbf{Z}$ is augmented with $\mathbf{\Omega}$ and $\mathbf{Y}$; and a large sample of observations will be sampled from $p(\boldsymbol{\theta}, \mathbf{\Omega}, \mathbf{Y}|\mathbf{Z})$ through the following Gibbs sampler (Geman and Geman, 1984). At the jth iteration with current values $\boldsymbol{\theta}^{(j)}$, $\mathbf{\Omega}^{(j)}$, and $\mathbf{Y}^{(j)}$:

A. Generate $\mathbf{\Omega}^{(j+1)}$ from $p(\mathbf{\Omega}|\boldsymbol{\theta}^{(j)}, \mathbf{Y}^{(j)}, \mathbf{Z})$.
B. Generate $\boldsymbol{\theta}^{(j+1)}$ from $p(\boldsymbol{\theta}|\mathbf{\Omega}^{(j+1)}, \mathbf{Y}^{(j)}, \mathbf{Z})$.
C. Generate $\mathbf{Y}^{(j+1)}$ from $p(\mathbf{Y}|\boldsymbol{\theta}^{(j+1)}, \mathbf{\Omega}^{(j+1)}, \mathbf{Z})$.

Conditional distributions relating to steps A and B can be obtained similarly to Section 5.2.3. For $p(\mathbf{Y}|\boldsymbol{\theta}, \mathbf{\Omega}, \mathbf{Z})$, as the $\mathbf{y}_i$ are mutually independent, it follows that

$$p(\mathbf{Y}|\boldsymbol{\theta}, \mathbf{\Omega}, \mathbf{Z}) = \prod_{i=1}^{n} p(\mathbf{y}_i|\boldsymbol{\theta}, \boldsymbol{\omega}_i, \mathbf{z}_i).$$

Moreover, it follows from the definition of the model and (5.8) that

$$[y_{ik}|\boldsymbol{\theta}, \boldsymbol{\omega}_i, \mathbf{z}_i] \stackrel{D}{=} \begin{cases} N\left[\mu_k + \mathbf{\Lambda}_k^T \boldsymbol{\omega}_i, 1\right] I_{(-\infty,0]}(y_{ik}), & \text{if } z_{ik} = 0, \\ N\left[\mu_k + \mathbf{\Lambda}_k^T \boldsymbol{\omega}_i, 1\right] I_{(0,\infty)}(y_{ik}), & \text{if } z_{ik} = 1, \end{cases} \tag{5.9}$$

where $I_A(y)$ is an indicator function that takes the value 1 if y is in A, and 0 otherwise.

Statistical inference on the model can be obtained on the basis of the simulated sample of observations from $p(\boldsymbol{\theta}, \mathbf{\Omega}, \mathbf{Y}|\mathbf{Z})$ as before. Note that for dichotomous data analysis, a vector of dichotomous observation $\mathbf{z}_i$ rather than $\mathbf{y}_i$ is observed; hence a lot of information about $\mathbf{y}$ is lost. As a result, it requires a large sample size to achieve accurate estimates. The PP p-value (Gelman *et al.*, 1996) for assessing the goodness of fit of a posited model, and the Bayes factor for model comparison can be obtained via developments similar to those presented in Chapter 4.

5.3 SEMs with variables from exponential family distributions

5.3.1 Introduction

The standard SEMs discussed so far require the crucial assumption that the conditional distribution of observed variables given latent variables is normal. For example, although we do not assume that $\mathbf{y}$ is normal in a nonlinear SEM, we assume that $\mathbf{y}|\boldsymbol{\omega}$ or $\boldsymbol{\epsilon}$ is normal.

In this section, we generalize the distribution of $\mathbf{y}|\boldsymbol{\omega}$ from normal to the exponential family distributions (EFDs). This family is very general: it includes discrete distributions such as binomial and Poisson, and continuous distributions such as normal and gamma, as special cases. The EFDs have been extensively used in many areas of statistics, particularly in relation to latent variable models such as the generalized linear models (McCullagh and Nelder, 1989) and generalized linear mixed models (Booth and Hobert, 1999). In contrast to SEMs, the main objective of these latent variable models is to assess the effects of covariates on the observed variables, and the latent variables in these models are usually used to model the random effects. Motivated by the above consideration, in this section we will consider a nonlinear SEM that can accommodate covariates, variables from the EFDs, and ordered categorical variables. The strategy that combines the data augmentation and MCMC methods is again used to develop the Bayesian methodologies.

5.3.2 The SEM framework with exponential family distributions

A nonlinear SEM with fixed covariates based on EFDs is defined as follows (see Song and Lee, 2007). For $i = 1, \ldots, n$, let $\mathbf{y}_i = (y_{i1}, \ldots, y_{ip})^T$ be a vector of observed variables measured on each of the n independently distributed individuals. For brevity, we assume that the dimension of $\mathbf{y}_i$ is the same for each i; however, this assumption can be relaxed without much difficulty. We wish to identify the relationship between the observed variables in $\mathbf{y}_i$ and the related latent vector $\boldsymbol{\omega}_i = (\omega_{i1}, \ldots, \omega_{iq})^T$ with fixed covariates. For $k = 1, \ldots, p$, we assume that y_{ik} given $\boldsymbol{\omega}_i$ are independent and the corresponding conditional distributions come from the following exponential family with a canonical parameter ϑ_{ik} (Sammel *et al.*, 1997):

$$\begin{aligned} p(y_{ik}|\boldsymbol{\omega}_i) &= \exp\{[y_{ik}\vartheta_{ik} - b(\vartheta_{ik})]/\psi_{\epsilon k} + c_k(y_{ik}, \psi_{\epsilon k})\}, \\ E(y_{ik}|\boldsymbol{\omega}_i) &= \dot{b}(\vartheta_{ik}), \quad \text{and} \quad \mathrm{Var}(y_{ik}|\boldsymbol{\omega}_i) = \psi_{\epsilon k}\ddot{b}(\vartheta_{ik}), \end{aligned} \tag{5.10}$$

where $b(\cdot)$ and $c_k(\cdot)$ are specific differentiable functions with the dots denoting the derivatives, and $\vartheta_{ik} = g_k(\mu_{ik})$ with a link function g_k. Let $\boldsymbol{\vartheta}_i = (\vartheta_{i1}, \ldots, \vartheta_{ip})^T$, $\mathbf{c}_{ik}$ $(m_k \times 1)$ be vectors of fixed covariates, $\mathbf{A}_k$ be a $m_k \times 1$ vector of unknown parameters, and $\boldsymbol{\Lambda} = (\boldsymbol{\Lambda}_1, \ldots, \boldsymbol{\Lambda}_p)^T$ is a matrix of unknown parameters. We use the following model to analyze the relation of ϑ_{ik} with $\mathbf{c}_{ik}$ and $\boldsymbol{\omega}_i$: for $k = 1, \ldots, p$,

$$\vartheta_{ik} = \mathbf{A}_k^T \mathbf{c}_{ik} + \boldsymbol{\Lambda}_k^T \boldsymbol{\omega}_i. \tag{5.11}$$

Note that equation (5.11) can accommodate an intercept μ_k by taking a component of $\mathbf{c}_{ik}$ as 1 and defining the corresponding component of $\mathbf{A}_k$ as μ_k. This equation can be viewed as a 'measurement' model. Its main purpose is to identify the latent variables via the corresponding observed variables in $\mathbf{y}$, with the help of the fixed covariates $\mathbf{c}_{ik}$. See Section 5.3.4 for a concrete example. Let $\boldsymbol{\omega}_i = (\boldsymbol{\eta}_i^T, \boldsymbol{\xi}_i^T)^T$, where $\boldsymbol{\eta}_i$ is the outcome latent vector and $\boldsymbol{\xi}_i$ is the explanatory latent vector. To assess how the latent variables affect each other, we introduce the following nonlinear structural equation with fixed covariates:

$$\boldsymbol{\eta}_i = \mathbf{B}\mathbf{d}_i + \boldsymbol{\Pi}\boldsymbol{\eta}_i + \boldsymbol{\Gamma}\mathbf{F}(\boldsymbol{\xi}_i) + \boldsymbol{\delta}_i, \tag{5.12}$$

where $\mathbf{d}_i$ is a vector of fixed covariates, $\mathbf{F}(\boldsymbol{\xi}_i) = (f_1(\boldsymbol{\xi}_i), \ldots, f_l(\boldsymbol{\xi}_i))^T$, $f_j(\boldsymbol{\xi}_i)$ is a nonzero differentiable function of $\boldsymbol{\xi}_i$, $\boldsymbol{\delta}_i$ is an error term, and $\mathbf{B}$, $\boldsymbol{\Pi}$, and $\boldsymbol{\Gamma}$ are unknown parameter matrices. Fixed covariates in $\mathbf{d}_i$ may or may not be equal to those in $\mathbf{c}_{ik}$. The distributions of $\boldsymbol{\xi}_i$ and $\boldsymbol{\delta}_i$ are $N[\mathbf{0}, \boldsymbol{\Phi}]$ and $N[\mathbf{0}, \boldsymbol{\Psi}_\delta]$, respectively, and $\boldsymbol{\xi}_i$ and $\boldsymbol{\delta}_i$ are uncorrelated. For computational efficiency and stability, the covariance matrix $\boldsymbol{\Psi}_\delta$ is assumed to be diagonal. We assume that

$\mathbf{I} - \mathbf{\Pi}$ is nonsingular and its determinant is independent of elements in $\mathbf{\Pi}$. Let $\mathbf{\Lambda}_\omega = (\mathbf{B}, \mathbf{\Pi}, \mathbf{\Gamma})$ and $\mathbf{G}(\boldsymbol{\omega}_i) = (\mathbf{d}_i^T, \boldsymbol{\eta}_i^T, \mathbf{F}(\boldsymbol{\xi}_i)^T)^T$; then (5.12) can be rewritten as $\boldsymbol{\eta}_i = \mathbf{\Lambda}_\omega \mathbf{G}(\boldsymbol{\omega}_i) + \boldsymbol{\delta}_i$.

To accommodate ordered categorical data, we allow any component y of $\mathbf{y}$ to be unobservable, and its information is given by an observable ordered categorical variable z as follows: $z = m$ if $\alpha_m \leq y < \alpha_{m+1}$, for $m = 0, \ldots, b$, where $\{-\infty = \alpha_0 < \alpha_1 < \ldots < \alpha_b < \alpha_{b+1} = \infty\}$ is the set of thresholds that defines the categories. This model can be identified as before. For instance, each ordered categorical variable can be identified by fixing α_1 and α_b at preassigned values; and the SEM can be identified by the common practice of restricting the appropriate elements in $\mathbf{\Lambda}$ and $\mathbf{\Lambda}_\omega$ to fixed known values. Dichotomous variables can be analyzed as a special case of ordered categorical variables with slight modifications.

5.3.3 Bayesian inference

Again, Bayesian methods are developed via the useful strategy that combines data augmentation and MCMC methods. In this subsection we present the full conditional distributions in the implementation of the Gibbs sampler for simulating observations of the parameters and the latent variables from their joint posterior distribution. These simulated observations are used to obtain the Bayesian estimates and their standard error estimates, and to compute the Bayes factor for model comparison.

Proper conjugate prior distributions are taken for various unknown parameters. More specifically, let $\mathbf{\Psi}_\epsilon$ be the diagonal covariance matrix of the error measurements that correspond to the ordered categorical variables

$$\begin{aligned}
&\mathbf{A}_k \stackrel{D}{=} N[\mathbf{A}_{0k}, \mathbf{H}_{0k}],\ \psi_{\epsilon k}^{-1} \stackrel{D}{=} \text{Gamma}[\alpha_{0\epsilon k}, \beta_{0\epsilon k}],\ [\mathbf{\Lambda}_k|\psi_{\epsilon k}] \stackrel{D}{=} N[\mathbf{\Lambda}_{0k}, \psi_{\epsilon k}\mathbf{H}_{0yk}],\\
&\mathbf{\Phi}^{-1} \stackrel{D}{=} W_{q_2}[\mathbf{R}_0, \rho_0],\ \psi_{\delta k}^{-1} \stackrel{D}{=} \text{Gamma}[\alpha_{0\delta k}, \beta_{0\delta k}],\ [\mathbf{\Lambda}_{\omega k}|\psi_{\delta k}] \stackrel{D}{=} N[\mathbf{\Lambda}_{0\omega k}, \psi_{\delta k}\mathbf{H}_{0\omega k}],
\end{aligned} \tag{5.13}$$

where $\psi_{\epsilon k}$ and $\psi_{\delta k}$ are the kth diagonal element of $\mathbf{\Psi}_\epsilon$ and $\mathbf{\Psi}_\delta$, respectively; $\mathbf{\Lambda}_k^T$ and $\mathbf{\Lambda}_{\omega k}^T$ are the kth rows of $\mathbf{\Lambda}$ and $\mathbf{\Lambda}_\omega$, respectively; and $\mathbf{A}_{0k}$, $\alpha_{0\epsilon k}$, $\beta_{0\epsilon k}$, $\mathbf{\Lambda}_{0k}$, $\alpha_{0\delta k}$, $\beta_{0\delta k}$, $\mathbf{\Lambda}_{0\omega k}$, ρ_0, and positive definite matrices $\mathbf{H}_{0k}$, $\mathbf{H}_{0yk}$, $\mathbf{H}_{0\omega k}$, and $\mathbf{R}_0$ are hyperparameters whose values are assumed to be given by the prior information. For $k \neq l$, it is assumed that prior distributions of $(\psi_{\epsilon k}, \mathbf{\Lambda}_k)$ and $(\psi_{\epsilon l}, \mathbf{\Lambda}_l)$, $(\psi_{\delta k}, \mathbf{\Lambda}_{\omega k})$ and $(\psi_{\delta l}, \mathbf{\Lambda}_{\omega l})$, as well as $\mathbf{A}_k$ and $\mathbf{A}_l$ are independent.

We first consider the situation in which components in $\mathbf{y}_i$ are neither dichotomous nor ordered categorical, but can be directly observed. Let $\mathbf{Y}$ be the observed data set. Based on the idea of data augmentation, we focus on the joint posterior distribution $[\mathbf{\Omega}, \boldsymbol{\theta}|\mathbf{Y}]$, where $\mathbf{\Omega}$ contains all the latent vectors, and $\boldsymbol{\theta}$ is the parameter vector that contains all the unknown parameters in the model. The Gibbs sampler (Geman and Geman, 1984) is used to simulate observations from the posterior distribution $[\mathbf{\Omega}, \boldsymbol{\theta}|\mathbf{Y}]$. The required full conditional distributions are given in Appendix 5.2.

To handle the ordered categorical data, let $\mathbf{y}_k^{*T}$ be the kth row of $\mathbf{Y}$ that is not directly observable. Let $\mathbf{z}_k$ be the corresponding observable ordered categorical vector, and $\boldsymbol{\alpha}_k = (\alpha_{k,2}, \ldots, \alpha_{k,b_k-1})$. It is natural to assume that the prior distribution of $\boldsymbol{\alpha}_k$ is independent of the prior distribution of $\boldsymbol{\theta}$. To deal with a general situation in which there is little or no information about the thresholds, the following noninformative prior distribution is used: $p(\boldsymbol{\alpha}_k) = p(\alpha_{k,2}, \ldots, \alpha_{k,b_k-1}) \propto C$ for $\alpha_{k,2} < \ldots < \alpha_{k,b_k-1}$, where C is a constant. Moreover, it is assumed that $\boldsymbol{\alpha}_k$ and $\boldsymbol{\alpha}_l$ are independent for $k \neq l$. Based on these assumptions, the full conditional distribution $[\boldsymbol{\alpha}_k, \mathbf{y}_k^*|\mathbf{z}_k, \mathbf{\Omega}, \boldsymbol{\theta}]$ is derived and presented in Appendix 5.2.

The Gibbs sampler algorithm proceeds by sampling $\boldsymbol{\omega}_i$, $(\boldsymbol{\alpha}_k, \mathbf{y}_k^*)$, and $\boldsymbol{\theta}$ from their full conditional distributions, most of which are nonstandard because of the assumption of EFDs. Various forms of the Metropolis–Hastings (MH) algorithm (Metropolis *et al.*, 1953; Hastings, 1970) are required to simulate observations from these nonstandard conditional distributions. Due to the complexity of the model and data structures considered, the implementation of the MH algorithm is not straightforward. Some details are also given in Appendix 5.2.

For model comparison, we use $\mathbf{D}_{\text{obs}}$ to denote the observed data, which include the directly observable data and the ordered categorical data, and use $\mathbf{D}_{\text{mis}}$ to denote the unobservable data, which include latent variables and unobserved data that underlie the ordered categorical data. Moreover, let $\boldsymbol{\theta}^* = (\boldsymbol{\theta}, \boldsymbol{\alpha})$ be the overall unknown parameter vector, where $\boldsymbol{\alpha}$ is a vector that includes all unknown thresholds. Suppose that $\mathbf{D}_{\text{obs}}$ has arisen under one of the two competing models M_0 and M_1. For $l = 0, 1$, let $p(\mathbf{D}_{\text{obs}}|M_l)$ be the probability density of $\mathbf{D}_{\text{obs}}$ under M_l. Recall that the Bayes factor is defined by $B_{10} = p(\mathbf{D}_{\text{obs}}|M_1)/p(\mathbf{D}_{\text{obs}}|M_0)$. Similarly, a path sampling procedure is presented to compute the Bayes factor for model comparison. Utilizing the idea of data augmentation, $\mathbf{D}_{\text{obs}}$ is augmented with $\mathbf{D}_{\text{mis}}$ in the computation. Let t be a continuous parameter in [0,1] to link the competing models M_0 and M_1, let $p(\mathbf{D}_{\text{mis}}, \mathbf{D}_{\text{obs}}|\boldsymbol{\theta}^*, t)$ be the complete-data likelihood, and $U(\boldsymbol{\theta}^*, \mathbf{D}_{\text{mis}}, \mathbf{D}_{\text{obs}}, t) = d \log p(\mathbf{D}_{\text{mis}}, \mathbf{D}_{\text{obs}}|\boldsymbol{\theta}^*, t)/dt$. Moreover, let S be the number of fixed grids $\{t_{(s)}\}_{s=1}^S$ between [0, 1] ordered as $0 = t_{(0)} < t_{(1)} < \ldots < t_{(S)} < t_{(S+1)} = 1$. Then $\log B_{10}$ can be computed as

$$\widehat{\log B_{10}} = \frac{1}{2} \sum_{s=0}^{S} (t_{(s+1)} - t_{(s)})(\bar{U}_{(s+1)} + \bar{U}_{(s)}), \tag{5.14}$$

where $\bar{U}_{(s)}$ is the average of the $U(\boldsymbol{\theta}^*, \mathbf{D}_{\text{mis}}, \mathbf{D}_{\text{obs}}, t)$ on the basis of all simulation draws at $t = t_{(s)}$, that is, $\bar{U}_{(s)} = J^{-1} \sum_{j=1}^J U(\boldsymbol{\theta}^{*(j)}, \mathbf{D}_{\text{mis}}^{(j)}, \mathbf{D}_{\text{obs}}, t_{(s)})$, in which $\{(\boldsymbol{\theta}^{*(j)}, \mathbf{D}_{\text{mis}}^{(j)}), j = 1, \ldots, J\}$ are observations simulated from the joint conditional distribution $p(\boldsymbol{\theta}^*, \mathbf{D}_{\text{mis}}| \mathbf{D}_{\text{obs}}, t_{(s)})$.

5.3.4 Simulation study

Recall that a dichotomous variable is an ordered categorical variable that is defined by two categories with a threshold of zero. It is usually coded with '0' and '1', and the probability of observing '0' and '1' is decided by an underlying normal distribution with a fixed threshold. Another kind of discrete variable which also has two categories and is usually coded with '0' and '1' is the binary variable. Although they have the same coding, binary variables are different from dichotomous variables. Binary variables are unordered, they do not associate with thresholds, and the probabilities of observing '0' and '1' are decided by a binomial distribution rather than the normal distribution. Hence, the methods for analyzing dichotomous variables should not be directly applied to analyze binary variables, otherwise misleading conclusions may be obtained. Given a variable coded '0' and '1', it is important to decide whether this variable is an ordered dichotomous variable or an unordered binary variable.

Results obtained from a simulation study (see Lee *et al.*, 2010) are presented here to illustrate the above idea. In this simulation study, a data set $\mathbf{V} = \{\mathbf{v}_i, i = 1, \ldots, n\}$ was generated with $\mathbf{v}_i = (z_{i1}, z_{i2}, z_{i3}, y_{i4}, \ldots, y_{i9})^T$. For $k = 1, 2, 3$, z_{ik} is dichotomous, while for $k = 4, \ldots, 9$, y_{ik} is binary with distribution $B(1, p_{ik})$. In the formulation of EFDs, we have $p(y_{ik}) \propto \exp\{y_{ik}\vartheta_{ik} - \log(1 + e^{\vartheta_{ik}})\}$, with $b(\vartheta_{ik}) = \log(1 + e^{\vartheta_{ik}})$ and $\vartheta_{ik} = \log(p_{ik}/(1 - p_{ik}))$. Note that for $k = 1, \ldots, 9$, $\psi_{\epsilon k} = 1.0$ is treated as fixed parameter. Let $\mathbf{y}_i = (y_{i1}, y_{i2}, y_{i3})^T$ be the latent continuous random vector corresponding to the dichotomous random vector $(z_{i1}, z_{i2}, z_{i3})^T$. We assume that

$$y_{ik} = \mu_k + \mathbf{\Lambda}_k^T \boldsymbol{\omega}_i + \epsilon_i, \; k = 1, 2, 3,$$
$$\vartheta_{ik} = \mu_k + \mathbf{\Lambda}_k^T \boldsymbol{\omega}_i, \qquad k = 4, \ldots, 9,$$

where $\mathbf{\Lambda}_k$ is the kth row of the loading matrix

$$\mathbf{\Lambda}^T = \begin{bmatrix} 1 & \lambda_{21} & \lambda_{31} & 0 & 0 & 0 & 0 & 0 & 0 \\ 0 & 0 & 0 & 1 & \lambda_{52} & \lambda_{62} & 0 & 0 & 0 \\ 0 & 0 & 0 & 0 & 0 & 0 & 1 & \lambda_{83} & \lambda_{93} \end{bmatrix},$$

in which the 1s and 0s are treated as fixed for identifying the model. The true values of elements in $\boldsymbol{\mu}$ and λ_{ij} are given by $\mu_1 = \ldots = \mu_9 = 1.0$, $\lambda_{21} = \lambda_{31} = 0.7$, $\lambda_{52} = \lambda_{62} = 0.8$, and $\lambda_{83} = \lambda_{93} = 0.7$. The relationships of the latent variables in $\boldsymbol{\omega}_i = (\eta_i, \xi_{i1}, \xi_{i2})^T$ are assessed by the nonlinear structural equation

$$\eta_i = bd_i + \gamma_1 \xi_{i1} + \gamma_2 \xi_{i2} + \gamma_3 \xi_{i1} \xi_{i2} + \delta_i, \tag{5.15}$$

where the fixed covariate d_i is assumed to come from $N[0, 1]$, and the true values of $b, \gamma_1, \gamma_2, \gamma_3$, and ψ_δ are chosen as 0.8, 0.6, 0.6, 0.8, and 0.3, respectively. The true values of ϕ_{11}, ϕ_{21}, and ϕ_{22} in $\mathbf{\Phi}$, the covariance matrix of $(\xi_{i1}, \xi_{i2})^T$, are 1.0, 0.3, and 1.0, respectively. The following prior inputs of the hyperparameter values in the conjugate prior distributions of the parameters are considered: elements in $\mathbf{A}_{0k}$, $\mathbf{\Lambda}_{0k}$, and $\mathbf{\Lambda}_{0\omega k}$ in (5.13) are set equal to the true values; $\mathbf{R}_0^{-1} = 7\mathbf{I}$; $\mathbf{H}_{0k}$, $\mathbf{H}_{0yk}$, and $\mathbf{H}_{0\omega k}$ are taken to be 0.25 times the identity matrices; $\alpha_{0\delta k} = 9$, $\beta_{0\delta k} = 3$, and $\rho_0 = 10$.

The purpose of this simulation study is to address the following questions in practical applications: (i) Does the Bayesian approach produce accurate results for samples with small sizes in analyzing binary or dichotomous data? (ii) What kind of bias will result from incorrectly treating dichotomous variables as binary variables? And vice versa.

The data were created on the basis of the model and the same true values as described above. In fitting the model, three sample sizes $n = 200$, 800, and 2000 were considered. For each sample size, simulated data were analyzed through the Bayesian approach in the following three cases: (A) correctly treating variables z_{i1}, z_{i2}, and z_{i3} as dichotomous variables, and $y_{i4}, \ldots, y_{i9}$ as binary variables; (B) incorrectly treating all the dichotomous variables as binary variables; and (C) incorrectly treating all the binary variables as dichotomous variables. Results were obtained on the basis of 100 replications.

The simulation studies were conducted using R2WinBUGS (Sturtz *et al.*, 2005). The WinBUGS and R2WinBUGS codes for conducting the current simulation study are given in Appendices 5.3 and 5.4 (see also Lee *et al.*, 2010). A few test runs were carried out to check convergence in order to decide the number of burn-in iterations required for achieving convergence. Results indicated that 15 000 burn-in iterations are sufficient. Hence, the Bayesian results were obtained from 20 000 simulated observations after 15 000 burn-in iterations.

Let $\theta(r)$ be the rth element of $\boldsymbol{\theta}$, $\theta_0(r)$ be the true value of $\theta(r)$, and $\hat{\theta}_j(r)$ be the estimate of $\theta(r)$ at the jth replication. Based on 100 replications, we obtain $\mathrm{M}(\hat{\theta}(r))$ and MC-SD($\hat{\theta}(r)$), the mean and the standard deviation of the parameter estimates of $\theta(r)$, respectively; and EST-SD($\hat{\theta}(r)$), the mean of the standard error estimates computed via the square root of

$\widehat{\text{Var}}(\boldsymbol{\theta}|\mathbf{V})$. The results are assessed through the following summary statistics:

$$\text{absolute bias (AB) of } \hat{\theta}(r) = |\text{M}(\hat{\theta}(r)) - \theta_0(r)|,$$

$$\text{root mean square (RMS) of } \hat{\theta}(r) = \left\{ 100^{-1} \sum_{j=1}^{100} [\hat{\theta}_j(r) - \theta_0(r)]^2 \right\}^{1/2},$$

$$\text{SE/SD of } \hat{\theta}(r) = \frac{\text{EST-SD}(\hat{\theta}(r))}{\text{MC-SD}(\hat{\theta}(r))}.$$

Results for case (A) and sample sizes of 200, 800, and 2000 are reported in Table 5.1. We observe that all AB values are quite small. However, for $n = 200$, the RMS values corresponding to parameters λ_{52}, λ_{62}, λ_{83}, λ_{93}, ϕ_{11}, and ϕ_{22} are larger than 0.200. It is expected that the empirical performance would be worse with smaller sample sizes. SE/SD results

Table 5.1 Simulation results for case (A).

		$n = 200$			$n = 800$			$n = 2000$		
Par	True	AB	SE/SD	RMS	AB	SE/SD	RMS	AB	SE/SD	RMS
μ_1	1.0	0.017	1.36	0.137	0.006	1.10	0.100	0.001	1.11	0.069
μ_2	1.0	0.056	1.25	0.150	0.007	0.98	0.096	0.011	1.02	0.061
μ_3	1.0	0.055	1.15	0.163	0.009	1.04	0.092	0.004	1.01	0.059
μ_4	1.0	0.031	1.06	0.163	0.011	1.09	0.087	0.020	1.10	0.060
μ_5	1.0	0.013	1.09	0.164	0.019	1.13	0.090	0.006	0.95	0.067
μ_6	1.0	0.010	1.14	0.155	0.005	1.18	0.083	0.008	0.99	0.065
μ_7	1.0	0.029	1.32	0.133	0.012	1.04	0.092	0.017	0.96	0.068
μ_8	1.0	0.021	1.15	0.152	0.005	1.12	0.085	0.012	0.97	0.064
μ_9	1.0	0.046	1.10	0.166	0.029	1.07	0.093	0.019	1.06	0.061
λ_{21}	0.7	0.105	1.37	0.165	0.041	1.12	0.109	0.019	1.02	0.076
λ_{31}	0.7	0.125	1.34	0.178	0.054	1.04	0.118	0.007	0.98	0.076
λ_{52}	0.8	0.084	1.50	0.234	0.170	1.29	0.226	0.092	1.06	0.166
λ_{62}	0.8	0.083	1.64	0.218	0.092	1.33	0.183	0.099	1.16	0.158
λ_{83}	0.7	0.109	1.58	0.223	0.165	1.20	0.215	0.128	1.04	0.170
λ_{93}	0.7	0.114	1.57	0.224	0.117	1.31	0.183	0.121	1.20	0.151
γ_1	0.6	0.050	1.73	0.128	0.029	1.43	0.106	0.071	1.21	0.101
γ_2	0.6	0.041	1.83	0.120	0.070	1.30	0.127	0.057	1.11	0.106
γ_3	0.8	0.004	2.22	0.112	0.084	1.81	0.128	0.115	1.31	0.149
b	0.8	0.035	1.13	0.137	0.003	1.06	0.083	0.012	1.06	0.059
ϕ_{11}	1.0	0.141	1.76	0.222	0.127	1.48	0.202	0.109	1.21	0.184
ϕ_{12}	0.3	0.007	1.30	0.135	0.055	0.93	0.113	0.085	1.04	0.074
ϕ_{22}	1.0	0.129	1.89	0.208	0.124	1.38	0.216	0.091	1.13	0.191
ψ_δ	0.3	0.180	3.79	0.062	0.129	2.30	0.058	0.088	1.64	0.057

Reproduced by permission of Taylor & Francis from Lee, S. Y., Song, X. Y. and Cai, J. H. (2010). A Bayesian approach for nonlinear structural equation models with dichotomous variables using logit and probit links. *Structural Equation Modeling – A Multidisciplinary Journal*, **17**, 280–302.

indicate that the standard error estimates overestimate the standard deviation of the estimates, even with $n = 800$.

Based on these simulation results, we have the following conclusions in analyzing nonlinear SEMs with binary and/or dichotomous variables: (i) It requires comparatively larger sample sizes than the analysis with continuous variables. To analyze a model with 23 unknown parameters, a sample size of about 800 is required to produce accurate result. (ii) Except for situations with large sample sizes, the standard error estimates obtained from the square roots of $\widehat{\text{Var}}(\boldsymbol{\theta}|\mathbf{V})$ overestimate the true standard deviations. The commonly used z-score that depends on these standard error estimates should not be used in hypothesis testing.

To study whether binary variables can be treated as ordinal variables, and vice versa, the same data sets were reanalyzed for cases (B) and (C). Results are presented in Tables 5.2 and 5.3. From Table 5.2, the AB and/or RMS values corresponding to μ_1, μ_2, μ_3, γ_1, γ_2, γ_3, b, ϕ_{11}, and ϕ_{22} are quite large. These parameters are related to the dichotomous variables z_{i1}, z_{i2}, and

Table 5.2 Simulation results for case (B).

		$n = 200$			$n = 800$			$n = 2000$		
Par	True	AB	SE/SD	RMS	AB	SE/SD	RMS	AB	SE/SD	RMS
μ_1	1.0	0.287	1.36	0.334	0.429	1.12	0.451	0.572	1.15	0.581
μ_2	1.0	0.492	1.45	0.520	0.613	1.00	0.632	0.689	1.08	0.696
μ_3	1.0	0.490	1.30	0.525	0.616	1.08	0.632	0.663	1.10	0.670
μ_4	1.0	0.033	1.07	0.167	0.001	1.12	0.086	0.011	1.05	0.061
μ_5	1.0	0.004	1.07	0.165	0.008	1.12	0.089	0.001	0.94	0.067
μ_6	1.0	0.026	1.12	0.159	0.006	1.17	0.082	0.000	1.00	0.062
μ_7	1.0	0.029	1.31	0.137	0.003	1.06	0.092	0.007	0.98	0.066
μ_8	1.0	0.009	1.15	0.152	0.006	1.10	0.086	0.006	0.96	0.063
μ_9	1.0	0.032	1.08	0.165	0.018	1.07	0.089	0.013	1.05	0.059
λ_{21}	0.7	0.307	1.62	0.257	0.232	1.21	0.197	0.123	1.07	0.118
λ_{31}	0.7	0.334	1.55	0.278	0.250	1.11	0.213	0.094	1.03	0.104
λ_{52}	0.8	0.002	1.38	0.233	0.074	1.13	0.200	0.027	1.01	0.149
λ_{62}	0.8	0.010	1.58	0.206	0.001	1.19	0.172	0.028	1.10	0.136
λ_{83}	0.7	0.037	1.50	0.212	0.048	1.11	0.184	0.057	0.96	0.153
λ_{93}	0.7	0.037	1.44	0.218	0.003	1.27	0.154	0.051	1.11	0.131
γ_1	0.6	0.136	1.74	0.162	0.315	1.35	0.235	0.565	1.18	0.364
γ_2	0.6	0.124	1.77	0.156	0.352	1.29	0.257	0.529	1.17	0.346
γ_3	0.8	0.144	1.84	0.184	0.358	1.63	0.319	0.588	1.45	0.493
b	0.8	0.390	1.20	0.353	0.467	1.08	0.392	0.605	1.07	0.492
ϕ_{11}	1.0	0.025	1.49	0.245	0.032	1.29	0.213	0.003	1.11	0.177
ϕ_{12}	0.3	0.504	1.19	0.237	0.263	0.89	0.158	0.085	0.98	0.083
ϕ_{22}	1.0	0.052	1.52	0.257	0.068	1.22	0.244	0.022	0.99	0.211
ψ_δ	0.3	0.300	4.01	0.097	0.511	2.26	0.169	1.257	1.46	0.401

Reproduced by permission of Taylor & Francis from Lee, S. Y., Song, X. Y. and Cai, J. H. (2010). A Bayesian approach for nonlinear structural equation models with dichotomous variables using logit and probit links. *Structural Equation Modeling – A Multidisciplinary Journal*, **17**, 280–302.

Table 5.3 Simulation results for case (C).

		$n = 200$			$n = 800$			$n = 2000$		
Par	True	AB	SE/SD	RMS	AB	SE/SD	RMS	AB	SE/SD	RMS
μ_1	1.0	0.023	1.26	0.133	0.010	1.15	0.085	0.005	1.09	0.063
μ_2	1.0	0.084	1.23	0.163	0.036	0.99	0.097	0.031	1.03	0.064
μ_3	1.0	0.086	1.14	0.175	0.039	1.06	0.094	0.015	1.06	0.055
μ_4	1.0	0.333	1.05	0.352	0.351	1.10	0.356	0.374	1.08	0.376
μ_5	1.0	0.355	0.97	0.374	0.380	1.08	0.384	0.394	0.94	0.396
μ_6	1.0	0.371	1.09	0.386	0.390	1.15	0.393	0.393	0.97	0.394
μ_7	1.0	0.327	1.28	0.340	0.350	1.04	0.355	0.369	0.95	0.372
μ_8	1.0	0.351	1.10	0.366	0.389	1.08	0.392	0.388	0.95	0.390
μ_9	1.0	0.334	1.05	0.351	0.373	1.02	0.377	0.384	1.05	0.386
λ_{21}	0.7	0.158	1.41	0.185	0.115	1.10	0.137	0.073	0.99	0.096
λ_{31}	0.7	0.186	1.33	0.206	0.130	1.06	0.148	0.044	1.02	0.083
λ_{52}	0.8	0.167	1.26	0.261	0.111	1.07	0.194	0.134	1.03	0.162
λ_{62}	0.8	0.167	1.35	0.247	0.181	1.19	0.204	0.128	1.08	0.156
λ_{83}	0.7	0.157	1.38	0.223	0.136	1.14	0.177	0.121	0.97	0.149
λ_{93}	0.7	0.144	1.30	0.230	0.167	1.15	0.185	0.126	1.17	0.136
γ_1	0.6	0.060	1.51	0.147	0.092	1.26	0.135	0.225	1.15	0.175
γ_2	0.6	0.036	1.58	0.138	0.114	1.25	0.145	0.177	1.22	0.148
γ_3	0.8	0.052	2.14	0.130	0.243	1.78	0.234	0.481	1.60	0.405
b	0.8	0.015	1.11	0.130	0.053	1.03	0.091	0.027	1.07	0.060
ϕ_{11}	1.0	0.370	1.73	0.390	0.458	1.37	0.468	0.517	1.25	0.522
ϕ_{12}	0.3	0.428	1.36	0.151	0.523	1.04	0.166	0.561	1.05	0.172
ϕ_{22}	1.0	0.346	2.11	0.362	0.447	1.52	0.457	0.492	1.08	0.501
ψ_δ	0.3	0.246	2.88	0.086	0.304	1.80	0.110	0.392	1.35	0.138

Reproduced by permission of Taylor & Francis from Lee, S. Y., Song, X. Y. and Cai, J. H. (2010). A Bayesian approach for nonlinear structural equation models with dichotomous variables using logit and probit links. *Structural Equation Modeling – A Multidisciplinary Journal*, **17**, 280–302.

z_{i3} that are incorrectly modeled as binary data through a logit link. From Table 5.3, we observe that the AB and/or RMS values corresponding to $\mu_4, \ldots, \mu_9, \lambda_{52}, \lambda_{62}, \lambda_{83}, \lambda_{93}, \gamma_3, \phi_{11}$, and ϕ_{22} are quite large. These parameters are related to the binary variables $y_{i4}, \ldots, y_{i9}$ that are incorrectly modeled as dichotomous data through a threshold specification. The general empirical performance does not improve with larger sample size. Again, standard error estimates overestimate the true standard deviations. Clearly, it can be concluded that incorrectly treating binary data as dichotomous, or vice versa, will produce misleading results.

5.4 SEMs with missing data

5.4.1 Introduction

Missing data are very common in substantive research. For example, missing data arise from situations where respondents in a household survey may refuse to report income, or individuals in an opinion survey may refuse to express their attitudes toward sensitive or embarrassing questions. Clearly, observations with missing entries need to be considered for better statistical inferences. In structural equation modeling, much attention has been devoted to analyzing models in the presence of missing data. For example, in analyzing standard SEMs, Arbuckle (1996) proposed a full information ML method which maximizes the casewise likelihood of observed continuous data. Recently, Bayesian methods for analyzing missing data in the context of more complex SEMs have been developed. For instance, Song and Lee (2002) and Lee and Song (2004) developed Bayesian methods for analyzing linear and nonlinear SEMs with mixed continuous and ordered categorical variables, on the basis of ignorable missing data that are missing at random (MAR); while Lee and Tang (2006) and Song and Lee (2007) developed Bayesian methods for analyzing nonlinear SEMs with nonignorable missing data.

The main objective of this section is to introduce the Bayesian approach for analyzing SEMs with ignorable missing data that are missing at random (MAR), and nonignorable missing data that are missing with a nonignorable missingness mechanism. According to Little and Rubin (2002), the missing data are regarded as MAR if the probability of missingness depends on the fully observed data but not on the missing data themselves. For nonignorable missing data, the probability of missingness depends not only on the observed data but also on the missing data, according to a nonignorable missing model. In the Bayesian approach, we employ the useful strategy that combines the idea of data augmentation and application of MCMC methods. We will show that Bayesian methods for analyzing SEMs with fully observed data can be extended to handle missing data without much theoretical and practical difficulty. Here, we regard observations with missing entries as partially observed data. We will present a Bayesian framework for analyzing general SEMs with missing data that are MAR, including Bayesian estimation, and model comparison via the Bayes factor. Then we present Bayesian methods to analyze nonlinear SEMs with missing data that are missing with a nonignorable mechanism. Finally, we demonstrate the use of WinBUGS to obtain the Bayesian solutions.

5.4.2 SEMs with missing data that are MAR

Let $\mathbf{V} = (\mathbf{v}_1, \ldots, \mathbf{v}_n)$ be a matrix of random vectors with $\mathbf{v}_i = (\mathbf{x}_i^T, \mathbf{y}_i^T)^T$, in which $\mathbf{x}_i$ and $\mathbf{y}_i$ are vectors of continuous variables whose exact measurements are observable and unobservable, respectively. Let $\mathbf{Z} = (\mathbf{z}_1, \ldots, \mathbf{z}_n)$ be observable ordered categorical data (or dichotomous data) that correspond to $\mathbf{Y} = (\mathbf{y}_1, \ldots, \mathbf{y}_n)$. Suppose $\mathbf{v}_i$ follows a general SEM with a vector of latent variables $\boldsymbol{\omega}_i$. Let $\boldsymbol{\Omega} = (\boldsymbol{\omega}_1, \ldots, \boldsymbol{\omega}_n)$ contain all the latent variables in the model. To deal with missing data that are MAR, let $\mathbf{X}_{\text{obs}}$ and $\mathbf{X}_{\text{mis}}$ be the observed and missing data sets corresponding to the continuous data $\mathbf{X} = (\mathbf{x}_1, \ldots, \mathbf{x}_n)$; $\mathbf{Z}_{\text{obs}}$ and $\mathbf{Z}_{\text{mis}}$ be the observed and missing data sets corresponding to the ordered categorical data $\mathbf{Z}$; and $\mathbf{Y}_{\text{obs}}$ and $\mathbf{Y}_{\text{mis}}$ be the hypothetical observed and missing data sets of $\mathbf{Y}$ corresponding to $\mathbf{Z}_{\text{obs}}$ and $\mathbf{Z}_{\text{mis}}$, respectively. Moreover, let $\mathbf{V}_{\text{obs}} = \{\mathbf{X}_{\text{obs}}, \mathbf{Y}_{\text{obs}}\}$ and $\mathbf{V}_{\text{mis}} = \{\mathbf{X}_{\text{mis}}, \mathbf{Y}_{\text{mis}}\}$. The main goal is to develop Bayesian methods for estimating the unknown parameter and threshold vector $\boldsymbol{\theta}^* = (\boldsymbol{\theta}, \boldsymbol{\alpha})$ of the model, and comparing competitive models on the basis of the observed data $\{\mathbf{X}_{\text{obs}}, \mathbf{Z}_{\text{obs}}\}$.

We first consider the Bayesian estimation by investigating the following posterior distribution of $\boldsymbol{\theta}^*$ with given $\mathbf{X}_{\text{obs}}$ and $\mathbf{Z}_{\text{obs}}$:

$$p(\boldsymbol{\theta}^* | \mathbf{X}_{\text{obs}}, \mathbf{Z}_{\text{obs}}) \propto p(\mathbf{X}_{\text{obs}}, \mathbf{Z}_{\text{obs}} | \boldsymbol{\theta}^*) p(\boldsymbol{\theta}^*),$$

where $p(\mathbf{X}_{\text{obs}}, \mathbf{Z}_{\text{obs}}|\boldsymbol{\theta}^*)$ is the observed-data likelihood and $p(\boldsymbol{\theta}^*)$ is the prior density of $\boldsymbol{\theta}^*$. As $p(\boldsymbol{\theta}^*|\mathbf{X}_{\text{obs}}, \mathbf{Z}_{\text{obs}})$ is usually very complicated, we utilize the idea of data augmentation (Tanner and Wong, 1987), and then perform the posterior simulation with the MCMC methods. Naturally, the observed data $\{\mathbf{X}_{\text{obs}}, \mathbf{Z}_{\text{obs}}\}$ are augmented with the latent and missing quantities $\{\boldsymbol{\Omega}, \mathbf{X}_{\text{mis}}, \mathbf{Y}_{\text{mis}}, \mathbf{Y}_{\text{obs}}\} = \{\boldsymbol{\Omega}, \mathbf{V}_{\text{mis}}, \mathbf{Y}_{\text{obs}}\}$. As $\mathbf{Y}_{\text{mis}}$ is included, it is not necessary to augment with the corresponding $\mathbf{Z}_{\text{mis}}$. A sufficiently large number of random observations will be simulated from the joint posterior distribution $[\boldsymbol{\theta}^*, \boldsymbol{\Omega}, \mathbf{V}_{\text{mis}}, \mathbf{Y}_{\text{obs}}|\mathbf{X}_{\text{obs}}, \mathbf{Z}_{\text{obs}}]$. This task can be completed by a hybrid algorithm that combines the Gibbs sampler (Geman and Geman, 1984) and the MH algorithm (Metropolis *et al.*, 1953; Hastings, 1970) as before. Bayesian estimates of parameters in $\boldsymbol{\theta}^*$ and the standard error estimates can be obtained through the sample of simulated observations, $\{(\boldsymbol{\theta}^{*(j)}, \boldsymbol{\Omega}^{(j)}, \mathbf{V}_{\text{mis}}^{(j)}, \mathbf{Y}_{\text{obs}}^{(j)}), j = 1, \ldots, J\}$, that are drawn from the joint posterior distribution.

The conditional distributions $p(\boldsymbol{\theta}|\boldsymbol{\Omega}, \mathbf{V}_{\text{mis}}, \mathbf{Y}_{\text{obs}}, \mathbf{X}_{\text{obs}}, \mathbf{Z}_{\text{obs}})$, $p(\boldsymbol{\Omega}|\boldsymbol{\theta}^*, \mathbf{V}_{\text{mis}}, \mathbf{Y}_{\text{obs}}, \mathbf{X}_{\text{obs}}, \mathbf{Z}_{\text{obs}})$, $p(\mathbf{V}_{\text{mis}}|\boldsymbol{\theta}^*, \boldsymbol{\Omega}, \mathbf{Y}_{\text{obs}}, \mathbf{X}_{\text{obs}}, \mathbf{Z}_{\text{obs}})$, and $p(\boldsymbol{\alpha}, \mathbf{Y}_{\text{obs}}|\boldsymbol{\theta}, \boldsymbol{\Omega}, \mathbf{V}_{\text{mis}}, \mathbf{X}_{\text{obs}}, \mathbf{Z}_{\text{obs}})$ are required in the implementation of the Gibbs sampler. With $\mathbf{Y} = (\mathbf{Y}_{\text{mis}}, \mathbf{Y}_{\text{obs}})$ and $\mathbf{V} = (\mathbf{V}_{\text{mis}}, \mathbf{V}_{\text{obs}})$ given, the conditional distributions corresponding to $\boldsymbol{\theta}$ and $\boldsymbol{\Omega}$ can be derived in exactly the same way as in the situation with fully observed data. Similarly, with $\boldsymbol{\theta}$, $\boldsymbol{\Omega}$, $\mathbf{V}_{\text{mis}}$, $\mathbf{X}_{\text{obs}}$, and $\mathbf{Z}_{\text{obs}}$ given, the conditional distribution corresponding to $(\boldsymbol{\alpha}, \mathbf{Y}_{\text{obs}})$ can be derived as before. We only need to derive the conditional distribution corresponding to $\mathbf{V}_{\text{mis}}$. Under the usual mild assumption that $\mathbf{v}_1, \ldots, \mathbf{v}_n$ are mutually independent, it follows that

$$p(\mathbf{V}_{\text{mis}}|\boldsymbol{\theta}^*, \boldsymbol{\Omega}, \mathbf{Y}_{\text{obs}}, \mathbf{X}_{\text{obs}}, \mathbf{Z}_{\text{obs}}) = \prod_{i=1}^{n} p(\mathbf{v}_{i,\text{mis}}|\boldsymbol{\theta}^*, \boldsymbol{\omega}_i, \mathbf{y}_{i,\text{obs}}, \mathbf{x}_{i,\text{obs}}, \mathbf{z}_{i,\text{obs}}), \tag{5.16}$$

where $\mathbf{v}_{i,\text{mis}} = (\mathbf{x}_{i,\text{mis}}, \mathbf{y}_{i,\text{mis}})$ is the ith data point in the random sample of size n. The individual $\mathbf{v}_{i,\text{mis}}$ can be separately simulated from the conditional distribution in (5.16). For most SEMs, the conditional distribution $p(\mathbf{v}_{i,\text{mis}}|\boldsymbol{\theta}^*, \boldsymbol{\omega}_i, \mathbf{y}_{i,\text{obs}}, \mathbf{x}_{i,\text{obs}}, \mathbf{z}_{i,\text{obs}})$ is usually simple. Consequently, the computational burden of sampling $\mathbf{V}_{\text{mis}}$ is light.

To address the model comparison problem, we let M_0 and M_1 be two competing models, and consider the computation of the Bayes factor

$$B_{10} = \frac{p(\mathbf{X}_{\text{obs}}, \mathbf{Z}_{\text{obs}}|M_1)}{p(\mathbf{X}_{\text{obs}}, \mathbf{Z}_{\text{obs}}|M_0)}.$$

Its logarithm $\log B_{10}$ can be similarly computed with path sampling (Gelman and Meng, 1998). Consider the following class of densities defined by a continuous parameter t in $[0, 1]$:

$$p(\boldsymbol{\theta}^*, \boldsymbol{\Omega}, \mathbf{V}_{\text{mis}}, \mathbf{Y}_{\text{obs}}|\mathbf{X}_{\text{obs}}, \mathbf{Z}_{\text{obs}}, t) = p(\boldsymbol{\theta}^*, \boldsymbol{\Omega}, \mathbf{V}_{\text{mis}}, \mathbf{Y}_{\text{obs}}, \mathbf{X}_{\text{obs}}, \mathbf{Z}_{\text{obs}}|t)/z(t),$$

where $z(t) = p(\mathbf{X}_{\text{obs}}, \mathbf{Z}_{\text{obs}}|t)$. The parameter t connects the competing models M_0 and M_1 such that $z(1) = p(\mathbf{X}_{\text{obs}}, \mathbf{Z}_{\text{obs}}|t = 1) = p(\mathbf{X}_{\text{obs}}, \mathbf{Z}_{\text{obs}}|M_1)$ and $z(0) = p(\mathbf{X}_{\text{obs}}, \mathbf{Z}_{\text{obs}}|t = 0) = p(\mathbf{X}_{\text{obs}}, \mathbf{Z}_{\text{obs}}|M_0)$, and $B_{10} = z(1)/z(0)$. Based on the reasoning given before, it can be similarly shown that

$$\widehat{\log B_{10}} = \frac{1}{2}\sum_{s=0}^{S}(t_{(s+1)} - t_{(s)})(\bar{U}_{(s+1)} + \bar{U}_{(s)}), \tag{5.17}$$

where $0 = t_{(0)} < t_{(1)} < \ldots < t_{(S)} < t_{(S+1)} = 1$, which are fixed grids at [0, 1], and

$$\bar{U}_{(s)} = J^{-1} \sum_{j=1}^{J} U\left(\boldsymbol{\theta}^{*(j)}, \boldsymbol{\Omega}^{(j)}, \mathbf{V}_{\text{mis}}^{(j)}, \mathbf{Y}_{\text{obs}}^{(j)}, \mathbf{X}_{\text{obs}}, \mathbf{Z}_{\text{obs}}, t_{(s)}\right), \tag{5.18}$$

in which $\{(\boldsymbol{\theta}^{*(j)}, \boldsymbol{\Omega}^{(j)}, \mathbf{V}_{\text{mis}}^{(j)}, \mathbf{Y}_{\text{obs}}^{(j)}), j = 1, \ldots, J\}$ is a sample of observations simulated from $p(\boldsymbol{\theta}^*, \boldsymbol{\Omega}, \mathbf{V}_{\text{mis}}, \mathbf{Y}_{\text{obs}}|\mathbf{X}_{\text{obs}}, \mathbf{Z}_{\text{obs}}, t_{(s)})$, and

$$U(\boldsymbol{\theta}^*, \boldsymbol{\Omega}, \mathbf{V}_{\text{mis}}, \mathbf{Y}_{\text{obs}}, \mathbf{X}_{\text{obs}}, \mathbf{Z}_{\text{obs}}, t) = \frac{d}{dt} \log p(\boldsymbol{\Omega}, \mathbf{V}_{\text{mis}}, \mathbf{Y}_{\text{obs}}, \mathbf{X}_{\text{obs}}, \mathbf{Z}_{\text{obs}}|\boldsymbol{\theta}^*, t),$$

where $p(\boldsymbol{\Omega}, \mathbf{V}_{\text{mis}}, \mathbf{Y}_{\text{obs}}, \mathbf{X}_{\text{obs}}, \mathbf{Z}_{\text{obs}}|\boldsymbol{\theta}^*, t)$ is the complete-data likelihood. Because a program for simulating $(\boldsymbol{\theta}^*, \boldsymbol{\Omega}, \mathbf{V}_{\text{mis}}, \mathbf{Y}_{\text{obs}})$ has already been developed in the Bayesian estimation, the implementation of the path sampling procedure does not require too much extra programming effort. Basically, the Bayesian methodologies for analyzing SEMs with fully observed data can be generalized to handle missing data that are MAR with only one additional simple component in the Gibbs sampler; see (5.16).

For instance, consider the linear SEM with mixed continuous and ordered categorical variables; see equations (5.1) and (5.2). Since $\boldsymbol{\Psi}_\epsilon$ is diagonal, $\mathbf{v}_{i,\text{mis}}$ is independent of $\mathbf{v}_{i,\text{obs}} = (\mathbf{x}_{i,\text{obs}}, \mathbf{y}_{i,\text{obs}})$. Let p_i be the dimension of $\mathbf{v}_{i,\text{mis}}$; it follows from (5.1) that

$$p(\mathbf{V}_{\text{mis}}|\mathbf{X}_{\text{obs}}, \mathbf{Z}_{\text{obs}}, \boldsymbol{\Omega}, \boldsymbol{\theta}, \boldsymbol{\alpha}, \mathbf{Y}_{\text{obs}}) = \prod_{i=1}^{n} p(\mathbf{v}_{i,\text{mis}}|\boldsymbol{\theta}, \boldsymbol{\omega}_i), \text{ and}$$

$$[\mathbf{v}_{i,\text{mis}}|\boldsymbol{\theta}, \boldsymbol{\omega}_i] \stackrel{D}{=} N[\boldsymbol{\mu}_{i,\text{mis}} + \boldsymbol{\Lambda}_{i,\text{mis}}\boldsymbol{\omega}_i, \boldsymbol{\Psi}_{i,\text{mis}}],$$

where $\boldsymbol{\mu}_{i,\text{mis}}$ is a $p_i \times 1$ subvector of $\boldsymbol{\mu}$ with elements corresponding to observed components deleted, $\boldsymbol{\Lambda}_{i,\text{mis}}$ is a $p_i \times q$ submatrix of $\boldsymbol{\Lambda}$ with rows corresponding to observed components deleted, and $\boldsymbol{\Psi}_{i,\text{mis}}$ is a $p_i \times p_i$ submatrix of $\boldsymbol{\Psi}_\epsilon$ with the appropriate rows and columns deleted. Hence, even though the form of $\mathbf{V}_{\text{mis}}$ is complicated with many distinct missingness patterns, its conditional distribution only involves a product of very simple univariate normal distributions.

5.4.3 An illustrative example

To illustrate the methodology, a portion of the data set obtained from a study (Morisky *et al.*, 1998) of the effects of establishment policies, knowledge, and attitudes toward condom use among Filipina commercial sex workers (CSWs) is analyzed. As commercial sex work promotes the spread of AIDS and other sexually transmitted diseases, promotion of safer sexual practices among CSWs is an important issue. In this example, we assume that there are no 'establishment' effects, so that observations obtained within the establishment are independently and identically distributed. A subtler two-level SEM will be introduced in Section 6.2 to relax this assumption. The data set was collected from female CSWs in 97 establishments (bars, night clubs, etc.) in cities of the Philippines. The entire questionnaire consists of 134 items, covering the areas of demographic knowledge, attitudes, beliefs, behaviors, self-efficacy for condom use, and social desirability. In our illustrative example, only six observed variables $(v_1, \ldots, v_6)$ are selected. Variables v_1 and v_2 are related to 'worry about getting AIDS', v_3 and v_4 are related to 'aggressiveness', while v_5 and v_6 are about 'attitude to the risk of getting AIDS'. Variables v_3 and v_4 are continuous, while the others are ordered categorical and

Table 5.4 Missingness patterns and their sample sizes, AIDS data set; '×' and 'o' indicate missing and observed entries, respectively.

		Observed variables								Observed variables					
Pattern	Sample size	1	2	3	4	5	6	Pattern	Sample size	1	2	3	4	5	6
1	784	o	o	o	o	o	o	11	7	×	o	o	o	×	o
2	100	×	o	o	o	o	o	12	7	×	o	o	o	o	×
3	57	o	×	o	o	o	o	13	9	o	×	o	o	×	o
4	6	o	o	×	o	o	o	14	3	o	×	o	o	o	×
5	4	o	o	o	×	o	o	15	1	o	×	o	×	o	o
6	25	o	o	o	o	×	o	16	1	o	×	×	o	o	o
7	26	×	o	o	o	o	×	17	4	o	×	o	o	×	×
8	17	×	×	o	o	o	o	18	2	×	o	o	o	×	×
9	23	o	o	o	o	×	×	19	1	o	o	×	o	×	×
10	2	×	o	×	o	o	o	20	1	×	×	o	o	×	×

Reproduced by permission of Taylor & Francis from Lee, S. Y., Song, X. Y. and Cai, J. H. (2010). A Bayesian approach for nonlinear structural equation models with dichotomous variables using logit and probit links. *Structural Equation Modeling – A Multidisciplinary Journal*, **17**, 280–302.

measured on a five-point scale. We assume that the missing values are MAR. After deleting obvious outliers, the data set contains 1080 observations, only 754 of which are fully observed. The missingness patterns are presented in Table 5.4. Note that some missingness patterns only have a very small number of observations. To unify the scales of the continuous variables, the corresponding continuous data are standardized. The sample means and sample standard deviations of the continuous variables are {1.58, 1203.74} and {1.84, 1096.32}, respectively. The cell frequencies of each individual ordered categorical variable range from 21 to 709. See Morisky *et al.* (1998) for other descriptive statistics.

To identify parameters associated with the ordered categorical variables, α_{11}, α_{14}, α_{21}, α_{24}, α_{31}, α_{34}, α_{41}, and α_{44} are fixed at -0.478, 1.034, -1.420, 0.525, -0.868, 0.559, -2.130, and -0.547, respectively. These fixed values are calculated via $\alpha_{kh} = \Phi^{*^{-1}}(f_{kh})$, where $\Phi^{*}(\cdot)$ is the distribution function of $N[0, 1]$, and f_{kh} are observed cumulative proportions of the categories with $z_k < h$. Based on the meanings of the questions corresponding to the selected observed variables, the data are analyzed through a model with three latent variables η, ξ_1, and ξ_2, together with the measurement equation as specified in (5.1), where $\mu = 0$ and

$$\Lambda^T = \begin{bmatrix} 1 & \lambda_{21} & 0 & 0 & 0 & 0 \\ 0 & 0 & 1 & \lambda_{42} & 0 & 0 \\ 0 & 0 & 0 & 0 & 1 & \lambda_{63} \end{bmatrix}.$$

Competing models associated with the following different structural equations but the same measurement equation are considered for the purposes of illustration:

$$M_1 : \eta = \gamma_1\xi_1 + \gamma_2\xi_2 + \delta,$$

$$M_2 : \eta = \gamma_1\xi_1 + \gamma_2\xi_2 + \gamma_3\xi_1^2 + \delta,$$

$$M_3 : \eta = \gamma_1\xi_1 + \gamma_2\xi_2 + \gamma_4\xi_1\xi_2 + \delta,$$

$$M_4 : \eta = \gamma_1\xi_1 + \gamma_2\xi_2 + \gamma_5\xi_2^2 + \delta.$$

Note that M_1 is nested in M_2, M_3, and M_4, whilst M_2, M_3, and M_4 are nonnested. Estimated log Bayes factors are obtained using the path sampling procedure with $S = 20$ and $J = 1000$. Assuming that we have no prior information from other sources, we conduct an initial Bayesian estimation based on M_1 with noninformative priors in order to get prior inputs of some hyperparameters. Here, we fixed $\mathbf{H}_{0yk} = \mathbf{I}$ and $\mathbf{H}_{0\omega k} = \mathbf{I}$; for other prior inputs, we take $\rho_0 = 10$, $\mathbf{R}_0^{-1} = 4\mathbf{I}$, $\alpha_{0\epsilon k} = \alpha_{0\delta k} = 8$, $\beta_{0\epsilon k} = \beta_{0\delta k} = 10$; and $\boldsymbol{\Lambda}_{0k}$ and $\boldsymbol{\Lambda}_{0\omega k}$ equal to the estimates of $\boldsymbol{\Lambda}_k$ and $\boldsymbol{\Lambda}_{\omega k}$ in the preliminary analysis.

We are interested in comparing the linear model M_1 with the nonlinear models. It is easy to construct a path to link the competing models. For example, the link model M_t for M_1 and M_2 is $M_t : \eta = \gamma_1\xi_1 + \gamma_2\xi_2 + t\gamma_3\xi_1^2 + \delta$. Hence, when $t = 0$, $M_t = M_1$; and when $t = 1$, $M_t = M_2$. We obtain the following results: $\{\widehat{\log B_{21}}, \widehat{\log B_{31}}, \widehat{\log B_{41}}\} = \{2.303, 0.340, 0.780\}$. In comparing M_2 and M_1, $\widehat{\log B_{21}} = 2.303$ clearly recommends the nonlinear model M_2. From $\widehat{\log B_{31}}$ and $\widehat{\log B_{41}}$, we see that the other nonlinear models are not significantly better than M_1. Hence, M_2 is the best model among $M_1, \ldots, M_4$.

To compare M_2 with more complex models, we consider the following models with more complicated structural equations:

$$M_5 : \eta = \gamma_1\xi_1 + \gamma_2\xi_2 + \gamma_3\xi_1^2 + \gamma_4\xi_1\xi_2 + \delta,$$

$$M_6 : \eta = \gamma_1\xi_1 + \gamma_2\xi_2 + \gamma_3\xi_1^2 + \gamma_5\xi_2^2 + \delta.$$

Here, M_2 is nested in M_5 and M_6. The estimated log Bayes factors are $\widehat{\log B_{52}} = 0.406$ and $\widehat{\log B_{62}} = 0.489$. We see that the more complex models are not significantly better than M_2; hence the simpler model M_2 is selected. We compute that the PP p-value (Gelman *et al*., 1996) corresponding to M_2 is 0.572. This indicates that M_2 fits the data well. For completeness, the estimates of the unknown parameters in M_2 are reported in Table 5.5.

Table 5.5 Bayesian estimates of parameters in M_2

Par	EST	Par	EST
λ_{21}	0.228	$\psi_{\epsilon 1}$	0.593
λ_{42}	0.353	$\psi_{\epsilon 2}$	0.972
λ_{63}	0.358	$\psi_{\epsilon 3}$	0.519
		$\psi_{\epsilon 4}$	0.943
γ_1	0.544	$\psi_{\epsilon 5}$	0.616
γ_2	−0.033	$\psi_{\epsilon 6}$	1.056
γ_3	−0.226		
		α_{12}	−0.030
ϕ_{11}	0.508	α_{13}	0.340
ϕ_{12}	−0.029	α_{22}	−0.961
ϕ_{22}	0.394	α_{23}	−0.620
		α_{32}	−0.394
ψ_δ	0.663	α_{33}	0.257
		α_{42}	−1.604
		α_{43}	−0.734

Reproduced by permission of Taylor & Francis from Lee, S. Y., Song, X. Y. and Cai, J. H. (2010). A Bayesian approach for nonlinear structural equation models with dichotomous variables using logit and probit links. *Structural Equation Modeling – A Multidisciplinary Journal*, **17**, 280–302.

Based on the results obtained, a nonlinear SEM has been chosen. Its specification of $\mathbf{\Lambda}$ in the measurement equation suggests that there are three non-overlapping latent factors η, ξ_1, and ξ_2, which can be roughly interpreted as 'worry about AIDS', 'aggressiveness' of CSWs, and 'attitude to the risk of getting AIDS'. These latent factors are related through the nonlinear structural equation $\eta = 0.544\xi_1 - 0.033\xi_2 - 0.226\xi_1^2$. Thus, 'aggressiveness' of the CSWs has both linear and quadratic effects on 'worry about AIDS'. Plotting the quadratic curve of η against ξ_1, we find that the maximum of η is roughly at $\xi_1 = 1.2$, and η decreases as ξ_1 moves away from both directions at 1.2. From the model comparison results, the model with the quadratic term of 'attitude to the risk of getting AIDS' or the corresponding interaction term with 'aggressiveness' is not as good. Thus, these nonlinear relationships are not important, and it is not necessary to consider the more complicated model involving both the interaction and quadratic terms.

5.4.4 Nonlinear SEMs with nonignorable missing data

Many missing data in behavioral, medical, social, and psychological research are nonignorable in the sense that the missing data depend on the observed data and the missing data themselves. For example, the side effects of the treatment may make the patients worse and thereby affect patients' participation. Non-ignorable missing data, which are more difficult to handle than ignorable missing data, have received considerable attention in statistics; see, for example, Ibrahim *et al.* (2001). In the field of SEM, not much work has been done to analyze nonignorable missing data. In this subsection we present a Bayesian approach (see Lee and Tang, 2006) for analyzing a nonlinear SEM with nonignorable missing data. For brevity, we focus on continuous data. However, the Bayesian development can be extended to ordered categorical data, and/or data from exponential family distributions based on the key ideas presented in this section and previous sections (see also Song and Lee, 2007). Again, the idea of data augmentation and the MCMC tools will be used to obtain the Bayesian estimates of the unknown parameters and the Bayes factor for model comparison. Although Ibrahim *et al.* (2001) pointed out that the parametric form of the assumed missingness mechanism itself is not 'testable' from the data, the Bayes factor provides a useful statistic for comparing different missing-data models. Moreover, in the context of a given nonignorable missing-data model, the Bayes factor can be used to select a better nonlinear SEM for fitting the data.

For each $p \times 1$ random vector $\mathbf{v}_i = (v_{i1}, \ldots, v_{ip})^T$ in the data set $\mathbf{V} = (\mathbf{v}_1, \ldots, \mathbf{v}_n)$, we define a missingness indicator $\mathbf{r}_i = (r_{i1}, \ldots, r_{ip})^T$ such that $r_{ij} = 1$ if v_{ij} is missing, and $r_{ij} = 0$ if v_{ij} is observed. Let $\mathbf{r} = (\mathbf{r}_1, \ldots, \mathbf{r}_n)$; and let $\mathbf{V}_{\text{mis}}$ and $\mathbf{V}_{\text{obs}}$ be the missing and observed data, respectively. If the distribution of $\mathbf{r}$ is independent of $\mathbf{V}_{\text{mis}}$, the missingness mechanism is defined to be MAR; otherwise the missingness mechanism is nonignorable (Little and Rubin, 2002). For the nonignorable missingness mechanism, it is necessary to investigate the conditional probability of $\mathbf{r}$ given $\mathbf{V}$, $p(\mathbf{r}|\mathbf{V}, \boldsymbol{\varphi})$, where $\boldsymbol{\varphi}$ is a parameter vector. If this probability does not contain unknown parameters in $\boldsymbol{\varphi}$, the missingness mechanism is called ignorable and known, otherwise it is called nonignorable and unknown. An example of a nonignorable and unknown mechanism is related to censored data with a known censoring point. For analyzing missing data with a nonignorable and unknown mechanism, the basic issues are specifying a reasonable model for $\mathbf{r}$ given $\mathbf{V}$, and developing statistical methods for analyzing this model together with the model in relation to $\mathbf{V}$.

Let $\mathbf{v}_i = (\mathbf{v}_{i,\text{obs}}^T, \mathbf{v}_{i,\text{mis}}^T)^T$, where $\mathbf{v}_{i,\text{obs}}$ is a $p_{i1} \times 1$ vector of observed components, $\mathbf{v}_{i,\text{mis}}$ is a $p_{i2} \times 1$ vector of missing components, and $p_{i1} + p_{i2} = p$. Here, we assume an arbitrary pattern of missing data in $\mathbf{v}_i$, and thus $\mathbf{v}_i = (\mathbf{v}_{i,\text{obs}}^T, \mathbf{v}_{i,\text{mis}}^T)^T$ may represent some permutation of the indices of the original $\mathbf{v}_i$. Let $[\mathbf{r}_i|\mathbf{v}_i, \boldsymbol{\omega}_i, \boldsymbol{\varphi}]$ be the conditional distribution of $\mathbf{r}_i$ given $\mathbf{v}_i$ and $\boldsymbol{\omega}_i$ with a probability density function $p(\mathbf{r}_i|\mathbf{v}_i, \boldsymbol{\omega}_i, \boldsymbol{\varphi})$. Let $\boldsymbol{\theta}$ be the structural parameter vector that contains all unknown distinct parameters in $\boldsymbol{\mu}$, $\boldsymbol{\Lambda}$, $\boldsymbol{\Lambda}_\omega$, $\boldsymbol{\Psi}_\epsilon$, $\boldsymbol{\Psi}_\delta$, and $\boldsymbol{\Phi}$. The main interest is in the posterior analyses of $\boldsymbol{\theta}$ and $\boldsymbol{\varphi}$ based on $\mathbf{r}$ and $\mathbf{V}_{\text{obs}} = \{\mathbf{v}_{i,\text{obs}}, i = 1, \ldots, n\}$. According to the definition of the model, the joint posterior density of $\boldsymbol{\theta}$ and $\boldsymbol{\varphi}$ based on $\mathbf{V}_{\text{obs}}$ and $\mathbf{r}$ is given by:

$$p(\boldsymbol{\theta}, \boldsymbol{\varphi}|\mathbf{V}_{\text{obs}}, \mathbf{r}) \propto \left\{\prod_{i=1}^{n} \int_{\boldsymbol{\omega}_i, \mathbf{v}_{i,\text{mis}}} p(\mathbf{v}_i|\boldsymbol{\omega}_i, \boldsymbol{\theta}) p(\mathbf{r}_i|\mathbf{v}_i, \boldsymbol{\omega}_i, \boldsymbol{\varphi}) p(\boldsymbol{\omega}_i|\boldsymbol{\theta}) d\boldsymbol{\omega}_i d\mathbf{v}_{i,\text{mis}}\right\} p(\boldsymbol{\theta}, \boldsymbol{\varphi}),$$

where $p(\boldsymbol{\theta}, \boldsymbol{\varphi})$ denotes the joint prior distribution of $\boldsymbol{\theta}$ and $\boldsymbol{\varphi}$. In general, the above integral does not have a closed form and its dimension is equal to the sum of the dimensions of $\boldsymbol{\omega}_i$ and $\mathbf{v}_{i,\text{mis}}$.

We consider the selection of a model for the nonignorable missingness mechanism. Theoretically, any general model can be taken. However, too complex a model will induce difficulty in deriving the corresponding conditional distributions of the missing responses given the observed data, and inefficient sampling from those conditional distributions. Now, since the observations are independent,

$$p(\mathbf{r}|\mathbf{V}, \boldsymbol{\Omega}, \boldsymbol{\varphi}) = \prod_{i=1}^{n} p(\mathbf{r}_i|\mathbf{v}_i, \boldsymbol{\omega}_i, \boldsymbol{\varphi}),$$

where $\boldsymbol{\Omega} = (\boldsymbol{\omega}_1, \ldots, \boldsymbol{\omega}_n)$. As the covariance matrix of the error measurement $\boldsymbol{\epsilon}_i$ is diagonal, it follows that when $\boldsymbol{\omega}_i$ is given, the components of $\mathbf{v}_i$ are independent. Hence, for $j \neq l$, it is reasonable to assume that the conditional distributions of r_{ij} and r_{il} given $\boldsymbol{\omega}_i$ are independent. Under this assumption, we use the following binomial model for the nonignorable missingness mechanism (see Ibrahim *et al.*, 2001; Lee and Tang, 2006; Song and Lee, 2007):

$$p(\mathbf{r}|\mathbf{V}, \boldsymbol{\Omega}, \boldsymbol{\varphi}) = \prod_{i=1}^{n}\prod_{j=1}^{p} \{\Pr(r_{ij} = 1|\mathbf{v}_i, \boldsymbol{\omega}_i, \boldsymbol{\varphi})\}^{r_{ij}} \{1 - \Pr(r_{ij} = 1|\mathbf{v}_i, \boldsymbol{\omega}_i, \boldsymbol{\varphi})\}^{1-r_{ij}}. \tag{5.19}$$

Ibrahim *et al.* (2001) pointed out that as r_{ij} is binary, one can use a sequence of logistic regressions for modeling $\Pr(r_{ij} = 1|\mathbf{v}_i, \boldsymbol{\omega}_i, \boldsymbol{\varphi})$ in (5.19). They also pointed out that this model has the potential for reducing the number of parameters in the missing-data mechanism, yields correlation structures between the r_{ij}, allows more flexibility in specifying the missing-data model, and facilitates efficient sampling from the conditional distribution of the missing response given the observed data. Following their suggestion, the following logistic regression model is used:

$$\begin{aligned} &\text{logit}\{\Pr(r_{ij} = 1|\mathbf{v}_i, \boldsymbol{\omega}_i, \boldsymbol{\varphi})\} \\ &= \varphi_0 + \varphi_1 v_{i1} + \ldots + \varphi_p v_{ip} + \varphi_{p+1}\omega_{i1} + \ldots + \varphi_{p+q}\omega_{iq} = \boldsymbol{\varphi}^T \mathbf{e}_i, \end{aligned} \tag{5.20}$$

where $\mathbf{e}_i = (1, v_{i1}, \ldots, v_{ip}, \omega_{i1}, \ldots, \omega_{iq})^T$ and $\boldsymbol{\varphi} = (\varphi_0, \varphi_1, \ldots, \varphi_{p+q})^T$. On the basis of the definition of the measurement equation and the basic concepts of latent variables and their indicators in SEMs, in which the characteristics of $\boldsymbol{\omega}_i$ are revealed by the observed variables in $\mathbf{v}_i$, it may be desirable to adopt the following special case of (5.20) which does not depend on $\boldsymbol{\omega}_i$:

$$\text{logit}\{\Pr(r_{ij} = 1|\mathbf{v}_i, \boldsymbol{\omega}_i, \boldsymbol{\varphi})\} = \varphi_0 + \varphi_1 v_{i1} + \ldots + \varphi_p v_{ip}. \tag{5.21}$$

However, for generality, the Bayesian approach will be presented on the basis of the more general model (5.20). As (5.21) is equivalent to specifying $\varphi_{p+1} = \ldots = \varphi_{p+q} = 0$ in (5.20), modifications of the general Bayesian development in handling this special case are straightforward. We do not recommend routinely using (5.20) or (5.21) for modeling the nonignorable missingness mechanism in every practical application. Other models may be preferable for situations where one is certain about the specific form of the missingness mechanism. However, the model specified in (5.20) or (5.21) is reasonable, and is useful for sensitivity analysis of the estimates with respect to missing data with other different missingness mechanisms.

Let $\boldsymbol{\Lambda}_k^T$ and $\boldsymbol{\Lambda}_{\omega k}^T$ be the kth rows of $\boldsymbol{\Lambda}$ and $\boldsymbol{\Lambda}_\omega$, respectively; and let $\psi_{\epsilon k}$ and $\psi_{\delta k}$ be the kth diagonal elements of $\boldsymbol{\Psi}_\epsilon$ and $\boldsymbol{\Psi}_\delta$, respectively. Let $\mathbf{V}_{\text{mis}} = \{\mathbf{v}_{i,\text{mis}}, i = 1, \ldots, n\}$ be the set of missing values associated with the observed variables. The observed data $\mathbf{V}_{\text{obs}}$ and the missing-data indicator $\mathbf{r}$ are augmented with the missing quantities $\{\mathbf{V}_{\text{mis}}, \boldsymbol{\Omega}\}$ in the posterior analysis. The Gibbs sampler (Geman and Geman, 1984) is used to generate a sequence of random observations from the joint posterior distribution $[\boldsymbol{\Omega}, \mathbf{V}_{\text{mis}}, \boldsymbol{\theta}, \boldsymbol{\varphi}|\mathbf{V}_{\text{obs}}, \mathbf{r}]$, and the Bayesian estimates are then obtained from the observations of this generated sequence. Specifically, observations $\{\boldsymbol{\Omega}, \mathbf{V}_{\text{mis}}, \boldsymbol{\theta}, \boldsymbol{\varphi}\}$ are sampled iteratively from the following conditional distributions: $p(\boldsymbol{\Omega}|\mathbf{V}_{\text{obs}}, \mathbf{V}_{\text{mis}}, \boldsymbol{\theta}, \boldsymbol{\varphi}, \mathbf{r}) = p(\boldsymbol{\Omega}|\mathbf{V}, \boldsymbol{\theta}, \boldsymbol{\varphi}, \mathbf{r})$, $p(\mathbf{V}_{\text{mis}}| \mathbf{V}_{\text{obs}}, \boldsymbol{\Omega}, \boldsymbol{\theta}, \boldsymbol{\varphi}, \mathbf{r})$, $p(\boldsymbol{\varphi}|\mathbf{V}_{\text{obs}}, \mathbf{V}_{\text{mis}}, \boldsymbol{\Omega}, \boldsymbol{\theta}, \mathbf{r}) = p(\boldsymbol{\varphi}|\mathbf{V}, \boldsymbol{\Omega}, \boldsymbol{\theta}, \mathbf{r})$, and $p(\boldsymbol{\theta}|\mathbf{V}_{\text{obs}}, \mathbf{V}_{\text{mis}}, \boldsymbol{\Omega}, \boldsymbol{\varphi}, \mathbf{r}) = p(\boldsymbol{\theta}|\mathbf{V}, \boldsymbol{\Omega})$. Note that because of the data augmentation, the last conditional distribution does not depend on $\mathbf{r}$, and can be obtained as before. Details of these conditional distributions are presented in Appendix 5.5.

We again use the Bayes factor for model comparison. For two competing models M_0 and M_1, the Bayes factor is defined as

$$B_{10} = \frac{p(\mathbf{V}_{\text{obs}}, \mathbf{r}|M_1)}{p(\mathbf{V}_{\text{obs}}, \mathbf{r}|M_0)},$$

where

$$p(\mathbf{V}_{\text{obs}}, \mathbf{r}|M_k) = \int p(\mathbf{V}_{\text{obs}}, \mathbf{r}|\boldsymbol{\theta}_k, \boldsymbol{\varphi}_k)p(\boldsymbol{\theta}_k, \boldsymbol{\varphi}_k)d\boldsymbol{\theta}_k d\boldsymbol{\varphi}_k, \quad k = 0, 1,$$

is the marginal density of M_k with parameter vectors $\boldsymbol{\theta}_k$ and $\boldsymbol{\varphi}_k$, and $p(\boldsymbol{\theta}_k, \boldsymbol{\varphi}_k)$ is the prior density of $\boldsymbol{\theta}_k$ and $\boldsymbol{\varphi}_k$. The log Bayes factor is computed using the path sampling procedure (Gelman and Meng, 1998) as follows. Let $U(\boldsymbol{\theta}, \boldsymbol{\varphi}, \boldsymbol{\Omega}, \mathbf{V}_{\text{mis}}, \mathbf{V}_{\text{obs}}, \mathbf{r}, t) = d \log p(\boldsymbol{\Omega}, \mathbf{V}_{\text{mis}}, \mathbf{V}_{\text{obs}}, \mathbf{r}|\boldsymbol{\theta}, \boldsymbol{\varphi}, t)/dt$, where $p(\boldsymbol{\Omega}, \mathbf{V}_{\text{mis}}, \mathbf{V}_{\text{obs}}, \mathbf{r}|\boldsymbol{\theta}, \boldsymbol{\varphi}, t)$ is the complete-data likelihood function defined with a continuous parameter $t \in [0, 1]$. Let $0 = t_{(0)} < t_{(1)} < t_{(2)} < \ldots < t_{(S)} < t_{(S+1)} = 1$ be fixed and ordered grids; $\log B_{10}$ is then estimated by

$$\widehat{\log B_{10}} = \frac{1}{2}\sum_{s=0}^{S}(t_{(s+1)} - t_{(s)})(\bar{U}_{(s+1)} + \bar{U}_s),$$

where

$$\bar{U}_{(s)} = J^{-1}\sum_{j=1}^{J} U\left(\boldsymbol{\theta}^{(j)}, \boldsymbol{\varphi}^{(j)}, \boldsymbol{\Omega}^{(j)}, \mathbf{V}_{\text{mis}}^{(j)}, \mathbf{V}_{\text{obs}}, \mathbf{r}, t_{(s)}\right),$$

and $\{(\boldsymbol{\theta}^{(j)}, \boldsymbol{\varphi}^{(j)}, \boldsymbol{\Omega}^{(j)}, \mathbf{V}_{\text{mis}}^{(j)}), j = 1, \ldots, J\}$ are observations that are simulated from $p(\boldsymbol{\theta}, \boldsymbol{\varphi}, \boldsymbol{\Omega}, \mathbf{V}_{\text{mis}}|\mathbf{V}_{\text{obs}}, \mathbf{r}, t_{(s)})$.

5.4.5 An illustrative real example

To give an illustration of the Bayesian methodology, a small portion of the ICPSR data set collected by the World Values Survey 1981–1984 and 1990–1993 (World Values Study Group, 1994) is analyzed in this example (see also Lee, 2007). Here, eight variables from the original data set (variables 116, 117, 252, 253, 254, 296, 298, 314; see Appendix 1.1) are taken as observed variables $\mathbf{v} = (v_1, \ldots, v_8)$. These variables are measured on a 10-point scale; for convenience, they are treated as continuous. We choose the data corresponding to females in Russia, who answered either question 116 or 117, or both. Under this choice, most of the data were obtained from working females. There are 712 random observations in the data set, of which only 451 (63.34%) are fully observed cases. The missing data are rather complicated, with 69 different missingness patterns. Considering that the questions are related to either personal attitudes or personal morality, the corresponding missing data are treated as nonignorable. To roughly unify the scales, the raw data are standardized using the sample mean and sample standard deviation obtained from the fully observed data.

Based on the meanings of the questions corresponding to the observed variables, we use a nonlinear SEM with the following specifications. For the measurement equation, we consider $\boldsymbol{\mu} = (\mu_1, \ldots, \mu_8)^T$, and the following factor loading matrix with a non-overlapping structure:

$$\boldsymbol{\Lambda}^T = \begin{bmatrix} 1 & \lambda_{21} & 0 & 0 & 0 & 0 & 0 & 0 \\ 0 & 0 & 1 & \lambda_{42} & \lambda_{52} & 0 & 0 & 0 \\ 0 & 0 & 0 & 0 & 0 & 1 & \lambda_{73} & \lambda_{83} \end{bmatrix},$$

which corresponds to latent variables η, ξ_1 and ξ_2. The 1s and 0s in $\boldsymbol{\Lambda}$ are fixed to identify the model and to achieve a clear interpretation of latent variables. The latent variable η can be roughly interpreted as 'job satisfaction', and the latent variables ξ_1 and ξ_2 can be roughly interpreted as 'job attitude' and 'morality (in relation to money)', respectively. We first consider the following model M_1, which involves an encompassing structural equation with all second-order terms of ξ_{i1} and ξ_{i2}:

$$M_1 : \eta_i = \gamma_1\xi_{i1} + \gamma_2\xi_{i2} + \gamma_3\xi_{i1}\xi_{i2} + \gamma_4\xi_{i1}^2 + \gamma_5\xi_{i2}^2 + \delta_i.$$

The following three models are considered for assessing the missing data in this example:

$$\begin{aligned} &M_a : \text{logit}\{\Pr(r_{ij} = 1|\mathbf{v}_i, \boldsymbol{\omega}_i, \boldsymbol{\varphi})\} = \varphi_0 + \varphi_1 v_{i1} + \ldots + \varphi_8 v_{i8}, \\ &M_b : \text{logit}\{\Pr(r_{ij} = 1|\mathbf{v}_i, \boldsymbol{\omega}_i, \boldsymbol{\varphi})\} = \varphi_0 + \varphi_1\eta_i + \varphi_2\xi_{i1} + \varphi_3\xi_{i2}, \\ &M_c : \text{MAR}. \end{aligned}$$

Note that M_a involves all the observed variables, while M_b involves all the latent variables.

The log Bayes factors for comparing the above models M_a, M_b, and M_c under M_1 are computed via the path sampling procedure. The prior inputs in the conjugate prior distributions are selected as before via an auxiliary estimation. The number of grids in the path sampling procedure for computing all the log Bayes factors is taken to be 10; and for each $t_{(s)}$, 5000 simulated observations collected after 5000 burn-in iterations are used to compute $\bar{U}_{(s)}$. The estimated log Bayes factors are equal to $\widehat{\log B_{ab}^1} = 47.34$, and $\widehat{\log B_{ac}^1} = 43.85$, where the

Table 5.6 The estimated log Bayes factors: $\log B^r_{ab}$ and $\log B^r_{ac}$, $r = 1, 2, 3, 4$.

SEM	$\log B^r_{ab}$	$\log B^r_{ac}$
M_1	47.34	43.85
M_2	48.56	46.66
M_3	50.40	44.04
M_4	50.38	44.69

Reproduced by permission of *Psychometrika* from Lee, S. Y. and Tang, N. S. (2006). Bayesian analysis of nonlinear structural equation models with nonignorable missing data. *Psychometrika*, **57**, 131–150.

superscript denotes M_1, and subscripts denote the competing models for the missingness mechanism. Clearly, based on these results, the data give strong evidence to support the missing-data model M_a, which is in the form of (5.21), for modeling the nonignorable missing data. In addition to the encompassing M_1, we also consider the following nonlinear SEMs:

$$M_2: \ \eta_i = \gamma_1\xi_{i1} + \gamma_2\xi_{i2} + \gamma_3\xi_{i1}^2 + \delta_i,$$

$$M_3: \ \eta_i = \gamma_1\xi_{i1} + \gamma_2\xi_{i2} + \gamma_3\xi_{i1}\xi_{i2} + \delta_i,$$

$$M_4: \ \eta_i = \gamma_1\xi_{i1} + \gamma_2\xi_{i2} + \gamma_3\xi_{i2}^2 + \delta_i.$$

Under each of the above models, we compare the missingness mechanism models M_a, M_b, and M_c. The estimated log Bayes factors under these models, together with those under M_1, are reported in Table 5.6; for example, $\widehat{\log B^2_{ab}} = 48.56$ and $\widehat{\log B^3_{ac}} = 44.04$. It is clear from the results in this table that for every M_r, $r = 1, \ldots, 4$, the data strongly support M_a. In each case, Bayesian estimates obtained under M_a are significantly different from those obtained under MAR. To save space, these estimates are not reported. Based on the above comparison results, model M_a is used for comparing M_1, M_2, M_3 and M_4. In this model comparison, the estimated log Bayes factors are equal to $\widehat{\log B_{12}} = -1.29$, $\widehat{\log B_{32}} = -2.59$, and $\widehat{\log B_{42}} = -1.51$. These results provide evidence that the data support M_2.

The Bayesian estimates (EST) and their standard error estimates (SE) of the unknown parameters in the selected model M_2 are presented in the left-hand columns of Table 5.7. We observe that the estimates of the coefficients $\varphi_0, \varphi_2, \varphi_3, \varphi_4, \varphi_5, \varphi_6$, and φ_8 are significantly different from zero. Hence, the nonignorable missing-data model that accounts for the nature of the missing data is necessary. The factor loading estimates indicate strong associations between the latent variables and their indicators. From $\hat{\phi}_{11}$, $\hat{\phi}_{12}$ and $\hat{\phi}_{22}$, the estimate of the correlation between ξ_1 and ξ_2 is 0.163. This estimate indicates that 'job attitude' (ξ_1) and 'morality' (ξ_2) are weakly correlated. The estimated nonlinear structural equation is

$$\eta = -0.103\xi_1 + 0.072\xi_2 + 0.306\xi_1^2.$$

The interpretation of this equation in relation to the effects of the explanatory latent variables ξ_1 and ξ_2 on the outcome latent variable η is similar to the interpretation of the ordinary nonlinear structural equation.

The WinBUGS software (Spiegelhalter *et al.*, 2003) can be used to produce Bayesian solutions for SEMs with missing data that are MAR or missing with a nonignorable mechanism.

Table 5.7 Bayesian estimates of M_2 with M_a and their standard error estimates.

	Our method		WinBUGS			Our method		WinBUGS	
Par	EST	SE	EST	SE	Par	EST	SE	EST	SE
φ_0	−2.791	0.043	−2.794	0.076	μ_1	−0.135	0.038	−0.139	0.065
φ_1	0.038	0.033	0.040	0.059	μ_2	−0.136	0.032	−0.129	0.058
φ_2	−0.280	0.037	−0.280	0.068	μ_3	0.018	0.023	0.015	0.039
φ_3	0.370	0.036	0.365	0.073	μ_4	0.004	0.023	0.005	0.041
φ_4	−0.265	0.041	−0.262	0.083	μ_5	−0.129	0.026	−0.139	0.045
φ_5	−0.455	0.070	−0.502	0.126	μ_6	−0.046	0.023	−0.040	0.041
φ_6	−0.405	0.073	−0.341	0.154	μ_7	0.053	0.026	0.045	0.046
φ_7	0.059	0.056	0.013	0.134	μ_8	0.144	0.026	0.141	0.045
φ_8	0.332	0.038	0.323	0.061	λ_{21}	0.917	0.129	0.830	0.168
					λ_{42}	0.307	0.060	0.317	0.123
					λ_{52}	0.328	0.068	0.320	0.119
					λ_{73}	1.244	0.122	0.955	0.203
					λ_{83}	0.455	0.071	0.388	0.114
					$\psi_{\epsilon 1}$	0.544	0.067	0.508	0.096
					$\psi_{\epsilon 2}$	0.637	0.060	0.673	0.080
					$\psi_{\epsilon 3}$	0.493	0.058	0.492	0.111
					$\psi_{\epsilon 4}$	0.935	0.033	0.932	0.059
					$\psi_{\epsilon 5}$	0.907	0.039	0.922	0.068
					$\psi_{\epsilon 6}$	0.640	0.042	0.548	0.095
					$\psi_{\epsilon 7}$	0.612	0.051	0.714	0.086
					$\psi_{\epsilon 8}$	1.065	0.040	1.065	0.069
					γ_1	−0.103	0.047	−0.103	0.085
					γ_2	0.072	0.052	0.044	0.081
					γ_3	0.306	0.083	0.317	0.139
					ϕ_{11}	0.459	0.057	0.459	0.113
					ϕ_{12}	0.062	0.016	0.071	0.033
					ϕ_{22}	0.316	0.041	0.405	0.096
					ψ_δ	0.413	0.056	0.463	0.105

Reproduced by permission of *Psychometrika* from Lee, S. Y. and Tang, N. S. (2006). Bayesian analysis of nonlinear structural equation models with nonignorable missing data. *Psychometrika*, **57**, 131–150.

As nonignorable missing data subsume MAR missing data, we focus on the discussion of nonignorable missing data. In writing the WinBUGS code, in addition to specifying the SEM of interest, we need to specify the nonignorable missing-data model and the prior distributions in relation to the parameters in the missing-data model, etc.

The data set in this illustrative example has been reanalyzed by using WinBUGS with the same settings, for example, the same model structure and same prior inputs. Results obtained on the basis of M_2 with the missing-data model M_a are reported in the right-hand columns of Table 5.7. The DIC value corresponding to this model is 16 961.2. We observe that the estimates obtained from WinBUGS are close to the estimates that are presented in the left-hand columns of Table 5.7. However, the numerical standard error (SE) estimates produced by this general software are larger than those produced by our tailor-made program for the specific SEM. The WinBUGS code and the data are provided in the following website:

`www.wiley.com/go/medical_behavioral_sciences`

Appendix 5.1 Conditional distributions and implementation of the MH algorithm for SEMs with continuous and ordered categorical variables

We first consider the conditional distribution in step A of the Gibbs sampler. We note that as the underlying continuous measurements in $\mathbf{Y}$ are given, $\mathbf{Z}$ gives no additional information on this conditional distribution. Moreover, as the $\mathbf{v}_i$ are conditionally independent, and the $\boldsymbol{\omega}_i$ are also conditionally independent among themselves and independent of $\mathbf{Z}$, we have

$$p(\boldsymbol{\Omega}|\boldsymbol{\alpha}, \boldsymbol{\theta}, \mathbf{Y}, \mathbf{X}, \mathbf{Z}) = \prod_{i=1}^{n} p(\boldsymbol{\omega}_i|\mathbf{v}_i, \boldsymbol{\theta}).$$

It can be shown that

$$[\boldsymbol{\omega}_i|\mathbf{v}_i, \boldsymbol{\theta}] \stackrel{D}{=} N\big[\boldsymbol{\Sigma}^* \boldsymbol{\Lambda}^T \boldsymbol{\Psi}_\epsilon^{-1}(\mathbf{v}_i - \boldsymbol{\mu}), \boldsymbol{\Sigma}^*\big], \tag{5.A1}$$

where $\boldsymbol{\Sigma}^* = (\boldsymbol{\Sigma}_\omega^{-1} + \boldsymbol{\Lambda}^T \boldsymbol{\Psi}_\epsilon^{-1} \boldsymbol{\Lambda})^{-1}$, in which

$$\boldsymbol{\Sigma}_\omega = \begin{bmatrix} \boldsymbol{\Pi}_0^{-1}(\boldsymbol{\Gamma\Phi\Gamma}^T + \boldsymbol{\Psi}_\delta)\boldsymbol{\Pi}_0^{-T} & \boldsymbol{\Pi}_0^{-1}\boldsymbol{\Gamma\Phi} \\ \boldsymbol{\Phi\Gamma}^T\boldsymbol{\Pi}_0^{-T} & \boldsymbol{\Phi} \end{bmatrix}, \quad \boldsymbol{\Pi}_0 = \mathbf{I} - \boldsymbol{\Pi},$$

is the covariance matrix of $\boldsymbol{\omega}_i$. An alternative expression for this conditional distribution can be obtained from the following result: $p(\boldsymbol{\omega}_i|\mathbf{v}_i, \boldsymbol{\theta}) \propto p(\mathbf{v}_i|\boldsymbol{\omega}_i, \boldsymbol{\theta})p(\boldsymbol{\eta}_i|\boldsymbol{\xi}_i, \boldsymbol{\theta})p(\boldsymbol{\xi}_i|\boldsymbol{\theta})$. Based on the definition of the model and assumptions, $p(\boldsymbol{\omega}_i|\mathbf{v}_i, \boldsymbol{\theta})$ is proportional to

$$\begin{aligned} \exp\Big\{ & -\tfrac{1}{2}\big[(\mathbf{v}_i - \boldsymbol{\mu} - \boldsymbol{\Lambda\omega}_i)^T \boldsymbol{\Psi}_\epsilon^{-1}(\mathbf{v}_i - \boldsymbol{\mu} - \boldsymbol{\Lambda\omega}_i) \\ & + (\boldsymbol{\eta}_i - \boldsymbol{\Pi\eta}_i - \boldsymbol{\Gamma\xi}_i)^T \boldsymbol{\Psi}_\delta^{-1}(\boldsymbol{\eta}_i - \boldsymbol{\Pi\eta}_i - \boldsymbol{\Gamma\xi}_i) + \boldsymbol{\xi}_i^T \boldsymbol{\Phi}^{-1}\boldsymbol{\xi}_i\big]\Big\}. \end{aligned} \tag{5.A2}$$

Based on the practical experience available so far, simulating observations on the basis of (5.A1) or (5.A2) gives similar and acceptable results for statistical inference.

To derive the conditional distributions with respect to the structural parameters in step B, let $\boldsymbol{\theta}_v$ be the unknown parameters in $\boldsymbol{\mu}$, $\boldsymbol{\Lambda}$, and $\boldsymbol{\Psi}_\epsilon$ associated with (5.1), and let $\boldsymbol{\theta}_\omega$ be the unknown parameters in $\boldsymbol{\Lambda}_\omega$, $\boldsymbol{\Phi}$, and $\boldsymbol{\Psi}_\delta$ associated with (5.2). It is natural to take prior distributions such that $p(\boldsymbol{\theta}) = p(\boldsymbol{\theta}_v)p(\boldsymbol{\theta}_\omega)$.

We first consider the conditional distributions corresponding to $\boldsymbol{\theta}_v$. As before, the following commonly used conjugate type prior distributions are used:

$$\boldsymbol{\mu} \stackrel{D}{=} N[\boldsymbol{\mu}_0, \boldsymbol{\Sigma}_0], \psi_{\epsilon k}^{-1} \stackrel{D}{=} \text{Gamma}[\alpha_{0\epsilon k}, \beta_{0\epsilon k}],$$

$$[\boldsymbol{\Lambda}_k|\psi_{\epsilon k}] \stackrel{D}{=} N[\boldsymbol{\Lambda}_{0k}, \psi_{\epsilon k}\mathbf{H}_{0vk}], \quad k = 1, \ldots, p,$$

where $\psi_{\epsilon k}$ is the kth diagonal element of $\boldsymbol{\Psi}_\epsilon$; $\boldsymbol{\Lambda}_k^T$ is a $1 \times l_k$ row vector that only contains the unknown parameters in the kth row of $\boldsymbol{\Lambda}$; and $\alpha_{0\epsilon k}$, $\beta_{0\epsilon k}$, $\boldsymbol{\mu}_0$, $\boldsymbol{\Lambda}_{0k}$, $\mathbf{H}_{0vk}$, and $\boldsymbol{\Sigma}_0$ are hyperparameters whose values are assumed to be given. For $k \neq h$, it is assumed that $(\psi_{\epsilon k}, \boldsymbol{\Lambda}_k)$ and $(\psi_{\epsilon h}, \boldsymbol{\Lambda}_h)$ are independent. To cope with the case with fixed known elements in $\boldsymbol{\Lambda}$, let $\mathbf{L} = (l_{kj})_{p\times q}$ be the index matrix such that $l_{kj} = 0$ if λ_{kj} is known and $l_{kj} = 1$ if λ_{kj} is unknown, and $l_k = \sum_{j=1}^{q} l_{kj}$. Let $\boldsymbol{\Omega}_k$ be a submatrix of $\boldsymbol{\Omega}$ such that the jth row with $l_{kj} = 0$ deleted, and let $\mathbf{v}_k^* = (v_{1k}^*, \ldots, v_{nk}^*)^T$ with

$$v_{ik}^* = v_{ik} - \mu_k - \sum_{j=1}^{q} \lambda_{kj}\omega_{ij}(1 - l_{kj}),$$

where v_{ik} is the kth element of $\mathbf{v}_i$, and μ_k is the kth element of $\boldsymbol{\mu}$. Let $\boldsymbol{\Sigma}_{vk} = (\mathbf{H}_{0vk}^{-1} + \boldsymbol{\Omega}_k\boldsymbol{\Omega}_k^T)^{-1}$, $\boldsymbol{\mu}_{vk} = \boldsymbol{\Sigma}_{vk}[\mathbf{H}_{0vk}^{-1}\boldsymbol{\Lambda}_{0k} + \boldsymbol{\Omega}_k\mathbf{v}_k^*]$, and $\beta_{\epsilon k} = \beta_{0\epsilon k} + 2^{-1}(\mathbf{v}_k^{*T}\mathbf{v}_k^* - \boldsymbol{\mu}_{vk}^T\boldsymbol{\Sigma}_{vk}^{-1}\boldsymbol{\mu}_{vk} + \boldsymbol{\Lambda}_{0k}^T\mathbf{H}_{0vk}^{-1}\boldsymbol{\Lambda}_{0k})$. Then it can be shown that for $k = 1, \ldots, p$,

$$\begin{aligned}
&[\psi_{\epsilon k}^{-1}|\boldsymbol{\mu}, \mathbf{V}, \boldsymbol{\Omega}] \stackrel{D}{=} \text{Gamma}[n/2 + \alpha_{0\epsilon k}, \beta_{\epsilon k}],\\
&[\boldsymbol{\Lambda}_k|\psi_{\epsilon k}, \boldsymbol{\mu}, \mathbf{V}, \boldsymbol{\Omega}] \stackrel{D}{=} N[\boldsymbol{\mu}_{vk}, \psi_{\epsilon k}\boldsymbol{\Sigma}_{vk}],\\
&[\boldsymbol{\mu}|\boldsymbol{\Lambda}, \boldsymbol{\Psi}_\epsilon, \mathbf{V}, \boldsymbol{\Omega}] \stackrel{D}{=} N\big[\big(\boldsymbol{\Sigma}_0^{-1} + n\boldsymbol{\Psi}_\epsilon^{-1}\big)^{-1}\big(n\boldsymbol{\Psi}_\epsilon^{-1}\widetilde{\mathbf{V}} + \boldsymbol{\Sigma}_0^{-1}\boldsymbol{\mu}_0\big), \big(\boldsymbol{\Sigma}_0^{-1} + n\boldsymbol{\Psi}_\epsilon^{-1}\big)^{-1}\big],
\end{aligned} \tag{5.A3}$$

where $\widetilde{\mathbf{V}} = \sum_{i=1}^n(\mathbf{v}_i - \boldsymbol{\Lambda}\boldsymbol{\omega}_i)/n$.

Now consider the conditional distribution of $\boldsymbol{\theta}_\omega$. As the parameters in $\boldsymbol{\theta}_\omega$ are only involved in the structural equation, this conditional distribution is proportional to $p(\boldsymbol{\Omega}|\boldsymbol{\theta}_\omega)\ p(\boldsymbol{\theta}_\omega)$, which is independent of $\mathbf{V}$ and $\mathbf{Z}$. Let $\boldsymbol{\Omega}_1 = (\boldsymbol{\eta}_1, \ldots, \boldsymbol{\eta}_n)$ and $\boldsymbol{\Omega}_2 = (\boldsymbol{\xi}_1, \ldots, \boldsymbol{\xi}_n)$. Since the distribution of $\boldsymbol{\xi}_i$ only involves $\boldsymbol{\Phi}$, $p(\boldsymbol{\Omega}_2|\boldsymbol{\theta}_\omega) = p(\boldsymbol{\Omega}_2|\boldsymbol{\Phi})$. Moreover, we take the prior distribution of $\boldsymbol{\Phi}$ such that it is independent of the prior distributions of $\boldsymbol{\Lambda}_\omega$ and $\boldsymbol{\Psi}_\delta$. It follows that $p(\boldsymbol{\Omega}|\boldsymbol{\theta}_\omega)p(\boldsymbol{\theta}_\omega) \propto [p(\boldsymbol{\Omega}_1|\boldsymbol{\Omega}_2, \boldsymbol{\Lambda}_\omega, \boldsymbol{\Psi}_\delta)p(\boldsymbol{\Lambda}_\omega, \boldsymbol{\Psi}_\delta)][p(\boldsymbol{\Omega}_2|\boldsymbol{\Phi})p(\boldsymbol{\Phi})]$. Hence, the marginal conditional densities of $(\boldsymbol{\Lambda}_\omega, \boldsymbol{\Psi}_\delta)$ and $\boldsymbol{\Phi}$ can be treated separately.

Consider a conjugate type prior distribution for $\boldsymbol{\Phi}$ with $\boldsymbol{\Phi}^{-1} \stackrel{D}{=} W_{q_2}[\mathbf{R}_0, \rho_0]$, where ρ_0 and the positive definite matrix $\mathbf{R}_0$ are the given hyperparameters. It can be shown that

$$[\boldsymbol{\Phi}|\boldsymbol{\Omega}_2] \stackrel{D}{=} \text{IW}_{q_2}\big[\big(\boldsymbol{\Omega}_2\boldsymbol{\Omega}_2^T + \mathbf{R}_0^{-1}\big), n + \rho_0\big]. \tag{5.A4}$$

The prior distributions of elements in $(\boldsymbol{\Psi}_\delta, \boldsymbol{\Lambda}_\omega)$ are taken as

$$\psi_{\delta k}^{-1} \stackrel{D}{=} \text{Gamma}[\alpha_{0\delta k}, \beta_{0\delta k}], \quad [\boldsymbol{\Lambda}_{\omega k}|\psi_{\delta k}] \stackrel{D}{=} N[\boldsymbol{\Lambda}_{0\omega k}, \psi_{\delta k}\mathbf{H}_{0\omega k}],$$

where $k = 1, \ldots, q_1$, $\boldsymbol{\Lambda}_{\omega k}^T$ is a $1 \times l_{\omega k}$ row vector that contains the unknown parameters in the kth row of $\boldsymbol{\Lambda}_\omega$; and $\alpha_{0\delta k}$, $\beta_{0\delta k}$, $\boldsymbol{\Lambda}_{0\omega k}$, and $\mathbf{H}_{0\omega k}$ are given hyperparameters. For $h \neq k$, $(\psi_{\delta k}, \boldsymbol{\Lambda}_{\omega k})$ and $(\psi_{\delta h}, \boldsymbol{\Lambda}_{\omega h})$ are assumed to be independent. Let $\mathbf{L}_\omega = (l_{\omega kj})_{q_1 \times q}$ be the index matrix associated with $\boldsymbol{\Lambda}_\omega$, and $l_{\omega k} = \sum_{j=1}^q l_{\omega kj}$. Let $\boldsymbol{\Omega}_k^*$ be the submatrix of $\boldsymbol{\Omega}$ such that all the jth rows corresponding to $l_{\omega kj} = 0$ are deleted; and $\boldsymbol{\Omega}_{\eta k}^* = (\eta_{1k}^*, \ldots, \eta_{nk}^*)^T$ with

$$\eta_{ik}^* = \eta_{ik} - \sum_{j=1}^{q} \lambda_{\omega kj}\omega_{ij}(1 - l_{\omega kj}),$$

where ω_{ij} is the jth element of $\boldsymbol{\omega}_i$. Then it can be shown that

$$[\psi_{\delta k}^{-1}|\boldsymbol{\Omega}] \stackrel{D}{=} \text{Gamma}[n/2 + \alpha_{0\delta k}, \beta_{\delta k}], \quad [\boldsymbol{\Lambda}_{\omega k}|\boldsymbol{\Omega}, \psi_{\delta k}] \stackrel{D}{=} N[\boldsymbol{\mu}_{\omega k}, \psi_{\delta k}\boldsymbol{\Sigma}_{\omega k}], \tag{5.A5}$$

where $\boldsymbol{\Sigma}_{\omega k} = (\mathbf{H}_{0\omega k}^{-1} + \boldsymbol{\Omega}_k^*\boldsymbol{\Omega}_k^{*T})^{-1}$, $\boldsymbol{\mu}_{\omega k} = \boldsymbol{\Sigma}_{\omega k}[\mathbf{H}_{0\omega k}^{-1}\boldsymbol{\Lambda}_{0\omega k} + \boldsymbol{\Omega}_k^*\boldsymbol{\Omega}_{\eta k}^*]$, and $\beta_{\delta k} = \beta_{0\delta k} + 2^{-1}(\boldsymbol{\Omega}_{\eta k}^{*T}\boldsymbol{\Omega}_{\eta k}^* - \boldsymbol{\mu}_{\omega k}^T\boldsymbol{\Sigma}_{\omega k}^{-1}\boldsymbol{\mu}_{\omega k} + \boldsymbol{\Lambda}_{0\omega k}^T\mathbf{H}_{0\omega k}^{-1}\boldsymbol{\Lambda}_{0\omega k})$.

Finally, we consider the joint conditional distribution of $(\boldsymbol{\alpha}, \mathbf{Y})$ given $\boldsymbol{\theta}$, $\boldsymbol{\Omega}$, $\mathbf{X}$, and $\mathbf{Z}$. Suppose that the model in relation to the subvector $\mathbf{y}_i = (y_{i1}, \ldots, y_{is})^T$ of $\mathbf{v}_i$ is given by

$$\mathbf{y}_i = \boldsymbol{\mu}_y + \boldsymbol{\Lambda}_y\boldsymbol{\omega}_i + \boldsymbol{\epsilon}_{yi},$$

where $\boldsymbol{\mu}_y(s \times 1)$ is a subvector of $\boldsymbol{\mu}$, $\boldsymbol{\Lambda}_y(s \times q)$ is a submatrix of $\boldsymbol{\Lambda}$, and $\boldsymbol{\epsilon}_{yi}(s \times 1)$ is a subvector of $\boldsymbol{\epsilon}_i$ with diagonal covariance submatrix $\boldsymbol{\Psi}_y$ of $\boldsymbol{\Psi}_\epsilon$. Let $\mathbf{z}_i = (z_{i1}, \ldots, z_{is})^T$ be the ordered categorical observation corresponding to $\mathbf{y}_i$, $i = 1, \ldots, n$. We use the following noninformative prior distribution for the unknown thresholds in $\boldsymbol{\alpha}_k$:

$$p(\alpha_{k,2}, \ldots, \alpha_{k,b_k-1}) \propto C, \quad \text{for } \alpha_{k,2} < \ldots < \alpha_{k,b_k-1}, \; k = 1, \ldots, s,$$

where C is a constant. Given $\boldsymbol{\Omega}$ and the fact that the covariance matrix $\boldsymbol{\Psi}_y$ is diagonal, the ordered categorical data $\mathbf{Z}$ and the thresholds corresponding to different rows are also conditionally independent. For $k = 1, \ldots, s$, let $\mathbf{Y}_k^T$ and $\mathbf{Z}_k^T$ be the kth rows of $\mathbf{Y}$ and $\mathbf{Z}$, respectively. It can be shown (Cowles, 1996) that

$$p(\boldsymbol{\alpha}_k, \mathbf{Y}_k|\mathbf{Z}_k, \boldsymbol{\theta}, \boldsymbol{\Omega}) = p(\boldsymbol{\alpha}_k|\mathbf{Z}_k, \boldsymbol{\theta}, \boldsymbol{\Omega})p(\mathbf{Y}_k|\boldsymbol{\alpha}_k, \mathbf{Z}_k, \boldsymbol{\theta}, \boldsymbol{\Omega}), \tag{5.A6}$$

where

$$p(\boldsymbol{\alpha}_k|\mathbf{Z}_k, \boldsymbol{\theta}, \boldsymbol{\Omega}) \propto \prod_{i=1}^n \Big[\Phi^*\left\{\psi_{yk}^{-1/2}(\alpha_{k,z_{ik}+1} - \mu_{yk} - \boldsymbol{\Lambda}_{yk}^T\boldsymbol{\omega}_i)\right\} - \Phi^*\left\{\psi_{yk}^{-1/2}(\alpha_{k,z_{ik}} - \mu_{yk} - \boldsymbol{\Lambda}_{yk}^T\boldsymbol{\omega}_i)\right\}\Big], \tag{5.A7}$$

and $p(\mathbf{Y}_k|\boldsymbol{\alpha}_k, \mathbf{Z}_k, \boldsymbol{\theta}, \boldsymbol{\Omega})$ is the product of $p(y_{ik}|\boldsymbol{\alpha}_k, \mathbf{Z}_k, \boldsymbol{\theta}, \boldsymbol{\Omega})$, where

$$[y_{ik}|\boldsymbol{\alpha}_k, \mathbf{Z}_k, \boldsymbol{\theta}, \boldsymbol{\Omega}] \stackrel{D}{=} N\big[\mu_{yk} + \boldsymbol{\Lambda}_{yk}^T\boldsymbol{\omega}_i, \psi_{yk}\big]I_{[\alpha_{k,z_{ik}}, \alpha_{k,z_{ik}+1})}(y_{ik}), \tag{5.A8}$$

in which ψ_{yk} is the kth diagonal element of $\boldsymbol{\Psi}_y$, μ_{yk} is the kth element of $\boldsymbol{\mu}_y$, $\boldsymbol{\Lambda}_{yk}^T$ is the kth row of $\boldsymbol{\Lambda}_y$, $I_A(y)$ is an index function which takes 1 if $y \in A$ and 0 otherwise, and $\Phi^*(\cdot)$ denotes the distribution function of $N[0, 1]$. As a result,

$$p(\boldsymbol{\alpha}_k, \mathbf{Y}_k|\mathbf{Z}_k, \boldsymbol{\theta}, \boldsymbol{\Omega}) \propto \prod_{i=1}^n \phi\left\{\psi_{yk}^{-1/2}(y_{ik} - \mu_{yk} - \boldsymbol{\Lambda}_{yk}^T\boldsymbol{\omega}_i)\right\} I_{[\alpha_{k,z_{ik}}, \alpha_{k,z_{ik}+1})}(y_{ik}), \tag{5.A9}$$

where $\phi(\cdot)$ is the standard normal density.

To sample from the conditional distributions (5.A2) and (5.A9), the MH algorithm is implemented as follows.

For $p(\boldsymbol{\omega}_i|\mathbf{v}_i, \boldsymbol{\theta})$, we choose $N[\mathbf{0}, \sigma^2\boldsymbol{\Sigma}^*]$ as the proposal distribution, where $\boldsymbol{\Sigma}^{*-1} = \boldsymbol{\Sigma}_\omega^{-1} + \boldsymbol{\Lambda}^T\boldsymbol{\Psi}_\epsilon^{-1}\boldsymbol{\Lambda}$, with

$$\boldsymbol{\Sigma}_\omega^{-1} = \begin{bmatrix} \boldsymbol{\Pi}_0^T\boldsymbol{\Psi}_\delta^{-1}\boldsymbol{\Pi}_0 & -\boldsymbol{\Pi}_0^T\boldsymbol{\Psi}_\delta^{-1}\boldsymbol{\Gamma} \\ -\boldsymbol{\Gamma}^T\boldsymbol{\Psi}_\delta^{-1}\boldsymbol{\Pi}_0 & \boldsymbol{\Phi}^{-1} + \boldsymbol{\Gamma}^T\boldsymbol{\Psi}_\delta^{-1}\boldsymbol{\Gamma} \end{bmatrix}.$$

Let $p(\cdot|\mathbf{0}, \sigma^2, \boldsymbol{\Sigma}^*)$ be the proposal density corresponding to $N[\mathbf{0}, \sigma^2\boldsymbol{\Sigma}^*]$, where σ^2 is an appropriate preassigned constant. The MH algorithm is implemented as follows: at the jth MH iteration with a current value $\boldsymbol{\omega}_i^{(j)}$, a new candidate $\boldsymbol{\omega}_i$ is generated from $p(\cdot|\boldsymbol{\omega}_i^{(j)}, \sigma^2, \boldsymbol{\Sigma}^*)$, and this new candidate is accepted with probability

$$\min\left\{1, \frac{p(\boldsymbol{\omega}_i|\mathbf{v}_i, \boldsymbol{\theta})}{p(\boldsymbol{\omega}_i^{(j)}|\mathbf{v}_i, \boldsymbol{\theta})}\right\},$$

where $p(\boldsymbol{\omega}_i|\mathbf{v}_i, \boldsymbol{\theta})$ is given by (5.A2).

For $p(\boldsymbol{\alpha}_k, \mathbf{Y}_k|\mathbf{Z}_k, \boldsymbol{\theta}, \boldsymbol{\Omega})$, we use equality (5.A6) to construct a joint proposal density for $\boldsymbol{\alpha}_k$, and $\mathbf{Y}_k$ in the MH algorithm for generating observations from it. At the jth MH iteration, we generate a vector of thresholds $(\alpha_{k,2}, \ldots, \alpha_{k,b_k-1})$ from the following univariate truncated normal distribution:

$$\alpha_{k,z} \stackrel{D}{=} N\left[\alpha_{k,z}^{(j)}, \sigma_{\alpha_k}^2\right] I_{(\alpha_{k,z-1}, \alpha_{k,z+1}^{(j)}]}(\alpha_{k,z}) \quad \text{for } z = 2, \ldots, b_k - 1,$$

where $\alpha_{k,z}^{(j)}$ is the current value of $\alpha_{k,z}$ at the jth iteration of the Gibbs sampler, and $\sigma_{\alpha_k}^2$ is an appropriate preassigned constant. Random observations from the above univariate truncated normal are simulated via the algorithm of Roberts (1995). Then, the acceptance probability for $(\boldsymbol{\alpha}_k, \mathbf{Y}_k)$ as a new observation is $\min\{1, R_k\}$, where

$$R_k = \prod_{z=2}^{b_k-1} \frac{\Phi^*\left\{\left(\alpha_{k,z+1}^{(j)} - \alpha_{k,z}^{(j)}\right)/\sigma_{\alpha_k}\right\} - \Phi^*\left\{\left(\alpha_{k,z-1} - \alpha_{k,z}^{(j)}\right)/\sigma_{\alpha_k}\right\}}{\Phi^*\left\{\left(\alpha_{k,z+1} - \alpha_{k,z}\right)/\sigma_{\alpha_k}\right\} - \Phi^*\left\{\left(\alpha_{k,z-1}^{(j)} - \alpha_{k,z}\right)/\sigma_{\alpha_k}\right\}}$$

$$\times \prod_{i=1}^{n} \frac{\Phi^*\left\{\psi_{yk}^{-1/2}\left(\alpha_{k,z_{ik}+1} - \mu_{yk} - \boldsymbol{\Lambda}_{yk}^T\boldsymbol{\omega}_i\right)\right\} - \Phi^*\left\{\psi_{yk}^{-1/2}\left(\alpha_{k,z_{ik}} - \mu_{yk} - \boldsymbol{\Lambda}_{yk}^T\boldsymbol{\omega}_i\right)\right\}}{\Phi^*\left\{\psi_{yk}^{-1/2}\left(\alpha_{k,z_{ik}+1}^{(j)} - \mu_{yk} - \boldsymbol{\Lambda}_{yk}^T\boldsymbol{\omega}_i\right)\right\} - \Phi^*\left\{\psi_{yk}^{-1/2}\left(\alpha_{k,z_{ik}}^{(j)} - \mu_{yk} - \boldsymbol{\Lambda}_{yk}^T\boldsymbol{\omega}_i\right)\right\}}.$$

As R_k only depends on the old and new values of $\boldsymbol{\alpha}_k$ and not on $\mathbf{Y}_k$, it does not require a new $\mathbf{Y}_k$ to be generated in any iteration in which the new value of $\boldsymbol{\alpha}_k$ is not accepted (see Cowles, 1996). For an accepted $\boldsymbol{\alpha}_k$, a new $\mathbf{Y}_k$ is simulated from (5.A8).

Appendix 5.2 Conditional distributions and implementation of MH algorithm for SEMs with EFDs

It can be shown that the full conditional distribution of $\mathbf{\Omega}$ is given by

$$p(\mathbf{\Omega}|\mathbf{Y}, \boldsymbol{\theta}) = \prod_{i=1}^{n} p(\boldsymbol{\omega}_i|\mathbf{y}_i, \boldsymbol{\theta}) \propto \prod_{i=1}^{n} p(\mathbf{y}_i|\boldsymbol{\omega}_i, \boldsymbol{\theta}) p(\boldsymbol{\eta}_i|\boldsymbol{\xi}_i, \boldsymbol{\theta}) p(\boldsymbol{\xi}_i|\boldsymbol{\theta}),$$

where $p(\boldsymbol{\omega}_i|\mathbf{y}_i, \boldsymbol{\theta})$ is proportional to

$$\exp\Bigg\{ \sum_{k=1}^{p} \Big[y_{ik}\vartheta_{ik} - b(\vartheta_{ik}) \Big] / \psi_{\epsilon k} \\ -\tfrac{1}{2}\Big[(\boldsymbol{\eta}_i - \mathbf{Bd}_i - \mathbf{\Pi}\boldsymbol{\eta}_i - \mathbf{\Gamma F}(\boldsymbol{\xi}_i))^T \mathbf{\Psi}_\delta^{-1} (\boldsymbol{\eta}_i - \mathbf{Bd}_i - \mathbf{\Pi}\boldsymbol{\eta}_i - \mathbf{\Gamma F}(\boldsymbol{\xi}_i)) + \boldsymbol{\xi}_i^T \mathbf{\Phi}^{-1} \boldsymbol{\xi}_i \Big] \Bigg\}. \tag{5.A10}$$

Under the conjugate prior distributions given in (5.13), it can be shown that the full conditional distributions of the components of $\boldsymbol{\theta}$ are given by

$$p(\mathbf{A}_k|\mathbf{Y}, \mathbf{\Omega}, \mathbf{\Lambda}_k, \psi_{\epsilon k}) \propto \exp\left\{ \sum_{i=1}^{n} \frac{y_{ik}\vartheta_{ik} - b(\vartheta_{ik})}{\psi_{\epsilon k}} - \frac{1}{2}(\mathbf{A}_k - \mathbf{A}_{0k})^T \mathbf{H}_{0k}^{-1} (\mathbf{A}_k - \mathbf{A}_{0k}) \right\},$$

$$p(\psi_{\epsilon k}|\mathbf{Y}, \mathbf{\Omega}, \mathbf{A}_k, \mathbf{\Lambda}_k) \propto \psi_{\epsilon k}^{-(\frac{n}{2}+\alpha_{0\epsilon k}-1)} \exp\left\{ \sum_{i=1}^{n} \left[\frac{y_{ik}\vartheta_{ik} - b(\vartheta_{ik})}{\psi_{\epsilon k}} + c_k(y_{ik}, \psi_{\epsilon k}) \right] - \frac{\beta_{0k}}{\psi_{\epsilon k}} \right\},$$

$$p(\mathbf{\Lambda}_k|\mathbf{Y}, \mathbf{\Omega}, \mathbf{A}_k, \psi_{\epsilon k}) \propto \exp\left\{ \sum_{i=1}^{n} \frac{y_{ik}\vartheta_{ik} - b(\vartheta_{ik})}{\psi_{\epsilon k}} - \frac{1}{2}\psi_{\epsilon k}^{-1} (\mathbf{\Lambda}_k - \mathbf{\Lambda}_{0k})^T \mathbf{H}_{0yk}^{-1} (\mathbf{\Lambda}_k - \mathbf{\Lambda}_{0k}) \right\},$$

$$[\psi_{\delta k}^{-1}|\mathbf{\Omega}, \mathbf{\Lambda}_{\omega k}] \stackrel{D}{=} \text{Gamma}[n/2 + \alpha_{0\delta k}, \beta_{\delta k}],$$

$$[\mathbf{\Lambda}_{\omega k}|\mathbf{\Omega}, \psi_{\delta k}] \stackrel{D}{=} N[\boldsymbol{\mu}_{\omega k}, \psi_{\delta k}\mathbf{\Sigma}_{\omega k}],$$

$$[\mathbf{\Phi}|\mathbf{\Omega}] \stackrel{D}{=} \text{IW}_{q_2}\left[\left(\mathbf{\Omega}_2\mathbf{\Omega}_2^T + \mathbf{R}_0^{-1} \right), n + \rho_0 \right], \tag{5.A11}$$

where $\mathbf{\Sigma}_{\omega k} = (\mathbf{H}_{0\omega k}^{-1} + \mathbf{G}\mathbf{G}^T)^{-1}$, $\boldsymbol{\mu}_{\omega k} = \mathbf{\Sigma}_{\omega k}(\mathbf{H}_{0\omega k}^{-1}\mathbf{\Lambda}_{0\omega k} + \mathbf{G}\mathbf{\Omega}_{1k})$, and $\beta_{\delta k} = \beta_{0\delta k} + (\mathbf{\Omega}_{1k}^T\mathbf{\Omega}_{1k} - \boldsymbol{\mu}_{\omega k}^T\mathbf{\Sigma}_{\omega k}^{-1}\boldsymbol{\mu}_{\omega k} + \mathbf{\Lambda}_{0\omega k}^T\mathbf{H}_{0\omega k}^{-1}\mathbf{\Lambda}_{0\omega k})/2$, in which $\mathbf{G} = (\mathbf{G}(\boldsymbol{\omega}_1), \ldots, \mathbf{G}(\boldsymbol{\omega}_n))$, $\mathbf{\Omega}_1 = (\boldsymbol{\eta}_1, \ldots, \boldsymbol{\eta}_n)$, $\mathbf{\Omega}_2 = (\boldsymbol{\xi}_1, \ldots, \boldsymbol{\xi}_n)$, and $\mathbf{\Omega}_{1k}^T$ is the kth row of $\mathbf{\Omega}_1$.

In simulating observations from $p(\boldsymbol{\omega}_i|\mathbf{y}_i, \boldsymbol{\theta})$ in (5.A10), we choose $N[\cdot, \sigma_\omega^2\mathbf{\Omega}_\omega]$ as the proposal distribution in the MH algorithm, where $\mathbf{\Omega}_\omega^{-1} = \mathbf{\Sigma}_\omega^* + \mathbf{\Lambda}^T\mathbf{\Psi}_\omega\mathbf{\Lambda}$, in which

$$\mathbf{\Sigma}_\omega^* = \begin{bmatrix} \mathbf{\Pi}_0^T\mathbf{\Psi}_\delta^{-1}\mathbf{\Pi}_0 & -\mathbf{\Pi}_0^T\mathbf{\Psi}_\delta^{-1}\mathbf{\Gamma\Delta} \\ -\mathbf{\Delta}^T\mathbf{\Gamma}^T\mathbf{\Psi}_\delta^{-1}\mathbf{\Pi}_0 & \mathbf{\Phi}^{-1} + \mathbf{\Delta}^T\mathbf{\Gamma}^T\mathbf{\Psi}_\delta^{-1}\mathbf{\Gamma\Delta} \end{bmatrix},$$

with $\mathbf{\Pi}_0 = \mathbf{I}_{q_1} - \mathbf{\Pi}$, $\mathbf{\Delta} = (\partial\mathbf{F}(\boldsymbol{\xi}_i)/\partial\boldsymbol{\xi}_i)^T|_{\boldsymbol{\xi}_i=\mathbf{0}}$, and $\mathbf{\Psi}_\omega = \text{diag}(\ddot{b}(\vartheta_{i1})/\psi_{\epsilon 1}, \ldots, \ddot{b}(\vartheta_{ip})/\psi_{\epsilon p})|_{\boldsymbol{\omega}_i=\mathbf{0}}$.

In simulating observations from the conditional distributions $p(\mathbf{A}_k|\mathbf{Y}, \mathbf{\Omega}, \mathbf{\Lambda}_k, \psi_{\epsilon k})$, $p(\psi_{\epsilon k}\ |\mathbf{Y}, \mathbf{\Omega}, \mathbf{A}_k, \mathbf{\Lambda}_k)$, and $p(\mathbf{\Lambda}_k|\mathbf{Y}, \mathbf{\Omega}, \mathbf{A}_k, \psi_{\epsilon k})$, the proposal distributions are $N[\cdot, \sigma_a^2\mathbf{\Omega}_{ak}]$,

$N[\cdot, \sigma_\psi^2 \Omega_{\psi k}]$, and $N[\cdot, \sigma_\lambda^2 \boldsymbol{\Omega}_{\lambda k}]$, respectively, where

$$\boldsymbol{\Omega}_{ak}^{-1} = \sum_{i=1}^{n} \ddot{b}(\vartheta_{ik}) \mathbf{c}_{ik} \mathbf{c}_{ik}^T / \psi_{\epsilon k} \Big|_{\mathbf{A}_k = \mathbf{0}} + \mathbf{H}_{0k}^{-1},$$

$$\Omega_{\psi k}^{-1} = 1 - n/2 - \alpha_{0\epsilon k} - 2 \sum_{i=1}^{n} [y_{ik}\vartheta_{ik} - b(\vartheta_{ik})] - \ddot{c}_k(y_{ik}, \psi_{\epsilon k}) \Big|_{\psi_{\epsilon k}=1} + 2\beta_{0\epsilon k},$$

$$\boldsymbol{\Omega}_{\lambda k}^{-1} = \sum_{i=1}^{n} \ddot{b}(\vartheta_{ik}) \boldsymbol{\omega}_i \boldsymbol{\omega}_i^T \Big|_{\boldsymbol{\Lambda}_k = \mathbf{0}} + \psi_{\epsilon k}^{-1} \mathbf{H}_{0yk}^{-1}.$$

To improve efficiency, we respectively use $N[\boldsymbol{\mu}_{ak}, \boldsymbol{\Omega}_{ak}]$, $N[\mu_{\psi k}, \boldsymbol{\Omega}_{\psi k}]$, and $N[\boldsymbol{\mu}_{\lambda k}, \boldsymbol{\Omega}_{\lambda k}]$ as initial proposal distributions in the first few iterations, where

$$\boldsymbol{\mu}_{ak} = \sum_{i=1}^{n} \left[y_{ik} - \dot{b}(\vartheta_{ik})|_{\mathbf{A}_k=\mathbf{0}} \right] \frac{\mathbf{c}_{ik}}{\psi_{\epsilon k}} + \mathbf{H}_{0k}^{-1} \mathbf{A}_{0k},$$

$$\mu_{\psi k} = 1 - n/2 - \alpha_{0\epsilon k} - \sum_{i=1}^{n} \left[y_{ik}\vartheta_{ik} - b(\vartheta_{ik}) \right] + \dot{c}_k(y_{ik}, \psi_{\epsilon k}) \Big|_{\psi_{\epsilon k}=1} + \beta_{0\epsilon k},$$

$$\boldsymbol{\mu}_{\lambda k} = \sum_{i=1}^{n} \left[y_{ik} - \dot{b}(\vartheta_{ik})|_{\boldsymbol{\Lambda}_k=\mathbf{0}} \right] \frac{\boldsymbol{\omega}_i}{\psi_{\epsilon k}} + \mathbf{H}_{0yk}^{-1} \boldsymbol{\Lambda}_{0k}.$$

Let $\mathbf{y}_k^{*T}$ be the kth row of $\mathbf{Y}$ which is not directly observable, $\mathbf{z}_k$ be the corresponding ordered categorical vector, and $\boldsymbol{\alpha}_k = (\alpha_{k,2}, \ldots, \alpha_{k,b_k-1})$. It can be shown by derivation similar to that in Appendix 5.1 that

$$\begin{aligned} p(\boldsymbol{\alpha}_k, \mathbf{y}_k^* | \mathbf{z}_k, \boldsymbol{\Omega}, \boldsymbol{\theta}) &= p(\boldsymbol{\alpha}_k | \mathbf{z}_k, \boldsymbol{\Omega}, \boldsymbol{\theta}) p(\mathbf{y}_k^* | \boldsymbol{\alpha}_k, \mathbf{z}_k, \boldsymbol{\Omega}, \boldsymbol{\theta}) \\ &\propto \prod_{i=1}^{n} \exp\left\{ [y_{ik}^* \vartheta_{ik} - b(\vartheta_{ik})]/\psi_{\epsilon k} + c_k(y_{ik}^*, \psi_{\epsilon k}) \right\} I_{[\alpha_{k,z_{ik}}, \alpha_{k,z_{ik}+1})}(y_{ik}^*), \end{aligned} \tag{5.A12}$$

where $I_A(y)$ is an indicator function which takes 1 if $y \in A$, and 0 otherwise. The treatment of dichotomous variables is similar.

A multivariate version of the MH algorithm is used to simulate observations from $p(\boldsymbol{\alpha}_k, \mathbf{y}_k^* | \mathbf{z}_k, \boldsymbol{\Omega}, \boldsymbol{\theta})$ in (5.A12). Following Cowles (1996), the joint proposal distribution of $\boldsymbol{\alpha}_k$ and $\mathbf{y}_k^*$ given $\mathbf{z}_k$, $\boldsymbol{\Omega}$, and $\boldsymbol{\theta}$ can be constructed according to the factorization $p(\boldsymbol{\alpha}_k, \mathbf{y}_k^* | \mathbf{z}_k, \boldsymbol{\Omega}, \boldsymbol{\theta}) = p(\boldsymbol{\alpha}_k | \mathbf{z}_k, \boldsymbol{\Omega}, \boldsymbol{\theta}) p(\mathbf{y}_k^* | \boldsymbol{\alpha}_k, \mathbf{z}_k, \boldsymbol{\Omega}, \boldsymbol{\theta})$. At the jth iteration, we generate a candidate vector of thresholds $(\alpha_{k,2}, \ldots, \alpha_{k,b_k-1})$ from the following univariate truncated normal distribution:

$$\alpha_{k,m} \sim N\left[\alpha_{k,m}^{(j)}, \sigma_{\alpha_k}^2\right] I_{(\alpha_{k,m-1}, \alpha_{k,m+1}^{(j)}]}(\alpha_{k,m}), \quad \text{for } m = 2, \ldots, b_k - 1,$$

where $\alpha_{k,m}^{(j)}$ is the current value of $\alpha_{k,m}$, and $\sigma_{\alpha_k}^2$ is chosen to obtain an average acceptance rate of approximately 0.25 or greater. The acceptance probability for a candidate vector $(\boldsymbol{\alpha}_k, \mathbf{y}_k^*)$ as a new observation $(\boldsymbol{\alpha}_k^{(j+1)}, \mathbf{y}_k^{*(j+1)})$ is $\min\{1, R_k\}$, where

$$R_k = \frac{p\left(\boldsymbol{\alpha}_k, \mathbf{y}_k^* | \mathbf{z}_k, \boldsymbol{\Omega}, \boldsymbol{\theta}\right) p\left(\boldsymbol{\alpha}_k^{(j)}, \mathbf{y}_k^{*(j)} | \boldsymbol{\alpha}_k, \mathbf{y}_k^*, \mathbf{z}_k, \boldsymbol{\Omega}, \boldsymbol{\theta}\right)}{p\left(\boldsymbol{\alpha}_k^{(j)}, \mathbf{y}_k^{*(j)} | \mathbf{z}_k, \boldsymbol{\Omega}, \boldsymbol{\theta}\right) p\left(\boldsymbol{\alpha}_k, \mathbf{y}_k^* | \boldsymbol{\alpha}_k^{(j)}, \mathbf{y}_k^{*(j)}, \mathbf{z}_k, \boldsymbol{\Omega}, \boldsymbol{\theta}\right)}.$$

For an accepted $\boldsymbol{\alpha}_k$, a new $\mathbf{y}_k^*$ is simulated from the following univariate truncated distribution:

$$[y_{ik}^*|\boldsymbol{\alpha}_k, z_{ik}, \boldsymbol{\omega}_i, \boldsymbol{\theta}] \stackrel{D}{=} \exp\{[y_{ik}^*\vartheta_{ik} - b(\vartheta_{ik})]/\psi_{\epsilon k} + c_k(y_{ik}^*, \psi_{\epsilon k})\} I_{[\alpha_{k,z_{ik}}, \alpha_{k,z_{ik}+1})}(y_{ik}^*),$$

where y_{ik}^* and z_{ik} are the ith components of $\mathbf{y}_k^*$ and $\mathbf{z}_k$, respectively, and $I_A(y)$ is an indicator function which takes 1 if y in A and zero otherwise.

Appendix 5.3 WinBUGS code related to section 5.3.4

```
model {
    for(i in 1:N){
        #Measurement equation model
        for(j in 1:3){
            y[i,j]~dnorm(mu[i,j],1)I(low[z[i,j]+1],high[z[i,j]+1])
        }
        for(j in 4:P){
            z[i,j]~dbin(pb[i,j],1)
            pb[i,j]<-exp(mu[i,j])/(1+exp(mu[i,j]))
        }
        mu[i,1]<-uby[1]+eta[i]
        mu[i,2]<-uby[2]+lam[1]*eta[i]
        mu[i,3]<-uby[3]+lam[2]*eta[i]
        mu[i,4]<-uby[4]+xi[i,1]
        mu[i,5]<-uby[5]+lam[3]*xi[i,1]
        mu[i,6]<-uby[6]+lam[4]*xi[i,1]
        mu[i,7]<-uby[7]+xi[i,2]
        mu[i,8]<-uby[8]+lam[5]*xi[i,2]
        mu[i,9]<-uby[9]+lam[6]*xi[i,2]

        #Structural equation model
        xi[i,1:2]~dmnorm(zero2[1:2],phi[1:2,1:2])
        eta[i]~dnorm(etamu[i],psd)
        etamu[i]<-ubeta*c[i]+gam[1]*xi[i,1]+gam[2]*xi[i,2]
                  +gam[3]*xi[i,1]*xi[i,2]
    } #End of i

    for(i in 1:2){ zero2[i]<-0 }

    #Priors inputs for loadings and coefficients
    for (i in 1:P){ uby[i]~dnorm(1.0,4.0) }
    lam[1]~dnorm(0.7,4.0);    lam[2]~dnorm(0.7,4.0)
    lam[3]~dnorm(0.8,4.0);    lam[4]~dnorm(0.8,4.0)
    lam[5]~dnorm(0.7,4.0);    lam[6]~dnorm(0.7,4.0)
    ubeta~dnorm(0.8,4.0)

    var.gam<-4.0*psd
    gam[1]~dnorm(0.6,var.gam);    gam[2]~dnorm(0.6,var.gam)
    gam[3]~dnorm(0.8,var.gam)

    #Priors inputs for precisions
    psd~dgamma(9,3);    sgd<-1/psd
    phi[1:2,1:2]~dwish(R[1:2,1:2], 10)
    phx[1:2,1:2]<-inverse(phi[1:2,1:2])
} #end
```

Appendix 5.4 R2WinBUGS code related to section 5.3.4

```
library(MASS)       #Load the MASS package
library(R2WinBUGS) #Load the R2WinBUGS package
library(boa)        #Load the boa package

N<-2000; P<-9

phi<-matrix(data=c(1.0,0.3,0.3,1.0),ncol=2) #The covariance matrix of xi
Ro<-matrix(data=c(7.0,2.1,2.1,7.0), ncol=2)
yo<-matrix(data=NA,nrow=N,ncol=P); p<-numeric(P); v<-numeric(P)

#Matrices save the Bayesian Estimates and Standard Errors
Eu<-matrix(data=NA,nrow=100,ncol=9)
SEu<-matrix(data=NA,nrow=100,ncol=9)
Elam<-matrix(data=NA,nrow=100,ncol=6)
SElam<-matrix(data=NA,nrow=100,ncol=6)
Egam<-matrix(data=NA,nrow=100,ncol=3)
SEgam<-matrix(data=NA,nrow=100,ncol=3)
Ephx<-matrix(data=NA,nrow=100,ncol=3)
SEphx<-matrix(data=NA,nrow=100,ncol=3)
Eb<-numeric(100); SEb<-numeric(100)
Esgd<-numeric(100); SEsgd<-numeric(100)

#Arrays save the HPD intervals
uby=array(NA, c(100,9,2))
ubeta=array(NA, c(100,2))
lam=array(NA, c(100,6,2))
gam=array(NA, c(100,3,2))
sgd=array(NA, c(100,2))
phx=array(NA, c(100,3,2))

DIC=numeric(100)    #DIC values

#Parameters to be estimated
parameters<-c(''uby'',''ubeta'',''lam'',''gam'',''sgd'',''phx'')

#Initial values for the MCMC in WinBUGS
init1<-list(uby=rep(1.0,9),ubeta=0.8,lam=c(0.7,0.7,0.8, 0.8,0.7,0.7),
gam=c(0.6,0.6,0.8),psd=3.33,phi=matrix(data=c (1.0989,-0.3267,-0.3267,
1.0989),ncol=2,byrow=TRUE), xi=matrix (data=rep(0.0,4000), ncol=2))

init2<-list(uby=rep(1.0,9),ubeta=1.0,lam=rep(1.0,6),gam=(1.0,3),
psd=3.0,phi=matrix(data=c(1.0,0.0,0.0,1.0),ncol=2,byrow=TRUE),
xi=matrix(data=rep(0.0,4000),ncol=2))

inits<-list(init1, init2)

#Do simulation for 100 replications
for (t in 1:100) {
    #Generate the data for the simulation study
    for (i in 1:N) {
        #Generate xi
        xi<-mvrnorm(1,mu=c(0,0),phi)
```

```
    #Generate the fixed covariates
    co<-rnorm(1,0,1)
    #Generate error term in structural equation
    delta<-rnorm(1,0,sqrt(0.3))
    #Generate eta according to the structural equation
    eta<-0.8*co[i]+0.6*xi[1]+0.6*xi[2]+0.8*xi[1]*xi[2]+delta
    #Generate error terms in measurement equations
    eps<-rnorm(3,0,1)

    #Generate theta according to measurement equations
    v[1]<-1.0+eta+eps[1]; v[2]<-1.0+0.7*eta+eps[2]
    v[3]<-1.0+0.7*eta+eps[3]
    v[4]<-1.0+xi[1]; v[5]<-1.0+0.8*xi[1]; v[6]<-1.0+0.8*xi[1]
    v[7]<-1.0+xi[2]; v[8]<-1.0+0.7*xi[2]; v[9]<-1.0+0.7*xi[2]

    #transform theta to orinal variables
    for (j in 1:3) { if (v[j]>0) yo[i,j]<-1 else yo[i,j]<-0 }

    #transform theta to binary variables
    for (j in 4:9) {
        p[j]<-exp(v[j])/(1+exp(v[j]))
        yo[i,j]<-rbinom(1,1,p[j])
    }
}

#Input data set for WinBUGS
data<-list(N=2000,P=9,R=Ro,z=yo,c=co,low=c(-2000,0),high=c(0,2000))

#Call WinBUGS
model<-bugs(data,inits,parameters,model.file=''D:/Run/model.txt'',
n.chains=2,n.iter=35000,n.burnin=15000,n.thin=1,DIC=True,
bugs.directory=''C:/Program Files/WinBUGS14/'',
working.directory=''D:/Run/'')

#Save Bayesian Estimates

Eu[t,]<-model$mean$uby; Elam[t,]<-model$mean$lam;
Egam[t,]<-model$mean$gam
Ephx[t,1]<-model$mean$phx[1,1]; Ephx[t,2]<-model$mean$phx[1,2]
Ephx[t,3]<-model$mean$phx[2,2]; Eb[t]<-model$mean$ubeta
Esgd[t]<-model$mean$sgd

#Save Standard Errors
SEu[t,]<-model$sd$uby; SElam[t,]<-model$sd$lam;
SEgam[t,]<-model$sd$gam
SEphx[t,1]<-model$sd$phx[1,1]; SEphx[t,2]<-model$sd$phx[1,2]
SEphx[t,3]<-model$sd$phx[2,2]; SEb[t]<-model$sd$ubeta
SEsgd[t]<-model$sd$sgd

#Save HPD intervals
for (i in 1:9) {
    temp=model$sims.array[,1,i];
    uby[t,i,]=boa.hpd (temp,0.05)
}
```

```
    temp=model$sims.array[,1,10]; ubeta[t,]=boa.hpd(temp,0.05)
    for (i in 1:6) {
        temp=model$sims.array[,1,10+i];
        lam[t,i,]=boa.hpd(temp,0.05)
    }
    for (i in 1:3) {
        temp=model$sims.array[,1,16+i];
        gam[t,i,]=boa.hpd(temp,0.05)
    }
    temp=model$sims.array[,1,20]; sgd[t,]=boa.hpd(temp,0.05)
    temp=model$sims.array[,1,21]; phx[t,1,]=boa.hpd(temp,0.05)
    temp=model$sims.array[,1,22]; phx[t,2,]=boa.hpd(temp,0.05)
    temp=model$sims.array[,1,24]; phx[t,3,]=boa.hpd(temp,0.05)

    #Save DIC value
    DIC[t]=model#DIC
}   #end
```

Appendix 5.5 Conditional distributions for SEMs with nonignorable missing data

Consider the conditional distribution $p(\boldsymbol{\Omega}|\mathbf{V}, \boldsymbol{\theta}, \boldsymbol{\varphi}, \mathbf{r})$. Note that when $\mathbf{V}_{\text{mis}}$ is given, the underlying model with missing data reduces to a nonlinear SEM with fully observed data. Thus, it follows that

$$p(\boldsymbol{\Omega}|\mathbf{V}, \boldsymbol{\theta}, \boldsymbol{\varphi}, \mathbf{r}) = \prod_{i=1}^{n} p(\boldsymbol{\omega}_i|\mathbf{v}_i, \boldsymbol{\theta}, \boldsymbol{\varphi}, \mathbf{r}_i) \propto \prod_{i=1}^{n} p(\mathbf{v}_i|\boldsymbol{\omega}_i, \boldsymbol{\theta}) p(\boldsymbol{\eta}_i|\boldsymbol{\xi}_i, \boldsymbol{\theta}) p(\boldsymbol{\xi}_i|\boldsymbol{\theta}) p(\mathbf{r}_i|\mathbf{v}_i, \boldsymbol{\omega}_i, \boldsymbol{\varphi}),$$

where $p(\boldsymbol{\omega}_i|\mathbf{v}_i, \boldsymbol{\theta}, \boldsymbol{\varphi}, \mathbf{r}_i)$ is proportional to

$$\exp\Big\{ -\frac{1}{2}\Big[(\mathbf{v}_i - \boldsymbol{\mu} - \boldsymbol{\Lambda}\boldsymbol{\omega}_i)^T \boldsymbol{\Psi}_\epsilon^{-1}(\mathbf{v}_i - \boldsymbol{\mu} - \boldsymbol{\Lambda}\boldsymbol{\omega}_i) + (\boldsymbol{\eta}_i - \boldsymbol{\Lambda}_\omega \mathbf{G}(\boldsymbol{\omega}_i))^T \boldsymbol{\Psi}_\delta^{-1}(\boldsymbol{\eta}_i - \boldsymbol{\Lambda}_\omega \mathbf{G}(\boldsymbol{\omega}_i)) \\ + \boldsymbol{\xi}_i^T \boldsymbol{\Phi}^{-1}\boldsymbol{\xi}_i\Big] + \left(\sum_{j=1}^{p} r_{ij}\right) \boldsymbol{\varphi}^T \mathbf{e}_i - p\log(1 + \exp(\boldsymbol{\varphi}^T \mathbf{e}_i))\Big\}. \tag{5.A13}$$

To derive $p(\mathbf{V}_{\text{mis}}|\mathbf{V}_{\text{obs}}, \boldsymbol{\Omega}, \boldsymbol{\theta}, \boldsymbol{\varphi}, \mathbf{r})$, we note that $\mathbf{r}_i$ is independent of $\boldsymbol{\theta}$. Moreover, as $\boldsymbol{\Psi}_\epsilon$ is diagonal, $\mathbf{v}_{i,\text{mis}}$ is independent of $\mathbf{v}_{i,\text{obs}}$. It can be shown that

$$p(\mathbf{V}_{\text{mis}}|\mathbf{V}_{\text{obs}}, \boldsymbol{\Omega}, \boldsymbol{\theta}, \boldsymbol{\varphi}, \mathbf{r}) = \prod_{i=1}^{n} p(\mathbf{v}_{i,\text{mis}}|\mathbf{v}_{i,\text{obs}}, \boldsymbol{\omega}_i, \boldsymbol{\theta}, \boldsymbol{\varphi}, \mathbf{r}_i) \propto \prod_{i=1}^{n} p(\mathbf{v}_{i,\text{mis}}|\boldsymbol{\omega}_i, \boldsymbol{\theta}) p(\mathbf{r}_i|\mathbf{v}_i, \boldsymbol{\omega}_i, \boldsymbol{\varphi}),$$

and $p(\mathbf{v}_{i,\text{mis}}|\mathbf{v}_{i,\text{obs}}, \boldsymbol{\omega}_i, \boldsymbol{\theta}, \boldsymbol{\varphi}, \mathbf{r}_i)$ is proportional to

$$\frac{\exp\left\{-\frac{1}{2}(\mathbf{v}_{i,\text{mis}} - \boldsymbol{\mu}_{i,\text{mis}} - \boldsymbol{\Lambda}_{i,\text{mis}}\boldsymbol{\omega}_i)^T \boldsymbol{\Psi}_{i,\text{mis}}^{-1}(\mathbf{v}_{i,\text{mis}} - \boldsymbol{\mu}_{i,\text{mis}} - \boldsymbol{\Lambda}_{i,\text{mis}}\boldsymbol{\omega}_i) + \left(\sum_{j=1}^{p} r_{ij}\right) \boldsymbol{\varphi}^T \mathbf{e}_i\right\}}{(1 + \exp(\boldsymbol{\varphi}^T \mathbf{e}_i))^p}, \tag{5.A14}$$

where $\boldsymbol{\mu}_{i,\text{mis}}$ is a $p_{i2} \times 1$ subvector of $\boldsymbol{\mu}$ with elements corresponding to missing components of $\mathbf{v}_i$, $\boldsymbol{\Lambda}_{i,\text{mis}}$ is a $p_{i2} \times q$ submatrix of $\boldsymbol{\Lambda}$ with rows corresponding to missing components of $\mathbf{v}_i$, and $\boldsymbol{\Psi}_{i,\text{mis}}$ is a $p_{i2} \times p_{i2}$ submatrix of $\boldsymbol{\Psi}_\epsilon$ with rows and columns corresponding to missing components of $\mathbf{v}_i$.

Finally, we consider the conditional distribution of $\boldsymbol{\varphi}$ given $\mathbf{V}$, $\boldsymbol{\Omega}$, $\boldsymbol{\theta}$, and $\mathbf{r}$. Let $p(\boldsymbol{\varphi})$ be the prior density of $\boldsymbol{\varphi}$, such that $\boldsymbol{\varphi} \stackrel{D}{=} N[\boldsymbol{\varphi}^0, \boldsymbol{\Sigma}_\varphi]$, where $\boldsymbol{\varphi}^0$ and $\boldsymbol{\Sigma}_\varphi$ are the hyperparameters whose values are assumed to be given by the prior information. Since the distribution of $\mathbf{r}$ only involves $\mathbf{V}$, $\boldsymbol{\Omega}$, and $\boldsymbol{\varphi}$, and it is assumed that the prior distribution of $\boldsymbol{\varphi}$ is independent if the prior distribution of $\boldsymbol{\theta}$, we have

$$p(\boldsymbol{\varphi}|\mathbf{V}, \boldsymbol{\Omega}, \boldsymbol{\theta}, \mathbf{r}) \propto p(\mathbf{r}|\mathbf{V}, \boldsymbol{\Omega}, \boldsymbol{\varphi})p(\boldsymbol{\varphi}).$$

Thus, it follows from (5.19) and (5.20) that $p(\boldsymbol{\varphi}|\mathbf{V}, \boldsymbol{\Omega}, \boldsymbol{\theta}, \mathbf{r})$ is proportional to

$$\frac{\exp\left\{\sum_{i=1}^{n}\left(\sum_{j=1}^{p} r_{ij}\right)\boldsymbol{\varphi}^T \mathbf{e}_i - \frac{1}{2}\left(\boldsymbol{\varphi} - \boldsymbol{\varphi}^0\right)^T \boldsymbol{\Sigma}_\varphi^{-1}\left(\boldsymbol{\varphi} - \boldsymbol{\varphi}^0\right)\right\}}{\prod_{i=1}^{n}(1 + \exp(\boldsymbol{\varphi}^T \mathbf{e}_i))^p}. \tag{5.A15}$$

This completes the derivation of the full conditional distributions that are required in the implementation of the Gibbs sampler. The conditional distributions $p(\boldsymbol{\omega}_i|\mathbf{v}_i, \boldsymbol{\theta}, \boldsymbol{\varphi}, \mathbf{r}_i)$, $p(\mathbf{v}_{i,\text{mis}}|\mathbf{v}_{i,\text{obs}}, \boldsymbol{\omega}_i, \boldsymbol{\theta}, \boldsymbol{\varphi}, \mathbf{r}_i)$, and $p(\boldsymbol{\varphi}|\mathbf{V}, \boldsymbol{\Omega}, \boldsymbol{\theta}, \mathbf{r})$ are nonstandard. Some details of the MH algorithm for simulating observations from these conditional distributions are presented in Appendix 12.1 in Lee (2007).

References

Arbuckle, J. L. (1996) Full information estimation in the presence of incomplete data. In G. A. Marcoulides and R. E. Schumacker (eds.), *Advanced Structural Equation Modeling*, Mahwah, NJ: Lawrence Erlbaum.

Bock, R. D. and Aitkin, M. (1981) Marginal maximum likelihood estimation of item parameters: Application of an EM algorithm. *Psychometrika*, **46**, 443–459.

Booth, J. G. and Hobert, J. P. (1999) Maximizing generalized linear mixed model likelihoods with an automated Monte Carlo EM algorithm. *Journal of the Royal Statistical Society, Series B*, **61**, 265–285.

Chib, S. and Greenberg, E. (1998) Analysis of multivariate probit models. *Biometrika*, **85**, 347–361.

Cowles, M. K. (1996) Accelerating Monte Carlo Markov chain convergence for cumulative-link generalized linear models. *Statistics and Computing*, **6**, 101–111.

Fayers, P. M. and Hand, D. J. (1997) Factor analysis, causal indicators and quality of life. *Quality of Life Research*, **6**, 139–150.

Fayers, P. M. and Machin, D. (1998) Factor analysis. In M. J. Staquet, R. D. Hays and P. M. Fayers (eds), *Quality of Life Assessment in Clinical Trials*. Oxford: Oxford University Press.

Gelman, A. (1996) Inference and monitoring convergence. In W. R. Gilks, S. Richardson and D. J. Spiegelhalter (eds), *Markov Chain Monte Carlo in Practice*, pp. 131–144. London: Chapman & Hall.

Gelman, A. and Meng, X. L. (1998) Simulating normalizing constants: From importance sampling to bridge sampling to path sampling. *Statistical Science*, **13**, 163–185.

Gelman, A., Meng, X. L. and Stern, H. (1996) Posterior predictive assessment of model fitness via realized discrepancies. *Statistica Sinica*, **6**, 733–759.

Geman, S. and Geman, D. (1984) Stochastic relaxation, Gibbs distribution and the Bayesian restoration of images. *IEEE Transactions on Pattern Analysis and Machine Intelligence*, **6**, 721–741.

Geyer, C. J. (1992) Practical Markov chain Monte Carlo. *Statistical Science*, **7**, 473–511.

Gibbons, R. D. and Wilcox-Gök, V. (1998) Health service utilization and insurance coverage: A multivariate probit model. *Journal of the American Statistical Association*, **93**, 63–72.

Glonek, G. F. V. and McCullagh, P. (1995) Multivariate logistic models. *Journal of the Royal Statistical Society, Series B*, **57**, 533–546.

Hastings, W. K. (1970) Monte Carlo sampling methods using Markov chains and their applications. *Biometrika*, **57**, 97–109.

Ibrahim, J. G., Chen, M. H. and Lipsitz, S. R. (2001). Missing responses in generalised linear mixed models when the missing data mechanism is nonignorable. *Biometrika*, **88**, 551–564.

Lee, S. Y. (2007) *Structural Equation Modeling: A Bayesian Approach*. Chichester: John Wiley & Sons, Ltd.

Lee, S. Y. and Song, X. Y. (2003) Bayesian analysis of structural equation models with dichotomous variables. *Statistics in Medicine*, **22**, 3073–3088.

Lee, S. Y. and Song, X. Y. (2004) Bayesian model comparison of nonlinear structural equation models with missing continuous and ordinal categorical data. *British Journal of Mathematical and Statistical Psychology*, **57**, 131–150.

Lee, S. Y. and Tang, N. S. (2006) Bayesian analysis of nonlinear structural equation models with nonignorable missing data. *Psychometrika*, **71**, 541–564.

Lee, S. Y., Poon, W. Y. and Bentler, P. M. (1990) Full maximum likelihood analysis of structural equation models with polytomous variables. *Statistics and Probability Letters*, **9**, 91–97.

Lee, S. Y., Song, X. Y., Skevington, S. and Hao, Y. T. (2005) Application of structural equation models to quality of life. *Structural Equation Modeling – A Multidisciplinary Journal*. **12**, 435–453.

Lee, S. Y., Song, X. Y. and Cai, J. H. (2010) A Bayesian approach for nonlinear structural equation models with dichotomous variables using logit and probit links. *Structural Equation Modeling – A Multidisciplinary Journal*, **17**, 280–302.

Little, R. J. A. and Rubin, D. B. (2002) *Statistical Analysis with Missing Data* (2nd edn). Hoboken, NJ: Wiley.

McCullagh, P. and Nelder, J. A. (1989) *Generalized Linear Models*. New York: Chapman & Hall.

Meng, X. L. and Schilling, S. (1996) Fitting full-information item factor models and an empirical investigation of bridge sampling. *Journal of the American Statistical Association*, **91**, 1254–1267.

Metropolis, N., Rosenbluth, A. W., Rosenbluth, M. N., Teller, A. H. and Teller, E. (1953) Equation of state calculations by fast computing machines. *Journal of Chemical Physics*, **21**, 1087–1091.

Morisky, D. E., Tiglao, T. V., Sneed, C. D., Tempongko, S. B., Baltazar, J. C., Detels, R. and Stein, J.A. (1998) The effects of establishment policies, knowledge and attitudes on condom use among Filipina sex workers. *AIDS Care*, **10**, 213–220.

Olschewski, M. and Schumacher, M. (1990) Statistical analysis of quality of life data in cancer clinical trials. *Statistics in Medicine*, **9**, 749–763.

Olsson, U. (1979) Maximum likelihood estimation of the polychoric correlation coefficient. *Psychometrika*, **44**, 443–460.

Power, M., Bullinger, M. and Harper, A. (1999) The World Health Organization WHOQOL-100: Tests of the universality of quality of life in 15 different cultural groups worldwide. *Health Psychology*, **18**, 495–505.

Roberts, C. P. (1995) Simulation of truncated normal variables. *Statistics and Computing*, **5**, 121–125.

Sammel, M. D., Ryan, L. M. and Legler, J. M. (1997) Latent variable models for mixed discrete and continuous outcomes. *Journal of the Royal Statistical Society, Series B*, **59**, 667–678.

Shi, J. Q. and Lee, S. Y. (1998) Bayesian sampling-based approach for factor analysis models with continuous and polytomous data. *British Journal of Mathematical and Statistical Psychology*, **51**, 233–252.

Shi, J. Q. and Lee, S. Y. (2000) Latent variable models with mixed continuous and polytomous data. *Journal of the Royal Statistical Society, Series B*, **62**, 77–87.

Song, X. Y. and Lee, S. Y. (2002) Analysis of structural equation model with ignorable missing continuous and polytomous data. *Psychometrika*, **67**, 261–288.

Song, X. Y. and Lee, S. Y. (2007) Bayesian analysis of latent variable models with non-ignorable missing outcomes from exponential family. *Statistics in Medicine*, **26**, 681–693.

Spiegelhalter, D. J., Thomas, A., Best, N. G. and Lunn, D. (2003) *WinBUGS User Manual. Version 1.4*. Cambridge: MRC Biostatistics Unit.

Staquet, M. J., Hays, R. D. and Fayers, P. M. (1998) *Quality of Life Assessment in Clinical Trials*. Oxford: Oxford University Press.

Sturtz, S., Ligges, U. and Gelman, A. (2005). R2WinBUGS: A package for running WinBUGS from R. *Journal of Statistical Software*, **12** 1–16.

Tanner, M. A. and Wong, W. H. (1987) The calculation of posterior distributions by data augmentation (with discussion). *Journal of the American statistical Association*, **82**, 528–550.

WHOQOL Group (1998) Development of the World Health Organization WHOQOL-BREF quality of life assessment. *Psychological Medicine*, **28**, 551–558.

World Values Study Group (1994) World Values Survey, 1981–1984 and 1990–1993. ICPSR version. Ann Arbor, MI: Institute for Social Research (producer). Ann Arbon, MI: Inter-university Consortium for Political and Social Research (distributor).

6

Structural equation models with hierarchical and multisample data

6.1 Introduction

The structural equation models and Bayesian methods described in previous chapters assume that the available data are obtained from a random sample from a single population. However, in much substantive research, the related data may exhibit at least two possible kinds of heterogeneity. The first kind is mixture data, which involve independent observations that come from one of the K populations with different distributions, where no information is available on which of the K populations an individual observation belongs to. Although K may be known or unknown, it is usually quite small. Mixture models, to be discussed in Chapter 7, are used to analyze this kind of heterogeneous data. The second kind of heterogeneous data are drawn from a number of different groups (clusters) with a known hierarchical structure. Examples are drawing of random samples of patients from within random samples of clinics or hospitals; individuals from within random samples of families; or students from within random samples of schools. In contrast to mixture data, these hierarchically structured data usually involve a large number of groups, and the group membership of each observation can be exactly specified. However, as individuals within a group share certain common influential factors, the random observations are correlated. Hence, the assumption of independence among observed data is violated. Clearly, ignoring the correlated structure of the data and analyzing them as observations from a single random sample will give erroneous results. Moreover, it is also desirable to establish a meaningful model for the between-group levels, and study the effects of the between-group latent variables on the within-group latent variables.

Basic and Advanced Bayesian Structural Equation Modeling: With Applications in the Medical and Behavioral Sciences, First Edition. Xin-Yuan Song and Sik-Yum Lee.

Multisample data also come from a number of distinct groups (populations). Usually, the number of groups is relatively small, while the number of observations within each group is large. For multisample data, we assume that the observations within each group are independent rather than correlated. Hence, multisample data do not have a hierarchical structure as two-level data. In addition, the number of groups is known, and the group membership of each observation can be specified exactly. In this sense, they can be regarded as a simple mixture data with given correct group label for every observation. As a result, compared to two-level data and/or mixture data, multisample data are easier to cope with.

The objectives of this chapter are to introduce two-level SEMs and multisample SEMs, as well as the associated Bayesian methodologies for analyzing two-level and multisample data.

6.2 Two-level structural equation models

The development of two-level SEMs for taking into consideration the correlated structure of the hierarchical data has received much attention; see, for example, McDonald and Goldstein (1989), Rabe-Hesketh *et al.* (2004), Skrondal and Rabe-Hesketh (2004), and Lee and Song (2005). Using a Bayesian approach, Song and Lee (2004) developed the MCMC methods for analyzing two-level nonlinear models with continuous and ordered categorical data, and Lee *et al.* (2007) considered two-level nonlinear SEMs with cross-level effects. For reasons stated in previous chapters, we will describe Bayesian methods for analyzing two-level SEMs in this chapter. To provide a comprehensive framework for analyzing two-level models, nonlinear structural equations are incorporated into the SEMs that are associated with within-group and between-group models. Moreover, the model can accommodate mixed types of continuous and ordered categorical data. In addition to Bayesian estimation, we will present a path sample procedure to compute the Bayes factor for model comparison. The generality of the model is important for providing a comprehensive framework for model comparison of different kinds of SEMs. Again, the idea of data augmentation is utilized. Here, the observed data are augmented with various latent variables at both levels, and the latent continuous random vectors that underlie the ordered categorical variables. An algorithm based on the Gibbs sampler (Geman and Geman, 1984) and the Metropolis–Hastings (MH) algorithm (Metropolis *et al.*, 1953; Hastings, 1970) is used for estimation. Observations generated with this algorithm will be used for the path sampling procedure in computing Bayes factors. Although we emphasize the two-level SEM, the methodology can be extended to higher-level SEMs. Finally, an application of WinBUGS to two-level nonlinear SEMs will be discussed.

6.2.1 Two-level nonlinear SEM with mixed type variables

Consider a collection of p-variate random vectors $\mathbf{u}_{gi}$, $i = 1, \ldots, N_g$, nested within groups $g = 1, \ldots, G$. The sample sizes N_g may differ from group to group so that the data set is unbalanced. At the first level, we assume that, conditional on the group mean $\mathbf{v}_g$, random observations in each group satisfy the following measurement equation:

$$\mathbf{u}_{gi} = \mathbf{v}_g + \mathbf{\Lambda}_{1g}\boldsymbol{\omega}_{1gi} + \boldsymbol{\epsilon}_{1gi}, \quad g = 1, \ldots, G, \ i = 1, \ldots, N_g, \tag{6.1}$$

where $\mathbf{\Lambda}_{1g}$ is a $p \times q_1$ matrix of factor loadings, $\boldsymbol{\omega}_{1gi}$ is a $q_1 \times 1$ random vector of latent factors, and $\boldsymbol{\epsilon}_{1gi}$ is a $p \times 1$ random vector of error measurements which is independent of $\boldsymbol{\omega}_{1gi}$ and is distributed as $N[\mathbf{0}, \mathbf{\Psi}_{1g}]$, where $\mathbf{\Psi}_{1g}$ is a diagonal matrix. Note that $\mathbf{u}_{gi}$ and $\mathbf{u}_{gj}$

are not independent due to the existence of $\mathbf{v}_g$. Hence, in the two-level SEM, the usual assumption on the independence of the observations is violated. To account for the structure at the between-group level, we assume that the group mean $\mathbf{v}_g$ satisfies the following factor analysis model:

$$\mathbf{v}_g = \boldsymbol{\mu} + \boldsymbol{\Lambda}_2\boldsymbol{\omega}_{2g} + \boldsymbol{\epsilon}_{2g}, \quad g = 1, \ldots, G, \tag{6.2}$$

where $\boldsymbol{\mu}$ is the vector of intercepts, $\boldsymbol{\Lambda}_2$ is a $p \times q_2$ matrix of factor loadings, $\boldsymbol{\omega}_{2g}$ is a $q_2 \times 1$ vector of latent variables, and $\boldsymbol{\epsilon}_{2g}$ is a $p \times 1$ random vector of error measurements which is independent of $\boldsymbol{\omega}_{2g}$ and is distributed as $N[\mathbf{0}, \boldsymbol{\Psi}_2]$, where $\boldsymbol{\Psi}_2$ is a diagonal matrix. Moreover, the first- and second-level measurement errors are assumed to be independent. It follows from equations (6.1) and (6.2) that

$$\mathbf{u}_{gi} = \boldsymbol{\mu} + \boldsymbol{\Lambda}_2\boldsymbol{\omega}_{2g} + \boldsymbol{\epsilon}_{2g} + \boldsymbol{\Lambda}_{1g}\boldsymbol{\omega}_{1gi} + \boldsymbol{\epsilon}_{1gi}. \tag{6.3}$$

In order to assess the interrelationships among the latent variables, latent vectors $\boldsymbol{\omega}_{1gi}$ and $\boldsymbol{\omega}_{2g}$ are partitioned as $\boldsymbol{\omega}_{1gi} = (\boldsymbol{\eta}_{1gi}^T, \boldsymbol{\xi}_{1gi}^T)^T$ and $\boldsymbol{\omega}_{2g} = (\boldsymbol{\eta}_{2g}^T, \boldsymbol{\xi}_{2g}^T)^T$, respectively, where $\boldsymbol{\eta}_{1gi}(q_{11} \times 1)$, $\boldsymbol{\xi}_{1gi}(q_{12} \times 1)$, $\boldsymbol{\eta}_{2g}(q_{21} \times 1)$, and $\boldsymbol{\xi}_{2g}(q_{22} \times 1)$ are latent vectors, with $q_{j1} + q_{j2} = q_j$, for $j = 1, 2$. The distributions of $\boldsymbol{\xi}_{1gi}$ and $\boldsymbol{\xi}_{2g}$ are $N[\mathbf{0}, \boldsymbol{\Phi}_{1g}]$ and $N[\mathbf{0}, \boldsymbol{\Phi}_2]$, respectively. The following nonlinear structural equations are incorporated into the between-group and within-group models of the two-level model:

$$\boldsymbol{\eta}_{1gi} = \boldsymbol{\Pi}_{1g}\boldsymbol{\eta}_{1gi} + \boldsymbol{\Gamma}_{1g}\mathbf{F}_1(\boldsymbol{\xi}_{1gi}) + \boldsymbol{\delta}_{1gi}, \tag{6.4}$$

$$\boldsymbol{\eta}_{2g} = \boldsymbol{\Pi}_2\boldsymbol{\eta}_{2g} + \boldsymbol{\Gamma}_2\mathbf{F}_2(\boldsymbol{\xi}_{2g}) + \boldsymbol{\delta}_{2g}, \tag{6.5}$$

where $\mathbf{F}_1(\boldsymbol{\xi}_{1gi}) = (f_{11}(\boldsymbol{\xi}_{1gi}), \ldots, f_{1a}(\boldsymbol{\xi}_{1gi}))^T$ and $\mathbf{F}_2(\boldsymbol{\xi}_{2g}) = (f_{21}(\boldsymbol{\xi}_{2g}), \ldots, f_{2b}(\boldsymbol{\xi}_{2g}))^T$ are vector-valued functions with nonzero differentiable functions f_{1k} and f_{2k}, and usually $a \geq q_{12}$ and $b \geq q_{22}$, $\boldsymbol{\Pi}_{1g}(q_{11} \times q_{11})$, $\boldsymbol{\Pi}_2(q_{21} \times q_{21})$, $\boldsymbol{\Gamma}_{1g}(q_{11} \times a)$, and $\boldsymbol{\Gamma}_2(q_{21} \times b)$ are unknown parameter matrices, $\boldsymbol{\delta}_{1gi}$ is a vector of error measurements which is distributed as $N[\mathbf{0}, \boldsymbol{\Psi}_{1g\delta}]$, $\boldsymbol{\delta}_{2g}$ is a vector of error measurements which is distributed as $N[\mathbf{0}, \boldsymbol{\Psi}_{2\delta}]$, and $\boldsymbol{\Psi}_{1g\delta}$ and $\boldsymbol{\Psi}_{2\delta}$ are diagonal matrices. Due to the nonlinearity induced by $\mathbf{F}_1$ and $\mathbf{F}_2$, the underlying distribution of $\mathbf{u}_{gi}$ is not normal. In the within-group structural equation, we assume as usual that $\boldsymbol{\xi}_{1gi}$ and $\boldsymbol{\delta}_{1gi}$ are independent. Similarly, in the between-group structural equation, we assume that $\boldsymbol{\xi}_{2g}$ and $\boldsymbol{\delta}_{2g}$ are independent. Moreover, we assume that the within-group latent vectors $\boldsymbol{\eta}_{1gi}$ and $\boldsymbol{\xi}_{1gi}$ are independent of the between-group latent vectors $\boldsymbol{\eta}_{2g}$ and $\boldsymbol{\xi}_{2g}$. Hence, it follows from (6.4) that $\boldsymbol{\eta}_{1gi}$ is independent of $\boldsymbol{\eta}_{2g}$ and $\boldsymbol{\xi}_{2g}$. That is, this two-level SEM does not accommodate the effects of the latent vectors in the between-group level on the latent vectors in the within-group level (see Lee, 2007, Section 9.6). However, in the within-group model or in the between-group model, nonlinear effects of explanatory latent variables on outcome latent variables can be assessed through (6.4) and (6.5); and the hierarchical structure of the data has been taken into account. Furthermore, we assume that $\mathbf{I}_1 - \boldsymbol{\Pi}_{1g}$ and $\mathbf{I}_2 - \boldsymbol{\Pi}_2$ are nonsingular, and their determinants are independent of the elements in $\boldsymbol{\Pi}_{1g}$ and $\boldsymbol{\Pi}_2$, respectively. The two-level SEM is not identified without imposing identification restrictions. The common method of fixing appropriate elements in $\boldsymbol{\Lambda}_{1g}$, $\boldsymbol{\Pi}_{1g}$, $\boldsymbol{\Gamma}_{1g}$, $\boldsymbol{\Lambda}_2$, $\boldsymbol{\Pi}_2$, and $\boldsymbol{\Gamma}_2$ at preassigned known values can be used to achieve an identified model.

To accommodate mixed ordered categorical and continuous variables, without loss of generality, we suppose that $\mathbf{u}_{gi} = (\mathbf{x}_{gi}^T, \mathbf{y}_{gi}^T)^T$, where $\mathbf{x}_{gi} = (x_{gi1}, \ldots, x_{gir})^T$ is an $r \times 1$ observable continuous random vector, and $\mathbf{y}_{gi} = (y_{gi1}, \ldots, y_{gis})^T$ is an $s \times 1$ unobservable continuous random vector. As in the previous chapters, a threshold specification is used to model the observable ordered categorical vector $\mathbf{z} = (z_1, \ldots, z_s)^T$ with its underlying continuous vector $\mathbf{y} = (y_1, \ldots, y_s)^T$ as described in (5.3), through integer values in $\{0, 1, \ldots, b_k\}$. Dichotomous variables are treated as an ordered categorical variable with a single threshold fixed at zero. The thresholds, mean and variance of an ordered categorical variable can be identified through the method given in Section 5.2.1.

The above model subsumes a number of important models in the recent developments of SEMs; for instance, the models discussed in Shi and Lee (1998, 2000) and Lee and Zhu (2000). Despite its generality, the two-level SEM introduced is defined by measurement and structural equations that describe the relationships among the observed and latent variables at both levels by conceptually simple regression models. Consider the following three major components of the model and data structure: (1) a two-level model for hierarchically structured data; (2) the discrete nature of the data; and (3) a nonlinear structural equation in the within-group model. The first two components are important for achieving correct statistical results. The last component is essential to the analysis of more complicated situations because nonlinear terms of latent variables have been found to be useful in establishing a better model. The between-group model is also defined with a nonlinear structural equation for the sake of generality. The development is useful for providing a general framework for analyzing a large number of its submodels. This is particularly true from a model comparison perspective. For example, even if a linear model is better than a nonlinear model in fitting a data set, such a conclusion cannot be reached without the model comparison under the more general nonlinear model framework. In practical situations where G is not large, it may not be worthwhile or feasible to consider a complicated between-group model. Moreover, most two-level SEMs in the literature assume that the within-group parameters are invariant over groups.

6.2.2 Bayesian inference

Motivated by its various advantages, we use the Bayesian approach to analyze the current two-level nonlinear SEM with mixed continuous, dichotomous, and/or ordered categorical data. Our basic strategy is to augment the observed data with the latent data that consist of the latent variables and/or latent measurements, and then apply MCMC tools to simulate observations in the posterior analysis.

Let $\boldsymbol{\theta}$ be the parameter vector that contains all the unknown structural parameters in $\boldsymbol{\Lambda}_{1g}$, $\boldsymbol{\Psi}_{1g}$, $\boldsymbol{\Pi}_{1g}$, $\boldsymbol{\Gamma}_{1g}$, $\boldsymbol{\Phi}_{1g}$, $\boldsymbol{\Psi}_{1g\delta}$, $\boldsymbol{\mu}$, $\boldsymbol{\Lambda}_2$, $\boldsymbol{\Psi}_2$, $\boldsymbol{\Pi}_2$, $\boldsymbol{\Gamma}_2$, $\boldsymbol{\Phi}_2$, and $\boldsymbol{\Psi}_{2\delta}$, and let $\boldsymbol{\alpha}$ be the parameter vector that contains all the unknown thresholds. The total number of unknown parameters in $\boldsymbol{\theta}$ and $\boldsymbol{\alpha}$ is usually large. In the following analysis, we assume that the two-level nonlinear model defined by $\boldsymbol{\theta}$ and $\boldsymbol{\alpha}$ is identified. Let $\mathbf{X}_g = (\mathbf{x}_{g1}, \ldots, \mathbf{x}_{gN_g})$ and $\mathbf{X} = (\mathbf{X}_1, \ldots, \mathbf{X}_G)$ be the observed continuous data, and $\mathbf{Z}_g = (\mathbf{z}_{g1}, \ldots, \mathbf{z}_{gN_g})$ and $\mathbf{Z} = (\mathbf{Z}_1, \ldots, \mathbf{Z}_G)$ be the observed ordered categorical data. Let $\mathbf{Y}_g = (\mathbf{y}_{g1}, \ldots, \mathbf{y}_{gN_g})$ and $\mathbf{Y} = (\mathbf{Y}_1, \ldots, \mathbf{Y}_G)$ be the latent continuous measurements associated with $\mathbf{Z}_g$ and $\mathbf{Z}$, respectively. The observed data will be augmented with $\mathbf{Y}$ in the posterior analysis. Once $\mathbf{Y}$ is given, all the data are continuous and the problem will be easier to cope with. Let $\mathbf{V} = (\mathbf{v}_1, \ldots, \mathbf{v}_G)$ be the matrix of between-group latent variables. If $\mathbf{V}$ is observed, the model is reduced to the single-level multisample model. Moreover, let $\boldsymbol{\Omega}_{1g} = (\boldsymbol{\omega}_{1g1}, \ldots, \boldsymbol{\omega}_{1gN_g})$, $\boldsymbol{\Omega}_1 = (\boldsymbol{\Omega}_{11}, \ldots, \boldsymbol{\Omega}_{1G})$, and $\boldsymbol{\Omega}_2 = (\boldsymbol{\omega}_{21}, \ldots, \boldsymbol{\omega}_{2G})$ be the matrices of latent variables at the within-group and between-group levels. If these matrices are observed, the complicated nonlinear structural equations (6.4) and (6.5) reduce to the regular simultaneous regression model. Difficulties due to the nonlinear relationships among the latent variables are greatly alleviated. Hence, problems associated with the complicated components of the model, such as the correlated structure of the observations induced by the two-level data, the discrete nature of the ordered categorical variables, and the nonlinearity of the latent variables at both levels, can be handled by data augmentation. In the posterior analysis, the observed data $(\mathbf{X}, \mathbf{Z})$ will be augmented with $(\mathbf{Y}, \mathbf{V}, \mathbf{\Omega}_1, \mathbf{\Omega}_2)$, and we will consider the joint posterior distribution $[\boldsymbol{\theta}, \boldsymbol{\alpha}, \mathbf{Y}, \mathbf{V}, \mathbf{\Omega}_1, \mathbf{\Omega}_2|\mathbf{X}, \mathbf{Z}]$. The Gibbs sampler (Geman and Geman, 1984) will be used to generate a sequence of observations from this joint posterior distribution. The Bayesian solution is then obtained using standard inferences based on the generated sample of observations. In applying the Gibbs sampler, we iteratively sample from the following conditional distributions: $[\mathbf{V}|\boldsymbol{\theta}, \boldsymbol{\alpha}, \mathbf{Y}, \mathbf{\Omega}_1, \mathbf{\Omega}_2, \mathbf{X}, \mathbf{Z}]$, $[\mathbf{\Omega}_1|\boldsymbol{\theta}, \boldsymbol{\alpha}, \mathbf{Y}, \mathbf{V}, \mathbf{\Omega}_2, \mathbf{X}, \mathbf{Z}]$, $[\mathbf{\Omega}_2|\boldsymbol{\theta}, \boldsymbol{\alpha}, \mathbf{Y}, \mathbf{V}, \mathbf{\Omega}_1, \mathbf{X}, \mathbf{Z}]$, $[\boldsymbol{\alpha}, \mathbf{Y}|\boldsymbol{\theta}, \mathbf{V}, \mathbf{\Omega}_1, \mathbf{\Omega}_2, \mathbf{X}, \mathbf{Z}]$, and $[\boldsymbol{\theta}|\boldsymbol{\alpha}, \mathbf{Y}, \mathbf{V}, \mathbf{\Omega}_1, \mathbf{\Omega}_2, \mathbf{X}, \mathbf{Z}]$.

For the two-level model defined, the conditional distribution $[\boldsymbol{\theta}|\boldsymbol{\alpha}, \mathbf{Y}, \mathbf{V}, \mathbf{\Omega}_1, \mathbf{\Omega}_2, \mathbf{X}, \mathbf{Z}]$ is further decomposed into components involving various structural parameters in the between-group and within-group models. These components are different under various special cases of the model. Some typical examples are as follows:

(a) Models with different within-group parameters across groups. In this case, the within-group structural parameters $\boldsymbol{\theta}_{1g} = \{\mathbf{\Lambda}_{1g}, \mathbf{\Psi}_{1g}, \mathbf{\Pi}_{1g}, \mathbf{\Gamma}_{1g}, \mathbf{\Phi}_{1g}, \mathbf{\Psi}_{1g\delta}\}$ and threshold parameters $\boldsymbol{\alpha}_g$ associated with the gth group are different from those associated with the hth group, for $g \neq h$. In practice, G and N_g should not be too small for drawing valid statistical conclusions for the between-group model and the gth within-group model.

(b) Models with some invariant within-group parameters. In this case, parameters $\boldsymbol{\theta}_{1g}$ and/or $\boldsymbol{\alpha}_g$ associated with the gth group are equal to those associated with some other groups.

(c) Models with all invariant within-group parameters. In this case, $\boldsymbol{\theta}_{11} = \ldots = \boldsymbol{\theta}_{1G}$ and $\boldsymbol{\alpha}_1 = \ldots = \boldsymbol{\alpha}_G$.

Conditional distributions in various special cases are similar but different. Moreover, prior distributions of the parameters are also involved. Based on the reasoning given in previous chapters, conjugate type prior distributions are used. The noninformative distribution is used for the prior distribution of the thresholds. The conditional distributions of the components in $[\boldsymbol{\theta}|\boldsymbol{\alpha}, \mathbf{Y}, \mathbf{V}, \mathbf{\Omega}_1, \mathbf{\Omega}_2, \mathbf{X}, \mathbf{Z}]$ as well as other conditional distributions required by the Gibbs sampler are briefly discussed in Appendix 6.1. As we can see in this appendix, these conditional distributions are generalizations of those that are associated with a single-level model; and most of them are standard distributions such as normal, gamma, and inverted Wishart distributions. Simulating observations from them requires little computation time. The MH algorithm will be used for simulating observations efficiently from the following three complicated conditional distributions: $[\mathbf{\Omega}_1|\boldsymbol{\theta}, \boldsymbol{\alpha}, \mathbf{Y}, \mathbf{V}, \mathbf{\Omega}_2, \mathbf{X}, \mathbf{Z}]$, $[\mathbf{\Omega}_2|\boldsymbol{\theta}, \boldsymbol{\alpha}, \mathbf{Y}, \mathbf{V}, \mathbf{\Omega}_1, \mathbf{X}, \mathbf{Z}]$, and $[\boldsymbol{\alpha}, \mathbf{Y}|\boldsymbol{\theta}, \mathbf{V}, \mathbf{\Omega}_1, \mathbf{\Omega}_2, \mathbf{X}, \mathbf{Z}]$. Some technical details on the implementation of the MH algorithm are given in Appendix 6.2.

The following Bayes factor (see Kass and Raftery, 1995) is used for comparing competing models M_0 and M_1:

$$B_{10} = \frac{p(\mathbf{X}, \mathbf{Z}|M_1)}{p(\mathbf{X}, \mathbf{Z}|M_0)}.$$

In the application of path sampling in computing B_{10}, we again use the data augmentation idea to augment $(\mathbf{X}, \mathbf{Z})$ with $(\mathbf{Y}, \mathbf{V}, \mathbf{\Omega}_1, \mathbf{\Omega}_2)$ in the analysis. It can be shown by reasoning similar to that in Chapter 4 that

$$\widehat{\log B_{10}} = \frac{1}{2}\sum_{s=0}^{S}\left(t_{(s+1)} - t_{(s)}\right)\left(\bar{U}_{(s+1)} + \bar{U}_{(s)}\right), \tag{6.6}$$

where $0 = t_{(0)} < t_{(1)} < \ldots < t_{(S)} < t_{(S+1)} = 1$ are fixed grids in [0, 1] and

$$\bar{U}_{(s)} = \frac{1}{J}\sum_{j=1}^{J} U\left(\boldsymbol{\theta}^{(j)}, \boldsymbol{\alpha}^{(j)}, \mathbf{Y}^{(j)}, \mathbf{V}^{(j)}, \boldsymbol{\Omega}_1^{(j)}, \boldsymbol{\Omega}_2^{(j)}, \mathbf{X}, \mathbf{Z}, t_{(s)}\right), \tag{6.7}$$

in which $\{(\boldsymbol{\theta}^{(j)}, \boldsymbol{\alpha}^{(j)}, \mathbf{Y}^{(j)}, \mathbf{V}^{(j)}, \boldsymbol{\Omega}_1^{(j)}, \boldsymbol{\Omega}_2^{(j)}), j = 1, \ldots, J\}$ is a sample of observations simulated from the joint posterior distribution $[\boldsymbol{\theta}, \boldsymbol{\alpha}, \mathbf{Y}, \mathbf{V}, \boldsymbol{\Omega}_1, \boldsymbol{\Omega}_2|\mathbf{X}, \mathbf{Z}, t_{(s)}]$, and

$$U(\boldsymbol{\theta}, \boldsymbol{\alpha}, \mathbf{Y}, \mathbf{V}, \boldsymbol{\Omega}_1, \boldsymbol{\Omega}_2, \mathbf{X}, \mathbf{Z}, t) = d\log p(\mathbf{Y}, \mathbf{V}, \boldsymbol{\Omega}_1, \boldsymbol{\Omega}_2, \mathbf{X}, \mathbf{Z}|\boldsymbol{\theta}, \boldsymbol{\alpha}, t)/dt, \tag{6.8}$$

where $p(\mathbf{Y}, \mathbf{V}, \boldsymbol{\Omega}_1, \boldsymbol{\Omega}_2, \mathbf{X}, \mathbf{Z}|\boldsymbol{\theta}, \boldsymbol{\alpha}, t)$ is the complete-data likelihood. Note that this complete-data likelihood is not complicated, thus obtaining the function $U(\cdot)$ through differentiation is not difficult. Moreover, the program implemented in the estimation can be used for simulating observations in equation (6.7), hence little additional programming effort is required. Usually, $S = 10$ grids are sufficient to prove a good approximation of $\log B_{10}$ for competing models that are not far apart. More grids are required for very different M_1 and M_0, and the issue should be approached on a problem-by-problem basis. In equation (6.7), a value of $J = 2000$ is sufficient for most practical applications.

An important step in applying path sampling for computing logarithm B_{12} is to find a good path t in [0, 1] to link the competing models M_1 and M_2. Because the two-level nonlinear SEM is rather complex, M_1 and M_2 can be quite different and finding a path to link them may require some insight. The following is an illustrative example.

The competing models M_1 and M_2 have the following within-group measurement and structural equations:

$$\mathbf{u}_{gi} = \mathbf{v}_g + \boldsymbol{\Lambda}_1\boldsymbol{\omega}_{1gi} + \boldsymbol{\epsilon}_{1gi}, \tag{6.9}$$

$$\boldsymbol{\eta}_{1gi} = \boldsymbol{\Pi}_1\boldsymbol{\eta}_{1gi} + \boldsymbol{\Gamma}_1\mathbf{F}_1(\boldsymbol{\xi}_{1gi}) + \boldsymbol{\delta}_{1gi}. \tag{6.10}$$

The difference between M_1 and M_2 is in the between-group models. Let

$$M_1 : \mathbf{v}_g = \boldsymbol{\mu} + \boldsymbol{\Lambda}_2^1\boldsymbol{\omega}_{2g} + \boldsymbol{\epsilon}_{2g}, \tag{6.11}$$

where $\boldsymbol{\omega}_{2g}$ is distributed as $N[\mathbf{0}, \boldsymbol{\Phi}_2]$. Thus, the between-group model in M_1 is a factor analysis model. In M_2, $\boldsymbol{\omega}_{2g} = (\boldsymbol{\eta}_{2g}^T, \boldsymbol{\xi}_{2g}^T)^T$, and the measurement and structural equations in the between-group model are as follows:

$$M_2 : \mathbf{v}_g = \boldsymbol{\mu} + \boldsymbol{\Lambda}_2^2\boldsymbol{\omega}_{2g} + \boldsymbol{\epsilon}_{2g}, \tag{6.12}$$

$$\boldsymbol{\eta}_{2g} = \boldsymbol{\Pi}_2^2\boldsymbol{\eta}_{2g} + \boldsymbol{\Gamma}_2^2\mathbf{F}_2(\boldsymbol{\xi}_{2g}) + \boldsymbol{\delta}_{2g}. \tag{6.13}$$

The between-group model in M_2 is a nonlinear SEM with a nonlinear structural equation. Note that M_1 and M_2 are nonnested. As there are two different models for $\boldsymbol{\omega}_{2g}$, it is rather difficult to directly link M_1 and M_2. This difficulty can be solved via an auxiliary model M_a which can be linked with both M_1 and M_2. We first compute $\log B_{1a}$ and $\log B_{2a}$, and then obtain $\log B_{12}$ via the following equation:

$$\log B_{12} = \log \frac{p(\mathbf{X}, \mathbf{Z}|M_1)/p(\mathbf{X}, \mathbf{Z}|M_a)}{p(\mathbf{X}, \mathbf{Z}|M_2)/p(\mathbf{X}, \mathbf{Z}|M_a)} = \log B_{1a} - \log B_{2a}. \tag{6.14}$$

For the above problem, one auxiliary model is M_a, in which the measurement and structural equations of the within-group model are given by (6.9) and (6.10), and the between-group model is defined by $\mathbf{v}_g = \boldsymbol{\mu} + \boldsymbol{\epsilon}_{2g}$. The link model M_{t1a} is defined by $M_{t1a} : \mathbf{u}_{gi} = \boldsymbol{\mu} + t\boldsymbol{\Lambda}_2^1\boldsymbol{\omega}_{2g} + \boldsymbol{\epsilon}_{2g} + \boldsymbol{\Lambda}_1\boldsymbol{\omega}_{1gi} + \boldsymbol{\epsilon}_{1gi}$, with the within-group structural equation given by (6.10), where $\boldsymbol{\omega}_{2g}$ is distributed as $N[\mathbf{0}, \boldsymbol{\Phi}_2]$ and without a between-group structural equation. Clearly, $t = 1$ and $t = 0$ correspond to M_1 and M_a, respectively. Hence, $\log B_{1a}$ can be computed under this setting via the path sampling procedure. The link model M_{t2a} is defined by $M_{t2a} : \mathbf{u}_{gi} = \boldsymbol{\mu} + t\boldsymbol{\Lambda}_2^2\boldsymbol{\omega}_{2g} + \boldsymbol{\epsilon}_{2g} + \boldsymbol{\Lambda}_1\boldsymbol{\omega}_{1gi} + \boldsymbol{\epsilon}_{1gi}$, with the within-group and between-group structural equations given by (6.10) and (6.13), respectively. Clearly, $t = 1$ and $t = 0$ correspond to M_2 and M_a, respectively. Hence, $\log B_{2a}$ can be obtained. Finally, $\log B_{12}$ can be obtained from $\log B_{1a}$ and $\log B_{2a}$ via (6.14).

In general, just one auxiliary model may not be adequate to link two very different models M_1 and M_2. However, based on the idea of the above example, the difficulty can be solved by using more than one appropriate auxiliary models $M_a, M_b, \ldots$ between M_1 and M_2. For example, suppose we use M_a and M_b to link M_1 and M_2, with M_a closer to M_1 and M_b closer to M_2. Then

$$\frac{p(\mathbf{X}, \mathbf{Z}|M_1)}{p(\mathbf{X}, \mathbf{Z}|M_2)} = \frac{p(\mathbf{X}, \mathbf{Z}|M_1)/p(\mathbf{X}, \mathbf{Z}|M_a)}{p(\mathbf{X}, \mathbf{Z}|M_2)/p(\mathbf{X}, \mathbf{Z}|M_a)} \quad \text{and} \quad \frac{p(\mathbf{X}, \mathbf{Z}|M_2)}{p(\mathbf{X}, \mathbf{Z}|M_a)} = \frac{p(\mathbf{X}, \mathbf{Z}|M_2)/p(\mathbf{X}, \mathbf{Z}|M_b)}{p(\mathbf{X}, \mathbf{Z}|M_a)/p(\mathbf{X}, \mathbf{Z}|M_b)};$$

hence, $\log B_{12} = \log B_{1a} + \log B_{ab} - \log B_{2b}$. Each log Bayes factor can be computed via path sampling.

Similar to the goodness of fit assessment in the context of single level nonlinear SEMs, it is rather difficult to find a saturated model for the two-level nonlinear SEMs. However, the goodness of fit of a proposed model can be assessed by means of the posterior predictive (PP) p-value and the estimated residual plots. The PP p-value (Gelman *et al.*, 1996a) can be used as a goodness of fit assessment for a hypothesized two-level nonlinear SEM with the mixed types data. A brief description of the PP p-values in the context of the current model is given in Appendix 6.3.

6.2.3 Application: Filipina CSWs study

As an illustration of the methodology, we use a small portion of the data set in the study of Morisky *et al.* (1998) on the effects of establishment policies, knowledge, and attitudes to condom use among Filipina commercial sex workers (CSWs). As commercial sex work promotes the spread of AIDS and other sexually transmitted diseases, the promotion of safer sexual practices among CSWs is important. The study of Morisky *et al.* (1998) was concerned with the development and preliminary findings from an AIDS preventative intervention for Filipina CSWs. The data set was collected from female CSWs in establishments (bars, night clubs, karaoke TV, and massage parlous) in cities in the Philippines. The whole questionnaire consisted of 134 items on areas of demographic knowledge, attitudes, beliefs, behaviors, self-efficacy for condom use, and social desirability. Latent psychological determinants such as CSWs' risk behaviors, knowledge and attitudes associated with AIDS and condom use are important issues to be assessed. For instance, a basic concern is to explore whether linear relationships among these latent variables are sufficient, or whether it is better to incorporate nonlinear relationships in the model. The observed variables that are used as indicators for latent quantities are measured on ordered categorical and continuous scales. Moreover, as emphasized by Morisky *et al.* (1998), establishment policies on their CSWs' condom use practices exert a strong influence on CSWs. Hence, it is interesting to study the influence of the establishment by incorporating a between-group model for the data. As observations within each establishment are correlated, the usual assumption of independence in the standard single-level SEMs is violated. Based on the above considerations, it is desirable to employ a two-level nonlinear SEM in the context of mixed ordered categorical and continuous data.

Nine observed variables, of which the seventh, eighth, and ninth are continuous and the rest ordered categorical on a five-point scale, are selected. Questions (1)–(9) corresponding to these variables are given in Appendix 1.1. For brevity, we delete those observations with missing entries in the analysis; the resulting sample size is 755. There are 97 establishments. The numbers of individuals in establishments varied from 1 to 58; this gives an unbalanced data set. The sample means and standard deviations of the continuous variables are {2.442, 1.180, 0.465} and {5.299, 2.208, 1.590}, respectively. The cell frequencies of the ordered categorical variables vary from 12 to 348. To unify the scales of variables, the raw continuous data are standardized.

After some preliminary studies and based on the meanings of the questions corresponding to the observed variables (see Appendix 1.1), in the measurement equations corresponding to the between-group and within-group models, we use the first three, the next three, and the last three observed variables as indicators for latent factors that can be roughly interpreted as 'worry about AIDS', 'attitude to the risk of getting AIDS', and 'aggressiveness'. For the between-group model we use a factor analysis model with the following specifications:

$$\mathbf{\Lambda}_2^T = \begin{bmatrix} 1 & \lambda_{2,21} & \lambda_{2,31} & 0 & 0 & 0 & 0 & 0 & 0 \\ 0 & 0 & 0 & 1 & \lambda_{2,52} & \lambda_{2,62} & 0 & 0 & 0 \\ 0 & 0 & 0 & 0 & 0 & 0 & 1 & \lambda_{2,83} & \lambda_{2,93} \end{bmatrix},$$

$$\mathbf{\Phi}_2 = \begin{bmatrix} \phi_{2,11} & & \text{sym} \\ \phi_{2,21} & \phi_{2,22} & \\ \phi_{2,31} & \phi_{2,32} & \phi_{2,33} \end{bmatrix},$$

$$\mathbf{\Psi}_2 = \text{diag}(0.3, 0.3, 0.3, 0.3, 0.3, 0.3, \psi_{27}, \psi_{28}, \psi_{29}),$$

where the unique variances corresponding to the ordered categorical variables are fixed at 0.3. Although other structure for $\mathbf{\Lambda}_2$ can be considered, we choose this common form in a confirmatory factor analysis that gives non-overlapping latent factors for clear interpretation. These latent factors are allowed to be correlated. For the within-group model with the latent factors $\{\eta_{1gi}, \xi_{1gi1}, \xi_{1gi2}\}$, we considered invariant within-group parameters such that $\mathbf{\Psi}_{1g} = \mathbf{\Psi}_1 = \text{diag}(\psi_{11}, \ldots, \psi_{19})$ and $\mathbf{\Lambda}_{1g} = \mathbf{\Lambda}_1$, where $\mathbf{\Lambda}_1$ has the same common structure as $\mathbf{\Lambda}_2$ with unknown loadings $\{\lambda_{1,21}, \lambda_{1,31}, \lambda_{1,52}, \lambda_{1,62}, \lambda_{1,83}, \lambda_{1,93}\}$. However, as the within-group model is directly related to the CSWs, we wish to consider a more subtle model with a structural equation that accounts for relationships among the latent factors. To assess the interaction effect of the explanatory latent factors, the following structural equation for the latent variables is taken:

$$\eta_{1gi} = \gamma_{11}\xi_{1gi1} + \gamma_{12}\xi_{1gi2} + \gamma_{13}\xi_{1gi1}\xi_{1gi2} + \delta_{1gi}. \tag{6.15}$$

To identify the model with respect to ordered categorical variables via the common method, α_{k1} and α_{k4}, $k = 1, \ldots, 6$ are fixed at $\alpha_{kj} = \Phi^{*^{-1}}(m_k)$, where Φ^* is the distribution function of $N[0, 1]$, and m_k is the observed cumulative marginal proportion of the categories with $z_{gk} < j$. There are a total of 49 parameters in this two-level nonlinear SEM.

In the Bayesian analysis, we need to specify hyperparameter values in the proper conjugate prior distributions of the unknown parameters. In this illustrative example, we use some data-dependent prior inputs, and *ad hoc* prior inputs that give rather vague but proper prior distributions. We emphasize that these prior inputs are used for the purpose of illustration only; we are not routinely recommending them for other substantive applications. The data-dependent prior inputs are obtained by conducting an auxiliary Bayesian estimation with proper vague conjugate prior distributions which gives estimates $\tilde{\mathbf{\Lambda}}_{01k}$, $\tilde{\mathbf{\Lambda}}^*_{01k}$, $\tilde{\mathbf{\Lambda}}_{02k}$, and $\tilde{\mathbf{\Lambda}}^*_{02k}$ for some hyperparameter values (according to the notation in Appendix 6.1). Then, results are obtained and compared on the basis of the following types of hyperparameter values:

(I) Hyperparameters $\mathbf{\Lambda}_{01k}$, $\mathbf{\Lambda}^*_{01k}$, $\mathbf{\Lambda}_{02k}$, and $\mathbf{\Lambda}^*_{02k}$ are equal to $\tilde{\mathbf{\Lambda}}_{01k}$, $\tilde{\mathbf{\Lambda}}^*_{01k}$, $\tilde{\mathbf{\Lambda}}_{02k}$, and $\tilde{\mathbf{\Lambda}}^*_{02k}$, respectively; $\mathbf{H}_{01k}$, $\mathbf{H}^*_{01k}$, $\mathbf{H}_{02k}$, and $\mathbf{H}^*_{02k}$ are equal to identity matrices of appropriate orders; $\alpha_{01k} = \alpha_{02k} = \alpha_{01\delta k} = \alpha_{02\delta k} = 10$, $\beta_{01k} = \beta_{02k} = \beta_{01\delta k} = \beta_{02\delta k} = 8$, $\rho_{01} = \rho_{02} = 6$, $\mathbf{R}_{01}^{-1} = 5\mathbf{I}_2$, and $\mathbf{R}_{02}^{-1} = 5\mathbf{I}_3$.

(II) Hyperparameter values in $\mathbf{\Lambda}_{01k}$, $\mathbf{\Lambda}^*_{01k}$, $\mathbf{\Lambda}_{02k}$, and $\mathbf{\Lambda}^*_{02k}$ are equal to zero, $\mathbf{H}_{01k}$, $\mathbf{H}^*_{01k}$, $\mathbf{H}_{02k}$, and $\mathbf{H}^*_{02k}$ are equal to 5 times the identity matrices of appropriate orders. Other hyperparameter values are equal to those given in (I). These prior inputs are not data-dependent.

Bayesian estimates are obtained using the MCMC algorithm that includes the Gibbs sampler and the MH algorithm. The convergence of this algorithm is monitored by plots of generated observations obtained with different starting values. We observe that the algorithm converges in less than 2000 iterations. Hence, we take a burn-in phase of 2000 iterations, and collect a further 3000 observations to produce the Bayesian estimates and their standard error estimates. Results obtained under prior inputs (I) and (II) are reported in Tables 6.1 and 6.2, respectively. We see that the estimates obtained under these different prior inputs are reasonably close. The PP p-values corresponding to these two sets of estimates are equal to 0.592 and 0.600, indicating that the proposed model fit the sample data, and that this statistic is quite robust to the selected prior inputs for the given sample size of 755.

In order to illustrate the path sampling in computing the Bayes factor for model comparison, we compare this two-level nonlinear model with some nonnested models. Let M_1 be the two-level nonlinear SEM with the above specifications and the nonlinear structural equation given in (6.15), and M_2 and M_3 be nonnested models with the same specifications except that the corresponding nonlinear structural equations are given by

$$M_2 : \eta_{1gi} = \gamma_{11}\xi_{1gi1} + \gamma_{12}\xi_{1gi2} + \gamma_{14}\xi^2_{1gi1} + \delta_{1gi}, \tag{6.16}$$

$$M_3 : \eta_{1gi} = \gamma_{11}\xi_{1gi1} + \gamma_{12}\xi_{1gi2} + \gamma_{15}\xi^2_{1gi2} + \delta_{1gi}. \tag{6.17}$$

To apply the path sampling to compute the Bayes factor for comparing M_1 and M_2, we link up M_1 and M_2 by M_t with the following structural equation:

$$\eta_{1gi} = \gamma_{11}\xi_{1gi1} + \gamma_{12}\xi_{1gi2} + (1-t)\gamma_{13}\xi_{1gi1}\xi_{1gi2} + t\gamma_{14}\xi^2_{1gi1} + \delta_{1gi}. \tag{6.18}$$

Table 6.1 Bayesian estimates of the structural parameters and thresholds under prior (I) for M_1: AIDS Data.

	Within group			Between group	
	EST	SE		EST	SE
Str. Par			Str. Par		
$\lambda_{1,21}$	0.238	0.081	$\lambda_{2,21}$	1.248	0.218
$\lambda_{1,31}$	0.479	0.112	$\lambda_{2,31}$	0.839	0.189
$\lambda_{1,52}$	1.102	0.213	$\lambda_{2,52}$	0.205	0.218
$\lambda_{1,62}$	0.973	0.185	$\lambda_{2,62}$	0.434	0.221
$\lambda_{1,83}$	0.842	0.182	$\lambda_{2,83}$	0.159	0.209
$\lambda_{1,93}$	0.885	0.192	$\lambda_{2,93}$	0.094	0.164
γ_{11}	0.454	0.147	$\phi_{2,11}$	0.212	0.042
γ_{12}	−0.159	0.159	$\phi_{2,12}$	−0.032	0.032
γ_{13}	−0.227	0.382	$\phi_{2,13}$	0.008	0.037
$\phi_{1,11}$	0.216	0.035	$\phi_{2,22}$	0.236	0.054
$\phi_{1,12}$	−0.031	0.017	$\phi_{2,23}$	0.006	0.041
$\phi_{1,22}$	0.202	0.037	$\phi_{2,33}$	0.257	0.063
ψ_{11}	0.558	0.087	ψ_{27}	0.378	0.070
ψ_{12}	0.587	0.049	ψ_{28}	0.349	0.053
ψ_{13}	0.725	0.063	ψ_{29}	0.259	0.039
ψ_{14}	0.839	0.084			
ψ_{15}	0.691	0.085			
ψ_{16}	0.730	0.081			
ψ_{17}	0.723	0.056			
ψ_{18}	0.629	0.053			
ψ_{19}	0.821	0.062			
$\psi_{1\delta}$	0.460	0.080			
Thresholds					
α_{12}	−1.163	0.054	α_{13}	−0.751	0.045
α_{22}	−0.083	0.033	α_{23}	0.302	0.035
α_{32}	−0.985	0.045	α_{33}	−0.589	0.044
α_{42}	−0.406	0.035	α_{43}	0.241	0.029
α_{52}	−1.643	0.063	α_{53}	−0.734	0.027
α_{62}	−1.038	0.043	α_{63}	−0.118	0.025

Source: Lee (2007).

Clearly, when $t = 1$, $M_t = M_2$; when $t = 0$, $M_t = M_1$. By differentiating the complete-data log-likelihood $\log p(\mathbf{Y}, \mathbf{V}, \mathbf{\Omega}_1, \mathbf{\Omega}_2, \mathbf{X}, \mathbf{Z}|\boldsymbol{\theta}, \boldsymbol{\alpha}, t)$ with respect to t, we obtain

$$U(\boldsymbol{\theta}, \boldsymbol{\alpha}, \mathbf{Y}, \mathbf{V}, \mathbf{\Omega}_1, \mathbf{\Omega}_2, \mathbf{X}, \mathbf{Z}, t) = -\sum_{i=1}^{n} \{\eta_{1gi} - \gamma_{11}\xi_{1gi1} - \gamma_{12}\xi_{1gi2} \\ -(1-t)\gamma_{13}\xi_{1gi1}\xi_{1gi2} - t\gamma_{14}\xi_{1gi1}^2\}\psi_{1\delta}^{-1}\{\gamma_{13}\xi_{1gi1}\xi_{1gi2} - \gamma_{14}\xi_{1gi1}^2\}.$$

Table 6.2 Bayesian estimates of the structural parameters and thresholds under prior (II) for M_1: AIDS data.

	Within group			Between group	
	EST	SE		EST	SE
Str. Par			Str. Par		
$\lambda_{1,21}$	0.239	0.080	$\lambda_{2,21}$	1.404	0.283
$\lambda_{1,31}$	0.495	0.119	$\lambda_{2,31}$	0.869	0.228
$\lambda_{1,52}$	1.210	0.284	$\lambda_{2,52}$	0.304	0.293
$\lambda_{1,62}$	1.083	0.250	$\lambda_{2,62}$	0.602	0.264
$\lambda_{1,83}$	0.988	0.215	$\lambda_{2,83}$	0.155	0.230
$\lambda_{1,93}$	0.918	0.197	$\lambda_{2,93}$	0.085	0.176
γ_{11}	0.474	0.157	$\phi_{2,11}$	0.196	0.043
γ_{12}	−0.232	0.165	$\phi_{2,12}$	−0.026	0.030
γ_{13}	−0.353	0.540	$\phi_{2,13}$	0.010	0.032
$\phi_{1,11}$	0.198	0.048	$\phi_{2,22}$	0.219	0.048
$\phi_{1,12}$	−0.022	0.015	$\phi_{2,23}$	0.008	0.037
$\phi_{1,22}$	0.181	0.035	$\phi_{2,33}$	0.251	0.060
ψ_{11}	0.562	0.100	ψ_{27}	0.376	0.068
ψ_{12}	0.587	0.049	ψ_{28}	0.350	0.055
ψ_{13}	0.715	0.066	ψ_{29}	0.256	0.039
ψ_{14}	0.849	0.091			
ψ_{15}	0.702	0.093			
ψ_{16}	0.697	0.079			
ψ_{17}	0.738	0.055			
ψ_{18}	0.601	0.056			
ψ_{19}	0.828	0.064			
$\psi_{1\delta}$	0.460	0.077			
Thresholds					
α_{12}	−1.170	0.060	α_{13}	−0.755	0.053
α_{22}	−0.084	0.029	α_{23}	0.303	0.033
α_{32}	−0.986	0.043	α_{33}	−0.589	0.042
α_{42}	−0.406	0.035	α_{43}	0.242	0.029
α_{52}	−1.656	0.066	α_{53}	−0.738	0.028
α_{62}	−1.032	0.044	α_{63}	−0.119	0.026

Source: Lee (2007).

Consequently, $\log B_{21}$ can be computed using (6.6) and (6.7) with a sample of observations simulated from the appropriate posterior distributions. The above procedure can be used similarly to compute $\log B_{23}$.

In this example, we take 20 grids in [0,1] and $J = 1000$ in computing log Bayes factors. The estimated $\log B_{21}$ and $\log B_{23}$ under prior inputs (I, II) are equal to (0.317, 0.018) and (0.176, 0.131), respectively. Hence, the values of the log Bayes factors are reasonably close with the given different prior inputs. According to the criterion given in Kass and Raftery

(1995) for comparing nonnested models, M_2 is slightly better than M_1 and M_3. To apply the procedure for comparing nested models, we further compare M_2 with a linear model M_0 and a more comprehensive model M_4. The competing models M_0 and M_4 have the same specifications as M_2, except that the corresponding structural equations are given by:

$$M_0: \ \eta_{1gi} = \gamma_{11}\xi_{1gi1} + \gamma_{12}\xi_{1gi2} + \delta_{1gi},$$

$$M_4: \ \eta_{1gi} = \gamma_{11}\xi_{1gi1} + \gamma_{12}\xi_{1gi2} + \gamma_{13}\xi_{1gi1}\xi_{1gi2} + \gamma_{14}\xi_{1gi1}^2 + \gamma_{15}\xi_{1gi2}^2 + \delta_{1gi}.$$

Note that M_0 is nested in M_2, and M_2 is nested in M_4. Using the path sampling procedure, the estimated $\log B_{40}$ and $\log B_{42}$ under prior inputs (I, II) are (1.181, 1.233) and (1.043, 1.071), respectively. Hence, M_4 is better than M_0 and M_2. The PP p-values corresponding to M_4 under prior inputs (I) and (II) are equal to 0.582 and 0.611, respectively. These two values are close and indicate the expected result that the selected model also fits the data. The Bayesian estimates and their standard error estimates under M_4 and prior inputs (I) are reported in Table 6.3. Results obtained under prior inputs (II) are similar. We also observe comparatively large variabilities for estimates of parameters in $\mathbf{\Lambda}_2$ corresponding to the between-group model and estimates of $\{\gamma_{13}, \gamma_{14}, \gamma_{15}\}$ corresponding to the nonlinear terms of the latent variables. This phenomenon may be due to the small sample size at the between-group level and the complicated nature of the parameters. Other straightforward interpretations are not presented. Based on the methodology mentioned above, more complicated or other combinations of nonlinear terms can be analyzed similarly.

To summarize, we have introduced a two-level nonlinear SEM with three non-overlapping factors, 'worry about AIDS', 'attitude to the risk of getting AIDS', and 'aggressiveness', in the within-group and between-group covariance structures. The significance of the establishments' influence is reflected by relatively large estimates of some between-group parameters.

The WinBUGS software (Spiegelhalter *et al.*, 2003) can produce Bayesian estimates of the parameters in some two-level nonlinear SEMs. To demonstrate this, we apply WinBUGS to analyze the current AIDS data based on M_4 and type (I) prior inputs. The WinBUGS code is given in Appendix 6.4.

6.3 Structural equation models with multisample data

In contrast to multilevel data, multisample data come from a comparatively smaller number of groups (populations); the number of observations within each group is usually large, and observations within each group are assumed independent. One of the main objectives in the analysis of multisample data is to investigate the similarities or differences among the models in the different groups. As a result, the statistical inferences emphasized in analyzing multisample SEMs are different from those in analyzing two-level SEMs. Analysis of multiple samples is a major topic in structural equation modeling. It is useful for investigating the behaviors of different groups of employees, different cultures, and different treatment groups, etc. The main interest lies in the testing of hypotheses about the different kinds of invariances among the models in different groups. This issue can be formulated as a model comparison problem, and can be effectively addressed by the Bayes factor or DIC in a Bayesian approach. Another advantage of the Bayesian model comparison through the

Table 6.3 Bayesian estimates of the structural parameters and thresholds under prior (I) for M_4: AIDS data.

	Within group			Between group	
	EST	SE		EST	SE
Str. Par			Str. Par		
$\lambda_{1,21}$	0.203	0.070	$\lambda_{2,21}$	1.261	0.233
$\lambda_{1,31}$	0.450	0.100	$\lambda_{2,31}$	0.842	0.193
$\lambda_{1,52}$	0.992	0.205	$\lambda_{2,52}$	0.189	0.227
$\lambda_{1,62}$	0.868	0.180	$\lambda_{2,62}$	0.461	0.209
$\lambda_{1,83}$	0.936	0.172	$\lambda_{2,83}$	0.157	0.230
$\lambda_{1,93}$	0.880	0.194	$\lambda_{2,93}$	0.074	0.167
γ_{11}	0.489	0.147	$\phi_{2,11}$	0.211	0.040
γ_{12}	−0.026	0.217	$\phi_{2,12}$	−0.029	0.033
γ_{13}	−0.212	0.265	$\phi_{2,13}$	0.010	0.035
γ_{14}	0.383	0.442	$\phi_{2,22}$	0.223	0.053
γ_{15}	−0.147	0.188	$\phi_{2,23}$	0.013	0.038
$\phi_{1,11}$	0.245	0.042	$\phi_{2,33}$	0.243	0.059
$\phi_{1,12}$	−0.029	0.020	ψ_{27}	0.377	0.068
$\phi_{1,22}$	0.186	0.031	ψ_{28}	0.351	0.055
ψ_{11}	0.546	0.093	ψ_{29}	0.258	0.040
ψ_{12}	0.591	0.047			
ψ_{13}	0.724	0.063			
ψ_{14}	0.826	0.081			
ψ_{15}	0.716	0.092			
ψ_{16}	0.731	0.077			
ψ_{17}	0.733	0.049			
ψ_{18}	0.610	0.048			
ψ_{19}	0.833	0.064			
$\psi_{1\delta}$	0.478	0.072			
Thresholds					
α_{12}	−1.163	0.058	α_{13}	−0.753	0.048
α_{22}	−0.088	0.032	α_{23}	0.299	0.036
α_{32}	−0.980	0.046	α_{33}	−0.583	0.047
α_{42}	−0.407	0.034	α_{43}	0.244	0.028
α_{52}	−1.650	0.063	α_{53}	−0.734	0.027
α_{62}	−1.034	0.043	α_{63}	−0.118	0.026

Source: Lee (2007).

Bayes factor or DIC is that nonnested models (hypotheses) can be compared, hence it is not necessary to follow a hierarchy of hypotheses to assess the invariance for the SEMs in different groups.

Bayesian methods for analyzing mutlisample SEMs are presented in this section. We will emphasize nonlinear SEMs with ordered categorical variables, although the general ideas can be applied to SEMs in other settings.

6.3.1 Bayesian analysis of a nonlinear SEM in different groups

Consider G independent groups of individuals that represent different populations. For $g = 1, \ldots, G$ and $i = 1, \ldots, N_g$, let $\mathbf{v}_i^{(g)}$ be the $p \times 1$ random vector of observed variables that correspond to the ith observation (subject) in the gth group. In contrast to two-level SEMs, for $i = 1, \ldots, N_g$ in the gth group, the $\mathbf{v}_i^{(g)}$ are assumed to be independent. For each $g = 1, \ldots, G$, $\mathbf{v}_i^{(g)}$ is related to latent variables in a $q \times 1$ random vector $\boldsymbol{\omega}_i^{(g)}$ through the measurement equation

$$\mathbf{v}_i^{(g)} = \boldsymbol{\mu}^{(g)} + \boldsymbol{\Lambda}^{(g)}\boldsymbol{\omega}_i^{(g)} + \boldsymbol{\epsilon}_i^{(g)}, \tag{6.19}$$

where $\boldsymbol{\mu}^{(g)}$, $\boldsymbol{\Lambda}^{(g)}$, $\boldsymbol{\omega}_i^{(g)}$, and $\boldsymbol{\epsilon}_i^{(g)}$ are defined as before. It is assumed that $\boldsymbol{\omega}_i^{(g)}$ and $\boldsymbol{\epsilon}_i^{(g)}$ are independent, and the distribution of $\boldsymbol{\epsilon}_i^{(g)}$ is $N[\mathbf{0}, \boldsymbol{\Psi}_\epsilon^{(g)}]$, where $\boldsymbol{\Psi}_\epsilon^{(g)}$ is diagonal. Let $\boldsymbol{\omega}_i^{(g)} = (\boldsymbol{\eta}_i^{(g)T}, \boldsymbol{\xi}_i^{(g)T})^T$. It is naturally assumed that the dimensions of $\boldsymbol{\xi}_i^{(g)}$ and $\boldsymbol{\eta}_i^{(g)}$ are independent of g; that is, they are the same for each group. To assess the effects of the nonlinear terms of latent variables in $\boldsymbol{\xi}_i^{(g)}(q_2 \times 1)$ on $\boldsymbol{\eta}_i^{(g)}(q_1 \times 1)$, we consider a nonlinear SEM with the nonlinear structural equation

$$\boldsymbol{\eta}_i^{(g)} = \boldsymbol{\Pi}^{(g)}\boldsymbol{\eta}_i^{(g)} + \boldsymbol{\Gamma}^{(g)}\mathbf{F}(\boldsymbol{\xi}_i^{(g)}) + \boldsymbol{\delta}_i^{(g)}, \tag{6.20}$$

where $\boldsymbol{\Pi}^{(g)}$, $\boldsymbol{\Gamma}^{(g)}$, $\mathbf{F}(\boldsymbol{\xi}_i^{(g)})$, and $\boldsymbol{\delta}_i^{(g)}$ are defined as before. It is assumed that $\boldsymbol{\xi}_i^{(g)}$ and $\boldsymbol{\delta}_i^{(g)}$ are independent, the distributions of $\boldsymbol{\xi}_i^{(g)}$ and $\boldsymbol{\delta}_i^{(g)}$ are $N[\mathbf{0}, \boldsymbol{\Phi}^{(g)}]$ and $N[\mathbf{0}, \boldsymbol{\Psi}_\delta^{(g)}]$, respectively, where $\boldsymbol{\Psi}_\delta^{(g)}$ is diagonal; and the vector-valued function $\mathbf{F}(\cdot)$ does not depend on g. However, different groups can have different linear or nonlinear terms of $\boldsymbol{\xi}_i^{(g)}$ by defining appropriate $\mathbf{F}(\cdot)$ and assigning zero values to appropriate elements in $\boldsymbol{\Gamma}^{(g)}$. Let $\boldsymbol{\Lambda}_\omega^{(g)} = (\boldsymbol{\Pi}^{(g)}, \boldsymbol{\Gamma}^{(g)})$ and $\mathbf{G}(\boldsymbol{\omega}_i^{(g)}) = (\boldsymbol{\eta}_i^{(g)^T}, \mathbf{F}(\boldsymbol{\xi}_i^{(g)})^T)^T$. Then equation (6.20) can be rewritten as

$$\boldsymbol{\eta}_i^{(g)} = \boldsymbol{\Lambda}_\omega^{(g)}\mathbf{G}(\boldsymbol{\omega}_i^{(g)}) + \boldsymbol{\delta}_i^{(g)}. \tag{6.21}$$

To handle the ordered categorical outcomes, suppose that $\mathbf{v}_i^{(g)} = (\mathbf{x}_i^{(g)T}, \mathbf{y}_i^{(g)T})^T$, where $\mathbf{x}_i^{(g)}$ is an $r \times 1$ subvector of observable continuous responses; while $\mathbf{y}_i^{(g)}$ is an $s \times 1$ subvector of unobservable continuous responses, the information of which is reflected by an observable ordered categorical vector $\mathbf{z}_i^{(g)}$. In a generic sense, an ordered categorical variable $z_m^{(g)}$ is defined with its underlying latent continuous random variable $y_m^{(g)}$ by

$$z_m^{(g)} = a, \quad \text{if} \alpha_{m,a}^{(g)} \le y_m^{(g)} < \alpha_{m,a+1}^{(g)}, \ a = 0, \ldots, b_m, \ m = 1, \ldots, s, \tag{6.22}$$

where $\{-\infty = \alpha_{m,0}^{(g)} < \alpha_{m,1}^{(g)} < \ldots < \alpha_{m,b_m}^{(g)} < \alpha_{m,b_m+1}^{(g)} = \infty\}$ is the set of threshold parameters that define the categories, and $b_m + 1$ is the number of categories for the ordered categorical variable $z_m^{(g)}$. For each ordered categorical variable, the number of thresholds is the same for each group. To tackle the identification problem related to the ordered categorical variables, we consider an ordered categorical variable $z_m^{(g)}$ that is defined by a set of thresholds $\alpha_{m,k}^{(g)}$ and an underlying latent continuous variable $y_m^{(g)}$ with a distribution $N[\mu_m^{(g)}, \sigma_m^{2(g)}]$. The indeterminacy is caused by the fact that $\alpha_{m,k}^{(g)}$, $\mu_m^{(g)}$, and $\sigma_m^{2(g)}$ are not simultaneously estimable. For a given group g, a common method to solve this identification problem with respect to each mth ordered categorical variable that corresponds to the gth group is to fix $\alpha_{m,1}^{(g)}$ and $\alpha_{m,b_m}^{(g)}$ at preassigned values (see Lee *et al.*, 2005). For example, we may fix $\alpha_{m,1}^{(g)} = \Phi^{*-1}(f_{m,1}^{(g)})$, and $\alpha_{m,b_m}^{(g)} = \Phi^{*-1}(f_{m,b_m}^{(g)})$, where $\Phi^*(\cdot)$ is the distribution function of $N[0, 1]$, and $f_{m,1}^{(g)}$ and $f_{m,b_m}^{(g)}$

are the frequencies of the first category and the cumulative frequencies of categories with $z_m^{(g)} < b_m$. For analyzing multisample models where group comparisons are of interest, it is important to impose conditions for identifying the ordered categorical variables such that the underlying latent continuous variables have the same scale among the groups. To achieve this, we can select the first group as the reference group, and identify its ordered categorical variables by fixing both end thresholds as above. Then, for any m, and $g \neq 1$, we impose the restrictions (see Lee *et al.*, 1989),

$$\alpha_{m,k}^{(g)} = \alpha_{m,k}^{(1)}, \quad k = 1, \ldots, b_m, \tag{6.23}$$

on the thresholds for every ordered categorical variable $z_m^{(g)}$. Under these identification conditions, the unknown parameters in the groups are interpreted in a relative sense, compared over groups. Note that when a different reference group is used, relations over groups are unchanged. Hence, the statistical inferences are unaffected by the choice of the reference group. Clearly, the compatibility of the groups is reflected in the differences between the parameter estimates.

Let $\boldsymbol{\theta}^{(g)}$ be the unknown parameter vector in an identified model and let $\boldsymbol{\alpha}^{(g)}$ be the vector of unknown thresholds that correspond to the gth group. In multisample analysis, a certain type of parameter in $\boldsymbol{\theta}^{(g)}$ is often hypothesized to be invariant over the group models. For example, restrictions on the thresholds, and the constraints $\boldsymbol{\Lambda}^{(1)} = \ldots = \boldsymbol{\Lambda}^{(G)}$, $\boldsymbol{\Phi}^{(1)} = \ldots = \boldsymbol{\Phi}^{(G)}$, and/or $\boldsymbol{\Gamma}^{(1)} = \ldots = \boldsymbol{\Gamma}^{(G)}$, are often imposed. Let $\boldsymbol{\theta}$ be the vector that contains all the unknown distinct parameters in $\boldsymbol{\theta}^{(1)}, \ldots, \boldsymbol{\theta}^{(G)}$, and let $\boldsymbol{\alpha}$ be the vector that contains all the unknown thresholds. Moreover, let $\mathbf{X}^{(g)} = (\mathbf{x}_1^{(g)}, \ldots, \mathbf{x}_{N_g}^{(g)})$ and $\mathbf{X} = (\mathbf{X}^{(1)}, \ldots, \mathbf{X}^{(G)})$ be the observed continuous data, let $\mathbf{Z}^{(g)} = (\mathbf{z}_1^{(g)}, \ldots, \mathbf{z}_{N_g}^{(g)})$ and $\mathbf{Z} = (\mathbf{Z}^{(1)}, \ldots, \mathbf{Z}^{(G)})$ be the observed ordered categorical data, and let $\mathbf{Y}^{(g)} = (\mathbf{y}_1^{(g)}, \ldots, \mathbf{y}_{N_g}^{(g)})$ and $\mathbf{Y} = (\mathbf{Y}^{(1)}, \ldots, \mathbf{Y}^{(G)})$ be the latent continuous measurement associated with $\mathbf{Z}^{(g)}$ and $\mathbf{Z}$, respectively. Finally, let $\boldsymbol{\Omega}^{(g)} = (\boldsymbol{\omega}_1^{(g)}, \ldots, \boldsymbol{\omega}_{N_g}^{(g)})$ and $\boldsymbol{\Omega} = (\boldsymbol{\Omega}^{(1)}, \ldots, \boldsymbol{\Omega}^{(G)})$ be the matrices of latent variables. In the posterior analysis, the observed data $(\mathbf{X}, \mathbf{Z})$ will be augmented with $(\mathbf{Y}, \boldsymbol{\Omega})$. The Gibbs sampler (Geman and Geman, 1984) will be used to generate a sequence of observations from the joint posterior distribution $[\boldsymbol{\theta}, \boldsymbol{\alpha}, \mathbf{Y}, \boldsymbol{\Omega}|\mathbf{X}, \mathbf{Z}]$. In applying the Gibbs sampler, we iteratively sample observations from the following conditional distributions: $[\boldsymbol{\Omega}|\boldsymbol{\theta}, \boldsymbol{\alpha}, \mathbf{Y}, \mathbf{X}, \mathbf{Z}]$, $[\boldsymbol{\alpha}, \mathbf{Y}|\boldsymbol{\theta}, \boldsymbol{\Omega}, \mathbf{X}, \mathbf{Z}]$, and $[\boldsymbol{\theta}|\boldsymbol{\alpha}, \mathbf{Y}, \boldsymbol{\Omega}, \mathbf{X}, \mathbf{Z}]$. As in our previous treatments of the thresholds, we assign a noninformative prior to $\boldsymbol{\alpha}$, so that the corresponding prior distribution is proportional to a constant. The first two conditional distributions can be derived by reasoning similar to Section 6.2 (Lee, 2007, Appendix 9.1). The conditional distribution $[\boldsymbol{\theta}|\boldsymbol{\alpha}, \mathbf{Y}, \boldsymbol{\Omega}, \mathbf{X}, \mathbf{Z}]$ is further decomposed into components involving various structural parameters in the different group models. These components are different under various hypotheses of interest or various competing models. Some examples of nonnested competing models (or hypotheses) are:

$$\begin{aligned} &M_A: \text{ No constraints}, M_1: \boldsymbol{\mu}^{(1)} = \ldots = \boldsymbol{\mu}^{(G)}, \quad M_2: \boldsymbol{\Lambda}^{(1)} = \ldots = \boldsymbol{\Lambda}^{(G)}, \\ &M_3: \boldsymbol{\Lambda}_\omega^{(1)} = \ldots = \boldsymbol{\Lambda}_\omega^{(G)}, \quad M_4: \boldsymbol{\Phi}^{(1)} = \ldots = \boldsymbol{\Phi}^{(G)}, \\ &M_5: \boldsymbol{\Psi}_\epsilon^{(1)} = \ldots = \boldsymbol{\Psi}_\epsilon^{(G)}, \quad M_6: \boldsymbol{\Psi}_\delta^{(1)} = \ldots = \boldsymbol{\Psi}_\delta^{(G)}. \end{aligned} \tag{6.24}$$

The components in the conditional distribution $[\boldsymbol{\theta}|\boldsymbol{\alpha}, \mathbf{Y}, \boldsymbol{\Omega}, \mathbf{X}, \mathbf{Z}]$ and the specification of prior distributions are slightly different under different M_k defined above. First, prior distributions for unconstrained parameters in different groups are naturally assumed to be independent. In estimating the unconstrained parameters, we need to separately specify the prior distributions of unconstrained parameters in each group, and the data in the corresponding group are used. For constrained parameters across groups, only one prior distribution for these constrained parameters is needed, and all the data in the groups should be combined in the estimation; see Song and Lee (2001). In this situation, we may not wish to take a joint prior distribution for the factor loading matrix and the unique variance of the error measurement. In the gth group model, let $\psi_{\epsilon k}^{(g)}$ and $\mathbf{\Lambda}_k^{(g)^T}$ be the kth diagonal element of $\mathbf{\Psi}_\epsilon^{(g)}$ and the kth row of $\mathbf{\Lambda}^{(g)}$, respectively. In the multisample analysis, if those parameters are not invariant over groups, their joint prior distribution could be taken as: $\psi_{\epsilon k}^{(g)-1} \stackrel{D}{=} \text{Gamma}[\alpha_{0\epsilon k}^{(g)}, \beta_{0\epsilon k}^{(g)}]$, $[\mathbf{\Lambda}_k^{(g)}|\psi_{\epsilon k}^{(g)}] \stackrel{D}{=} N[\mathbf{\Lambda}_{0k}^{(g)}, \psi_{\epsilon k}^{(g)}\mathbf{H}_{0yk}^{(g)}]$, where $\alpha_{0\epsilon k}^{(g)}$, $\beta_{0\epsilon k}^{(g)}$, $\mathbf{\Lambda}_{0k}^{(g)}$, and $\mathbf{H}_{0yk}^{(g)}$ are hyperparameters. This kind of joint prior distribution may cause problems under the constrained situation where $\mathbf{\Lambda}^{(1)} = \ldots = \mathbf{\Lambda}^{(G)} = \mathbf{\Lambda}$ and $\mathbf{\Psi}_\epsilon^{(1)} \neq \ldots \neq \mathbf{\Psi}_\epsilon^{(G)}$, because it is difficult to select $p(\mathbf{\Lambda}_k|\cdot)$ based on a set of different $\psi_{\epsilon k}^{(g)}$. Hence, for convenience, and following the suggestion of Song and Lee (2001), we select independent prior distributions for $\mathbf{\Lambda}^{(g)}$ and $\mathbf{\Psi}_\epsilon^{(g)}$, such that $p(\mathbf{\Lambda}^{(g)}, \mathbf{\Psi}_\epsilon^{(g)}) = p(\mathbf{\Lambda}^{(g)})p(\mathbf{\Psi}_\epsilon^{(g)})$, for $g = 1, 2, \ldots, G$. Under this choice, the prior distribution of $\mathbf{\Lambda}$ under the constraint $\mathbf{\Lambda}^{(1)} = \ldots = \mathbf{\Lambda}^{(G)} = \mathbf{\Lambda}$ is given by $\mathbf{\Lambda}_k \stackrel{D}{=} N[\mathbf{\Lambda}_{0k}, \mathbf{H}_{0yk}]$, which is independent of $\psi_{\epsilon k}^{(g)}$. Here, $\mathbf{\Lambda}_k^T$ is the kth row of $\mathbf{\Lambda}$. In the situation where $\mathbf{\Lambda}^{(1)} \neq \ldots \neq \mathbf{\Lambda}^{(G)}$, the prior distribution of each $\mathbf{\Lambda}_k^{(g)}$ is given by $N[\mathbf{\Lambda}_{0k}^{(g)}, \mathbf{H}_{0yk}^{(g)}]$. The prior distribution of $\psi_{\epsilon k}^{(g)-1}$ is again $\text{Gamma}[\alpha_{0\epsilon k}^{(g)}, \beta_{0\epsilon k}^{(g)}]$. Similarly, we select the prior distributions for $\mathbf{\Lambda}_\omega^{(g)}$ and $\mathbf{\Psi}_\delta^{(g)}$ such that $p(\mathbf{\Lambda}_\omega^{(g)}, \mathbf{\Psi}_\delta^{(g)}) = p(\mathbf{\Lambda}_\omega^{(g)})p(\mathbf{\Psi}_\delta^{(g)})$, for $g = 1, \ldots, G$. Let $\mathbf{\Lambda}_{\omega k}^T$ and $\mathbf{\Lambda}_{\omega k}^{(g)^T}$ be the kth rows of $\mathbf{\Lambda}_\omega$ and $\mathbf{\Lambda}_\omega^{(g)}$, respectively. The prior distributions of $\mathbf{\Lambda}_\omega$ are given by

(i) $\mathbf{\Lambda}_{\omega k} \stackrel{D}{=} N[\mathbf{\Lambda}_{0\omega k}, \mathbf{H}_{0\omega k}]$, if $\mathbf{\Lambda}_\omega^{(1)} = \ldots = \mathbf{\Lambda}_\omega^{(G)} = \mathbf{\Lambda}_\omega$,

(ii) $\mathbf{\Lambda}_{\omega k}^{(g)} \stackrel{D}{=} N[\mathbf{\Lambda}_{0\omega k}^{(g)}, \mathbf{H}_{0\omega k}^{(g)}]$, if $\mathbf{\Lambda}_\omega^{(1)} \neq \ldots \neq \mathbf{\Lambda}_\omega^{(G)}$,

with the hyperparameters $\mathbf{\Lambda}_{0\omega k}$, $\mathbf{\Lambda}_{0\omega k}^{(g)}$, $\mathbf{H}_{0\omega k}$, and $\mathbf{H}_{0\omega k}^{(g)}$. Let $\psi_{\delta k}^{(g)}$ be the kth diagonal element of $\mathbf{\Psi}_\delta^{(g)}$. The prior distribution of $\psi_{\delta k}^{(g)-1}$ is $\text{Gamma}[\alpha_{0\delta k}^{(g)}, \beta_{0\delta k}^{(g)}]$, with hyperparamters $\alpha_{0\delta k}^{(g)}$ and $\beta_{0\delta k}^{(g)}$. The prior distributions of $\boldsymbol{\mu}^{(g)}$ and $\mathbf{\Phi}^{(g)}$ are given by:

$$\boldsymbol{\mu}^{(g)} \stackrel{D}{=} N\left[\boldsymbol{\mu}_0^{(g)}, \mathbf{\Sigma}_0^{(g)}\right], \quad \mathbf{\Phi}^{(g)-1} \stackrel{D}{=} W_{q_2}\left[\mathbf{R}_0^{(g)}, \rho_0^{(g)}\right], g = 1, \ldots, G,$$

where $\boldsymbol{\mu}_0^{(g)}$, $\mathbf{\Sigma}_0^{(g)}$, $\mathbf{R}_0^{(g)}$, and $\rho_0^{(g)}$ are hyperparameters. Similar adjustments are made under various combinations of constraints. Based on the above understanding, and the reasoning given in Section 6.2, the conditional distribution $[\boldsymbol{\theta}|\boldsymbol{\alpha}, \mathbf{Y}, \mathbf{\Omega}, \mathbf{X}, \mathbf{Z}]$ under various competing models can be obtained. Some results are given in Appendix 6.5.

In the analysis of multisample SEMs, one important statistical inference is the test of whether some types of parameters are invariant over the groups. In Bayesian analysis, each hypothesis of interest is associated with a model, and the problem is approached through model comparison. In contrast to the traditional approach using the likelihood ratio test, it is not necessary to carry out the model comparison with a hierarchy of hypotheses (see Bollen, 1989). For instance, depending on the matter of interest within a substantive problem, we can compare any two nonnested models M_k and M_h, as given in (6.24); or compare any M_k with any combination of the models given in (6.24). Similarly, M_k and M_h can be compared using the Bayes factor

$$B_{kh} = \frac{p(\mathbf{X}, \mathbf{Z}|M_k)}{p(\mathbf{X}, \mathbf{Z}|M_h)},$$

where $(\mathbf{X}, \mathbf{Z})$ is the observed data set. Let t be a path in $[0, 1]$ to link M_h and M_k, and $0 = t_{(0)} < t_{(1)} < \ldots < t_{(S)} < t_{(S+1)} = 1$ be fixed grids in $[0, 1]$. Let $p(\mathbf{Y}, \boldsymbol{\Omega}, \mathbf{X}, \mathbf{Z}|\boldsymbol{\theta}, \boldsymbol{\alpha}, t)$ be the complete-data likelihood, $\boldsymbol{\theta}$ the vector of unknown parameters in the link model, and

$$U(\boldsymbol{\theta}, \boldsymbol{\alpha}, \mathbf{Y}, \boldsymbol{\Omega}, \mathbf{X}, \mathbf{Z}, t) = d \log p(\mathbf{Y}, \boldsymbol{\Omega}, \mathbf{X}, \mathbf{Z}|\boldsymbol{\theta}, \boldsymbol{\alpha}, t)/dt.$$

Then,

$$\widehat{\log B_{kh}} = \frac{1}{2} \sum_{s=0}^{S} (t_{(s+1)} - t_{(s)})(\bar{U}_{(s+1)} + \bar{U}_{(s)}),$$

where

$$\bar{U}_{(s)} = \frac{1}{J} \sum_{j=1}^{J} U(\boldsymbol{\theta}^{(j)}, \boldsymbol{\alpha}^{(j)}, \mathbf{Y}^{(j)}, \boldsymbol{\Omega}^{(j)}, \mathbf{X}, \mathbf{Z}, t_{(s)}),$$

in which $\{\boldsymbol{\theta}^{(j)}, \boldsymbol{\alpha}^{(j)}, \mathbf{Y}^{(j)}, \boldsymbol{\Omega}^{(j)} : j = 1, 2, \ldots, J\}$ is a sample of observations simulated from the joint posterior distribution $[\boldsymbol{\theta}, \boldsymbol{\alpha}, \mathbf{Y}, \boldsymbol{\Omega}|\mathbf{X}, \mathbf{Z}, t_{(s)}]$.

Finding a good path to link the competing models M_k and M_h is a crucial step in the path sampling procedure for computing $\log B_{kh}$. As an illustrative example, suppose that the competing models M_1 and M_2 are defined as follows: for $g = 1, 2$ and $i = 1, \ldots, N_g$,

$$\begin{aligned} M_1 : \ \mathbf{v}_i^{(g)} &= \boldsymbol{\mu}^{(g)} + \boldsymbol{\Lambda}\boldsymbol{\omega}_i^{(g)} + \boldsymbol{\epsilon}_i^{(g)}, \\ \boldsymbol{\eta}_i^{(g)} &= \boldsymbol{\Gamma}^{(g)}\mathbf{F}(\boldsymbol{\xi}_i^{(g)}) + \boldsymbol{\delta}_i^{(g)}, \\ M_2 : \ \mathbf{v}_i^{(g)} &= \boldsymbol{\mu}^{(g)} + \boldsymbol{\Lambda}^{(g)}\boldsymbol{\omega}_i^{(g)} + \boldsymbol{\epsilon}_i^{(g)}, \\ \boldsymbol{\eta}_i^{(g)} &= \boldsymbol{\Gamma}\mathbf{F}(\boldsymbol{\xi}_i^{(g)}) + \boldsymbol{\delta}_i^{(g)}. \end{aligned}$$

In M_1, $\boldsymbol{\Lambda}$ is invariant over the two groups, while in M_2, $\boldsymbol{\Gamma}$ is invariant over the groups. Note that in both models, the form of the nonlinear terms is the same. Due to the constraints imposed on the parameters, it is rather difficult to find a path t in $[0, 1]$ that directly links M_1 and M_2. This difficulty can be solved through the use of the following auxiliary model M_a:

$$M_a : \mathbf{v}_i^{(g)} = \boldsymbol{\mu}^{(g)} + \boldsymbol{\epsilon}_i^{(g)}, \quad g = 1, 2, i = 1, \ldots, N_g.$$

The link model M_{ta1} for linking M_1 and M_a is defined as follows: for $g = 1, 2$ and $i = 1, \ldots, N_g$,

$$\begin{aligned} M_{ta1} : \ \mathbf{v}_i^{(g)} &= \boldsymbol{\mu}^{(g)} + t\boldsymbol{\Lambda}\boldsymbol{\omega}_i^{(g)} + \boldsymbol{\epsilon}_i^{(g)}, \\ \boldsymbol{\eta}_i^{(g)} &= \boldsymbol{\Gamma}^{(g)}\mathbf{F}(\boldsymbol{\xi}_i^{(g)}) + \boldsymbol{\delta}_i^{(g)}. \end{aligned}$$

When $t = 1$, M_{ta1} reduces to M_1, and when $t = 0$, M_{ta1} reduces to M_a. The parameter vector $\boldsymbol{\theta}$ in M_{ta1} contains $\boldsymbol{\mu}^{(1)}$, $\boldsymbol{\mu}^{(2)}$, $\boldsymbol{\Lambda}$, $\boldsymbol{\Psi}_\epsilon^{(1)}$, $\boldsymbol{\Psi}_\epsilon^{(2)}$, $\boldsymbol{\Gamma}^{(1)}$, $\boldsymbol{\Gamma}^{(2)}$, $\boldsymbol{\Phi}^{(1)}$, $\boldsymbol{\Phi}^{(2)}$, $\boldsymbol{\Psi}_\delta^{(1)}$, and $\boldsymbol{\Psi}_\delta^{(2)}$. The link model M_{ta2} for linking M_2 and M_a is defined as follows:

$$\begin{aligned} M_{ta2}: \ \mathbf{v}_i^{(g)} &= \boldsymbol{\mu}^{(g)} + t\boldsymbol{\Lambda}^{(g)}\boldsymbol{\omega}_i^{(g)} + \boldsymbol{\epsilon}_i^{(g)}, \\ \boldsymbol{\eta}_i^{(g)} &= \boldsymbol{\Gamma}\mathbf{F}(\boldsymbol{\xi}_i^{(g)}) + \boldsymbol{\delta}_i^{(g)}. \end{aligned}$$

Clearly, when $t = 1$ and $t = 0$, M_{ta2} reduces to M_2 and M_a, respectively. The parameter vector in M_{ta2} contains $\boldsymbol{\mu}^{(1)}$, $\boldsymbol{\mu}^{(2)}$, $\boldsymbol{\Lambda}^{(1)}$, $\boldsymbol{\Lambda}^{(2)}$, $\boldsymbol{\Psi}_\epsilon^{(1)}$, $\boldsymbol{\Psi}_\epsilon^{(2)}$, $\boldsymbol{\Gamma}$, $\boldsymbol{\Phi}^{(1)}$, $\boldsymbol{\Phi}^{(2)}$, $\boldsymbol{\Psi}_\delta^{(1)}$, and $\boldsymbol{\Psi}_\delta^{(2)}$. We first compute $\log B_{1a}$ and $\log B_{2a}$, and then obtain $\log B_{12}$ via the equation

$$\log B_{12} = \log \frac{p(\mathbf{X}, \mathbf{Z}|M_1)/p(\mathbf{X}, \mathbf{Z}|M_a)}{p(\mathbf{X}, \mathbf{Z}|M_2)/p(\mathbf{X}, \mathbf{Z}|M_a)} = \log B_{1a} - \log B_{2a}.$$

Model comparison can also be conducted with DIC through the use of WinBUGS. See the illustrative example in Section 6.3.2.

6.3.2 Analysis of multisample quality of life data via WinBUGS

Analysis of single-group quality of life (QOL) data was considered in Section 5.2.4. Here, we describe the Bayesian methods for analyzing multisample QOL data. The WHOQOL-BREF (Power *et al.*, 1999) instrument was taken from the WHOQOL-100 instrument by selecting 26 ordered categorical items out of the 100 original items. The observations were taken from 15 international field centers, one of which is China, and the rest are Western countries, such as the United Kingdom, Italy, and Germany. The first two items are the overall QOL and general health, the next seven items measure physical health, the next six items measure psychological health, the three items that follow are for social relationships, and the last eight items measure the environment. All of the items are measured on a five-point scale (1 = 'not at all/very dissatisfied'; 2 = 'a little/dissatisfied'; 3 = 'moderate/neither'; 4 = 'very much/satisfied'; and 5 = 'extremely/very satisfied'). To illustrate the Bayesian methodology, we use a synthetic two-sample data set that mimics the QOL study with the same items as mentioned above for each sample (see Lee *et al.*, 2005; Lee, 2007). That is, we consider a two-sample SEM on the basis of a simulated data set of randomly drawn observations from two populations. The sample sizes are $N_1 = 338$ and $N_2 = 247$. In the Bayesian analysis, we identify the ordered categorical variables by the method described in Section 6.3.1, using the first group ($g = 1$) as the reference group. Based on the meaning of the questions, we use the following non-overlapping $\boldsymbol{\Lambda}^{(g)}$ for clear interpretation of latent variables: for $g = 1, 2$,

$$\boldsymbol{\Lambda}^{(g)T} = \begin{bmatrix} 1 & \lambda_{2,1}^{(g)} & 0 & 0 & \cdots & 0 & 0 & 0 & \cdots & 0 & 0 & 0 & 0 & 0 & 0 & \cdots & 0 \\ 0 & 0 & 1 & \lambda_{4,2}^{(g)} & \cdots & \lambda_{9,2}^{(g)} & 0 & 0 & \cdots & 0 & 0 & 0 & 0 & 0 & 0 & \cdots & 0 \\ 0 & 0 & 0 & 0 & \cdots & 0 & 1 & \lambda_{11,3}^{(g)} & \cdots & \lambda_{15,3}^{(g)} & 0 & 0 & 0 & 0 & 0 & \cdots & 0 \\ 0 & 0 & 0 & 0 & \cdots & 0 & 0 & 0 & \cdots & 0 & 1 & \lambda_{17,4}^{(g)} & \lambda_{18,4}^{(g)} & 0 & 0 & \cdots & 0 \\ 0 & 0 & 0 & 0 & \cdots & 0 & 0 & 0 & \cdots & 0 & 0 & 0 & 0 & 1 & \lambda_{20,5}^{(g)} & \cdots & \lambda_{26,5}^{(g)} \end{bmatrix},$$

where the 1s and 0s are fixed parameters. The latent variables in $\boldsymbol{\omega}_i^{(g)T} = (\eta_i^{(g)}, \xi_{i1}^{(g)}, \xi_{i2}^{(g)}, \xi_{i3}^{(g)}, \xi_{i4}^{(g)})$ are interpreted as 'health-related QOL' (η), 'physical health' (ξ_1), 'psychological health' (ξ_2), 'social relationships' (ξ_3), and 'environment' (ξ_4). The measurement equation in the model is given by

$$\mathbf{v}_i^{(g)} = \boldsymbol{\mu}^{(g)} + \boldsymbol{\Lambda}^{(g)}\boldsymbol{\omega}_i^{(g)} + \boldsymbol{\epsilon}_i^{(g)}, \quad g = 1, 2,$$

Table 6.4 Bayesian estimates of unknown parameters in the two-group SEM with no constraints.

	Group			Group			Group	
	$g=1$	$g=2$		$g=1$	$g=2$		$g=1$	$g=2$
μ_1	0.021	−0.519	$\lambda_{2,1}$	0.859	0.804	γ_1	0.847	0.539
μ_2	0.001	0.059	$\lambda_{4,2}$	0.952	0.754	γ_2	0.334	0.139
μ_3	0.002	−0.240	$\lambda_{5,2}$	1.112	1.016	γ_3	0.167	0.026
μ_4	0.009	−0.300	$\lambda_{6,2}$	1.212	0.976	γ_4	−0.068	0.241
μ_5	−0.004	−0.188	$\lambda_{7,2}$	0.820	0.805	ψ_1	0.400	0.248
μ_6	0.008	−0.382	$\lambda_{8,2}$	1.333	1.123	ψ_2	0.422	0.268
μ_7	−0.002	−0.030	$\lambda_{9,2}$	1.203	0.961	ψ_3	0.616	0.584
μ_8	0.008	−0.070	$\lambda_{11,3}$	0.799	0.827	ψ_4	0.628	0.445
μ_9	0.003	0.108	$\lambda_{12,3}$	0.726	0.987	ψ_5	0.462	0.214
μ_{10}	0.004	−0.358	$\lambda_{13,3}$	0.755	0.669	ψ_6	0.401	0.184
μ_{11}	0.003	−0.286	$\lambda_{14,3}$	1.011	0.762	ψ_7	0.709	0.253
μ_{12}	0.001	−0.087	$\lambda_{15,3}$	0.874	0.719	ψ_8	0.271	0.202
μ_{13}	0.004	−0.373	$\lambda_{17,4}$	0.273	0.627	ψ_9	0.393	0.191
μ_{14}	0.003	0.031	$\lambda_{18,4}$	0.954	0.961	ψ_{10}	0.471	0.288
μ_{15}	0.002	0.079	$\lambda_{20,5}$	0.804	1.108	ψ_{11}	0.654	0.262
μ_{16}	0.012	−0.404	$\lambda_{21,5}$	0.772	0.853	ψ_{12}	0.707	0.428
μ_{17}	0.000	0.037	$\lambda_{22,5}$	0.755	0.815	ψ_{13}	0.698	0.348
μ_{18}	0.010	−0.596	$\lambda_{23,5}$	0.723	0.672	ψ_{14}	0.453	0.269
μ_{19}	0.005	−0.183	$\lambda_{24,5}$	0.984	0.647	ψ_{15}	0.575	1.137
μ_{20}	0.004	−0.543	$\lambda_{25,5}$	0.770	0.714	ψ_{16}	0.462	0.267
μ_{21}	0.003	−0.571	$\lambda_{26,5}$	0.842	0.761	ψ_{17}	0.962	0.297
μ_{22}	0.002	−0.966	ϕ_{11}	0.450	0.301	ψ_{18}	0.522	0.301
μ_{23}	0.001	−0.220	ϕ_{12}	0.337	0.279	ψ_{19}	0.530	0.559
μ_{24}	0.017	−1.151	ϕ_{13}	0.211	0.162	ψ_{20}	0.679	0.565
μ_{25}	−0.001	−0.837	ϕ_{14}	0.299	0.207	ψ_{21}	0.708	0.392
μ_{26}	0.007	−0.982	ϕ_{22}	0.579	0.537	ψ_{22}	0.714	0.386
			ϕ_{23}	0.390	0.251	ψ_{23}	0.736	0.493
			ϕ_{24}	0.393	0.290	ψ_{24}	0.577	0.451
			ϕ_{33}	0.599	0.301	ψ_{25}	0.719	0.482
			ϕ_{34}	0.386	0.210	ψ_{26}	0.670	0.408
			ϕ_{44}	0.535	0.386			
			ψ_δ	0.246	0.234			

with $\mathbf{\Lambda}^{(g)}$ defined as above. The following structural equation is used to assess the effects of the latent constructs in $\boldsymbol{\xi}_i^{(g)}$ on the health-related QOL, $\eta_i^{(g)}$:

$$\eta_i^{(g)} = \gamma_1^{(g)}\xi_{i1}^{(g)} + \gamma_2^{(g)}\xi_{i2}^{(g)} + \gamma_3^{(g)}\xi_{i3}^{(g)} + \gamma_4^{(g)}\xi_{i4}^{(g)} + \delta_i^{(g)}.$$

In the Bayesian analysis, the prior inputs of the hyperparameters in the conjugate prior distributions are taken as follows: $\alpha_{0\epsilon k}^{(g)} = \alpha_{0\delta k}^{(g)} = 10$, $\beta_{0\epsilon k}^{(g)} = \beta_{0\delta k}^{(g)} = 8$, elements in $\mathbf{\Lambda}_{0k}^{(g)}$ are taken as 0.8, elements in $\mathbf{\Lambda}_{0\omega k}^{(g)}$ are taken as 0.6, $\mathbf{H}_{0yk}^{(g)}$ and $\mathbf{H}_{0\omega k}^{(g)}$ are diagonal matrices with diagonal elements 0.25, $\mathbf{R}_0^{(g)^{-1}} = 8\mathbf{I}_4$, and $\rho_0^{(g)} = 30$. Three multisample models M_1, M_2, and M_3 that are respectively associated with following hypotheses are considered: H_1 : no constraints; $H_2 : \mathbf{\Lambda}^{(1)} = \mathbf{\Lambda}^{(2)}$; and $H_3 : \mathbf{\Lambda}^{(1)} = \mathbf{\Lambda}^{(2)}$, $\mathbf{\Phi}^{(1)} = \mathbf{\Phi}^{(2)}$. The WinBUGS software was applied to obtain the Bayesian results. In the analysis, the number of burn-in iterations was taken as 10 000, and an additional 10 000 observations were collected to produce the results. The DIC values corresponding to M_1, M_2, and M_3 are 32 302.6, 32 321.7, and 32 341.9, respectively. Hence, model M_1, with the smallest DIC value, is selected. The Bayesian estimates and their standard error estimates produced by WinBUGS under M_1 are presented in Table 6.4. The WinBUGS codes for analyzing models M_1, M_2, and M_3 are given in the following website:

`www.wiley.com/go/medical_behavioral_sciences`

Appendix 6.1 Conditional distributions: Two-level nonlinear SEM

Owing to the complexity of the model, it is very tedious to derive all the conditional distributions required by the Gibbs sampler, hence only a brief discussion is given. For brevity, we will use $p(\cdot|\cdot)$ to denote the conditional distribution if the context is clear. Moreover, we only consider the case where all parameters in $\mathbf{\Lambda}_{1g}$, $\mathbf{\Lambda}_2$, $\mathbf{\Pi}_{1g}$, $\mathbf{\Gamma}_{1g}$, $\mathbf{\Pi}_2$, and $\mathbf{\Gamma}_2$ are not fixed. Conditional distributions for the case with fixed parameters can be obtained by slight modifications as given in previous chapters.

Conditional Distribution $p(\mathbf{V}|\boldsymbol{\theta}, \boldsymbol{\alpha}, \mathbf{Y}, \mathbf{\Omega}_1, \mathbf{\Omega}_2, \mathbf{X}, \mathbf{Z})$

Since the $\mathbf{v}_g$ are independent and do not depend on $\boldsymbol{\alpha}$, this conditional distribution is equal to a product of $p(\mathbf{v}_g|\boldsymbol{\theta}, \boldsymbol{\alpha}, \mathbf{Y}_g, \mathbf{\Omega}_{1g}, \boldsymbol{\omega}_{2g}, \mathbf{X}_g, \mathbf{Z}_g)$ with $g = 1, \ldots, G$. For each gth term in this product,

$$p(\mathbf{v}_g|\boldsymbol{\theta}, \boldsymbol{\alpha}, \mathbf{Y}_g, \mathbf{\Omega}_{1g}, \boldsymbol{\omega}_{2g}, \mathbf{X}_g, \mathbf{Z}_g) \propto p(\mathbf{v}_g|\boldsymbol{\theta}, \boldsymbol{\omega}_{2g}) \prod_{i=1}^{N_g} p(\mathbf{u}_{gi}|\boldsymbol{\theta}, \mathbf{v}_g, \boldsymbol{\omega}_{1gi}) \tag{6.A1}$$

$$\propto \exp\left[-\frac{1}{2}\left\{\mathbf{v}_g^T\left(N_g\mathbf{\Psi}_{1g}^{-1} + \mathbf{\Psi}_2^{-1}\right)\mathbf{v}_g - 2\mathbf{v}_g^T\left[\mathbf{\Psi}_{1g}^{-1}\sum_{i=1}^{N_g}(\mathbf{u}_{gi} - \mathbf{\Lambda}_{1g}\boldsymbol{\omega}_{1gi}) + \mathbf{\Psi}_2^{-1}(\boldsymbol{\mu} + \mathbf{\Lambda}_2\boldsymbol{\omega}_{2g})\right]\right\}\right].$$

Hence, for each $\mathbf{v}_g$, its conditional distribution $p(\mathbf{v}_g|\cdot)$ is $N[\boldsymbol{\mu}_g^*, \mathbf{\Sigma}_g^*]$, where

$$\boldsymbol{\mu}_g^* = \mathbf{\Sigma}_g^*\left[\mathbf{\Psi}_{1g}^{-1}\sum_{i=1}^{N_g}(\mathbf{u}_{gi} - \mathbf{\Lambda}_{1g}\boldsymbol{\omega}_{1gi}) + \mathbf{\Psi}_2^{-1}(\boldsymbol{\mu} + \mathbf{\Lambda}_2\boldsymbol{\omega}_{2g})\right] \quad \text{and} \quad \mathbf{\Sigma}_g^* = \left(N_g\mathbf{\Psi}_{1g}^{-1} + \mathbf{\Psi}_2^{-1}\right)^{-1}.$$

Conditional Distribution $p(\mathbf{\Omega}_1|\boldsymbol{\theta}, \boldsymbol{\alpha}, \mathbf{Y}, \mathbf{V}, \mathbf{\Omega}_2, \mathbf{X}, \mathbf{Z})$

Since the $\boldsymbol{\omega}_{1gi}$ are mutually independent, $\mathbf{u}_{gi}$ is independent of $\mathbf{u}_{hi}$ for all $h \neq g$, and they do not depend on $\boldsymbol{\alpha}$ and $\mathbf{Y}$, we have

$$p(\mathbf{\Omega}_1|\cdot) = \prod_{g=1}^{G}\prod_{i=1}^{N_g} p(\boldsymbol{\omega}_{1gi}|\boldsymbol{\theta}, \mathbf{v}_g, \boldsymbol{\omega}_{2g}, \mathbf{u}_{gi}) \propto \prod_{g=1}^{G}\prod_{i=1}^{N_g} p(\mathbf{u}_{gi}|\boldsymbol{\theta}, \mathbf{v}_g, \boldsymbol{\omega}_{1gi})p(\boldsymbol{\eta}_{1gi}|\boldsymbol{\xi}_{1gi}, \boldsymbol{\theta})p(\boldsymbol{\xi}_{1gi}|\boldsymbol{\theta}).$$

It follows that $p(\boldsymbol{\omega}_{1gi}|\cdot)$ is proportional to

$$\exp\left[-\frac{1}{2}\{\boldsymbol{\xi}_{1gi}^T\mathbf{\Phi}_{1g}^{-1}\boldsymbol{\xi}_{1gi} + (\mathbf{u}_{gi} - \mathbf{v}_g - \mathbf{\Lambda}_{1g}\boldsymbol{\omega}_{1gi})^T\mathbf{\Psi}_{1g}^{-1}(\mathbf{u}_{gi} - \mathbf{v}_g - \mathbf{\Lambda}_{1g}\boldsymbol{\omega}_{1gi})\right.$$
$$\left. + [\boldsymbol{\eta}_{1gi} - \mathbf{\Pi}_{1g}\boldsymbol{\eta}_{1gi} - \mathbf{\Gamma}_{1g}\mathbf{F}_1(\boldsymbol{\xi}_{1gi})]^T\mathbf{\Psi}_{1g\delta}^{-1}[\boldsymbol{\eta}_{1gi} - \mathbf{\Pi}_{1g}\boldsymbol{\eta}_{1gi} - \mathbf{\Gamma}_{1g}\mathbf{F}_1(\boldsymbol{\xi}_{1gi})]\}\right]. \tag{6.A2}$$

The conditional distribution $p(\mathbf{\Omega}_2|\boldsymbol{\theta}, \boldsymbol{\alpha}, \mathbf{Y}, \mathbf{V}, \mathbf{\Omega}_1, \mathbf{X}, \mathbf{Z})$ has a very similar form to $p(\mathbf{\Omega}_1|\cdot)$ and (6.A2), hence it is omitted.

Conditional Distribution $p(\boldsymbol{\alpha}, \mathbf{Y}|\boldsymbol{\theta}, \mathbf{V}, \mathbf{\Omega}_1, \mathbf{\Omega}_2, \mathbf{X}, \mathbf{Z})$

We only consider the case where all the thresholds corresponding to each within group are different. The other cases can be similarly derived. To deal with the situation with little or no information about these parameters, the following noninformative prior distribution is used:

$$p(\boldsymbol{\alpha}_{gk}) = p(\alpha_{gk,2}, \ldots, \alpha_{gk,b_k-1}) \propto C, \quad g = 1, \ldots, G, \ k = 1, \ldots, s,$$

where C is a constant. Now, since $(\boldsymbol{\alpha}_g, \mathbf{Y}_g)$ is independent of $(\boldsymbol{\alpha}_h, \mathbf{Y}_h)$ for $g \neq h$, and $\boldsymbol{\Psi}_{1g}$ is diagonal,

$$p(\boldsymbol{\alpha}, \mathbf{Y}|\cdot) = \prod_{g=1}^{G} p(\boldsymbol{\alpha}_g, \mathbf{Y}_g|\cdot) = \prod_{g=1}^{G}\prod_{k=1}^{s} p(\boldsymbol{\alpha}_{gk}, \mathbf{Y}_{gk}|\cdot), \tag{6.A3}$$

where $\mathbf{Y}_{gk} = (y_{g1k}, \ldots, y_{gN_gk})^T$. Let $\boldsymbol{\Psi}_{1gy}$, $\boldsymbol{\Lambda}_{1gy}$, and $\mathbf{v}_{gy}$ be the submatrices and subvector of $\boldsymbol{\Psi}_{1g}$, $\boldsymbol{\Lambda}_{1g}$, and $\mathbf{v}_g$ corresponding to the ordered categorical variables in $\mathbf{Y}$; let ψ_{1gyk} be the kth diagonal element of $\boldsymbol{\Psi}_{1gy}$, $\boldsymbol{\Lambda}_{1gyk}^T$ be the kth row of $\boldsymbol{\Lambda}_{1gy}$, v_{gyk} be the kth element of $\mathbf{v}_{gy}$, and $I_A(y)$ be an indicator function with value 1 if y in A and zero otherwise. Then $p(\boldsymbol{\alpha}, \mathbf{Y}|\cdot)$ can be obtained from (6.A3) and

$$p(\boldsymbol{\alpha}_{gk}, \mathbf{Y}_{gk}|\cdot) \propto \prod_{i=1}^{N_g} \phi\{\psi_{1gyk}^{-1/2}(y_{gik} - v_{gyk} - \boldsymbol{\Lambda}_{1gyk}^T\boldsymbol{\omega}_{1gi})\} I_{(\alpha_{gk,z_{gik}}, \alpha_{gk,z_{gik}+1}]}(y_{gik}), \tag{6.A4}$$

where ϕ is the probability density function of $N[0, 1]$.

Conditional Distribution $p(\boldsymbol{\theta}|\boldsymbol{\alpha}, \mathbf{Y}, \mathbf{V}, \boldsymbol{\Omega}_1, \boldsymbol{\Omega}_2, \mathbf{X}, \mathbf{Z})$

This conditional distribution is different under different special cases as discussed in Section 6.2.2. We first consider the situation with distinct within-group parameters, that is, $\boldsymbol{\theta}_{11} \neq \ldots \neq \boldsymbol{\theta}_{1G}$. Let $\boldsymbol{\theta}_2$ be the vector of unknown parameters in $\boldsymbol{\mu}$, $\boldsymbol{\Lambda}_2$, and $\boldsymbol{\Psi}_2$; and $\boldsymbol{\theta}_{2\omega}$ be the vector of unknown parameters in $\boldsymbol{\Pi}_2$, $\boldsymbol{\Gamma}_2$, $\boldsymbol{\Phi}_2$, and $\boldsymbol{\Psi}_{2\delta}$. These between-group parameters are the same for each g. For the within-group parameters, let $\boldsymbol{\theta}_{1gy}$ be the vector of unknown parameters in $\boldsymbol{\Lambda}_{1g}$ and $\boldsymbol{\Psi}_{1g}$; and $\boldsymbol{\theta}_{1g\omega}$ be the vector of unknown parameters in $\boldsymbol{\Pi}_{1g}$, $\boldsymbol{\Gamma}_{1g}$, $\boldsymbol{\Phi}_{1g}$, and $\boldsymbol{\Psi}_{1g\delta}$. It is natural to assume the prior distributions of these parameter vectors in different independent groups are independent of each other, and hence they can be treated separately.

For $\boldsymbol{\theta}_{1gy}$, the following commonly used conjugate type prior distributions are used:

$$\psi_{1gk}^{-1} \stackrel{D}{=} \text{Gamma}[\alpha_{01gk}, \beta_{01gk}], \ [\boldsymbol{\Lambda}_{1gk}|\psi_{1gk}] \stackrel{D}{=} N[\boldsymbol{\Lambda}_{01gk}, \psi_{1gk}\mathbf{H}_{01gk}], \quad k = 1, \ldots, p,$$

where ψ_{1gk} is the kth diagonal element of $\boldsymbol{\Psi}_{1g}$, $\boldsymbol{\Lambda}_{1gk}^T$ is the kth row of $\boldsymbol{\Lambda}_{1g}$, and α_{01gk}, β_{01gk}, $\boldsymbol{\Lambda}_{01gk}$, and $\mathbf{H}_{01gk}$ are given hyperparameter values. For $k \neq h$, it is assumed that $(\psi_{1gk}, \boldsymbol{\Lambda}_{1gk})$ and $(\psi_{1gh}, \boldsymbol{\Lambda}_{1gh})$ are independent. Let $\mathbf{U}_g^* = \{\mathbf{u}_{gi} - \mathbf{v}_g, \ i = 1, \ldots, N_g\}$ and $\mathbf{U}_{gk}^{*T}$ be the kth row of $\mathbf{U}_g^*$, $\boldsymbol{\Sigma}_{1gk} = (\mathbf{H}_{01gk}^{-1} + \boldsymbol{\Omega}_{1g}\boldsymbol{\Omega}_{1g}^T)^{-1}$, $\mathbf{m}_{1gk} = \boldsymbol{\Sigma}_{1gk}(\mathbf{H}_{01gk}^{-1}\boldsymbol{\Lambda}_{01gk} + \boldsymbol{\Omega}_{1g}\mathbf{U}_{gk}^*)$, $\boldsymbol{\Omega}_{1g} = (\boldsymbol{\omega}_{1g1}, \ldots, \boldsymbol{\omega}_{1gN_g})$, and $\beta_{1gk} = \beta_{01gk} + (\mathbf{U}_{gk}^{*T}\mathbf{U}_{gk}^* - \mathbf{m}_{1gk}^T\boldsymbol{\Sigma}_{1gk}^{-1}\mathbf{m}_{1gk} + \boldsymbol{\Lambda}_{01gk}^T\mathbf{H}_{01gk}^{-1}\boldsymbol{\Lambda}_{01gk})/2$. It can be shown that

$$[\psi_{1gk}^{-1}|\cdot] \stackrel{D}{=} \text{Gamma}\,(N_g/2 + \alpha_{01gk}, \beta_{1gk}), \quad [\boldsymbol{\Lambda}_{1gk}|\psi_{1gk}, \cdot] \stackrel{D}{=} N[\mathbf{m}_{1gk}, \psi_{1gk}\boldsymbol{\Sigma}_{1gk}]. \tag{6.A5}$$

For $\boldsymbol{\theta}_{1g\omega}$, it is assumed that $\boldsymbol{\Phi}_{1g}$ is independent of $(\boldsymbol{\Lambda}_{1g}^*, \boldsymbol{\Psi}_{1g\delta})$, where $\boldsymbol{\Lambda}_{1g}^* = (\boldsymbol{\Pi}_{1g}, \boldsymbol{\Gamma}_{1g})$. Also, $(\boldsymbol{\Lambda}_{1gk}^*, \psi_{1g\delta k})$ and $(\boldsymbol{\Lambda}_{1gh}^*, \psi_{1g\delta h})$ are independent, where $\boldsymbol{\Lambda}_{1gk}^{*T}$ and $\psi_{1g\delta k}$ are the kth row and diagonal element of $\boldsymbol{\Lambda}_{1g}^*$ and $\boldsymbol{\Psi}_{1g\delta}$, respectively. The associated prior distribution of $\boldsymbol{\Phi}_{1g}$ is $\boldsymbol{\Phi}_{1g}^{-1} \stackrel{D}{=} W_{q_{12}}[\mathbf{R}_{01g}, \rho_{01g}]$, where ρ_{01g} and the positive definite matrix $\mathbf{R}_{01g}$ are given hyperparameters. Moreover, the prior distributions of $\psi_{1g\delta k}$ and $\mathbf{\Lambda}_{1gk}^*$ are

$$\psi_{1g\delta k}^{-1} \stackrel{D}{=} \text{Gamma}[\alpha_{01g\delta k}, \beta_{01g\delta k}],\ [\mathbf{\Lambda}_{1gk}^*|\psi_{1g\delta k}] \stackrel{D}{=} N[\mathbf{\Lambda}_{01gk}^*, \psi_{1g\delta k}\mathbf{H}_{01gk}^*], \quad k = 1, \ldots, q_{11},$$

where $\alpha_{01g\delta k}$, $\beta_{01g\delta k}$, $\mathbf{\Lambda}_{01gk}^*$, and $\mathbf{H}_{01gk}^*$ are given hyperparameters. Let $\mathbf{\Omega}_{1g}^* = \{\boldsymbol{\eta}_{1g1}, \ldots, \boldsymbol{\eta}_{1gN_g}\}$, $\mathbf{\Omega}_{1gk}^{*T}$ be the kth row of $\mathbf{\Omega}_{1g}^*$, $\Xi_{1g} = \{\boldsymbol{\xi}_{1g1}, \ldots, \boldsymbol{\xi}_{1gN_g}\}$ and $\mathbf{F}_{1g}^* = \{\mathbf{F}_1^*(\boldsymbol{\omega}_{1g1}), \ldots, \mathbf{F}_1^*(\boldsymbol{\omega}_{1gN_g})\}$, in which $\mathbf{F}_1^*(\boldsymbol{\omega}_{1gi}) = (\boldsymbol{\eta}_{1gi}^T, \mathbf{F}_1(\boldsymbol{\xi}_{1gi})^T)^T$, $i = 1, \ldots, N_g$. It can be shown that

$$[\psi_{1g\delta k}^{-1}|\cdot] \stackrel{D}{=} \text{Gamma}\,[N_g/2 + \alpha_{01g\delta k}, \beta_{1g\delta k}], \quad [\mathbf{\Lambda}_{1gk}^*|\psi_{1g\delta k}^{-1}, \cdot] \stackrel{D}{=} N[\mathbf{m}_{1gk}^*, \psi_{1g\delta k}\mathbf{\Sigma}_{1gk}^*], \quad (6.A6)$$

where $\mathbf{\Sigma}_{1gk}^* = (\mathbf{H}_{01gk}^{*-1} + \mathbf{F}_{1g}^*\mathbf{F}_{1g}^{*T})^{-1}$, $\mathbf{m}_{1gk}^* = \mathbf{\Sigma}_{1gk}^*(\mathbf{H}_{01gk}^{*-1}\mathbf{\Lambda}_{01gk}^* + \mathbf{F}_{1g}^*\mathbf{\Omega}_{1gk}^*)$, and $\beta_{1g\delta k} = \beta_{01g\delta k} + (\mathbf{\Omega}_{1gk}^{*T}\mathbf{\Omega}_{1gk}^* - \mathbf{m}_{1gk}^{*T}\mathbf{\Sigma}_{1gk}^{*-1}\mathbf{m}_{1gk}^* + \mathbf{\Lambda}_{01gk}^{*T}\mathbf{H}_{01gk}^{*-1}\mathbf{\Lambda}_{01gk}^*)/2$. The conditional distribution related to $\mathbf{\Phi}_{1g}$ is given by

$$[\mathbf{\Phi}_{1g}|\Xi_{1g}] \stackrel{D}{=} \text{IW}_{q_{12}}\left[\left(\Xi_{1g}\Xi_{1g}^T + \mathbf{R}_{01g}^{-1}\right), N_g + \rho_{01g}\right]. \quad (6.A7)$$

Conditional distributions involved in $\boldsymbol{\theta}_2$ are derived similarly on the basis of the following independent conjugate type prior distributions: for $k = 1, \ldots, p$,

$$\boldsymbol{\mu} \stackrel{D}{=} N[\boldsymbol{\mu}_0, \mathbf{\Sigma}_0], \quad \psi_{2k}^{-1} \stackrel{D}{=} \text{Gamma}[\alpha_{02k}, \beta_{02k}], \quad [\mathbf{\Lambda}_{2k}|\psi_{2k}] \stackrel{D}{=} N[\mathbf{\Lambda}_{02k}, \psi_{2k}\mathbf{H}_{02k}].$$

where $\mathbf{\Lambda}_{2k}^T$ is the kth row of $\mathbf{\Lambda}_2$, ψ_{2k} is the kth diagonal element of $\mathbf{\Psi}_2$, and α_{02k}, β_{02k}, $\boldsymbol{\mu}_0$, $\mathbf{\Sigma}_0$, $\mathbf{\Lambda}_{02k}$, and $\mathbf{H}_{02k}$ are given hyperparameters.

Similarly, conditional distributions involved in $\boldsymbol{\theta}_{2\omega}$ are derived on the basis of the following conjugate type prior distributions: for $k = 1, \ldots, q_{21}$,

$$\mathbf{\Phi}_2^{-1} \stackrel{D}{=} W_{q_{22}}[\mathbf{R}_{02}, \rho_{02}], \quad \psi_{2\delta k}^{-1} \stackrel{D}{=} \text{Gamma}[\alpha_{02\delta k}, \beta_{02\delta k}], \quad [\mathbf{\Lambda}_{2k}^*|\psi_{2\delta k}] \stackrel{D}{=} N[\mathbf{\Lambda}_{02k}^*, \psi_{2\delta k}\mathbf{H}_{02k}^*],$$

where $\mathbf{\Lambda}_2^* = (\mathbf{\Pi}_2, \mathbf{\Gamma}_2)$, $\mathbf{\Lambda}_{2k}^{*T}$ is the vector that contains the unknown parameters in the kth row of $\mathbf{\Lambda}_2^*$, and $\psi_{2\delta k}$ is the kth diagonal element of $\mathbf{\Psi}_{2\delta}$. As these conditional distributions are similar to those in (6.A5)–(6.A7), they are omitted.

In the situation where $\boldsymbol{\theta}_{11} = \ldots = \boldsymbol{\theta}_{1G}(= \boldsymbol{\theta}_1)$, the prior distributions corresponding to components of $\boldsymbol{\theta}_1$ do not depend on g, and all the data in the within groups should be combined in deriving the conditional distributions for the estimation. Conditional distributions can be derived with the following conjugate type prior distributions: in notation similar to the foregoing,

$$\psi_{1k}^{-1} \stackrel{D}{=} \text{Gamma}[\alpha_{01k}, \beta_{01k}], \quad [\mathbf{\Lambda}_{1k}|\psi_{1k}] \stackrel{D}{=} N[\mathbf{\Lambda}_{01k}, \psi_{1k}\mathbf{H}_{01k}], \quad \mathbf{\Phi}_1^{-1} \stackrel{D}{=} W_{q_{12}}[\mathbf{R}_{01}, \rho_{01}],$$

$$\psi_{1\delta k}^{-1} \stackrel{D}{=} \text{Gamma}[\alpha_{01\delta k}, \beta_{01\delta k}], \quad [\mathbf{\Lambda}_{1k}^*|\psi_{1\delta k}] \stackrel{D}{=} N[\mathbf{\Lambda}_{01k}^*, \psi_{1\delta k}\mathbf{H}_{01k}^*], \quad (6.A8)$$

and the prior distributions and conditional distributions corresponding to structural parameters in the between-group covariance matrix are the same as before.

Appendix 6.2 The MH algorithm: Two-level nonlinear SEM

Simulating observations from the gamma, normal and inverted Wishart distributions is straightforward and fast. However, the conditional distributions, $p(\mathbf{\Omega}_1|\cdot)$, $p(\mathbf{\Omega}_2|\cdot)$, and $p(\boldsymbol{\alpha}, \mathbf{Y}|\cdot)$, are complex, hence it is necessary to implement the MH algorithm for efficient simulation of observations from these conditional distributions.

For the conditional distribution $p(\mathbf{\Omega}_1|\cdot)$, we need to simulate observations from the target density $p(\boldsymbol{\omega}_{1gi}|\cdot)$ as given in (6.A2). Similar to the method of Zhu and Lee (1999) and Lee and Zhu (2000), we choose $N[\cdot, \sigma_1^2\mathbf{D}_{1g}]$ as the proposal distribution, where $\mathbf{D}_{1g}^{-1} = \mathbf{D}_{1g\omega}^{-1} + \mathbf{\Lambda}_{1g}^T\mathbf{\Psi}_{1g}^{-1}\mathbf{\Lambda}_{1g}$, and $\mathbf{D}_{1g\omega}^{-1}$ is given by

$$\mathbf{D}_{1g\omega}^{-1} = \begin{bmatrix} \mathbf{\Pi}_{1g0}^T\mathbf{\Psi}_{1g\delta}^{-1}\mathbf{\Pi}_{1g0} & -\mathbf{\Pi}_{1g0}^T\mathbf{\Psi}_{1g\delta}^{-1}\mathbf{\Gamma}_{1g}\mathbf{\Delta}_{1g} \\ -\mathbf{\Delta}_{1g}^T\mathbf{\Gamma}_{1g}^T\mathbf{\Psi}_{1g\delta}^{-1}\mathbf{\Pi}_{1g0} & \mathbf{\Phi}_{1g}^{-1} + \mathbf{\Delta}_{1g}^T\mathbf{\Gamma}_{1g}^T\mathbf{\Psi}_{1g\delta}^{-1}\mathbf{\Gamma}_{1g}\mathbf{\Delta}_{1g} \end{bmatrix},$$

where $\mathbf{\Pi}_{1g0} = \mathbf{I}_{q11} - \mathbf{\Pi}_{1g}$ with an identity matrix $\mathbf{I}_{q11}$ of order q_{11}, and $\mathbf{\Delta}_{1g} = (\partial\mathbf{F}_1(\boldsymbol{\xi}_{1gi})/\partial\boldsymbol{\xi}_{1gi})^T|_{\boldsymbol{\xi}_{1gi}=\mathbf{0}}$. Let $p(\cdot|\boldsymbol{\omega}^*, \sigma_1^2\mathbf{D}_{1g})$ be the density function corresponding to the proposal distribution $N[\boldsymbol{\omega}^*, \sigma_1^2\mathbf{D}_{1g}]$. The MH algorithm is implemented as follows: at the mth iteration with current value $\boldsymbol{\omega}_{1gi}^{(m)}$, a new candidate $\boldsymbol{\omega}_i^*$ is generated from $p(\cdot|\boldsymbol{\omega}_{1gi}^{(m)}, \sigma_1^2\mathbf{D}_{1g})$ and accepted with probability $\min\{1, p(\boldsymbol{\omega}_i^*|\cdot)/p(\boldsymbol{\omega}_{1gi}^{(m)}|\cdot)\}$. The variance σ_1^2 can be chosen such that the average acceptance rate is approximately 0.25 or more; see Gelman *et al.* (1996b).

Observations from the conditional distribution $p(\mathbf{\Omega}_2|\cdot)$ with target density similar to (6.A2) can be simulated via an MH algorithm similar to that described above. To save space, the details are omitted.

An MH type algorithm is necessary for simulating observations from the complex distribution $p(\boldsymbol{\alpha}, \mathbf{Y}|\cdot)$. Here, the target density is given in (6.A4). According to the factorization recommended by Cowles (1996); see also Lee and Zhu (2000), the joint proposal density of $\boldsymbol{\alpha}_{gk}$ and $\mathbf{Y}_{gk}$ is constructed as

$$p(\boldsymbol{\alpha}_{gk}, \mathbf{Y}_{gk}|\cdot) = p(\boldsymbol{\alpha}_{gk}|\cdot)p(\mathbf{Y}_{gk}|\boldsymbol{\alpha}_{gk}, \cdot). \tag{6.A9}$$

Then the algorithm is implemented as follows: at the mth iteration with $(\boldsymbol{\alpha}_{gk}^{(m)}, \mathbf{Y}_{gk}^{(m)})$, the acceptance probability for a new observation $(\boldsymbol{\alpha}_{gk}^{(m+1)}, \mathbf{Y}_{gk}^{(m+1)})$ of $(\boldsymbol{\alpha}_{gk}, \mathbf{Y}_{gk})$ is $\min\{1, R_{gk}\}$, where

$$R_{gk} = \frac{p(\boldsymbol{\alpha}_{gk}, \mathbf{Y}_{gk}|\boldsymbol{\theta}, \mathbf{Z}_{gk}, \mathbf{\Omega}_{1g})p(\boldsymbol{\alpha}_{gk}^{(m)}, \mathbf{Y}_{gk}^{(m)}|\boldsymbol{\alpha}_{gk}, \mathbf{Y}_{gk}, \boldsymbol{\theta}, \mathbf{Z}_{gk}, \mathbf{\Omega}_{1g})}{p(\boldsymbol{\alpha}_{gk}^{(m)}, \mathbf{Y}_{gk}^{(m)}|\boldsymbol{\theta}, \mathbf{Z}_{gk}, \mathbf{\Omega}_{1g})p(\boldsymbol{\alpha}_{gk}, \mathbf{Y}_{gk}|\boldsymbol{\alpha}_{gk}^{(m)}, \mathbf{Y}_{gk}^{(m)}, \boldsymbol{\theta}, \mathbf{Z}_{gk}, \mathbf{\Omega}_{1g})}.$$

To search for a new observation via the proposal density (6.A9), we first generate a vector of thresholds $(\alpha_{gk,2}, \ldots, \alpha_{gk,b_k-1})$ from the truncated normal distribution

$$\alpha_{gk,z} \stackrel{D}{=} N[\alpha_{gk,z}^{(m)}, \sigma_{\alpha gk}^2]I_{(\alpha_{gk,z-1}, \alpha_{gk,z+1}^{(m)}]}(\alpha_{gk,z}), \quad z = 2, \ldots, b_k - 1,$$

where $\sigma^2_{\alpha gk}$ is a preassigned value to give an approximate acceptance rate of 0.44; see Cowles (1996). It follows from (6.A4) and the above result that

$$R_{gk} = \prod_{z=2}^{b_k-1} \frac{\Phi^*\{(\alpha^{(m)}_{gk,z+1} - \alpha^{(m)}_{gk,z})/\sigma_{\alpha gk}\} - \Phi^*\{(\alpha_{gk,z-1} - \alpha^{(m)}_{gk,z})/\sigma_{\alpha gk}\}}{\Phi^*\{(\alpha_{gk,z+1} - \alpha_{gk,z})/\sigma_{\alpha gk}\} - \Phi^*\{(\alpha^{(m)}_{gk,z-1} - \alpha_{gk,z})/\sigma_{\alpha gk}\}}$$

$$\times \prod_{i=1}^{N_g} \frac{\Phi^*\{\psi^{-1/2}_{1gyk}(\alpha_{gk,z_{gik}+1} - \nu_{gyk} - \mathbf{\Lambda}^T_{1gyk}\boldsymbol{\omega}_{1gi})\} - \Phi^*\{\psi^{-1/2}_{1gyk}(\alpha_{gk,z_{gik}} - \nu_{gyk} - \mathbf{\Lambda}^T_{1gyk}\boldsymbol{\omega}_{1gi})\}}{\Phi^*\{\psi^{-1/2}_{1gyk}(\alpha^{(m)}_{gk,z_{gik}+1} - \nu_{gyk} - \mathbf{\Lambda}^T_{1gyk}\boldsymbol{\omega}_{1gi})\} - \Phi^*\{\psi^{-1/2}_{1gyk}(\alpha^{(m)}_{gk,z_{gik}} - \nu_{gyk} - \mathbf{\Lambda}^T_{1gyk}\boldsymbol{\omega}_{1gi})\}},$$

where Φ^* is the distribution function of $N[0, 1]$. Since R_{gk} only depends on the old and new values of $\boldsymbol{\alpha}_{gk}$ but not on $\mathbf{Y}_{gk}$, all that is necessary is to generate a new $\mathbf{Y}_{gk}$ for an accepted $\boldsymbol{\alpha}_{gk}$. This new $\mathbf{Y}_{gk}$ is simulated from the truncated normal distribution $p(\mathbf{Y}_{gk}|\boldsymbol{\alpha}_{gk}, \cdot)$ via the algorithm given in Robert (1995).

Appendix 6.3 PP p-value for two-level nonlinear SEM with mixed continuous and ordered categorical variables

Suppose null hypothesis H_0 is that the model defined in (6.1) and (6.2) is plausible, the PP p-value is defined as

$$p_B(\mathbf{X}, \mathbf{Z}) = \Pr\{D(\mathbf{U}^{\text{rep}}|\boldsymbol{\theta}, \boldsymbol{\alpha}, \mathbf{Y}, \mathbf{V}, \boldsymbol{\Omega}_1, \boldsymbol{\Omega}_2) \geq D(\mathbf{U}|\boldsymbol{\theta}, \boldsymbol{\alpha}, \mathbf{Y}, \mathbf{V}, \boldsymbol{\Omega}_1, \boldsymbol{\Omega}_2)|\mathbf{X}, \mathbf{Z}, H_0\},$$

where $\mathbf{U}^{\text{rep}}$ denotes a replication of $\mathbf{U} = \{\mathbf{u}_{gi}, i = 1, \ldots, N_g, \ g = 1, \ldots, G\}$, with $\mathbf{u}_{gi}$ satisfying the model defined by equation (6.3) that involves structural parameters and latent variables satisfying (6.4) and (6.5), and $D(\cdot|\cdot)$ is a discrepancy variable. Here, the following χ^2 discrepancy variable is used:

$$D(\mathbf{U}^{\text{rep}}|\boldsymbol{\theta}, \boldsymbol{\alpha}, \mathbf{Y}, \mathbf{V}, \boldsymbol{\Omega}_1, \boldsymbol{\Omega}_2) = \sum_{g=1}^{G}\sum_{i=1}^{N_g}\left(\mathbf{u}_{gi}^{\text{rep}} - \mathbf{v}_g - \boldsymbol{\Lambda}_{1g}\boldsymbol{\omega}_{1gi}\right)^T \boldsymbol{\Psi}_{1g}^{-1}\left(\mathbf{u}_{gi}^{\text{rep}} - \mathbf{v}_g - \boldsymbol{\Lambda}_{1g}\boldsymbol{\omega}_{1gi}\right),$$

which is distributed as $\chi^2(pn)$, a χ^2 distribution with pn degrees of freedom. Here, $n = N_1 + \ldots + N_G$. The PP p-value on the basis of this discrepancy variable is

$$P_B(\mathbf{X}, \mathbf{Z}) = \int \Pr\{\chi^2(pn) \geq D(\mathbf{U}|\boldsymbol{\theta}, \boldsymbol{\alpha}, \mathbf{Y}, \mathbf{V}, \boldsymbol{\Omega}_1, \boldsymbol{\Omega}_2)\}$$
$$\times p(\boldsymbol{\theta}, \boldsymbol{\alpha}, \mathbf{Y}, \mathbf{V}, \boldsymbol{\Omega}_1, \boldsymbol{\Omega}_2|\mathbf{X}, \mathbf{Z})d\boldsymbol{\theta}d\boldsymbol{\alpha}d\mathbf{Y}d\mathbf{V}d\boldsymbol{\Omega}_1 d\boldsymbol{\Omega}_2.$$

A Rao-Blackwellized type estimate of the PP p-value is given by

$$\hat{P}_B(\mathbf{X}, \mathbf{Z}) = T^{-1}\sum_{t=1}^{T}\Pr\left\{\chi^2(pn) \geq D\left(\mathbf{U}|\boldsymbol{\theta}^{(t)}, \boldsymbol{\alpha}^{(t)}, \mathbf{Y}^{(t)}, \mathbf{V}^{(t)}, \boldsymbol{\Omega}_1^{(t)}, \boldsymbol{\Omega}_2^{(t)}\right)\right\},$$

where $D(\mathbf{U}|\boldsymbol{\theta}^{(t)}, \boldsymbol{\alpha}^{(t)}, \mathbf{Y}^{(t)}, \mathbf{V}^{(t)}, \boldsymbol{\Omega}_1^{(t)}, \boldsymbol{\Omega}_2^{(t)})$ is calculated at each iteration, and the tail area of a χ^2 distribution can be obtained via standard statistical software. The hypothesized model is rejected if $\hat{P}_B(\mathbf{X}, \mathbf{Z})$ is not close to 0.5.

Appendix 6.4 WinBUGS code

```
model {
for (g in 1:G) {
#second level
for (j in 1:P) { vg[g,j]~dnorm(u2[g,j],psi2[j])}

u2[g,1]<-1.0*xi2[g,1]
u2[g,2]<-lb[1]*xi2[g,1]
u2[g,3]<-lb[2]*xi2[g,1]

u2[g,4]<-1.0*xi2[g,2]
u2[g,5]<-lb[3]*xi2[g,2]
u2[g,6]<-lb[4]*xi2[g,2]

u2[g,7]<-1.0*xi2[g,3]
u2[g,8]<-lb[5]*xi2[g,3]
u2[g,9]<-lb[6]*xi2[g,3]

xi2[g,1:3]~dmnorm(ux2[1:3],phip[1:3,1:3])

#first model
for (i in 1:N[g]) {

for (j in 1:6) {
w[kk[g]+i,j] dcat(p[kk[g]+i,j,1:C])
p[kk[g]+i,j,1]<-Q[kk[g]+i,j,1]
for (t in 2:C-1) { p[kk[g]+i,j,t]<-Q[kk[g]+i,j,t]-Q[kk[g]+i,j,t-1]}
p[kk[g]+i,j,C]<-1-Q[kk[g]+i,j,C-1]
for (t in 1:C-1)
{ Q[kk[g]+i,j,t]<-phi((alph[j,t]-u1[kk[g]+i,j])*sqrt(psi11[j]))}
}
#Note: the coding for the ordered categorical variable is 1,2,...,C

for (j in 7:9) { w[kk[g]+i,j]~dnorm(u1[kk[g]+i,j],psi1[j])}

u1[kk[g]+i,1]<-vg[g,1]+1.0*eta1[g,i]
u1[kk[g]+i,2]<-vg[g,2]+lw[1]*eta1[g,i]
u1[kk[g]+i,3]<-vg[g,3]+lw[2]*eta1[g,i]

u1[kk[g]+i,4]<-vg[g,4]+1.0*xi1[g,i,1]
u1[kk[g]+i,5]<-vg[g,5]+lw[3]*xi1[g,i,1]
u1[kk[g]+i,6]<-vg[g,6]+lw[4]*xi1[g,i,1]

u1[kk[g]+i,7]<-vg[g,7]+1.0*xi1[g,i,2]
u1[kk[g]+i,8]<-vg[g,8]+lw[5]*xi1[g,i,2]
u1[kk[g]+i,9]<-vg[g,9]+lw[6]*xi1[g,i,2]

#Structural Equation model
eta1[g,i]~dnorm(nu1[g,i], psd)
nu1[g,i]<-gam[1]*xi1[g,i,1]+gam[2]*xi1[g,i,2]+gam[3]*xi1[g,i,1]*xi1[g,i,2]
        +gam[4]*xi1[g,i,1]*xi1[g,i,1]+gam[5]*xi1[g,i,2]*xi1[g,i,2]

xi1[g,i,1:2]~dmnorm(ux1[1:2],phi1[1:2,1:2])
```

```
} # end of i

} # end of g

for (i in 1:2) { ux1[i]<-0.0}
for (i in 1:3) { ux2[i]<-0.0}

    # priors on loadings and coefficients
    lb[1] dnorm(lbp[1],psi2[2]) lb[2]~dnorm(lbp[2],psi2[3])
    lb[3] dnorm(lbp[3],psi2[5]) lb[4]~dnorm(lbp[4],psi2[6])
    lb[5] dnorm(lbp[5],psi2[8]) lb[6]~dnorm(lbp[6],psi2[9])

    lw[1] dnorm(lwp[1],psi1[2]) lw[2]~dnorm(lwp[2],psi1[3])
    lw[3] dnorm(lwp[3],psi1[5]) lw[4]~dnorm(lwp[4],psi1[6])
    lw[5] dnorm(lwp[5],psi1[8]) lw[6]~dnorm(lwp[6],psi1[9])

for (i in 1:5) { gam[i]~dnorm(gamp[i], psd)}

# priors on thresholds
for (j in 1:6) {
alph[j,1]<-a
alph[j,2]~dnorm(0,0.01)I(alph[j,1],alph[j,3])
alph[j,3]~dnorm(0,0.01)I(alph[j,2],alph[j,4])
alph[j,4]<-b
}
# a, b are fixed to identify the ordered categorical variable

# priors on precisions

for (j in 1:9) {
psi1[j]~dgamma(10.0,8.0)
sgm1[j]<-1/psi1[j]
}

for (j in 1:6) { psi2[j]<-1.0/0.3}

for (j in 7:9) {
psi2[j]~dgamma(10.0,8.0)
sgm2[j]<-1/psi2[j]
}

   psd~dgamma(10.0,8.0)
   sgd<-1/psd

   phi1[1:2,1:2]~dwish(R1[1:2,1:2],5)
   phx1[1:2,1:2]<-inverse(phi1[1:2,1:2])

   phi2[1:3,1:3] dwish(R2[1:2,1:2],5)
   phx2[1:3,1:3]<-inverse(phi2[1:3,1:3])

} # end of model
```

Appendix 6.5 Conditional distributions: Multisample SEMs

The conditional distributions $[\boldsymbol{\Omega}|\boldsymbol{\theta}, \boldsymbol{\alpha}, \mathbf{Y}, \mathbf{X}, \mathbf{Z}]$, $[\boldsymbol{\alpha}, \mathbf{Y}|\boldsymbol{\theta}, \boldsymbol{\Omega}, \mathbf{X}, \mathbf{Z}]$, and $[\boldsymbol{\theta}|\boldsymbol{\alpha}, \mathbf{Y}, \boldsymbol{\Omega}, \mathbf{X}, \mathbf{Z}]$ that are required in the implementation of the Gibbs sampler are presented in this appendix. Note that the results on the first two conditional distributions are natural extension of those given in Section 5.2, but they can be regarded as special cases of those given in Section 6.2. Also note that we allow common parameters in $\boldsymbol{\theta}$ according to the constraints under the competing models.

The conditional distribution of $[\boldsymbol{\Omega}|\boldsymbol{\theta}, \boldsymbol{\alpha}, \mathbf{Y}, \mathbf{X}, \mathbf{Z}]$ can be obtained as follows:

$$p[\boldsymbol{\Omega}|\boldsymbol{\theta}, \boldsymbol{\alpha}, \mathbf{Y}, \mathbf{X}, \mathbf{Z}] = \prod_{g=1}^{G}\prod_{i=1}^{N_g} p\big(\boldsymbol{\omega}_i^{(g)}|\mathbf{v}_i^{(g)}, \boldsymbol{\theta}^{(g)}\big),$$

where

$$p(\boldsymbol{\omega}_i^{(g)}|\mathbf{v}_i^{(g)}, \boldsymbol{\theta}^{(g)}) \propto \exp\Big\{-\frac{1}{2}\Big[\big(\mathbf{v}_i^{(g)} - \boldsymbol{\mu}^{(g)} - \boldsymbol{\Lambda}^{(g)}\boldsymbol{\omega}_i^{(g)}\big)^T \boldsymbol{\Psi}_\epsilon^{(g)-1}\big(\mathbf{v}_i^{(g)} - \boldsymbol{\mu}^{(g)} - \boldsymbol{\Lambda}^{(g)}\boldsymbol{\omega}_i^{(g)}\big)$$
$$+ \big(\boldsymbol{\eta}_i^{(g)} - \boldsymbol{\Lambda}_\omega^{(g)}\mathbf{G}(\boldsymbol{\omega}_i^{(g)})\big)^T \boldsymbol{\Psi}_\delta^{(g)-1}\big(\boldsymbol{\eta}_i^{(g)} - \boldsymbol{\Lambda}_\omega^{(g)}\mathbf{G}(\boldsymbol{\omega}_i^{(g)})\big) + \boldsymbol{\xi}_i^{(g)T}\boldsymbol{\Phi}^{(g)-1}\boldsymbol{\xi}_i^{(g)}\Big]\Big\}. \quad (6.A10)$$

Since the conditional distribution of (6.A10) is not standard, the Metropolis–Hastings algorithm can be used to draw random observations from this distribution.

In the multisample situation, the notation in the conditional distribution $[\boldsymbol{\alpha}, \mathbf{Y}|\boldsymbol{\theta}, \boldsymbol{\Omega}, \mathbf{X}, \mathbf{Z}]$ is very tedious. The derivation is similar to the two-level case as given in Appendix 6.1, equations (6.A3) and (6.A4). As $(\boldsymbol{\alpha}^{(g)}, \mathbf{Y}^{(g)})$ is independent of $(\boldsymbol{\alpha}^{(h)}, \mathbf{Y}^{(h)})$ for $g \neq h$, and $\boldsymbol{\Psi}_\delta^{(g)}$ is diagonal,

$$p(\boldsymbol{\alpha}, \mathbf{Y}|\cdot) = \prod_{g=1}^{G} p(\boldsymbol{\alpha}^{(g)}, \mathbf{Y}^{(g)}|\cdot) = \prod_{g=1}^{G}\prod_{k=1}^{s} p(\boldsymbol{\alpha}_k^{(g)}, \mathbf{Y}_k^{(g)}|\cdot), \quad (6.A11)$$

where $\mathbf{Y}_k^{(g)} = (y_{1k}^{(g)}, \ldots, y_{N_g k}^{(g)})^T$. Let $\boldsymbol{\Psi}_{\epsilon y}^{(g)}$, $\boldsymbol{\Lambda}_y^{(g)}$, and $\boldsymbol{\mu}_y^{(g)}$ be the submatrices and subvector of $\boldsymbol{\Psi}_\epsilon^{(g)}$, $\boldsymbol{\Lambda}^{(g)}$, and $\boldsymbol{\mu}^{(g)}$ corresponding to the ordered categorical variables in $\mathbf{Y}$; let $\psi_{\epsilon yk}^{(g)}$ be the kth diagonal element of $\boldsymbol{\Psi}_{\epsilon y}^{(g)}$, $\mu_{yk}^{(g)}$ be the kth element of $\boldsymbol{\mu}_y^{(g)}$, $\boldsymbol{\Lambda}_{yk}^{(g)T}$ be the kth row of $\boldsymbol{\Lambda}_y^{(g)}$, and $I_A(y)$ be an indicator function with value 1 if y in A and zero otherwise. Then $p(\boldsymbol{\alpha}, \mathbf{Y}|\cdot)$ can be obtained from (6.A11) and

$$p(\boldsymbol{\alpha}_k^{(g)}, \mathbf{Y}_k^{(g)}|\cdot) \propto \prod_{i=1}^{N_g} \phi\big\{\psi_{\epsilon yk}^{(g)-1/2}\big(y_{ik}^{(g)} - \mu_{yk}^{(g)} - \boldsymbol{\Lambda}_{yk}^{(g)T}\boldsymbol{\omega}_i^{(g)}\big)\big\} I_{[\alpha_{k,z_{ik}^{(g)}}^{(g)}, \alpha_{k,z_{ik}^{(g)}+1}^{(g)}]}(y_{ik}^{(g)}), \quad (6.A12)$$

where ϕ is the probability density function of $N[0, 1]$.

Under the prior distributions of components in $\boldsymbol{\theta}$ as given in Section 6.3, the conditional distribution $[\boldsymbol{\theta}|\boldsymbol{\alpha}, \mathbf{Y}, \boldsymbol{\Omega}, \mathbf{X}, \mathbf{Z}]$ is presented. Note that as $\mathbf{Y}$ is given, the model is defined with continuous data; hence, the conditional distribution is independent of $\boldsymbol{\alpha}$ and $\mathbf{Z}$.

The conditional distributions of some components in $\boldsymbol{\theta}^{(g)}$, $g = 1, \ldots, G$, in the situation of no parameter constraints are given as follows. Let $\boldsymbol{\Lambda}_k^{(g)T}$ be the kth row of $\boldsymbol{\Lambda}^{(g)}$, and $\psi_{\epsilon k}^{(g)}$ be the kth diagonal element of $\boldsymbol{\Psi}_\epsilon^{(g)}$, $\mathbf{V}_k^{*(g)T}$ be the kth row of $\mathbf{V}^{*(g)} = (\mathbf{v}_1^{(g)} - \boldsymbol{\mu}^{(g)}, \ldots, \mathbf{v}_{N_g}^{(g)} - \boldsymbol{\mu}^{(g)})$, and $\boldsymbol{\Omega}_2^{(g)} = (\boldsymbol{\xi}_1^{(g)}, \ldots, \boldsymbol{\xi}_{N_g}^{(g)})$. It can be shown that:

$$\begin{aligned}
&[\boldsymbol{\mu}^{(g)}|\boldsymbol{\Lambda}^{(g)}, \boldsymbol{\Psi}_\epsilon^{(g)}, \mathbf{Y}, \boldsymbol{\Omega}, \mathbf{X}] \stackrel{D}{=} N(\mathbf{a}_\mu^{(g)}, \mathbf{A}_\mu^{(g)}),\\
&[\boldsymbol{\Lambda}_k^{(g)}|\boldsymbol{\Psi}_\epsilon^{(g)}, \boldsymbol{\mu}^{(g)}, \mathbf{Y}, \boldsymbol{\Omega}, \mathbf{X}] \stackrel{D}{=} N(\mathbf{a}_k^{(g)}, \mathbf{A}_k^{(g)}),\\
&[\psi_{\epsilon k}^{(g)-1}|\boldsymbol{\Lambda}_k^{(g)}, \boldsymbol{\mu}^{(g)}, \mathbf{Y}, \boldsymbol{\Omega}, \mathbf{X}] \stackrel{D}{=} \text{Gamma}(N_g/2 + \alpha_{0\epsilon k}^{(g)}, \beta_{\epsilon k}^{(g)}),\\
&[\boldsymbol{\Phi}^{(g)}|\boldsymbol{\Omega}_2^{(g)}] \stackrel{D}{=} \text{IW}_{q_2}[(\boldsymbol{\Omega}_2^{(g)}\boldsymbol{\Omega}_2^{(g)T} + \mathbf{R}_0^{(g)-1}), N_g + \rho_0^{(g)}],
\end{aligned} \tag{6.A13}$$

where

$$\mathbf{a}_\mu^{(g)} = \mathbf{A}_\mu^{(g)}[\boldsymbol{\Sigma}_0^{(g)-1}\boldsymbol{\mu}_0^{(g)} + N_g\boldsymbol{\Psi}_\epsilon^{(g)-1}(\bar{\mathbf{v}}^{(g)} - \boldsymbol{\Lambda}^{(g)}\bar{\boldsymbol{\omega}}^{(g)})], \quad \mathbf{A}_\mu^{(g)} = (\boldsymbol{\Sigma}_0^{(g)-1} + N_g\boldsymbol{\Psi}_\epsilon^{(g)-1})^{-1},$$

$$\mathbf{a}_k^{(g)} = \mathbf{A}_k^{(g)}[\mathbf{H}_{0yk}^{(g)-1}\boldsymbol{\Lambda}_{0k}^{(g)} + \psi_{\epsilon k}^{(g)-1}\boldsymbol{\Omega}^{(g)}\mathbf{V}_k^{*(g)}], \quad \mathbf{A}_k^{(g)} = [\psi_{\epsilon k}^{(g)-1}\boldsymbol{\Omega}^{(g)}\boldsymbol{\Omega}^{(g)T} + \mathbf{H}_{0yk}^{(g)-1}]^{-1}$$

$$\beta_{\epsilon k}^{(g)} = \beta_{0\epsilon k}^{(g)} + [\boldsymbol{\Lambda}_k^{(g)T}\boldsymbol{\Omega}^{(g)}\boldsymbol{\Omega}^{(g)T}\boldsymbol{\Lambda}_k^{(g)} - 2\boldsymbol{\Lambda}_k^{(g)T}\boldsymbol{\Omega}^{(g)}\mathbf{V}_k^{*(g)} + \mathbf{V}_k^{*(g)T}\mathbf{V}_k^{*(g)}]/2,$$

in which $\bar{\mathbf{v}}^{(g)} = \sum_{i=1}^{N_g}\mathbf{v}_i^{(g)}/N_g$ and $\bar{\boldsymbol{\omega}}^{(g)} = \sum_{i=1}^{N_g}\boldsymbol{\omega}_i^{(g)}/N_g$ are the means of $\mathbf{v}_i^{(g)}$ and $\boldsymbol{\omega}_i^{(g)}$ within the gth group.

As we mentioned, slight modifications are required to handle models with parameter constraints (see Section 6.3). Under the constraints $\boldsymbol{\Lambda}_k^{(1)} = \ldots = \boldsymbol{\Lambda}_k^{(G)} = \boldsymbol{\Lambda}_k$, the conjugate prior distribution of $\boldsymbol{\Lambda}_k$ is $N[\boldsymbol{\Lambda}_{0k}, \mathbf{H}_{0yk}]$, and the conditional distribution is

$$[\boldsymbol{\Lambda}_k|\psi_{\epsilon k}^{(1)}, \ldots, \psi_{\epsilon k}^{(G)}, \boldsymbol{\mu}^{(1)}, \ldots, \boldsymbol{\mu}^{(G)}, \mathbf{Y}, \boldsymbol{\Omega}, \mathbf{X}] \stackrel{D}{=} N[\mathbf{a}_k, \mathbf{A}_k], \tag{6.A14}$$

where $\mathbf{a}_k = \mathbf{A}_k(\mathbf{H}_{0yk}^{-1}\boldsymbol{\Lambda}_{0k} + \sum_{g=1}^G \psi_{\epsilon k}^{(g)-1}\boldsymbol{\Omega}^{(g)}\mathbf{V}_k^{*(g)})$, and $\mathbf{A}_k = (\sum_{g=1}^G \psi_{\epsilon k}^{(g)-1}\boldsymbol{\Omega}^{(g)}\boldsymbol{\Omega}^{(g)T} + \mathbf{H}_{0yk}^{-1})^{-1}$. Under the constraints $\psi_{\epsilon k}^{(1)} = \ldots = \psi_{\epsilon k}^{(G)} = \psi_{\epsilon k}$, the conjugate prior distribution of $\psi_{\epsilon k}^{-1}$ is Gamma$(\alpha_{0\epsilon k}, \beta_{0\epsilon k})$, and the conditional distribution is

$$[\psi_{\epsilon k}^{-1}|\boldsymbol{\Lambda}_k^{(1)}, \ldots, \boldsymbol{\Lambda}_k^{(G)}, \boldsymbol{\mu}^{(1)}, \ldots, \boldsymbol{\mu}^{(G)}, \mathbf{Y}, \boldsymbol{\Omega}, \mathbf{X}] \stackrel{D}{=} \text{Gamma}(n/2 + \alpha_{0\epsilon k}, \beta_{\epsilon k}), \tag{6.A15}$$

where $n = N_1 + \ldots + N_G$,

$$\beta_{\epsilon k} = \beta_{0\epsilon k} + \sum_{g=1}^G [\boldsymbol{\Lambda}_k^{(g)T}(\boldsymbol{\Omega}^{(g)}\boldsymbol{\Omega}^{(g)T})\boldsymbol{\Lambda}_k^{(g)} - 2\boldsymbol{\Lambda}_k^{(g)T}\boldsymbol{\Omega}^{(g)}\mathbf{V}_k^{*(g)} + \mathbf{V}_k^{*(g)T}\mathbf{V}_k^{*(g)}]/2.$$

Under the constraints $\boldsymbol{\Phi}^{(1)} = \ldots = \boldsymbol{\Phi}^{(G)} = \boldsymbol{\Phi}$, the conjugate prior distribution of $\boldsymbol{\Phi}^{-1}$ is $W_{q_2}[\mathbf{R}_0, \rho_0]$, and the conditional distribution is

$$[\boldsymbol{\Phi}|\boldsymbol{\Omega}_2^{(1)}, \ldots, \boldsymbol{\Omega}_2^{(G)}] \stackrel{D}{=} \text{IW}_{q_2}\left[\left(\sum_{g=1}^G \boldsymbol{\Omega}_2^{(g)}\boldsymbol{\Omega}_2^{(g)T} + \mathbf{R}_0^{-1}\right), n + \rho_0\right]. \tag{6.A16}$$

The conditional distributions of $\boldsymbol{\Lambda}_{\omega k}^{(g)}$ and $\psi_{\delta k}^{(g)}$ are similar, and thus omitted.

As the conditional distributions involved in (6.A13) or (6.A14)–(6.A16) are standard distributions, drawing observations from them is straightforward. Simulating observations from the conditional distributions that are given in (6.A12) involves the univariate truncated normal distribution, and this is done by the inverse distribution method proposed by Robert (1995). A Metropolis–Hastings algorithm is used to simulate observations from the more complex conditional distribution (6.A10).

References

Bollen, K. A. (1989) *Structural Equations with Latent Variables*. New York: John Wiley & Sons, Inc.

Cowles, M. K. (1996) Accelerating Monte Carlo Markov chain convergence for cumulative-link generalized linear models. *Statistics and Computing*, **6**, 101–111.

Gelman, A., Meng, X. L. and Stern, H. (1996a) Posterior predictive assessment of model fitness via realized discrepancies. *Statistica Sinica*, **6**, 733–760.

Gelman, A., Roberts, G. O. and Gilks, W. R. (1996b) Efficient Metropolis jumping rules. In J. M. Bernardo, J. O. Berger, A. P. Dawid and A. F. M. Smith (eds), *Bayesian Statistics 5*, pp. 599–607. Oxford: Oxford University Press.

Geman, S. and Geman, D. (1984) Stochastic relaxation, Gibbs distributions, and the Bayesian restoration of images. *IEEE Transactions on Pattern Analysis and Machine Intelligence*, **6**, 721–741.

Hastings, W. K. (1970) Monte Carlo sampling methods using Markov chains and their applications. *Biometrika*, **57**, 97–109.

Kass, R. E. and Raftery, A. E. (1995) Bayes factors. *Journal of the American Statistical Association*, **90**, 773–795.

Lee, S. Y. (2007) *Structural Equation Modeling: A Bayesian Approach*. Chichester: John Wiley & Sons, Ltd.

Lee, S. Y. and Song, X. Y. (2005) Maximum likelihood analysis of a two-level nonlinear structural equation model with fixed covariates. *Journal of Educational and Behavioral Statistics*, **30**, 1–26.

Lee, S. Y. and Zhu, H. T. (2000) Statistical analysis of nonlinear structural equation models with continuous and polytomous data. *British Journal of Mathematical and Statistical Psychology*, **53**, 209–232.

Lee, S. Y., Poon, W. Y. and Bentler, P. M. (1989) Simultaneous analysis of multivariate polytomous variates in several groups. *Psychometrika*, **54**, 63–73.

Lee, S. Y., Song, X. Y., Skevington, S. and Hao, Y. T. (2005) Application of structural equation models to quality of life. *Structural Equation Modeling – A Multidisciplinary Journal*, **12**, 43–453.

Lee, S. Y., Song, X. Y. and Tang, N. S. (2007) Bayesian methods for analyzing structural equation models with covariates, interaction, and quadratic latent variables. *Structural Equation Modeling – A Multidisciplinary Journal*, **14**, 404–434.

McDonald, R. P. and Goldstein, H. (1989) Balanced versus unbalanced designs for linear structural relations in two-level data. *British Journal of Mathematical and Statistical Psychology*, **42**, 215–232.

Metropolis, N., Rosenbluth, A. W., Rosenbluth, M. N., Teller, A. H. and Teller, E. (1953) Equation of state calculations by fast computing machines. *Journal of Chemical Physics*, **21**, 1087–1092.

Morisky, D. E., Tiglao, T. V., Sneed, C. D., Tempongko, S. B., Baltazar, J. C., Detels, R. and Stein, J.A. (1998) The effects of establishment practices, knowledge and attitudes on condom use among Filipina sex workers. *AIDS Care*, **10**, 213–220.

Power, M., Bullinger, M., Harper, A. and WHOQOL Group (1999) The World Health Organization WHOQOL-100: Tests of the universality of quality of life in 15 different cultural groups worldwide. *Health Psychology*, **18**, 495–505.

Rabe-Hesketh, S., Skrondal, A. and Pickles, A. (2004) Generalized multilevel structural equation modeling. *Psychometrika*, **69**, 167–190.

Robert, C. P. (1995) Simulation of truncated normal variables. *Statistics and Computing*, **5**, 121–125.

Shi, J. Q. and Lee, S. Y. (1998) Bayesian sampling-based approach for factor analysis models with continuous and polytomous data. *British Journal of Mathematical and Statistical Psychology*, **51**, 233–252.

Shi, J. Q. and Lee, S. Y. (2000) Latent variable models with mixed continuous and polytomous data. *Journal of the Royal Statistical Society, Series B*, **62**, 77–87.

Skrondal, A. and Rabe-Hesketh, S. (2004) *Generalized Latent Variable Modeling: Multilevel, Longitudinal, and Structural Equation Models*. Boca Raton, FL: Chapman & Hall/CRC.

Song, X. Y. and Lee, S. Y. (2001) Bayesian estimation and test for factor analysis model with continuous and polytomous data in several populations. *British Journal of Mathematical and Statistical Psychology*, **54** 237–263.

Song, X. Y. and Lee, S. Y. (2004) Bayesian analysis of two-level nonlinear structural equation models with continuous and polytomous data. *British Journal of Mathematical and Statistical Psychology*, **57**, 29–52.

Spiegelhalter, D. J., Thomas, A., Best, N. G. and Lunn, D. (2003) *WinBUGS User Manual. Version 1.4*. Cambridge: MRC Biostatistics Unit.

Zhu, H. T. and Lee, S. Y. (1999) Statistical analysis of nonlinear factor analysis models. *British Journal of Mathematical and Statistical Psychology*, **52**, 225–242.

7

Mixture structural equation models

7.1 Introduction

In Chapter 6 we discussed two-level SEMs and multisample SEMs, which are useful tools for analyzing hierarchical data and multiple-group data. In this chapter we focus on another kind of heterogeneous data which involve independent observations that come from one of the K populations with different distributions, and no information is available on which of the K populations an individual observation belongs to. In general, a finite mixture model arises with a population which is a mixture of K components with probability densities $\{f_k, k = 1, \ldots, K\}$ and mixing proportions $\{\pi_k, k = 1, \ldots, K\}$. Models of this kind arise in many fields, including behavioral, medical, and environmental sciences. They have been used in handling outliers (Pettit and Smith, 1985) and density estimation (Roeder and Wasserman, 1997). Statistical analysis of mixture models is not straightforward. For the estimation of mixture models with a fixed number of components, a variety of methods have been proposed. Examples are the method of moments (Lindsay and Basak, 1993), Bayesian methods with MCMC techniques (Diebolt and Robert, 1994; Robert, 1996), and the ML method (Hathaway, 1985). For mixture models with K treated as random, Richardson and Green (1997) developed a full Bayesian analysis with a reversible jump MCMC method. For the challenging problem of testing the number of components, the classical likelihood-based inference encountered serious difficulties due to nonregularity problems: some standard asymptotic properties associated with the likelihood ratio test are not valid. In contrast, as pointed out by Richardson and Green (1997), the Bayes paradigm is particularly suitable for analyzing mixture models with an unknown K.

In the field of SEM, Jedidi *et al.* (1997) considered the estimation of a finite mixtures of SEMs with a fixed number of components, and gave a brief discussion on model selection via the Bayesian information criterion (BIC). Yung (1997) investigated finite mixtures of

Basic and Advanced Bayesian Structural Equation Modeling: With Applications in the Medical and Behavioral Sciences,
First Edition. Xin-Yuan Song and Sik-Yum Lee.

confirmatory factor analysis models, while Dolan and van der Maas (1998) applied a quasi-Newton algorithm to finite mixtures and inferred the estimation by changing the degree of separation and the sample size. Arminger *et al.* (1999) discussed ML analysis for mixtures of conditional mean- and covariance-structure models, and established three estimation strategies based on the Expectation-Maximization (EM) algorithm. Zhu and Lee (2001) set out a Bayesian analysis of finite mixtures in the LISREL model, using the idea of data augmentation and some MCMC methods. Lee and Song (2003) developed a path sampling procedure to compute the observed-data log-likelihood, for evaluating the BIC in selecting the appropriate number of components for a mixture SEM with missing data. A Bayesian approach for analyzing mixtures of SEMs with an unknown number of components was developed by Lee and Song (2002), based on the Bayes factor computed via a path sampling procedure. Spiegelhalter *et al.* (2003) pointed out that the DIC may not be appropriate for model comparison in the context of mixture models. Hence, WinBUGS does not give DIC results for mixture models. In Section 7.3.3 we present a modified DIC for the comparison of mixture SEMs using our tailor-made R code.

For a mixture SEM with K components, the model is invariant with respect to permutation of the labels $k = 1, \ldots, K$. Thus, the model is not identified, and adoption of a unique labeling for identifiability is important. In the literature, a common method is to use some constraints on the components of the mean vector to force a unique labeling. In a Bayesian approach, arbitrary constraints may not be able to solve the problem. We apply the permutation sampler (Frühwirth-Schnatter, 2001) to find the appropriate identifiability constraints.

The objectives of this chapter are to introduce finite mixture SEMs and a modified mixture SEM. The Bayesian methodologies for analyzing heterogeneous data through these models are also discussed. Section 7.2 presents a general finite mixture SEM, in which the probabilities of component memberships, $\pi_1, \ldots, \pi_K$, are unknown and estimated together with other parameters. Section 7.3 extends the general mixture SEM to a modified mixture SEM, in which the probabilities of component memberships are modeled through a multinomial logit model. With this extension, the effects of some important covariates on individuals' component memberships are incorporated to achieve better results. In addition, the modified mixture SEM can accommodate component-specific nonlinear interrelationships among latent variables, as well as nonignorable missing responses and covariates.

7.2 Finite mixture SEMs

7.2.1 The model

Let $\mathbf{y}_i$ be a $p \times 1$ random vector corresponding to the ith observation, and suppose that its distribution is given by the probability density function

$$f(\mathbf{y}_i|\boldsymbol{\theta}) = \sum_{k=1}^{K} \pi_k f_k(\mathbf{y}_i|\boldsymbol{\mu}_k, \boldsymbol{\theta}_k), \quad i = 1, \ldots, n, \tag{7.1}$$

where K is a given integer, π_k is the unknown mixing proportion such that $\pi_k > 0$ and $\pi_1 + \cdots + \pi_K = 1$, and $f_k(\mathbf{y}_i|\boldsymbol{\mu}_k, \boldsymbol{\theta}_k)$ is the multivariate normal density function with an unknown mean vector $\boldsymbol{\mu}_k$ and a general covariance structure $\boldsymbol{\Sigma}_k = \boldsymbol{\Sigma}_k(\boldsymbol{\theta}_k)$ that depends on an unknown parameter vector $\boldsymbol{\theta}_k$. Let $\boldsymbol{\theta}$ be the parameter vector that contains all unknown parameters in π_k, $\boldsymbol{\mu}_k$, and $\boldsymbol{\theta}_k$, $k = 1, \ldots, K$. For the kth component, the measurement equation of the model is given by

$$\mathbf{y}_i = \boldsymbol{\mu}_k + \boldsymbol{\Lambda}_k\boldsymbol{\omega}_i + \boldsymbol{\epsilon}_i, \tag{7.2}$$

where $\boldsymbol{\mu}_k$ is the mean vector, $\boldsymbol{\Lambda}_k$ is the $p \times q$ factor loading matrix, $\boldsymbol{\omega}_i$ is a random vector of latent variables, and $\boldsymbol{\epsilon}_i$ is a random vector of residuals which is distributed as $N[\mathbf{0}, \boldsymbol{\Psi}_k]$, where $\boldsymbol{\Psi}_k$ is a diagonal matrix. It is assumed that $\boldsymbol{\omega}_i$ and $\boldsymbol{\epsilon}_i$ are independent. Let $\boldsymbol{\omega}_i = (\boldsymbol{\eta}_i^T, \boldsymbol{\xi}_i^T)^T$ be a partition of $\boldsymbol{\omega}_i$ into an outcome latent vector $\boldsymbol{\eta}_i$ and an explanatory latent vector $\boldsymbol{\xi}_i$. The structural equation of the model is defined as

$$\boldsymbol{\eta}_i = \boldsymbol{\Pi}_k\boldsymbol{\eta}_i + \boldsymbol{\Gamma}_k\boldsymbol{\xi}_i + \boldsymbol{\delta}_i, \tag{7.3}$$

where $\boldsymbol{\eta}_i$ and $\boldsymbol{\xi}_i$ are $q_1 \times 1$ and $q_2 \times 1$ subvectors of $\boldsymbol{\omega}_i$ respectively, $\boldsymbol{\delta}_i$ is a random vector of residuals that is independent of $\boldsymbol{\xi}_i$, $\boldsymbol{\Pi}_k$ and $\boldsymbol{\Gamma}_k$ are unknown parameter matrices such that $\boldsymbol{\Pi}_{0k}^{-1} = (\mathbf{I} - \boldsymbol{\Pi}_k)^{-1}$ exists, and $|\boldsymbol{\Pi}_{0k}|$ is independent of the elements in $\boldsymbol{\Pi}_k$. Let the distributions of $\boldsymbol{\xi}_i$ and $\boldsymbol{\delta}_i$ in the kth component be $N[\mathbf{0}, \boldsymbol{\Phi}_k]$ and $N[\mathbf{0}, \boldsymbol{\Psi}_{\delta k}]$, respectively, where $\boldsymbol{\Psi}_{\delta k}$ is a diagonal matrix. The parameter vector $\boldsymbol{\theta}_k$ contains the free unknown parameters in $\boldsymbol{\Lambda}_k$, $\boldsymbol{\Pi}_k$, $\boldsymbol{\Gamma}_k$, $\boldsymbol{\Phi}_k$, $\boldsymbol{\Psi}_k$, and $\boldsymbol{\Psi}_{\delta k}$. The covariance structure of $\boldsymbol{\omega}_i$ in the kth component is given by

$$\boldsymbol{\Sigma}_{\omega k} = \begin{bmatrix} \boldsymbol{\Pi}_{0k}^{-1}\left(\boldsymbol{\Gamma}_k\boldsymbol{\Phi}_k\boldsymbol{\Gamma}_k^T + \boldsymbol{\Psi}_{\delta k}\right)\left(\boldsymbol{\Pi}_{0k}^{-1}\right)^T & \boldsymbol{\Pi}_{0k}^{-1}\boldsymbol{\Gamma}_k\boldsymbol{\Phi}_k \\ \boldsymbol{\Phi}_k\boldsymbol{\Gamma}_k^T\left(\boldsymbol{\Pi}_{0k}^{-1}\right)^T & \boldsymbol{\Phi}_k \end{bmatrix},$$

and $\boldsymbol{\Sigma}_k(\boldsymbol{\theta}_k) = \boldsymbol{\Lambda}_k\boldsymbol{\Sigma}_{\omega k}\boldsymbol{\Lambda}_k^T + \boldsymbol{\Psi}_k$. Any of these unknown parameter matrices can be invariant across components. However, it is important to assign a different $\boldsymbol{\mu}_k$ in the measurement equation of each component in order to effectively analyze data from the heterogeneous populations that differ by their mean vectors.

As the mixture model defined in (7.1) is invariant with respect to permutation of labels $k = 1, \ldots, K$, adoption of a unique labeling for identifiability is important. Our method is to impose the ordering $\mu_{1,1} < \ldots < \mu_{K,1}$ for solving the label switching problem (jumping between various labeling subspaces), where $\mu_{k,1}$ is the first element of the mean vector $\boldsymbol{\mu}_k$. This works fine if $\mu_{1,1} < \ldots < \mu_{K,1}$ are well separated. However, if $\mu_{1,1} < \ldots < \mu_{K,1}$ are close to each other, it may not be able to eliminate the label switching problem, and may give biased results. Hence, it is important to find an appropriate identifiability constraint. Here, the random permutation sampler developed by Frühwirth-Schnatter (2001) will be used to find suitable identifiability constraints. Moreover, for each $k = 1, \ldots K$, structural parameters in the covariance matrix $\boldsymbol{\Sigma}_k$ corresponding to the model defined by (7.2) and (7.3) are not identified. This problem is solved by the common method in structural equation modeling of fixing appropriate elements in $\boldsymbol{\Lambda}_k$, $\boldsymbol{\Pi}_k$, and/or $\boldsymbol{\Gamma}_k$ at preassigned values that are chosen on a problem-by-problem basis. For the sake of a clear presentation of the Bayesian method, we assume that all the unknown parameters in the model are identified.

7.2.2 Bayesian estimation

Let $\boldsymbol{\theta}_{yk}$ be the vector of unknown parameters in $\boldsymbol{\Lambda}_k$ and $\boldsymbol{\Psi}_k$, and let $\boldsymbol{\theta}_{\omega k}$ be the vector of unknown parameters in $\boldsymbol{\Pi}_k$, $\boldsymbol{\Gamma}_k$, $\boldsymbol{\Phi}_k$, and $\boldsymbol{\Psi}_{\delta k}$. Let $\boldsymbol{\mu}$, $\boldsymbol{\pi}$, $\boldsymbol{\theta}_y$, and $\boldsymbol{\theta}_\omega$ be the vectors that contain the unknown parameters in $\{\boldsymbol{\mu}_1, \ldots, \boldsymbol{\mu}_K\}$, $\{\pi_1, \ldots, \pi_K\}$, $\{\boldsymbol{\theta}_{y1}, \ldots, \boldsymbol{\theta}_{yK}\}$, and $\{\boldsymbol{\theta}_{\omega 1}, \ldots, \boldsymbol{\theta}_{\omega K}\}$, respectively; and let $\boldsymbol{\theta} = (\boldsymbol{\mu}, \boldsymbol{\pi}, \boldsymbol{\theta}_y, \boldsymbol{\theta}_\omega)$ be the overall parameter vector. Inspired by other work on finite mixture models, we introduce a group label w_i for the ith observation $\mathbf{y}_i$ as a latent allocation variable, and assume that it is independently drawn from the distribution

$$p(w_i = k) = \pi_k, \quad \text{for } k = 1, \ldots, K. \tag{7.4}$$

Moreover, let $\mathbf{Y} = (\mathbf{y}_1, \ldots, \mathbf{y}_n)$ be the observed data matrix, $\boldsymbol{\Omega} = (\boldsymbol{\omega}_1, \ldots, \boldsymbol{\omega}_n)$ be the matrix of latent vectors, and $\mathbf{W} = (w_1, \ldots, w_n)$ be the vector of allocation variables.

In a standard Bayesian analysis, we need to evaluate the posterior distribution of the unknown parameters, $p[\boldsymbol{\theta}|\mathbf{Y}]$. Due to the nature of the mixture model, this posterior distribution is complicated. However, if $\mathbf{W}$ is observed, the component of every $\mathbf{y}_i$ can be identified and the mixture model becomes the more familiar multiple-group model. In addition, if $\boldsymbol{\Omega}$ is observed, the underlying SEM will become the linear simultaneous equation model which is comparatively easy to handle. Hence, the observed data $\mathbf{Y}$ are augmented with the latent quantities $\boldsymbol{\Omega}$ and $\mathbf{W}$ in the posterior analysis, and the posterior analysis is based on $p(\boldsymbol{\theta}, \boldsymbol{\Omega}, \mathbf{W}|\mathbf{Y})$.

The label switching problem has to be solved in the posterior analysis. For general mixture models with K components, the unconstrained parameter space contains $K!$ subspaces, each one corresponding to a different way to label the states. In the current mixture of SEM, the likelihood is invariant to relabeling the states. If the prior distributions of $\boldsymbol{\pi}$ and other parameters in $\boldsymbol{\theta}$ are also invariant, the unconstrained posterior is invariant to relabeling the states and identical on all labeling subspaces. This induces a multimodal posterior and a serious problem in Bayesian estimation.

We will use the MCMC approach proposed by Frühwirth-Schnatter (2001) to deal with the above label switching problem. In this approach, an unidentified model is first estimated by sampling from the unconstrained posterior using the random permutation sampler, where each sweep is concluded by a random permutation of the current labeling of the components. The random permutation sampler delivers a sample that explores the whole unconstrained parameter space and jumps between various labeling subspaces in a balanced fashion. As pointed out by Frühwirth-Schnatter (2001), although the model is unidentified, the output of the random permutation sampler can be used to estimate unknown parameters that are invariant to relabeling the states, and can be explored to find suitable identifiability constraints. Then the model is reestimated by sampling from the posterior distribution under the imposed identifiability constraints, again using the permutation sampler. The implementation of the permutation sampler in relation to the mixture of SEMs, and the method of selecting the identifiability constraint are briefly described in Appendices 7.1 and 7.2, respectively.

The main task in the Bayesian estimation is to simulate a sufficiently large sample of observations from $[\boldsymbol{\theta}, \boldsymbol{\Omega}, \mathbf{W}|\mathbf{Y}]$. Similar to many Bayesian analyses of SEMs, this is done by the Gibbs sampler (Geman and Geman, 1984) as follows. At the rth iteration with current values $\boldsymbol{\theta}^{(r)}$, $\boldsymbol{\Omega}^{(r)}$, and $\mathbf{W}^{(r)}$:

A. Generate $(\mathbf{W}^{(r+1)}, \boldsymbol{\Omega}^{(r+1)})$ from $p(\boldsymbol{\Omega}, \mathbf{W}|\mathbf{Y}, \boldsymbol{\theta}^{(r)})$.

B. Generate $\boldsymbol{\theta}^{(r+1)}$ from $p(\boldsymbol{\theta}|\mathbf{Y}, \boldsymbol{\Omega}^{(r+1)}, \mathbf{W}^{(r+1)})$.

B. Reorder the labels through the permutation sampler to achieve the identifiability.

As $p(\boldsymbol{\Omega}, \mathbf{W}|\mathbf{Y}, \boldsymbol{\theta}) = p(\mathbf{W}|\mathbf{Y}, \boldsymbol{\theta})p(\boldsymbol{\Omega}|\mathbf{Y}, \mathbf{W}, \boldsymbol{\theta})$, step A can be further decomposed into the following two steps:

A1. Generate $\mathbf{W}^{(r+1)}$ from $p(\mathbf{W}|\mathbf{Y}, \boldsymbol{\theta}^{(r)})$.

A2. Generate $\boldsymbol{\Omega}^{(r+1)}$ from $p(\boldsymbol{\Omega}|\mathbf{Y}, \boldsymbol{\theta}^{(r)}, \mathbf{W}^{(r+1)})$.

Simulating observations $(\mathbf{W}, \boldsymbol{\Omega})$ through steps A1 and A2 is more efficient than using step A. Conditional distributions required for implementing the Gibbs sampler are discussed below.

We first consider the conditional distribution associated with step A1. As the w_i are independent,

$$p(\mathbf{W}|\mathbf{Y}, \boldsymbol{\theta}) = \prod_{i=1}^{n} p(w_i|\mathbf{y}_i, \boldsymbol{\theta}). \tag{7.5}$$

Moreover,

$$p(w_i = k|\mathbf{y}_i, \boldsymbol{\theta}) = \frac{p(w_i = k, \mathbf{y}_i|\boldsymbol{\theta})}{p(\mathbf{y}_i|\boldsymbol{\theta})} = \frac{p(w_i = k|\boldsymbol{\pi})p(\mathbf{y}_i|w_i = k, \boldsymbol{\theta})}{p(\mathbf{y}_i|\boldsymbol{\theta})} = \frac{\pi_k f_k(\mathbf{y}_i|\boldsymbol{\mu}_k, \boldsymbol{\theta}_k)}{f(\mathbf{y}_i|\boldsymbol{\theta})}, \tag{7.6}$$

where $f_k(\mathbf{y}_i|\boldsymbol{\mu}_k, \boldsymbol{\theta}_k)$ is the probability density function of $N[\boldsymbol{\mu}_k, \boldsymbol{\Sigma}_k(\boldsymbol{\theta}_k)]$. Hence, the conditional distribution of $\mathbf{W}$ given $\mathbf{Y}$ and $\boldsymbol{\theta}$ can be derived from (7.5) and (7.6).

Consider the conditional distribution involved in step A2. Because the $\boldsymbol{\omega}_i$ are mutually independent, we have

$$\begin{aligned}\prod_{i=1}^{n} p(\boldsymbol{\omega}_i|\mathbf{y}_i, w_i, \boldsymbol{\theta}) &= p(\boldsymbol{\Omega}|\mathbf{Y}, \boldsymbol{\theta}, \mathbf{W}) \propto p(\mathbf{Y}|\boldsymbol{\Omega}, \mathbf{W}, \boldsymbol{\mu}, \boldsymbol{\theta}_y)p(\boldsymbol{\Omega}|\mathbf{W}, \boldsymbol{\theta}_\omega) \\ &= \prod_{i=1}^{n} p(\mathbf{y}_i|\boldsymbol{\omega}_i, w_i, \boldsymbol{\mu}, \boldsymbol{\theta}_y)p(\boldsymbol{\omega}_i|w_i, \boldsymbol{\theta}_\omega).\end{aligned} \tag{7.7}$$

Let $\mathbf{C}_k = \boldsymbol{\Sigma}_{\omega k}^{-1} + \boldsymbol{\Lambda}_k^T \boldsymbol{\Psi}_k^{-1} \boldsymbol{\Lambda}_k$, where $\boldsymbol{\Sigma}_{\omega k}$ is the covariance matrix of $\boldsymbol{\omega}_i$ in the kth component. Moreover, as the conditional distribution of $\boldsymbol{\omega}_i$ given $\boldsymbol{\theta}_\omega$ and '$w_i = k$' is $N[\mathbf{0}, \boldsymbol{\Sigma}_{\omega k}]$, and the conditional distribution of $\mathbf{y}_i$ given $\boldsymbol{\omega}_i, \boldsymbol{\mu}, \boldsymbol{\theta}_y$, and '$w_i = k$' is $N[\boldsymbol{\mu}_k + \boldsymbol{\Lambda}_k \boldsymbol{\omega}_i, \boldsymbol{\Psi}_k]$, it can be shown (see Lindley and Smith, 1972) that

$$[\boldsymbol{\omega}_i|\mathbf{y}_i, w_i = k, \boldsymbol{\theta}] \stackrel{D}{=} N\left[\mathbf{C}_k^{-1}\boldsymbol{\Lambda}_k^T\boldsymbol{\Psi}_k^{-1}(\mathbf{y}_i - \boldsymbol{\mu}_k), \mathbf{C}_k^{-1}\right]. \tag{7.8}$$

The conditional distribution of $p(\boldsymbol{\Omega}|\mathbf{Y}, \boldsymbol{\theta}, \mathbf{W})$ can be obtained from (7.7) and (7.8). Drawing observations from this familiar normal distribution is fast.

We now consider the conditional distribution $p(\boldsymbol{\theta}|\mathbf{Y}, \boldsymbol{\Omega}, \mathbf{W})$ in step B of the Gibbs sampler. This conditional distribution is quite complicated. However, the difficulty can be reduced by assuming the following mild conditions on the prior distribution of $\boldsymbol{\theta}$. We assume that the prior distribution of the mixing proportion $\boldsymbol{\pi}$ is independent of the prior distributions of $\boldsymbol{\mu}, \boldsymbol{\theta}_y$, and $\boldsymbol{\theta}_\omega$. Like many Bayesian SEM analyses, the prior distribution of the mean vector $\boldsymbol{\mu}$ can be taken to be independent of the prior distributions of the parameters $\boldsymbol{\theta}_y$ and $\boldsymbol{\theta}_\omega$ in the covariance structures. Moreover, when $\boldsymbol{\Omega}$ is given, the parameters in $\boldsymbol{\theta}_{yk} = \{\boldsymbol{\Lambda}_k, \boldsymbol{\Psi}_k\}$ are the parameters involved in the linear regression model with the observed variables in $\mathbf{y}$ (see (7.2)), and the parameters in $\boldsymbol{\theta}_{\omega k} = \{\boldsymbol{\Pi}_k, \boldsymbol{\Gamma}_k, \boldsymbol{\Phi}_k, \boldsymbol{\Psi}_{\delta k}\}$ are the parameters involved in the other simultaneous equation model with the latent variables (see (7.3)). Hence, we assume that the prior distributions of $\boldsymbol{\theta}_y$ and $\boldsymbol{\theta}_\omega$ are independent. As a result, $p(\boldsymbol{\theta}) = p(\boldsymbol{\pi}, \boldsymbol{\mu}, \boldsymbol{\theta}_y, \boldsymbol{\theta}_\omega) = p(\boldsymbol{\pi})p(\boldsymbol{\mu})p(\boldsymbol{\theta}_y)p(\boldsymbol{\theta}_\omega)$. Moreover, from the definition of the model and the properties of $\mathbf{W}, \boldsymbol{\Omega}$, and $\boldsymbol{\theta}$, we have $p(\mathbf{W}|\boldsymbol{\theta}) = p(\mathbf{W}|\boldsymbol{\pi})$ and $p(\boldsymbol{\Omega}, \mathbf{Y}|\mathbf{W}, \boldsymbol{\theta}) = p(\mathbf{Y}|\boldsymbol{\Omega}, \mathbf{W}, \boldsymbol{\mu}, \boldsymbol{\theta}_y)p(\boldsymbol{\Omega}|\mathbf{W}, \boldsymbol{\theta}_\omega)$. Hence, the joint conditional distribution of

$\boldsymbol{\theta} = (\boldsymbol{\pi}, \boldsymbol{\mu}, \boldsymbol{\theta}_y, \boldsymbol{\theta}_\omega)$ can be expressed as

$$\begin{aligned} p(\boldsymbol{\theta}|\mathbf{W}, \boldsymbol{\Omega}, \mathbf{Y}) &= p(\boldsymbol{\pi}, \boldsymbol{\mu}, \boldsymbol{\theta}_y, \boldsymbol{\theta}_\omega|\mathbf{W}, \boldsymbol{\Omega}, \mathbf{Y}) \\ &\propto p(\boldsymbol{\pi})p(\boldsymbol{\mu})p(\boldsymbol{\theta}_y)p(\boldsymbol{\theta}_\omega)p(\mathbf{W}, \boldsymbol{\Omega}, \mathbf{Y}|\boldsymbol{\theta}) \\ &\propto p(\boldsymbol{\pi})p(\boldsymbol{\mu})p(\boldsymbol{\theta}_y)p(\boldsymbol{\theta}_\omega)p(\mathbf{W}|\boldsymbol{\theta})p(\boldsymbol{\Omega}, \mathbf{Y}|\boldsymbol{\theta}, \mathbf{W}) \\ &\propto p(\boldsymbol{\pi})p(\boldsymbol{\mu})p(\boldsymbol{\theta}_y)p(\boldsymbol{\theta}_\omega)p(\mathbf{W}|\boldsymbol{\pi})p(\boldsymbol{\Omega}|\mathbf{W}, \boldsymbol{\theta}_\omega)p(\mathbf{Y}|\mathbf{W}, \boldsymbol{\Omega}, \boldsymbol{\mu}, \boldsymbol{\theta}_y) \\ &= [p(\boldsymbol{\pi})p(\mathbf{W}|\boldsymbol{\pi})][p(\boldsymbol{\mu})p(\boldsymbol{\theta}_y)p(\mathbf{Y}|\mathbf{W}, \boldsymbol{\Omega}, \boldsymbol{\mu}, \boldsymbol{\theta}_y)][p(\boldsymbol{\theta}_\omega)p(\boldsymbol{\Omega}|\mathbf{W}, \boldsymbol{\theta}_\omega)]. \end{aligned} \tag{7.9}$$

Using this result, the marginal densities $p(\boldsymbol{\pi}|\cdot)$, $p(\boldsymbol{\mu}, \boldsymbol{\theta}_y|\cdot)$, and $p(\boldsymbol{\theta}_\omega|\cdot)$ can be treated separately.

The prior distribution of $\boldsymbol{\pi}$ is taken as the symmetric Dirichlet distribution, that is, $\boldsymbol{\pi} \stackrel{D}{=} D(\alpha, \ldots, \alpha)$ with probability density function given by

$$p(\boldsymbol{\pi}) = \frac{\Gamma(K\alpha)}{\Gamma(\alpha)^K}\pi_1^\alpha \ldots \pi_K^\alpha,$$

where $\Gamma(\cdot)$ is the gamma function. Since $p(\mathbf{W}|\boldsymbol{\pi}) \propto \prod_{k=1}^K \pi_k^{n_k}$, it follows from (7.9) that the full conditional distribution of $\boldsymbol{\pi}$ remains Dirichlet in the following form:

$$p(\boldsymbol{\pi}|\cdot) \propto p(\boldsymbol{\pi})p(\mathbf{W}|\boldsymbol{\pi}) \propto \prod_{k=1}^K \pi_k^{n_k+\alpha}, \tag{7.10}$$

where n_k is the total number of i such that $w_i = k$. Thus, $p(\boldsymbol{\pi}|\cdot)$ is distributed as $D(\alpha + n_1, \ldots, \alpha + n_K)$.

Let $\mathbf{Y}_k$ and $\boldsymbol{\Omega}_k$ be the respective submatrices of $\mathbf{Y}$ and $\boldsymbol{\Omega}$, such that all the ith columns with $w_i \neq k$ are deleted. It is natural to assume that for $k \neq h$, $(\boldsymbol{\mu}_k, \boldsymbol{\theta}_{yk}, \boldsymbol{\theta}_{\omega k})$ and $(\boldsymbol{\mu}_h, \boldsymbol{\theta}_{yh}, \boldsymbol{\theta}_{\omega h})$ are independent. Hence, given $\mathbf{W}$, we have

$$p(\boldsymbol{\mu}, \boldsymbol{\theta}_y, \boldsymbol{\theta}_\omega|\mathbf{Y}, \boldsymbol{\Omega}, \mathbf{W}) \propto \prod_{k=1}^K p(\boldsymbol{\mu}_k)p(\boldsymbol{\theta}_{yk})p(\boldsymbol{\theta}_{\omega k})p(\mathbf{Y}_k|\boldsymbol{\Omega}_k, \boldsymbol{\mu}_k, \boldsymbol{\theta}_{yk})p(\boldsymbol{\Omega}_k|\boldsymbol{\theta}_{\omega k}), \tag{7.11}$$

and we can treat the product in (7.11) separately with each k. When $\mathbf{W}$ is given, the original complicated problem of finite mixtures reduces to a much simpler multisample problem. Here, for brevity, we assume that there are no cross-group constraints, and the analysis can be carried out separately with each individual sample. Situations with cross-group constraints can be handled similarly to multiple-group analysis.

For mixture models, Roeder and Wasserman (1997) pointed out that using fully noninformative prior distributions may lead to improper posterior distributions. Thus, most Bayesian analyses involving normal mixtures have used conjugate type prior distributions. Here we make use of this type of prior distributions for various components of $\boldsymbol{\theta}$. Let $\boldsymbol{\Lambda}_{\omega k} = (\boldsymbol{\Pi}_k, \boldsymbol{\Gamma}_k)$; for $m = 1, \ldots, p$ and $l = 1, \ldots, q_1$, we take

$$\begin{aligned} &[\boldsymbol{\Lambda}_{km}|\psi_{km}] \stackrel{D}{=} N[\boldsymbol{\Lambda}_{0km}, \psi_{km}\mathbf{H}_{0ykm}], \ \psi_{km}^{-1} \stackrel{D}{=} \text{Gamma}[\alpha_{0\epsilon k}, \beta_{0\epsilon k}], \\ &[\boldsymbol{\Lambda}_{\omega kl}|\psi_{\delta kl}] \stackrel{D}{=} N[\boldsymbol{\Lambda}_{0\omega kl}, \psi_{\delta kl}\mathbf{H}_{0\omega kl}], \ \psi_{\delta kl}^{-1} \stackrel{D}{=} \text{Gamma}[\alpha_{0\delta k}, \beta_{0\delta k}], \\ &\boldsymbol{\mu}_k \stackrel{D}{=} N[\boldsymbol{\mu}_{0k}, \boldsymbol{\Sigma}_{0k}], \ \boldsymbol{\Phi}_k^{-1} \stackrel{D}{=} W_{q_2}[\mathbf{R}_{0k}, \rho_{0k}], \end{aligned} \tag{7.12}$$

where ψ_{km} and $\psi_{\delta kl}$ are the mth diagonal element of $\mathbf{\Psi}_k$ and the lth diagonal element of $\mathbf{\Psi}_{\delta k}$, respectively; $\mathbf{\Lambda}_{km}^T$ and $\mathbf{\Lambda}_{\omega kl}^T$ are vectors that contain unknown parameters in the mth row of $\mathbf{\Lambda}_k$ and the lth row of $\mathbf{\Lambda}_{\omega k}$, respectively; and $\alpha_{0\epsilon k}$, $\beta_{0\epsilon k}$, $\mathbf{\Lambda}_{0km}$, $\alpha_{0\delta k}$, $\beta_{0\delta k}$, $\mathbf{\Lambda}_{0\omega kl}$, $\boldsymbol{\mu}_{0k}$, ρ_{0k}, and positive definite matrices $\mathbf{H}_{0ykm}$, $\mathbf{H}_{0\omega kl}$, $\mathbf{\Sigma}_{0k}$, and $\mathbf{R}_{0k}$ are hyperparameters whose values are assumed given. Moreover, we also make the mild assumptions that $(\psi_{km}, \mathbf{\Lambda}_{km})$ is independent of $(\psi_{kh}, \mathbf{\Lambda}_{kh})$ for $m \neq h$, and $(\psi_{\delta kl}, \mathbf{\Lambda}_{\omega kl})$ is independent of $(\psi_{\delta kh}, \mathbf{\Lambda}_{\omega kh})$ for $l \neq h$.

Let $\mathbf{\Omega}_1 = (\boldsymbol{\eta}_1, \ldots, \boldsymbol{\eta}_n)$, $\mathbf{\Omega}_2 = (\boldsymbol{\xi}_1, \ldots, \boldsymbol{\xi}_n)$, and let $\mathbf{\Omega}_{1k}$ and $\mathbf{\Omega}_{2k}$ be the submatrices of $\mathbf{\Omega}_1$ and $\mathbf{\Omega}_2$ respectively such that all the ith columns with $w_i \neq k$ are deleted. It can be shown by derivations similar to those in previous chapters that the conditional distributions of components of $\boldsymbol{\theta}_k$ are the following familiar normal, gamma, and inverted Wishart distributions:

$$[\boldsymbol{\mu}_k|\mathbf{Y}_k, \mathbf{\Omega}_k, \mathbf{\Lambda}_k, \mathbf{\Psi}_k] \stackrel{D}{=} N\left[\left(\mathbf{\Sigma}_{0k}^{-1} + n_k\mathbf{\Psi}_k^{-1}\right)^{-1}\left(n_k\mathbf{\Psi}_k^{-1}\bar{\mathbf{Y}}_k + \mathbf{\Sigma}_{0k}^{-1}\boldsymbol{\mu}_{0k}\right), \left(\mathbf{\Sigma}_{0k}^{-1} + n_k\mathbf{\Psi}_k^{-1}\right)^{-1}\right],$$

$$[\mathbf{\Lambda}_{km}|\mathbf{Y}_k, \mathbf{\Omega}_k, \psi_{km}] \stackrel{D}{=} N\left[\mathbf{a}_{ykm}, \psi_{km}\mathbf{A}_{ykm}\right],$$

$$\left[\psi_{km}^{-1}|\mathbf{Y}_k, \mathbf{\Omega}_k, \mu_{km}\right] \stackrel{D}{=} \text{Gamma}\left[n_k/2 + \alpha_{0\epsilon k}, \beta_{\epsilon km}\right],$$

$$[\mathbf{\Lambda}_{\omega kl}|\mathbf{Y}_k, \mathbf{\Omega}_k, \psi_{\delta kl}] \stackrel{D}{=} N\left[\mathbf{a}_{\delta kl}, \psi_{\delta kl}\mathbf{A}_{\omega kl}\right],$$

$$\left[\psi_{\delta kl}^{-1}|\mathbf{Y}_k, \mathbf{\Omega}_k\right] \stackrel{D}{=} \text{Gamma}\left[n_k/2 + \alpha_{0\delta k}, \beta_{\delta kl}\right],$$

$$[\mathbf{\Phi}_k|\mathbf{\Omega}_{2k}] \stackrel{D}{=} \text{IW}_{q_2}\left[\left(\mathbf{\Omega}_{2k}\mathbf{\Omega}_{2k}^T + \mathbf{R}_{0k}^{-1}\right), n_k + \rho_{0k}\right],$$

where $\bar{\mathbf{Y}}_k = \sum_{i:w_i=k}(\mathbf{y}_i - \mathbf{\Lambda}_k\boldsymbol{\omega}_i)/n_k$, with $\sum_{i:w_i=k}$ denoting summation with respect to those i such that $w_i = k$, and

$$\mathbf{a}_{ykm} = \mathbf{A}_{ykm}\left(\mathbf{H}_{0ykm}^{-1}\mathbf{\Lambda}_{0km} + \mathbf{\Omega}_k\tilde{\mathbf{Y}}_{km}\right), \quad \mathbf{A}_{ykm} = \left(\mathbf{H}_{0ykm}^{-1} + \mathbf{\Omega}_k\mathbf{\Omega}_k^T\right)^{-1},$$

$$\beta_{\epsilon km} = \beta_{0\epsilon k} + \left[\tilde{\mathbf{Y}}_{km}^T\tilde{\mathbf{Y}}_{km} - \mathbf{a}_{ykm}^T\mathbf{A}_{ykm}^{-1}\mathbf{a}_{ykm} + \mathbf{\Lambda}_{0km}^T\mathbf{H}_{0ykm}^{-1}\mathbf{\Lambda}_{0km}\right]/2,$$

$$\mathbf{a}_{\delta kl} = \mathbf{A}_{\omega kl}\left(\mathbf{H}_{0\omega kl}^{-1}\mathbf{\Lambda}_{0\omega kl} + \mathbf{\Omega}_k\mathbf{\Omega}_{1kl}\right), \quad \mathbf{A}_{\omega kl} = \left(\mathbf{H}_{0\omega kl}^{-1} + \mathbf{\Omega}_k\mathbf{\Omega}_k^T\right)^{-1},$$

$$\beta_{\delta kl} = \beta_{0\delta k} + \left[\mathbf{\Omega}_{1kl}^T\mathbf{\Omega}_{1kl} - \mathbf{a}_{\delta kl}^T\mathbf{A}_{\omega kl}^{-1}\mathbf{a}_{\delta kl} + \mathbf{\Lambda}_{0\omega kl}^T\mathbf{H}_{0\omega kl}^{-1}\mathbf{\Lambda}_{0\omega kl}\right]/2,$$

in which $\tilde{\mathbf{Y}}_{km}^T$ is the mth row of $\tilde{\mathbf{Y}}_k$, which is a matrix whose columns are equal to the columns of $\mathbf{Y}_k$ minus $\boldsymbol{\mu}_k$, and $\mathbf{\Omega}_{1kl}^T$ is the lth row of $\mathbf{\Omega}_{1k}$. The computational burden in simulating observations from these conditional distributions is light. The situation with fixed parameters in $\mathbf{\Lambda}_k$ or $\mathbf{\Lambda}_{\omega k}$ can be handled as in Zhu and Lee (2001); see also Appendix 3.3 above. The conditional distributions given above are familiar and simple distributions. The computational burden required in simulating observations from these distributions is not heavy.

In addition to their role in facilitating estimation, the allocation variables in $\mathbf{W}$ also form a coherent basis for Bayesian classification of the observations. Classification can be addressed either on a within-sample basis or on a predictive basis. See Lee (2007a, Chapter 12) for more details.

7.2.3 Analysis of an artificial example

An important issue in the analysis of mixture SEMs is the separation of the components. Yung (1997) and Dolan and van der Maas (1998) pointed out that some of their statistical results cannot be trusted when the separation is poor. Yung (1997) considered $d_{kh} = \max_{l\in\{k,h\}}$

$\{(\boldsymbol{\mu}_k - \boldsymbol{\mu}_h)^T \boldsymbol{\Sigma}_l^{-1} (\boldsymbol{\mu}_k - \boldsymbol{\mu}_h)\}^{1/2}$ as a measure of separation and suggested that d_{kh} should be about 3.8 or over. In view of this, one objective of this artificial example is to investigate the performance of the Bayesian approach in analyzing a mixture of SEMs with two components that are not well separated. Another objective is to demonstrate the random permutation sampler for finding suitable identifiability constraints. Random observations are simulated from a mixture SEM with two components defined by (7.1)–(7.3). The model for each $k = 1, 2$ involves nine observed variables that are indicators of three latent variables η, ξ_1, and ξ_2. The structure of the factor loading matrix in each component is

$$\boldsymbol{\Lambda}_k^T = \begin{bmatrix} 1 & \lambda_{k,21} & \lambda_{k,31} & 0 & 0 & 0 & 0 & 0 & 0 \\ 0 & 0 & 0 & 1 & \lambda_{k,52} & \lambda_{k,62} & 0 & 0 & 0 \\ 0 & 0 & 0 & 0 & 0 & 0 & 1 & \lambda_{k,83} & \lambda_{k,93} \end{bmatrix},$$

where the 1s and 0s are parameters fixed in order to obtain an identified model. In the kth component, the structural equation is given by: $\eta = \gamma_{k,1}\xi_1 + \gamma_{k,2}\xi_2 + \delta$. The true population values of the unknown parameters are given by $\pi_1 = \pi_2 = 0.5$, $\boldsymbol{\mu}_1 = (0.0, 0.0, 0.0, 0.0, 0.0, 1.0, 1.0, 1.0, 1.0)^T$, $\boldsymbol{\mu}_2 = (0.0, 0.0, 0.0, 0.5, 1.5, 0.0, 1.0, 1.0, 1.0)^T$, $\lambda_{1,21} = \lambda_{1,31} = \lambda_{1,83} = \lambda_{1,93} = 0.4$, $\lambda_{1,52} = \lambda_{1,62} = 0.8$, $\lambda_{2,21} = \lambda_{2,31} = \lambda_{2,83} = \lambda_{2,93} = 0.8$, $\lambda_{2,52} = \lambda_{2,62} = 0.4$, $\gamma_{1,1} = 0.2$, $\gamma_{1,2} = 0.7$, $\gamma_{2,1} = 0.7$, $\gamma_{2,2} = 0.2$, $\phi_{1,11} = \phi_{1,22} = \phi_{2,11} = \phi_{2,22} = 1.0$, $\phi_{1,12} = \phi_{2,12} = 0.3$, $\psi_{11} = \ldots = \psi_{19} = \psi_{21} = \ldots = \psi_{29} = \psi_{\delta 11} = \psi_{\delta 21} = 0.5$. In this two-component mixture SEM, the total number of unknown parameters is 62. The separation d_{12} is equal to 2.56, which is less than the value suggested in Yung (1997).

Based on the above settings, we simulate 400 observations from each component, and the total sample size is 800. We focus on $\boldsymbol{\mu}_1$ (or $\boldsymbol{\mu}_2$) in finding a suitable identifiability constraint. The first step is to apply the random permutation sampler to produce an MCMC sample from the unconstrained posterior with size 5000 after a burn-in phase of 500 simulations. This random permutation sampler delivers a sample that explores a whole unconstrained parameter space and jumps between the various labeling subspaces in a balanced fashion. For a mixture of SEMs with two components, we have only 2! labeling subspaces. In the random permutation sampler, after each sweep the first state (1s) and the second state (2s) are permuted randomly; that is, with probability 0.5, the 1s stay as 1s, and with probability 0.5 they become 2s. The output can be explored to find a suitable identifiability constraint. Based on the reasoning given in Appendix 7.2, it suffices to consider the parameters in $\boldsymbol{\mu}_1$. To search for an appropriate identifiability constraint, we look at the scatter plots of $\mu_{1,1}$ versus $\mu_{1,l}$, $l = 2, \ldots, 9$, to obtain information on aspects of the states that are most different. These scatter plots are presented in Figure 7.1, which clearly indicates that the most two significant differences between the two components are sampled values corresponding to $\mu_{1,5}$ and $\mu_{1,6}$. If permutation sampling is based on the constraint $\mu_{1,5} < \mu_{2,5}$ or $\mu_{1,6} > \mu_{2,6}$, the label switching will not appear.

Bayesian estimates are obtained using the permutation sampler with the identifiability constraint $\mu_{1,5} < \mu_{2,5}$. Values of hyperparameters in the conjugate prior distributions (see (7.12)) are taken as follows. For $m = 1, \ldots, 9$, $\mu_{0k,m}$, the mth element of $\boldsymbol{\mu}_{0k}$, equals the sample mean $\bar{y}_m$, $\boldsymbol{\Sigma}_{0k} = 10^2\mathbf{I}$, elements in $\boldsymbol{\Lambda}_{0km}$, and $\boldsymbol{\Lambda}_{0\omega kl}$ (which only involves the γs) are taken to be true parameter values, $\mathbf{H}_{0ykm}$ and $\mathbf{H}_{0\omega kl}$ are the identity matrices, $\alpha_{0\epsilon k} = \alpha_{0\delta k} = 10$, $\beta_{0\epsilon k} = \beta_{0\delta k} = 8$, $\rho_{0k} = 6$, and $\mathbf{R}_{0k}^{-1} = 5\mathbf{I}$. The α in the Dirichlet distribution of $\boldsymbol{\pi}$ is taken as 1. A few test runs show that the algorithm converges in less than 500 iterations. Hence,

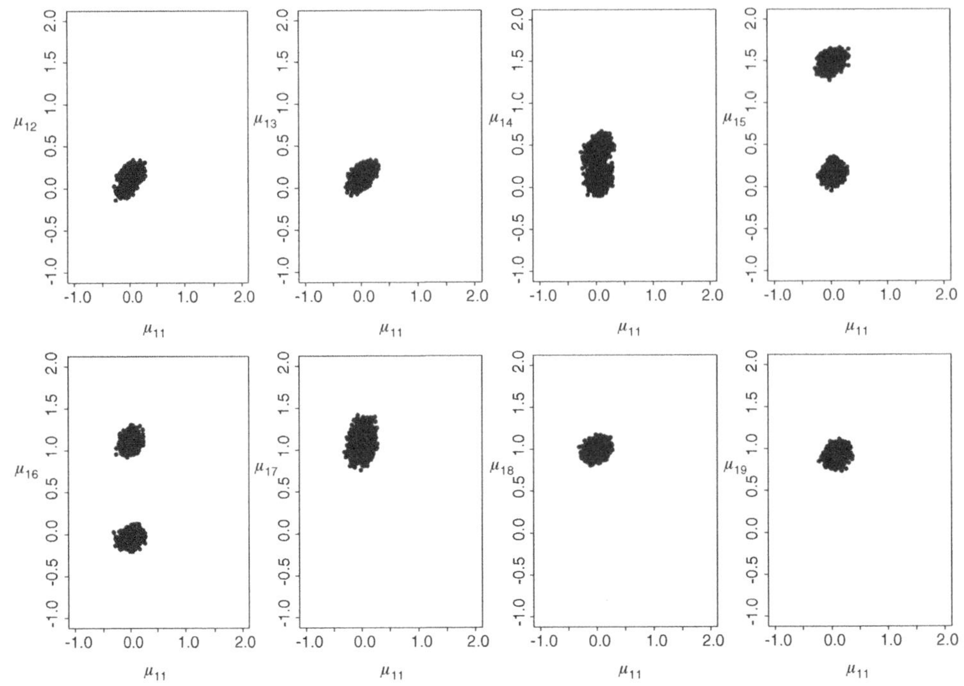

Figure 7.1 Scatter plots of MCMC output for components of $\boldsymbol{\mu}_1$.

Bayesian estimates are obtained using a burn-in phase of 500 iterations and a total of 2000 observations collected after the burn-in phase. Results are reported in Table 7.1. We observe that the Bayesian estimates are pretty close to their true parameter values.

This artificial data set has also been analyzed using WinBUGS (Spiegelhalter, *et al.*, 2003). First, an initial Bayesian estimation was conducted without the identifiability constraints to determine the appropriate identifiability constraint $\mu_{1,5} < \mu_{2,5}$ from the output as before. The model was then reestimated with this identifiability constraint, and three starting values of the parameters that are obtained from the sample mean, 5th, and 95th percentiles of the corresponding simulated samples. Bayesian estimates are obtained using the permutation samples with the identifiability constraint and the hyperparameter values given above. Results are presented in Table 7.2. The WinBUGS code under the identifiability constraint $\mu_{1,5} < \mu_{2,5}$, and the data are respectively given in the following website:

`www.wiley.com/go/medical_behavioral_sciences`

7.2.4 Example from the world values survey

A small portion of the ICPSR data set collected in the project World Values Survey 1981–1984 and 1990–1993 (World Values Study Group, 1994) is analyzed. The whole data set was collected in 45 societies around the world on broad topics such as work, the meaning and purpose of life, family life, and contemporary social issues. As an illustration, only the data obtained from the United Kingdom, with sample size 1484, are used. Eight variables in the

Table 7.1 Bayesian estimates in the artificial example.

Component 1			Component 2		
Par	EST	SE	Par	EST	SE
$\pi_1 = 0.5$	0.504	0.208	$\pi_2 = 0.5$	0.496	0.028
$\mu_{1,1} = 0.0$	0.070	0.082	$\mu_{2,1} = 0.0$	0.030	0.084
$\mu_{1,2} = 0.0$	0.056	0.046	$\mu_{2,2} = 0.0$	−0.056	0.061
$\mu_{1,3} = 0.0$	0.036	0.045	$\mu_{2,3} = 0.0$	−0.014	0.061
$\mu_{1,4} = 0.0$	0.108	0.075	$\mu_{2,4} = 0.5$	0.430	0.071
$\mu_{1,5} = 0.0$	0.209	0.061	$\mu_{2,5} = 1.5$	1.576	0.057
$\mu_{1,6} = 1.0$	1.101	0.062	$\mu_{2,6} = 0.0$	−0.084	0.052
$\mu_{1,7} = 1.0$	1.147	0.112	$\mu_{2,7} = 1.0$	0.953	0.110
$\mu_{1,8} = 1.0$	1.033	0.046	$\mu_{2,8} = 1.0$	1.041	0.056
$\mu_{1,9} = 1.0$	0.974	0.046	$\mu_{2,9} = 1.0$	0.941	0.057
$\lambda_{1,21} = 0.4$	0.322	0.052	$\lambda_{2,21} = 0.8$	0.851	0.060
$\lambda_{1,31} = 0.4$	0.411	0.052	$\lambda_{2,31} = 0.8$	0.810	0.060
$\lambda_{1,52} = 0.8$	0.712	0.060	$\lambda_{2,52} = 0.4$	0.498	0.067
$\lambda_{1,62} = 0.8$	0.695	0.066	$\lambda_{2,62} = 0.4$	0.480	0.064
$\lambda_{1,83} = 0.4$	0.386	0.075	$\lambda_{2,83} = 0.8$	0.738	0.077
$\lambda_{1,93} = 0.4$	0.428	0.079	$\lambda_{2,93} = 0.8$	0.826	0.083
$\gamma_{1,1} = 0.2$	0.236	0.104	$\gamma_{2,1} = 0.7$	0.817	0.104
$\gamma_{1,2} = 0.7$	0.740	0.074	$\gamma_{2,2} = 0.2$	0.210	0.074
$\phi_{1,11} = 1.0$	1.017	0.121	$\phi_{2,11} = 1.0$	0.820	0.118
$\phi_{1,12} = 0.3$	0.249	0.090	$\phi_{2,12} = 0.3$	0.283	0.074
$\phi_{1,22} = 1.0$	0.900	0.185	$\phi_{2,22} = 1.0$	0.982	0.163
$\psi_{11} = 0.5$	0.535	0.092	$\psi_{21} = 0.5$	0.588	0.080
$\psi_{12} = 0.5$	0.558	0.046	$\psi_{22} = 0.5$	0.489	0.053
$\psi_{13} = 0.5$	0.510	0.045	$\psi_{23} = 0.5$	0.565	0.057
$\psi_{14} = 0.5$	0.483	0.067	$\psi_{24} = 0.5$	0.620	0.085
$\psi_{15} = 0.5$	0.492	0.056	$\psi_{25} = 0.5$	0.556	0.056
$\psi_{16} = 0.5$	0.554	0.063	$\psi_{26} = 0.5$	0.507	0.050
$\psi_{17} = 0.5$	0.696	0.126	$\psi_{27} = 0.5$	0.569	0.108
$\psi_{18} = 0.5$	0.563	0.052	$\psi_{28} = 0.5$	0.578	0.062
$\psi_{19} = 0.5$	0.566	0.053	$\psi_{29} = 0.5$	0.508	0.065
$\psi_{\delta 11} = 0.5$	0.549	0.094	$\psi_{\delta 21} = 0.5$	0.549	0.082

original data set (variables 116, 117, 180, 132, 96, 255, 254, and 252) that are related to respondents' job and home life are taken as observed variables in $\mathbf{y}$. A description of these variables in the questionnaire is given in Appendix 1.1 (see also Lee, 2007a, Section 12.4.3). For simplicity, we delete the cases with missing data, reducing the sample size to 824. The data set is analyzed with a mixture SEM with two components. In each component, three latent variables, which can be roughly interpreted as 'job satisfaction' (η), 'home life' (ξ_1), and 'job attitude' (ξ_2), are considered. For $k = 1, 2$, the parameter matrices in the model formulation

Table 7.2 Bayesian estimates in the artificial example using WinBUGS.

Component 1			Component 2		
Par	EST	SE	Par	EST	SE
$\pi_1 = 0.5$	0.503	0.027	$\pi_2 = 0.5$	0.498	0.027
$\mu_{1,1} = 0.0$	0.035	0.068	$\mu_{2,1} = 0.0$	0.028	0.070
$\mu_{1,2} = 0.0$	0.050	0.046	$\mu_{2,2} = 0.0$	−0.043	0.062
$\mu_{1,3} = 0.0$	0.034	0.046	$\mu_{2,3} = 0.0$	−0.008	0.062
$\mu_{1,4} = 0.0$	0.124	0.067	$\mu_{2,4} = 0.5$	0.435	0.066
$\mu_{1,5} = 0.0$	0.192	0.060	$\mu_{2,5} = 1.5$	1.590	0.056
$\mu_{1,6} = 1.0$	1.089	0.061	$\mu_{2,6} = 0.0$	−0.065	0.053
$\mu_{1,7} = 1.0$	1.068	0.067	$\mu_{2,7} = 1.0$	0.961	0.066
$\mu_{1,8} = 1.0$	1.024	0.046	$\mu_{2,8} = 1.0$	1.053	0.056
$\mu_{1,9} = 1.0$	0.974	0.047	$\mu_{2,9} = 1.0$	0.916	0.057
$\lambda_{1,21} = 0.4$	0.355	0.047	$\lambda_{2,21} = 0.8$	0.850	0.053
$\lambda_{1,31} = 0.4$	0.428	0.047	$\lambda_{2,31} = 0.8$	0.817	0.053
$\lambda_{1,52} = 0.8$	0.723	0.062	$\lambda_{2,52} = 0.4$	0.507	0.065
$\lambda_{1,62} = 0.8$	0.741	0.068	$\lambda_{2,62} = 0.4$	0.495	0.064
$\lambda_{1,83} = 0.4$	0.403	0.058	$\lambda_{2,83} = 0.8$	0.741	0.061
$\lambda_{1,93} = 0.4$	0.385	0.061	$\lambda_{2,93} = 0.8$	0.837	0.064
$\gamma_{1,1} = 0.2$	0.208	0.071	$\gamma_{2,1} = 0.7$	0.873	0.103
$\gamma_{1,2} = 0.7$	0.740	0.094	$\gamma_{2,2} = 0.2$	0.152	0.068
$\phi_{1,11} = 1.0$	0.953	0.115	$\phi_{2,11} = 1.0$	0.785	0.110
$\phi_{1,12} = 0.3$	0.278	0.071	$\phi_{2,12} = 0.3$	0.305	0.067
$\phi_{1,22} = 1.0$	0.932	0.133	$\phi_{2,22} = 1.0$	0.988	0.117
$\psi_{11} = 0.5$	0.496	0.072	$\psi_{21} = 0.5$	0.519	0.059
$\psi_{12} = 0.5$	0.536	0.043	$\psi_{22} = 0.5$	0.512	0.052
$\psi_{13} = 0.5$	0.504	0.042	$\psi_{23} = 0.5$	0.566	0.054
$\psi_{14} = 0.5$	0.517	0.067	$\psi_{24} = 0.5$	0.620	0.076
$\psi_{15} = 0.5$	0.492	0.056	$\psi_{25} = 0.5$	0.536	0.052
$\psi_{16} = 0.5$	0.542	0.063	$\psi_{26} = 0.5$	0.518	0.051
$\psi_{17} = 0.5$	0.636	0.093	$\psi_{27} = 0.5$	0.533	0.066
$\psi_{18} = 0.5$	0.536	0.045	$\psi_{28} = 0.5$	0.574	0.054
$\psi_{19} = 0.5$	0.586	0.048	$\psi_{29} = 0.5$	0.487	0.054
$\psi_{\delta 11} = 0.5$	0.479	0.077	$\psi_{\delta 21} = 0.5$	0.510	0.072

are given by $\mathbf{\Pi}_k = \mathbf{0}$, $\mathbf{\Psi}_{\delta k} = \psi_{\delta k}$, $\mathbf{\Gamma}_k = (\gamma_{k,1}, \gamma_{k,2})$,

$$\mathbf{\Lambda}_k^T = \begin{bmatrix} 1 & \lambda_{k,21} & 0 & 0 & 0 & 0 & 0 & 0 \\ 0 & 0 & 1 & \lambda_{k,42} & \lambda_{k,52} & 0 & 0 & 0 \\ 0 & 0 & 0 & 0 & 0 & 1 & \lambda_{k,73} & \lambda_{k,83} \end{bmatrix}, \quad \mathbf{\Phi}_k = \begin{bmatrix} \phi_{k,11} & \phi_{k,12} \\ \phi_{k,21} & \phi_{k,22} \end{bmatrix}, \tag{7.13}$$

and $\mathbf{\Psi}_k = \text{diag}(\psi_{k1}, \ldots, \psi_{k8})$. To identify the model, the 1s and 0s in $\mathbf{\Lambda}_k$ are fixed. The total number of unknown parameters is 56.

Bayesian estimates of the structural parameters and the factor scores are obtained via the Gibbs sampler. The following hyperparameters are used: $\alpha = 1$, $\boldsymbol{\mu}_{0k} = \bar{\mathbf{y}}$, $\boldsymbol{\Sigma}_{0k} = \mathbf{S}_y^2/2.0$, $\rho_{0k} = 5$, and $\mathbf{R}_{0k}^{-1} = 5\mathbf{I}_2$, where $\bar{\mathbf{y}}$ and $\mathbf{S}_y^2$ are the sample mean and sample covariance matrix calculated using the observed data; $\alpha_{0\epsilon k} = \alpha_{0\delta k} = \beta_{0\epsilon k} = \beta_{0\delta k} = 6$ for all k; $\mathbf{H}_{0ykm} = \mathbf{I}$, $\mathbf{H}_{0\omega kl} = \mathbf{I}$; and $\boldsymbol{\Lambda}_{0km} = \tilde{\boldsymbol{\Lambda}}_{0km}$ and $\boldsymbol{\Lambda}_{0\omega kl} = \tilde{\boldsymbol{\Lambda}}_{0\omega kl}$ for all k, m, and l, where $\tilde{\boldsymbol{\Lambda}}_{0km}$ and $\tilde{\boldsymbol{\Lambda}}_{0\omega kl}$ are the initial estimates of $\boldsymbol{\Lambda}_{0km}$ and $\boldsymbol{\Lambda}_{0\omega kl}$ obtained using noninformative prior distributions. We first use MCMC samples simulated by the random permutation sampler to find an identifiability constraint, and observe that $\mu_{1,1} < \mu_{2,1}$ is a suitable one. Based on different starting values of the parameters, three parallel sequences of observations are generated and the EPSR values are calculated. We observe that the Gibbs sampler algorithm converges within 1000 iterations. After the convergence of the Gibbs sampler, a total of 1000 observations with a spacing of 10 are collected for analysis. The Bayesian estimates of the structural parameters and their standard error estimates are reported in Table 7.3. From this table, it can be seen that there are at least two components which have different sets of Bayesian parameter estimates.

7.2.5 Bayesian model comparison of mixture SEMs

The objective of this subsection is to consider the Bayesian model selection problem in selecting one of the two mixtures of SEMs with different numbers of components. An approach based on the Bayes factor (Kass and Raftery, 1995), together with the path sampling procedure, will be introduced. The underlying finite mixture of SEMs is again defined by equations (7.1)–(7.3), except that K is not fixed and the π_k are nonnegative component probabilities that sum to 1.0. Note that some π_k may be equal to zero. When using the likelihood ratio test, some unknown parameters may be on the boundary of the parameter space, and this causes serious difficulty in developing the test statistics for the hypothesis testing of the number of components. In contrast, the Bayesian approach for model comparison with the Bayes factor does not have this problem.

Let M_1 be a mixture SEM with K components, and M_0 be a mixture SEM with c components, where $c < K$. The Bayes factor for selection between M_0 and M_1 is defined by

$$B_{10} = \frac{P(\mathbf{Y}|M_1)}{P(\mathbf{Y}|M_0)}. \tag{7.14}$$

In computing the Bayes factor through path sampling, the observed data set $\mathbf{Y}$ is augmented with the matrix of latent variables $\boldsymbol{\Omega}$. Based on reasoning and derivation similar to those given in previous chapters, $\log B_{10}$ can be estimated as follows. Let

$$U(\mathbf{Y}, \boldsymbol{\Omega}, \boldsymbol{\theta}, t) = \frac{d}{dt}\log\{p(\mathbf{Y}, \boldsymbol{\Omega}|\boldsymbol{\theta}, t)\},$$

where $p(\mathbf{Y}, \boldsymbol{\Omega}|\boldsymbol{\theta}, t)$ is the complete-data likelihood function. Then

$$\widehat{\log B_{10}} = \frac{1}{2}\sum_{s=0}^{S}\left(t_{(s+1)} - t_{(s)}\right)\left(\bar{U}_{(s+1)} + \bar{U}_{(s)}\right), \tag{7.15}$$

Table 7.3 Bayesian estimates and standard error estimates of the ICPSR example.

	Component 1		Component 2	
Par	EST	SE	EST	SE
π_k	0.56	0.03	0.44	0.03
$\mu_{k,1}$	6.91	0.11	8.09	0.09
$\mu_{k,2}$	6.30	0.14	7.90	0.14
$\mu_{k,3}$	5.87	0.14	7.83	0.11
$\mu_{k,4}$	7.83	0.10	8.70	0.07
$\mu_{k,5}$	7.10	0.11	8.07	0.09
$\mu_{k,6}$	5.41	0.14	4.01	0.15
$\mu_{k,7}$	4.06	0.13	3.61	0.14
$\mu_{k,8}$	5.59	0.14	4.61	0.14
$\lambda_{k,11}$	1*	–	1*	–
$\lambda_{k,21}$	0.49	0.11	0.86	0.13
$\lambda_{k,32}$	1*	–	1*	–
$\lambda_{k,42}$	1.30	0.17	0.94	0.10
$\lambda_{k,52}$	1.58	0.20	1.02	0.11
$\lambda_{k,63}$	1*	–	1*	–
$\lambda_{k,73}$	2.05	0.44	0.98	0.07
$\lambda_{k,83}$	1.08	0.27	0.74	0.08
$\gamma_{k,1}$	0.68	0.14	0.77	0.11
$\gamma_{k,2}$	−0.02	0.15	−0.09	0.04
$\phi_{k,11}$	1.18	0.26	0.90	0.18
$\phi_{k,21}$	−0.12	0.09	−0.28	0.15
$\phi_{k,22}$	0.92	0.30	4.30	0.52
ψ_{k1}	1.56	0.65	0.56	0.11
ψ_{k2}	6.92	0.50	2.80	0.34
ψ_{k3}	4.86	0.37	1.35	0.18
ψ_{k4}	2.51	0.27	0.45	0.07
ψ_{k5}	1.29	0.27	0.55	0.08
ψ_{k6}	6.31	0.50	1.25	0.35
ψ_{k7}	2.43	0.76	1.07	0.23
ψ_{k8}	6.39	0.57	3.15	0.40
$\psi_{\delta k}$	3.38	0.72	0.70	0.12

Source: Zhu and Lee (2001).

where the $t_{(s)}$ are fixed grids in [0, 1] such that $0 = t_{(0)} < t_{(1)} < t_{(2)} < \ldots < t_{(S)} < t_{(S+1)} = 1$, and

$$\bar{U}_{(s)} = J^{-1} \sum_{j=1}^{J} U\left(\mathbf{Y}, \boldsymbol{\Omega}^{(j)}, \boldsymbol{\theta}^{(j)}, t_{(s)}\right), \tag{7.16}$$

in which $\{(\boldsymbol{\Omega}^{(j)}, \boldsymbol{\theta}^{(j)}), j = 1, \ldots, J\}$ are simulated observations drawn from $p(\boldsymbol{\Omega}, \boldsymbol{\theta}|\mathbf{Y}, t_{(s)})$.

The implementation of path sampling is straightforward. Drawing observations $\{(\mathbf{\Omega}^{(j)}, \boldsymbol{\theta}^{(j)}) : j = 1, \ldots, J\}$ from the posterior distribution $p(\mathbf{\Omega}, \boldsymbol{\theta}|\mathbf{Y}, t_{(s)})$ is the major task in the proposed procedure. Similar to estimation, we further utilize the idea of data augmentation to augment the observed data $\mathbf{Y}$ with the latent matrix $\mathbf{W}$ of the allocation variables. As a consequence, the Gibbs sampler described in Section 7.2.2 can be applied to simulate observations from $p(\mathbf{\Omega}, \boldsymbol{\theta}|\mathbf{Y}, t_{(s)})$. In computing Bayes factors, the inclusion of an identifiability constraint in simulating $\{(\mathbf{\Omega}^{(j)}, \boldsymbol{\theta}^{(j)}), j = 1, \ldots, J\}$ is not necessary. As the likelihood is invariant to relabeling the states, the inclusion of such a constraint will not change the values of $U(\mathbf{Y}, \mathbf{\Omega}, \boldsymbol{\theta}, t)$. As a result, the log Bayes factor estimated through (7.15) and (7.16) is not changed.

Finding a good path to link the competing models M_1 and M_0 is important in applying path sampling. We give an illustrative example. Consider the following competing models:

$$M_1 : [\mathbf{Y}|\boldsymbol{\theta}, \boldsymbol{\pi}] \stackrel{D}{=} \sum_{k=1}^{K} \pi_k f_k(\mathbf{Y}|\boldsymbol{\mu}_k, \boldsymbol{\theta}_k), \tag{7.17}$$

corresponding to a model of K components with positive component probabilities π_k, and

$$M_0 : [\mathbf{Y}|\boldsymbol{\theta}, \boldsymbol{\pi}^*] \stackrel{D}{=} \sum_{k=1}^{c} \pi_k^* f_k(\mathbf{Y}|\boldsymbol{\mu}_k, \boldsymbol{\theta}_k), \tag{7.18}$$

corresponding to a model of c components with positive component probabilities π_k^*, where $1 \leq c < K$. Clearly, these competing models are linked by a path $M_t : t \in [0, 1]$ as follows:

$$\begin{aligned} M_t : [\mathbf{y}|\boldsymbol{\theta}, \boldsymbol{\pi}, t] \stackrel{D}{=} & [\pi_1 + (1-t)a_1(\pi_{c+1} + \ldots + \pi_K)] f_1(\mathbf{y}|\boldsymbol{\mu}_1, \boldsymbol{\theta}_1) + \ldots \\ & + [\pi_c + (1-t)a_c(\pi_{c+1} + \ldots + \pi_K)] f_c(\mathbf{y}|\boldsymbol{\mu}_c, \boldsymbol{\theta}_c) \\ & + t\pi_{c+1} f_{c+1}(\mathbf{y}|\boldsymbol{\mu}_{c+1}, \boldsymbol{\theta}_{c+1}) + \ldots + t\pi_K f_K(\mathbf{y}|\boldsymbol{\mu}_K, \boldsymbol{\theta}_K), \end{aligned} \tag{7.19}$$

where $a_1, \ldots, a_c$ are given positive weights such that $a_1 + \ldots + a_c = 1$. When $t = 1$, M_t reduces to M_1; and when $t = 0$, M_t reduces to M_0 with $\pi_k^* = \pi_k + a_k(\pi_{c+1} + \ldots + \pi_K)$, $k = 1, \ldots, c$. The weights $a_1, \ldots, a_c$ represent the increases in the corresponding component probabilities from a K-component SEM to a c-component SEM. A natural and simple suggestion for practical applications is to take $a_k = c^{-1}$.

The complete-data log-likelihood function can be written as

$$\begin{aligned} \log p(\mathbf{Y}, \mathbf{\Omega}|\boldsymbol{\theta}, t) = \sum_{i=1}^{n} \log \Bigg\{ & \sum_{k=1}^{c} \left[\pi_k + (1-t)a_k \sum_{h=c+1}^{K} \pi_h \right] \\ & \times f_k(\mathbf{y}_i, \boldsymbol{\omega}_i|\boldsymbol{\mu}_k, \boldsymbol{\theta}_k) + \sum_{k=c+1}^{K} t\pi_k f_k(\mathbf{y}_i, \boldsymbol{\omega}_i|\boldsymbol{\mu}_k, \boldsymbol{\theta}_k) \Bigg\}. \end{aligned} \tag{7.20}$$

By differentiation with respect to t, we have

$$U(\mathbf{Y}, \mathbf{\Omega}, \boldsymbol{\theta}, t) =$$

$$\sum_{i=1}^{n} \frac{-\sum_{h=c+1}^{K} \pi_h \sum_{k=1}^{c} a_k f_k(\mathbf{y}_i, \boldsymbol{\omega}_i|\boldsymbol{\mu}_k, \boldsymbol{\theta}_k) + \sum_{k=c+1}^{K} \pi_k f_k(\mathbf{y}_i, \boldsymbol{\omega}_i|\boldsymbol{\mu}_k, \boldsymbol{\theta}_k)}{\sum_{k=1}^{c} \left[\pi_k + (1-t)a_k \sum_{h=c+1}^{K} \pi_h\right] f_k(\mathbf{y}_i, \boldsymbol{\omega}_i|\boldsymbol{\mu}_k, \boldsymbol{\theta}_k) + \sum_{k=c+1}^{K} t\pi_k f_k(\mathbf{y}_i, \boldsymbol{\omega}_i|\boldsymbol{\mu}_k, \boldsymbol{\theta}_k)}, \tag{7.21}$$

where

$$f_k(\mathbf{y}_i, \boldsymbol{\omega}_i|\boldsymbol{\mu}_k, \boldsymbol{\theta}_k) = (2\pi)^{-p/2}|\boldsymbol{\Psi}_k|^{-1/2}\exp\left[-\frac{1}{2}(\mathbf{y}_i - \boldsymbol{\mu}_k - \boldsymbol{\Lambda}_k\boldsymbol{\omega}_i)^T\boldsymbol{\Psi}_k^{-1}(\mathbf{y}_i - \boldsymbol{\mu}_k - \boldsymbol{\Lambda}_k\boldsymbol{\omega}_i)\right]$$
$$\times(2\pi)^{-q_1/2}|\mathbf{I}_{q_1} - \boldsymbol{\Pi}_k||\boldsymbol{\Psi}_{\delta k}|^{-1/2}\exp\left[-\frac{1}{2}(\boldsymbol{\eta}_i - \boldsymbol{\Lambda}_{\omega k}\boldsymbol{\omega}_i)^T\boldsymbol{\Psi}_{\delta k}^{-1}(\boldsymbol{\eta}_i - \boldsymbol{\Lambda}_{\omega k}\boldsymbol{\omega}_i)\right]$$
$$\times(2\pi)^{-q_2/2}|\boldsymbol{\Phi}_k|^{-1/2}\exp\left(-\frac{1}{2}\boldsymbol{\xi}_i^T\boldsymbol{\Phi}_k^{-1}\boldsymbol{\xi}_i\right),$$

and $\boldsymbol{\Lambda}_{\omega k} = (\boldsymbol{\Pi}_k, \boldsymbol{\Gamma}_k)$. Thus, the Bayes factor can be estimated with

$$\bar{U}_{(s)} = J^{-1}\sum_{j=1}^{J} U\left(\mathbf{Y}, \boldsymbol{\Omega}^{(j)}, \boldsymbol{\theta}^{(j)}, t_{(s)}\right),$$

where $\{(\boldsymbol{\Omega}^{(j)}, \boldsymbol{\theta}^{(j)}) : j = 1, \ldots, J\}$ are observations drawn from $p(\boldsymbol{\Omega}, \boldsymbol{\theta}|\mathbf{Y}, t_{(s)})$.

7.2.6 An illustrative example

The same portion of the ICPSR data set as described in Section 7.2.4 is reanalyzed to illustrate the path sampling procedure. We wish to find out whether there are some mixture models that are better than the mixture SEM with two components presented in Section 7.2.4. For each component, the specification of the model is the same as before. However, the number of components, K, is not fixed.

The hyperparameter values are assigned as follows. First $\alpha = 1$; $\boldsymbol{\mu}_{0k} = \bar{\mathbf{y}}$, $\boldsymbol{\Sigma}_{0k} = \mathbf{S}_y^2/2$, where $\bar{\mathbf{y}}$ and $\mathbf{S}_y^2$ are the sample mean and sample covariance matrix calculated using the observed data; $\rho_{0k} = 6$ and $\mathbf{R}_{0k}^{-1} = 5\mathbf{I}$; and $\mathbf{H}_{0ykm} = \mathbf{I}$ and $\mathbf{H}_{0\omega kl} = \mathbf{I}$ are selected for each k, $m = 1, \ldots, p$, and $l = 1, \ldots, q_1$. Moreover, $\{\alpha_{0\epsilon k}, \beta_{0\epsilon k}\}$, and $\{\alpha_{0\delta k}, \beta_{0\delta k}\}$ are selected such that the means and standard deviations of the prior distributions associated with ψ_{km} and $\psi_{\delta kl}$ are equal to 5. Finally, we take $\boldsymbol{\Lambda}_{0km} = \tilde{\boldsymbol{\Lambda}}_{0km}$, $\boldsymbol{\Lambda}_{0\omega kl} = \tilde{\boldsymbol{\Lambda}}_{0\omega kl}$ for all k, m, and l, where $\tilde{\boldsymbol{\Lambda}}_{0km}$ and $\tilde{\boldsymbol{\Lambda}}_{0\omega kl}$ are the corresponding Bayesian estimates obtained through a single-component model with noninformative prior distributions. Again, for each $t_{(s)}$, the convergence of the Gibbs sampler algorithm is monitored by parallel sequences of observations generated from very different starting values. We observe that the algorithm converges quickly within 200 iterations. A total of $J = 1000$ additional observations are collected after a burn-in phase of 200 iterations to compute $\bar{U}_{(s)}$ in (7.16), and then the log Bayes factors are estimated via (7.15), using 20 fixed grids in [0,1]. Let M_k denotes the mixture model with k components. The estimated log Bayes factors are $\widehat{\log B_{21}} = 75.055$, $\widehat{\log B_{32}} = 4.381$, $\widehat{\log B_{43}} = -0.824$, and $\widehat{\log B_{53}} = -1.395$. Based on the criterion of the log Bayes factor, the one-component model is significantly worse than the two-component model which is significantly worse than the three-component model; while the three-component model is almost as good as the more complicated four- and five-component models. Hence, a mixture model with three components should be chosen. Although the two-component model suggested in Section 7.2.4 is plausible, it does not give as strong evidence of support as the three-component model.

In estimation based on the MCMC samples simulated by the random permutation sampler, we find $\mu_{1,1} < \mu_{2,1} < \mu_{3,1}$ is a suitable identifiability constraint. Bayesian estimates of the selected three-component mixture model obtained under the constraint $\mu_{1,1} < \mu_{2,1} < \mu_{3,1}$ are presented in Table 7.4, together with the corresponding standard error estimates. For

Table 7.4 Bayesian estimates of parameters and standard errors for the selected model with three components in the analysis of the ICPSR data set.

	Component 1		Component 2		Component 3	
Par	EST	SE	EST	SE	EST	SE
π_k	0.51	0.03	0.23	0.03	0.26	0.03
$\mu_{k,1}$	6.75	0.13	8.05	0.15	8.25	0.15
$\mu_{k,2}$	5.95	0.12	7.53	0.21	8.63	0.17
$\mu_{k,3}$	5.76	0.18	7.67	0.18	7.87	0.14
$\mu_{k,4}$	7.74	0.13	8.65	0.12	8.77	0.12
$\mu_{k,5}$	7.05	0.12	8.06	0.12	8.04	0.11
$\mu_{k,6}$	5.50	0.25	2.70	0.18	5.20	0.15
$\mu_{k,7}$	4.12	0.23	2.60	0.16	4.35	0.14
$\mu_{k,8}$	5.66	0.24	3.08	0.23	5.94	0.15
$\lambda_{k,21}$	0.31	0.12	1.10	0.21	0.66	0.08
$\lambda_{k,42}$	1.38	0.18	0.84	0.13	0.87	0.16
$\lambda_{k,52}$	1.67	0.19	0.92	0.15	1.10	0.18
$\lambda_{k,73}$	2.15	0.31	0.98	0.09	1.94	0.22
$\lambda_{k,83}$	0.88	0.22	0.97	0.11	0.64	0.20
$\gamma_{k,1}$	0.62	0.16	0.52	0.15	0.69	0.14
$\gamma_{k,2}$	0.01	0.11	−0.37	0.12	−0.12	0.14
$\phi_{k,11}$	1.07	0.21	1.30	0.33	0.81	0.20
$\phi_{k,21}$	−0.13	0.13	−0.59	0.20	0.07	0.07
$\phi_{k,22}$	1.10	0.49	1.45	0.38	1.57	0.21
ψ_{k1}	1.08	0.12	0.87	0.19	0.56	0.35
ψ_{k2}	6.79	0.17	2.02	0.45	0.83	0.46
ψ_{k3}	4.75	0.38	1.71	0.40	1.17	0.37
ψ_{k4}	2.54	0.13	0.45	0.08	0.69	0.27
ψ_{k5}	1.11	0.16	0.55	0.09	0.71	0.23
ψ_{k6}	5.75	0.55	0.55	0.13	4.71	0.46
ψ_{k7}	1.36	0.35	0.60	0.11	1.13	0.47
ψ_{k8}	6.10	0.52	1.05	0.50	4.52	0.47
$\psi_{\delta k}$	3.80	0.13	0.63	0.15	0.68	0.51

parameters directly associated with observed variables $y_1, \ldots, y_5$, we observe from this table that their Bayesian estimates under component 2 are close to those under component 3, but these estimates are quite different from those under component 1. In contrast, for parameters directly associated with observed variables y_6, y_7, and y_8, estimates under component 1 are close to those under component 3, but are quite different from those under component 2. Hence, it is reasonable to select a three-component model for this data set. The estimated separations of these components are $d_{12} = 2.257$, $d_{13} = 2.590$, and $d_{23} = 2.473$. These results indicate that the introduced procedure is able to select the appropriate three-component model whose components are not well separated.

7.3 A modified mixture SEM

In the analysis of mixture SEMs, it is of interest to examine the effects of covariates on the probability of component membership, which plays an extremely important role in a mixture model. This kind of modeling has been discussed in latent class models and latent growth mixture models (Muthén and Shedden, 1999; Elliott *et al.*, 2005; Guo *et al.*, 2006). Another important issue in the analysis of mixture SEMs is related to missing data. Lee and Song (2003) pointed out that the case deletion method which deleted observations with missing entries would produce less accurate estimation results. Specifically, the bias and the root mean square values of parameter estimates and their true population values are larger compared with those obtained by the methods that include observations with missing entries. Lee (2007b) further demonstrated that the selection of the number of components in mixture SEMs would result in misleading conclusions if observations with missing entries are ignored. Moreover, the assumption of data missing at random (MAR) may not be realistic for heterogeneous data because the probability of missingness for an individual may strongly depend on its associated component with some special characteristics. Here, we present statistical methods to handle missing responses and covariates with a nonignorable missingness mechanism.

In this section, we introduce a modified mixture SEM which extends the previous mixture SEMs in three respects. First, a multinomial logit model with covariates is incorporated to predict the unknown component membership. Second, a nonlinear structural equation is introduced in each component to capture the component-specific nonlinear effects of explanatory latent variables and covariates on outcome latent variables. Third, nonignorable missing data are considered for both responses and covariates. Again, Bayesian methods are used to conduct the analysis. The methodologies are illustrated through a longitudinal study of polydrug use conducted in five California counties in 2004.

7.3.1 Model description

The modified mixture SEM for a $p \times 1$ random vector $\mathbf{y}_i$, $i = 1, \ldots, n$ is defined as follows (Cai *et al.*, 2010):

$$f(\mathbf{y}_i) = \sum_{k=1}^{K} \pi_{ik} f_k(\mathbf{y}_i|\boldsymbol{\theta}_k), \quad i = 1, \ldots, n, \tag{7.22}$$

where K is the number of mixture components, π_{ik} is the subject probability of component membership for $\mathbf{y}_i$ such that $\sum_{k=1}^{K} \pi_{ik} = 1$, and $f_k(\cdot)$ is the density function of $\mathbf{y}_i$ with a parameter vector $\boldsymbol{\theta}_k$. The component probabilities of the $\mathbf{y}_i$, π_{ik}, are further related to an $m_1 \times 1$ vector of covariates $\mathbf{x}_i$ via the following multinomial logit model: for $k = 1, \ldots, K$,

$$\pi_{ik} = p(z_i = k|\mathbf{x}_i) = \frac{\exp\left\{\boldsymbol{\tau}_k^T \mathbf{x}_i\right\}}{\sum_{j=1}^{K} \exp\left\{\boldsymbol{\tau}_j^T \mathbf{x}_i\right\}}, \tag{7.23}$$

where z_i is a latent allocation variable of $\mathbf{y}_i$, $\boldsymbol{\tau}_k$ $(m_1 \times 1)$ is an unknown vector of coefficients, and the elements in $\boldsymbol{\tau}_K$ are fixed at zero for identification purposes. The elements of $\boldsymbol{\tau}_k$ carry the information about the probability of component membership present in $\mathbf{x}_i$, which includes covariates that may come from continuous or discrete distributions with a parameter vector $\boldsymbol{\tau}_x$. In contrast to conventional mixture models, the subject probability of unknown component membership in the current mixture SEM is modeled by incorporating explanatory covariates

$\mathbf{x}_i$ through a multinomial logit model. Alternative terms in $\mathbf{x}_i$ can be concomitant variables, grouping variables, external variables, and exogenous variables. In substantive research, $\mathbf{x}_i$ and $\mathbf{y}_i$ may or may not have common variables. For example, $\mathbf{x}_i$ can be considered as the same set or a subset of $\mathbf{y}_i$ to help explain differences in component-specific parameters (Muthén and Shedden, 1999; Guo *et al.*, 2006). In contrast, Elliott *et al.* (2005) considered $\mathbf{x}_i$ to include an intercept and an indicator of baseline depression, which were excluded in $\mathbf{y}_i$. The main purpose of equation (7.23) is to provide an improved model with some covariates for predicting unknown component probabilities.

In order to group observed variables in $\mathbf{y}_i$ into latent factors, the measurement equation is defined as follows. Conditional on the kth component,

$$\mathbf{y}_i = \boldsymbol{\mu}_k + \boldsymbol{\Lambda}_k \boldsymbol{\omega}_i + \boldsymbol{\epsilon}_i, \tag{7.24}$$

where $\boldsymbol{\mu}_k$ is a $p \times 1$ intercept vector, $\boldsymbol{\Lambda}_k$ is a $p \times q$ factor loading matrix, $\boldsymbol{\omega}_i$ is a $q \times 1$ random vector of latent variables, $\boldsymbol{\epsilon}_i$ is a $p \times 1$ random vector of error measurements with distribution $N[\mathbf{0}, \boldsymbol{\Psi}_k]$, $\boldsymbol{\epsilon}_i$ is independent of $\boldsymbol{\omega}_i$, and $\boldsymbol{\Psi}_k$ is a diagonal matrix. Furthermore, we consider a partition of $\boldsymbol{\omega}_i$ into a $q_1 \times 1$ outcome latent vector $\boldsymbol{\eta}_i$ and a $q_2 \times 1$ explanatory latent vector $\boldsymbol{\xi}_i$. To assess the interrelationships among $\boldsymbol{\eta}_i$, $\boldsymbol{\xi}_i$, and some fixed covariates, a general structural equation is defined as follows:

$$\boldsymbol{\eta}_i = \mathbf{B}_k \mathbf{d}_i + \boldsymbol{\Pi}_k \boldsymbol{\eta}_i + \boldsymbol{\Gamma}_k \mathbf{F}(\boldsymbol{\xi}_i) + \boldsymbol{\delta}_i, \tag{7.25}$$

where $\mathbf{d}_i$ is an $m_2 \times 1$ vector of fixed covariates, conditional on the kth component which may come from continuous or discrete distributions with a parameter vector $\boldsymbol{\tau}_{kd}$; $\mathbf{F}(\boldsymbol{\xi}_i) = (f_1(\boldsymbol{\xi}_i), \ldots, f_r(\boldsymbol{\xi}_i))^T$ $(r \geq q_2)$ is a vector of general differentiable functions $f_1, \ldots, f_r$ that are linearly independent; $\mathbf{B}_k(q_1 \times m_2)$, $\boldsymbol{\Pi}_k(q_1 \times q_1)$, and $\boldsymbol{\Gamma}_k(q_1 \times r)$ are unknown parameter matrices; and $\boldsymbol{\xi}_i$ and $\boldsymbol{\delta}_i$ are independently distributed as $N[\mathbf{0}, \boldsymbol{\Phi}_k]$ and $N[\mathbf{0}, \boldsymbol{\Psi}_{\delta k}]$ with a diagonal matrix $\boldsymbol{\Psi}_{\delta k}$, respectively. Similar to many SEMs, we assume that $|\mathbf{I} - \boldsymbol{\Pi}_k|$ is nonzero and independent of the elements in $\boldsymbol{\Pi}_k$. Let $\boldsymbol{\Lambda}_{\omega k} = (\mathbf{B}_k, \boldsymbol{\Pi}_k, \boldsymbol{\Gamma}_k)$ and $\mathbf{G}(\boldsymbol{\omega}_i) = (\mathbf{d}_i^T, \boldsymbol{\eta}_i^T, \mathbf{F}(\boldsymbol{\xi}_i)^T)^T$; then (7.25) can be rewritten as

$$\boldsymbol{\eta}_i = \boldsymbol{\Lambda}_{\omega k} \mathbf{G}(\boldsymbol{\omega}_i) + \boldsymbol{\delta}_i. \tag{7.26}$$

For each $k = 1, \ldots, K$, the measurement and structural equations defined by equations (7.24) and (7.26) are not identified. A common method in structural equation modeling for model identification is to fix the appropriate elements in $\boldsymbol{\Lambda}_k$ and/or $\boldsymbol{\Lambda}_{\omega k}$ at preassigned values. In the subsequent analysis, let $\boldsymbol{\theta}_k$ be the parameter vector that includes all unknown parameters in $\boldsymbol{\mu}_k$, $\boldsymbol{\Lambda}_k$, $\boldsymbol{\Lambda}_{\omega k}$, $\boldsymbol{\Phi}_k$, $\boldsymbol{\Psi}_k$, and $\boldsymbol{\Psi}_{\delta k}$, and $\boldsymbol{\theta} = \{\boldsymbol{\theta}_1, \ldots, \boldsymbol{\theta}_K\}$ be the vector including all unknown structural parameters that define an identified model.

To deal with the missing data in mixture SEMs, we define the missingness indicator vector $\mathbf{r}_i^y = (r_{i1}^y, \ldots, r_{ip}^y)^T$ of $\mathbf{y}_i$ such that $r_{ij}^y = 1$ if y_{ij} is missing, and $r_{ij}^y = 0$ otherwise. Similarly, the missingness indicator vector of $\mathbf{d}_i$ is defined by $\mathbf{r}_i^d = (r_{i1}^d, \ldots, r_{im_2}^d)^T$. To cope with the nonignorable missing data in both responses and covariates, we need to define appropriate mechanisms to model the conditional distributions of $\mathbf{r}_i^y$ given $\mathbf{y}_i$ and $\boldsymbol{\omega}_i$, as well as $\mathbf{r}_i^d$ given $\boldsymbol{\omega}_i$ and $\mathbf{d}_i$. We assume that the conditional distributions of r_{ij}^y $(j = 1, \ldots, p)$ given $\mathbf{y}_i$ and $\boldsymbol{\omega}_i$ are independent (Song and Lee, 2007), and the conditional distributions of r_{ij}^d $(j = 1, \ldots, m_2)$

given $\mathbf{d}_i$ and $\boldsymbol{\omega}_i$ are independent. Thus, conditional on the kth component,

$$p(\mathbf{r}_i^y|\mathbf{y}_i, \boldsymbol{\omega}_i, \boldsymbol{\varphi}_{ky}) = \prod_{j=1}^{p} \{p(r_{ij}^y = 1|\mathbf{y}_i, \boldsymbol{\omega}_i, \boldsymbol{\varphi}_{ky})\}^{r_{ij}^y}\{1 - p(r_{ij}^y = 1|\mathbf{y}_i, \boldsymbol{\omega}_i, \boldsymbol{\varphi}_{ky})\}^{1-r_{ij}^y},$$

$$p(\mathbf{r}_i^d|\mathbf{d}_i, \boldsymbol{\omega}_i, \boldsymbol{\varphi}_{kd}) = \prod_{j=1}^{m_2} \{p(r_{ij}^d = 1|\mathbf{d}_i, \boldsymbol{\omega}_i, \boldsymbol{\varphi}_{kd})\}^{r_{ij}^d}\{1 - p(r_{ij}^d = 1|\mathbf{d}_i, \boldsymbol{\omega}_i, \boldsymbol{\varphi}_{kd})\}^{1-r_{ij}^d},$$

where $\boldsymbol{\varphi}_{ky}$ and $\boldsymbol{\varphi}_{kd}$ are the component-specific parameter vectors associated with $\mathbf{r}_i^y$ and $\mathbf{r}_i^d$, respectively. For simplicity, we further assume that $p(r_{ij}^y|\mathbf{y}_i, \boldsymbol{\omega}_i, \boldsymbol{\varphi}_{ky}) = p(r_{ij}^y|\mathbf{y}_i, \boldsymbol{\varphi}_{ky})$ and $p(r_{ij}^d|\mathbf{d}_i, \boldsymbol{\omega}_i, \boldsymbol{\varphi}_{kd}) = p(r_{ij}^d|\mathbf{d}_i, \boldsymbol{\varphi}_{kd})$, and propose the following logistic regression models:

$$\text{logit}\{p(r_{ij}^y = 1|\mathbf{y}_i, \boldsymbol{\varphi}_{ky})\} = \varphi_{k0}^y + \varphi_{k1}^y y_{i1} + \cdots + \varphi_{kp}^y y_{ip} = \boldsymbol{\varphi}_{ky}^T \mathbf{u}_i^y, \tag{7.27}$$

$$\text{logit}\{p(r_{ij}^d = 1|\mathbf{d}_i, \boldsymbol{\varphi}_{kd})\} = \varphi_{k0}^d + \varphi_{k1}^d d_{i1} + \cdots + \varphi_{km_2}^d d_{im_2} = \boldsymbol{\varphi}_{kd}^T \mathbf{u}_i^d, \tag{7.28}$$

where $\mathbf{u}_i^y = (1, \mathbf{y}_i^T)^T$, $\boldsymbol{\varphi}_{ky} = (\varphi_{k0}^y, \varphi_{k1}^y, \ldots, \varphi_{kp}^y)^T$, $\mathbf{u}_i^d = (1, \mathbf{d}_i^T)^T$, and $\boldsymbol{\varphi}_{kd} = (\varphi_{k0}^d, \varphi_{k1}^d, \ldots, \varphi_{km_2}^d)^T$. To deal with the missing covariates in the multinomial logit model (7.23), we use $\mathbf{r}_i^x = (r_{i1}^x, \ldots, r_{im_1}^x)^T$ to represent the missingness indicator vectors of $\mathbf{x}_i$, where r_{ij}^x is defined similarly to r_{ij}^y. The following mechanism is used to model the conditional distribution of $\mathbf{r}_i^x$ given $\mathbf{x}_i$ and $\boldsymbol{\varphi}_x$:

$$p(\mathbf{r}_i^x|\mathbf{x}_i, \boldsymbol{\varphi}_x) = \prod_{j=1}^{m_1} \{p(r_{ij}^x = 1|\mathbf{x}_i, \boldsymbol{\varphi}_x)\}^{r_{ij}^x}\{1 - p(r_{ij}^x = 1|\mathbf{x}_i, \boldsymbol{\varphi}_x)\}^{1-r_{ij}^x},$$

$$\text{logit}\{p(r_{ij}^x = 1|\mathbf{x}_i, \boldsymbol{\varphi}_x)\} = \varphi_0^x + \varphi_1^x x_{i1} + \ldots + \varphi_{m_1}^x x_{im_1} = \boldsymbol{\varphi}_x^T \mathbf{u}_i^x, \tag{7.29}$$

where $\mathbf{u}_i^x = (1, \mathbf{x}_i^T)^T$, and $\boldsymbol{\varphi}_x = (\varphi_0^x, \ldots, \varphi_{m_1}^x)^T$ is a parameter vector.

The above binomial modeling with logistic regressions is not the only choice for modeling the nonignorable missingness mechanisms. For instance, one can also use probit regression models to model $p(r_{ij}^y|\cdot)$, $p(r_{ij}^d|\cdot)$, and/or $p(r_{ij}^x|\cdot)$. We use the current modeling strategy because (i) conditional distributions associated with the missing components can easily be derived, (ii) not too many nuisance parameters are involved, and (iii) the logistic regression model is a natural way to model the probability of missingness (Ibrahim *et al.*, 2001). As the true missingness mechanism is unknown, a comparison of modeling strategies can be viewed as a sensitivity analysis for model misspecification of the missing-data mechanisms. Note that unknown parameters $\boldsymbol{\varphi}_{ky}$ and $\boldsymbol{\varphi}_{kd}$ in the missingness mechanisms (7.27) and (7.28) are different across distinct components. Hence, the possible heterogeneity in relation to the missingness mechanisms can be addressed.

7.3.2 Bayesian estimation

Let $\mathbf{Y} = \{\mathbf{y}_i, \ i = 1, \ldots, n\}$, $\mathbf{D} = \{\mathbf{d}_i, \ i = 1, \ldots, n\}$, $\mathbf{X} = \{\mathbf{x}_i, \ i = 1, \ldots, n\}$, $\mathbf{y}_i = \{\mathbf{y}_{i,\text{obs}}, \mathbf{y}_{i,\text{mis}}\}$, $\mathbf{d}_i = \{\mathbf{d}_{i,\text{obs}}, \mathbf{d}_{i,\text{mis}}\}$, $\mathbf{x}_i = \{\mathbf{x}_{i,\text{obs}}, \mathbf{x}_{i,\text{mis}}\}$, where $\{\mathbf{y}_{i,\text{obs}}, \mathbf{d}_{i,\text{obs}}, \mathbf{x}_{i,\text{obs}}\}$ and $\{\mathbf{y}_{i,\text{mis}}, \mathbf{d}_{i,\text{mis}}, \mathbf{x}_{i,\text{mis}}\}$ denote the observed elements and missing elements in $\mathbf{y}_i$, $\mathbf{d}_i$, and $\mathbf{x}_i$, respectively. Let $\mathbf{Y}_{\text{obs}} = \{\mathbf{y}_{i,\text{obs}}, \ i = 1, \ldots, n\}$, $\mathbf{R}^y = \{\mathbf{r}_i^y, \ i = 1, \ldots, n\}$, $\mathbf{D}_{\text{obs}} = \{\mathbf{d}_{i,\text{obs}}, \ i = 1, \ldots, n\}$, $\mathbf{R}^d = \{\mathbf{r}_i^d, \ i = 1, \ldots, n\}$, $\mathbf{X}_{\text{obs}} = \{\mathbf{x}_{i,\text{obs}}, \ i = 1, \ldots, n\}$, $\mathbf{R}^x = \{\mathbf{r}_i^x, \ i = 1, \ldots, n\}$, and $\mathbf{F}_{\text{obs}} = \{\mathbf{Y}_{\text{obs}}, \mathbf{D}_{\text{obs}}, \mathbf{X}_{\text{obs}}, \mathbf{R}^y, \mathbf{R}^d, \mathbf{R}^x\}$. Let $\boldsymbol{\pi}_k = \{\pi_{ik}, \ i = 1, \ldots, n\}$, $\boldsymbol{\pi} = \{\boldsymbol{\pi}_1, \ldots, \boldsymbol{\pi}_{K-1}\}$,

$\boldsymbol{\tau} = \{\boldsymbol{\tau}_1, \ldots, \boldsymbol{\tau}_{K-1}\}$, $\boldsymbol{\tau}_d = \{\boldsymbol{\tau}_{1d}, \ldots, \boldsymbol{\tau}_{Kd}\}$, $\boldsymbol{\varphi}_y = \{\boldsymbol{\varphi}_{1y}, \ldots, \boldsymbol{\varphi}_{Ky}\}$, $\boldsymbol{\varphi}_d = \{\boldsymbol{\varphi}_{1d}, \ldots, \boldsymbol{\varphi}_{Kd}\}$, $\boldsymbol{\vartheta}_s = \{\boldsymbol{\varphi}_y, \boldsymbol{\varphi}_d, \boldsymbol{\varphi}_x, \boldsymbol{\tau}, \boldsymbol{\tau}_x, \boldsymbol{\tau}_d\}$, and $\boldsymbol{\theta}_* = \{\boldsymbol{\theta}, \boldsymbol{\pi}, \boldsymbol{\vartheta}_s\}$, where $\boldsymbol{\vartheta}_s$ contains the parameters in logistic regression models (7.27)–(7.29) and those involved in the probability distributions of $\mathbf{x}_i$ and $\mathbf{d}_i$ in models (7.23) and (7.25). As all the components in $\boldsymbol{\vartheta}_s$ are associated with the missingness mechanisms rather than the modified mixture SEM, they are considered as a nuisance parameter vector in Bayesian analysis. To obtain the Bayesian estimate of $\boldsymbol{\theta}_*$, the main task is to draw observations from the posterior distribution $p(\boldsymbol{\theta}_* |\mathbf{F}_{\text{obs}})$. Due to the complexity of the model and the existence of nonignorable missing data, this posterior distribution involves high-dimensional integrals and does not have a closed form. We utilize the idea of data augmentation with the help of a latent allocation variable z_i for each $\mathbf{y}_i$. Here, we assume that z_i follows a multinomial distribution $\text{Multi}(\pi_{i1}, \ldots, \pi_{iK})$ with

$$p(z_i = k|\mathbf{x}_i) = \pi_{ik}, \quad k = 1, \ldots, K. \tag{7.30}$$

Let $\mathbf{Z} = \{z_1, \ldots, z_n\}$. If $\mathbf{Z}$ is given, the allocation of each $\mathbf{y}_i$ is identified, and the mixture model becomes a familiar multiple-group model. Furthermore, let $\mathbf{Y}_{\text{mis}} = \{\mathbf{y}_{i,\text{mis}},\ i = 1, \ldots, n\}$, $\mathbf{D}_{\text{mis}} = \{\mathbf{d}_{i,\text{mis}}\ i = 1, \ldots, n\}$, $\mathbf{X}_{\text{mis}} = \{\mathbf{x}_{i,\text{mis}},\ i = 1, \ldots, n\}$, and $\boldsymbol{\Omega} = \{\boldsymbol{\omega}_i,\ i = 1, \ldots, n\}$. The observed data $\mathbf{F}_{\text{obs}}$ will be augmented with the latent quantities $\mathbf{F}_{\text{mis}} = \{\mathbf{Y}_{\text{mis}}, \mathbf{D}_{\text{mis}}, \mathbf{X}_{\text{mis}}, \boldsymbol{\Omega}, \mathbf{Z}\}$ in the posterior analysis. Hence, the Bayesian estimate of $\boldsymbol{\theta}_*$ can be obtained by drawing samples from the joint posterior distribution $p(\boldsymbol{\theta}_*, \mathbf{F}_{\text{mis}}|\mathbf{F}_{\text{obs}})$ through MCMC methods, such as the Gibbs sampler (Geman and Geman, 1984) and the Metropolis–Hastings algorithm (Metropolis *et al.*, 1953; Hastings, 1970). The random permutation sampler proposed by Frühwirth-Schnatter (2001) is used to deal with the label switching problem in the MCMC algorithm (for details, see Section 7.2.2).

The full conditional distributions in implementing the MCMC algorithm involve the prior distributions of unknown parameters in $\boldsymbol{\theta}_*$. As suggested in the literature (Lee, 2007a; Lee and Song, 2003), the following conjugate prior distributions are used. Let $\boldsymbol{\Lambda}_{kj}^T$ and $\boldsymbol{\Lambda}_{\omega kl}^T$ be the jth and lth rows of $\boldsymbol{\Lambda}_k$ and $\boldsymbol{\Lambda}_{\omega k}$, and ψ_{kj} and $\psi_{\delta kl}$ be the jth and the lth diagonal elements of $\boldsymbol{\Psi}_k$ and $\boldsymbol{\Psi}_{\delta k}$, respectively. The prior distributions of the unknown parameters in $\boldsymbol{\theta}_k$, $k = 1, \ldots, K$ are given as follows: for $j = 1, \ldots, p$ and $l = 1, \ldots, q_1$,

$$\begin{aligned}
[\boldsymbol{\Lambda}_{kj}|\psi_{kj}] &\stackrel{D}{=} N[\boldsymbol{\Lambda}_{0kj}, \psi_{kj}\mathbf{H}_{0kj}], & \psi_{kj}^{-1} &\stackrel{D}{=} \text{Gamma}[\alpha_{0kj}, \beta_{0kj}],\\
[\boldsymbol{\Lambda}_{\omega kl}|\psi_{\delta kl}] &\stackrel{D}{=} N[\tilde{\boldsymbol{\Lambda}}_{0kl}, \psi_{\delta kl}\tilde{\mathbf{H}}_{0kl}], & \psi_{\delta kl}^{-1} &\stackrel{D}{=} \text{Gamma}[\tilde{\alpha}_{0kl}, \tilde{\beta}_{0kl}],\\
\boldsymbol{\mu}_k &\stackrel{D}{=} N[\boldsymbol{\mu}_{0k}, \boldsymbol{\Sigma}_{0k}], & \boldsymbol{\Phi}_k^{-1} &\stackrel{D}{=} W_{q_2}[\mathbf{V}_{0k}, \rho_{0k}].
\end{aligned} \tag{7.31}$$

The prior distributions of $\boldsymbol{\tau}_k$, $\boldsymbol{\varphi}_x$, $\boldsymbol{\varphi}_{ky}$, and $\boldsymbol{\varphi}_{kd}$ are given as follows:

$$\begin{aligned}
\boldsymbol{\tau}_k &\stackrel{D}{=} N[\boldsymbol{\mu}_{0k\tau}, \boldsymbol{\Sigma}_{0k\tau}], & \boldsymbol{\varphi}_x &\stackrel{D}{=} N[\boldsymbol{\varphi}_{0x}, \boldsymbol{\Sigma}_{0x}],\\
\boldsymbol{\varphi}_{ky} &\stackrel{D}{=} N[\boldsymbol{\varphi}_{0ky}, \boldsymbol{\Sigma}_{0ky}], & \boldsymbol{\varphi}_{kd} &\stackrel{D}{=} N[\boldsymbol{\varphi}_{0kd}, \boldsymbol{\Sigma}_{0kd}].
\end{aligned} \tag{7.32}$$

Moreover, the conjugate prior distributions of $\boldsymbol{\tau}_x$ and $\boldsymbol{\tau}_d$ can be related on the basis of the distributions of $\mathbf{x}_i$ and $\mathbf{d}_i$. The hyperparameters in (7.31) and (7.32) include $\boldsymbol{\Lambda}_{0kj}$, $\tilde{\boldsymbol{\Lambda}}_{0kl}$, α_{0kj}, β_{0kj}, $\tilde{\alpha}_{0kl}$, $\tilde{\beta}_{0kl}$, $\boldsymbol{\mu}_{0k}$, ρ_{0k}, $\boldsymbol{\mu}_{0k\tau}$, $\boldsymbol{\varphi}_{0x}$, $\boldsymbol{\varphi}_{0ky}$, $\boldsymbol{\varphi}_{0kd}$, and positive definite matrices $\mathbf{H}_{0kj}$, $\tilde{\mathbf{H}}_{0kl}$, $\boldsymbol{\Sigma}_{0k}$, $\boldsymbol{\Sigma}_{0k\tau}$, $\boldsymbol{\Sigma}_{0x}$, $\boldsymbol{\Sigma}_{0ky}$, $\boldsymbol{\Sigma}_{0kd}$, and $\mathbf{V}_{0k}$, whose values are assumed to be given according to prior information. With the above prior distributions, the full conditional distributions of the unknown parameters in $\boldsymbol{\theta}_*$ are derived in Appendix 7.3.

7.3.3 Bayesian model selection using a modified DIC

For the modified mixture SEM with missing data, competing models are compared with respect to (i) the different numbers of components involved in the mixture model; and (ii) the different missingness mechanisms for the missing data. In this section, a modified deviance information criterion (DIC; Spiegelhalter *et al.*, 2002) is considered for model selection. It is well known that directly applying the DIC to the model selection of mixture models with incomplete data is problematic (Spiegelhalter *et al.*, 2003). Recently, Celeux *et al.* (2006) explored a wide range of options for constructing an appropriate DIC for mixture models. Here, we use one of these adaptations, namely, a modified DIC, as follows:

$$\begin{aligned}\mathrm{DIC} = &-4E_{\boldsymbol{\theta}*,\mathbf{F}_{\mathrm{mis}}}\{\log p(\mathbf{F}_{\mathrm{obs}}, \mathbf{F}_{\mathrm{mis}}|\boldsymbol{\theta}_*)|\mathbf{F}_{\mathrm{obs}}\}\\ &+2E_{\mathbf{F}_{\mathrm{mis}}}\{\log p(\mathbf{F}_{\mathrm{obs}}, \mathbf{F}_{\mathrm{mis}}|E_{\boldsymbol{\theta}_*}[\boldsymbol{\theta}_*|\mathbf{F}_{\mathrm{obs}}, \mathbf{F}_{\mathrm{mis}}])|\mathbf{F}_{\mathrm{obs}}\},\end{aligned} \quad (7.33)$$

where $\log p(\mathbf{F}_{\mathrm{obs}}, \mathbf{F}_{\mathrm{mis}}|\boldsymbol{\theta}_*)$ is the complete-data log-likelihood function, which can be written as

$$\log p(\mathbf{F}_{\mathrm{obs}}, \mathbf{F}_{\mathrm{mis}}|\boldsymbol{\theta}_*) = \sum_{i=1}^{n} \log p\big(\mathbf{y}_i, \boldsymbol{\omega}_i, \mathbf{d}_i, z_i, \mathbf{x}_i, \mathbf{r}_i^y, \mathbf{r}_i^d, \mathbf{r}_i^x|\boldsymbol{\theta}_*\big),$$

in which

$$\begin{aligned}
&\log p\big(\mathbf{y}_i, \boldsymbol{\omega}_i, \mathbf{d}_i, z_i, \mathbf{x}_i, \mathbf{r}_i^y, \mathbf{r}_i^d, \mathbf{r}_i^x|\boldsymbol{\theta}_*\big)\\
&= \log(\mathbf{y}_i|\boldsymbol{\omega}_i, \boldsymbol{\mu}_k, \boldsymbol{\Lambda}_k, \boldsymbol{\Psi}_k, z_i = k) + \log p(\boldsymbol{\eta}_i|\boldsymbol{\xi}_i, \mathbf{d}_i, \boldsymbol{\Lambda}_{\omega k}, \boldsymbol{\Psi}_{\delta k}, z_i = k) + \log p(\boldsymbol{\xi}_i|\boldsymbol{\Phi}_k, z_i = k)\\
&\quad + \log p(\mathbf{d}_i|\boldsymbol{\tau}_{kd}, z_i = k) + \log p(z_i = k|\boldsymbol{\tau}, \mathbf{x}_i) + \log p(\mathbf{x}_i|\boldsymbol{\tau}_x)\\
&\quad + \log p\big(\mathbf{r}_i^y|\mathbf{y}_i, \boldsymbol{\varphi}_{ky}, z_i = k\big) + \log p\big(\mathbf{r}_i^d|\mathbf{d}_i, \boldsymbol{\varphi}_{kd}, z_i = k\big) + \log p\big(\mathbf{r}_i^x|\boldsymbol{\varphi}_x, \mathbf{x}_i\big)\\
&= -\frac{1}{2}\{p\log(2\pi) + \log|\boldsymbol{\Psi}_k| + (\mathbf{y}_i - \boldsymbol{\mu}_k - \boldsymbol{\Lambda}_k\boldsymbol{\omega}_i)^T\boldsymbol{\Psi}_k^{-1}(\mathbf{y}_i - \boldsymbol{\mu}_k - \boldsymbol{\Lambda}_k\boldsymbol{\omega}_i)\}\\
&\quad -\frac{1}{2}\{q_1\log(2\pi) + \log|\boldsymbol{\Psi}_{\delta k}| + (\boldsymbol{\eta}_i - \boldsymbol{\Lambda}_{\omega k}\mathbf{G}(\boldsymbol{\omega}_i))^T\boldsymbol{\Psi}_{\delta k}^{-1}(\boldsymbol{\eta}_i - \boldsymbol{\Lambda}_{\omega k}\mathbf{G}(\boldsymbol{\omega}_i))\}\\
&\quad -\frac{1}{2}\{q_2\log(2\pi) + \log|\boldsymbol{\Phi}_k| + \boldsymbol{\xi}_i^T\boldsymbol{\Phi}_k^{-1}\boldsymbol{\xi}_i\}\\
&\quad + \log p(\mathbf{d}_i|\boldsymbol{\tau}_{kd}, z_i = k) + \boldsymbol{\tau}_k^T\mathbf{x}_i - \log\left\{\sum_{j=1}^{K}\exp\left(\boldsymbol{\tau}_j^T\mathbf{x}_i\right)\right\} + \log p(\mathbf{x}_i|\boldsymbol{\tau}_x)\\
&\quad + \left(\sum_{j=1}^{p} r_{ij}^y\right)\left(\boldsymbol{\varphi}_{ky}^T\mathbf{u}_i^y\right) - p\log\left\{1 + \exp\left(\boldsymbol{\varphi}_{ky}^T\mathbf{u}_i^y\right)\right\}\\
&\quad + \left(\sum_{j=1}^{m_2} r_{ij}^d\right)\left(\boldsymbol{\varphi}_{kd}^T\mathbf{u}_i^d\right) - m_2\log\left\{1 + \exp\left(\boldsymbol{\varphi}_{kd}^T\mathbf{u}_i^d\right)\right\}\\
&\quad + \left(\sum_{j=1}^{m_1} r_{ij}^x\right)\left(\boldsymbol{\varphi}_x^T\mathbf{u}_i^x\right) - m_1\log\left\{1 + \exp\left(\boldsymbol{\varphi}_x^T\mathbf{u}_i^x\right)\right\}.
\end{aligned}$$

Hence, the first expectation in (7.33) can be obtained using the following approximation with the MCMC output $\{(\mathbf{F}_{\text{mis}}^{(j)}, \boldsymbol{\theta}_*^{(j)}), j = 1, \ldots, J\}$:

$$E_{\boldsymbol{\theta}_*,\mathbf{F}_{\text{mis}}}\{\log p(\mathbf{F}_{\text{obs}}, \mathbf{F}_{\text{mis}}|\boldsymbol{\theta}_*)|\mathbf{F}_{\text{obs}}\} \approx \frac{1}{J}\sum_{j=1}^{J} \log p\big(\mathbf{F}_{\text{obs}}, \mathbf{F}_{\text{mis}}^{(j)}|\boldsymbol{\theta}_*^{(j)}\big).$$

Furthermore, let $\boldsymbol{\theta}_*^{(j,l)}$, $l = 1, \ldots, L$ be the observations generated from $p(\boldsymbol{\theta}_*|\mathbf{F}_{\text{obs}}, \mathbf{F}_{\text{mis}}^{(j)})$ via the MCMC method described above. We have

$$E_{\boldsymbol{\theta}_*}\big[\boldsymbol{\theta}_*|\mathbf{F}_{\text{obs}}, \mathbf{F}_{\text{mis}}^{(j)}\big] \approx \bar{\boldsymbol{\theta}}_*^{(j)} = \frac{1}{L}\sum_{l=1}^{L} \boldsymbol{\theta}_*^{(j,l)}.$$

Thus, the second expectation in (7.33) can be approximated by

$$E_{\mathbf{F}_{\text{mis}}}\{\log p(\mathbf{F}_{\text{obs}}, \mathbf{F}_{\text{mis}}|E_{\boldsymbol{\theta}_*}[\boldsymbol{\theta}_*|\mathbf{F}_{\text{obs}}, \mathbf{F}_{\text{mis}}])|\mathbf{F}_{\text{obs}}\} \approx \frac{1}{J}\sum_{j=1}^{J} \log p\big(\mathbf{F}_{\text{obs}}, \mathbf{F}_{\text{mis}}^{(j)}|\bar{\boldsymbol{\theta}}_*^{(j)}\big).$$

Finally, we can obtain the approximation of the modified DIC as follows:

$$\text{DIC} = -\frac{4}{J}\sum_{j=1}^{J} \log p\big(\mathbf{F}_{\text{obs}}, \mathbf{F}_{\text{mis}}^{(j)}|\boldsymbol{\theta}_*^{(j)}\big) + \frac{2}{J}\sum_{j=1}^{J} \log p\big(\mathbf{F}_{\text{obs}}, \mathbf{F}_{\text{mis}}^{(j)}|\bar{\boldsymbol{\theta}}_*^{(j)}\big).$$

7.3.4 An illustrative example

The methodology is illustrated through a longitudinal study of polydrug use conducted in five California counties in 2004 (Cai *et al.*, 2010). Data were collected from self-reported and administrative questionnaires about the retention of drug treatment, drug use history, drug-related crime history, motivation for drug treatment, and received service and test for 1588 participants at intake, 3-month, and 12-month follow-up interviews (see Appendix 1.1). The modified mixture SEM is applied to examine the possible explanatory effects on treatment retention, and to explore possible heterogeneity in the data. Our primary interest is 'retention' (denoted by Retent in Appendix 1.1, and y_1 here), which was collected at 12-month follow-up interview and which indicated the number of days' stay in treatment. Other observed variables include 'drug use in past 30 days at intake' (Drgday30, y_2), 'drug problems in past 30 days at intake' (Drgplm30, y_3), 'the number of arrests in lifetime at intake' (ArrN, y_4), 'the number of incarcerations in lifetime at intake' (Incar, y_5), and 'the age of first arrest' (Agefirstarrest, y_6). These variables are treated as continuous. As $\{y_2, y_3\}$ are associated with the severity of drug use, they were grouped into a latent variable, 'drug severity' (ξ_1), and as $\{y_4, y_5, y_6\}$ are associated with drug-related crime history, they were grouped into a latent variable, 'crime' (ξ_2). Therefore, an SEM is adopted in which a measurement equation is used to identify two latent variables, 'drug severity' and 'crime', and a structural equation is used to study the influence of these latent variables on the outcome variable 'retention' (η). In addition, variables for treatment motivation (Mtsum01, Mtsum02, and Mtsum03) were collected at intake. They were treated as fixed covariates in the structural equation to incorporate their possible effects on retention. Moreover, some variables were collected at 3-month follow-up interview, including 'services received in the past 3 months at TSI 3-month interview' (Servicem), 'the number of drug tests by TX in the past 3 months at TSI 3-month interview' (DrugtestTX), and 'the number of drug tests by criminal justice in the past 3 months at TSI 3-month interview'

(DrugtestCJ). As these variables are related to the service and test received, they are likely to affect the pattern of influence of 'drug severity', 'crime', and treatment motivation on 'retention'. Thus, they were used to predict the component probability (see equation (7.23)). In this study, there are 1588 random observations, many of which have missing entries. Because most of variables in polydrug use data were nonnormal, the logarithm and square root transformations were applied to the nonnormal variables. Furthermore, the continuous measurements were standardized to unify the scale.

According to the above description, the model was formulated as follows. The six observed variables $y_1, \ldots, y_6$ were grouped into three latent variables η, ξ_1, and ξ_2, which were interpreted as 'retention', 'drug severity', and 'crime', respectively. In order to obtain a clear interpretation of each latent variable, the following non-overlapping loading matrix $\mathbf{\Lambda}_k$ was used in each component:

$$\mathbf{\Lambda}_k^T = \begin{bmatrix} 1 & 0 & 0 & 0 & 0 & 0 \\ 0 & 1 & \lambda_{k,32} & 0 & 0 & 0 \\ 0 & 0 & 0 & 1 & \lambda_{k,53} & \lambda_{k,63} \end{bmatrix},$$

where the 1s and 0s were fixed for model identification. Furthermore, because there was only one indicator corresponding to the latent variable 'retention' ($\eta = y_1$), we fixed $\psi_{k1} = 0.0$ to identify the model. In each component, a structural equation was used to assess the effects of 'drug severity' and 'crime', together with covariates of treatment motivations (d_1, d_2, d_3), on 'retention' as follows:

$$\eta_i = b_{k1}d_{i1} + b_{k2}d_{i2} + b_{k3}d_{i3} + \gamma_{k1}\xi_{i1} + \gamma_{k2}\xi_{i2} + \delta_i.$$

The component probabilities π_{ik} were determined by the following multinomial logit model:

$$\pi_{ik} = \frac{\exp\{\tau_{k0} + \tau_{k1}x_{i1} + \tau_{k2}x_{i2} + \tau_{k3}x_{i3}\}}{\sum_{j=1}^{K} \exp\{\tau_{j0} + \tau_{j1}x_{i1} + \tau_{j2}x_{i2} + \tau_{j3}x_{i3}\}}, \quad k = 1, \ldots, K.$$

Based on the nature of the questionnaires, we assumed that d_j, $j = 1, 2, 3$, came from multinomial distributions Multi$(p_{j1}, \ldots, p_{j5})$, x_1 came from a normal distribution, and x_2 and x_3 came from Poisson distributions.

The first step was to check the heterogeneity of the data using the modified DIC. For $k = 1, 2, 3$, let M_k be the k-component mixture SEM with nonignorable missingness mechanisms defined by (7.27)–(7.29). In the following analysis, a vague prior was taken as follows: $\boldsymbol{\mu}_{0k} = \bar{\mathbf{y}}$, $\mathbf{\Sigma}_{0k} = 4\mathbf{S}_y^2$, where $\bar{\mathbf{y}}$ and $\mathbf{S}_y^2$ are the sample mean and sample covariance matrix calculated from the fully observed data; the elements in $\mathbf{\Lambda}_{0kj}$, $\tilde{\mathbf{\Lambda}}_{0kl}$, $\boldsymbol{\mu}_{0k\tau}$, $\boldsymbol{\varphi}_{0x}$, $\boldsymbol{\varphi}_{0ky}$, and $\boldsymbol{\varphi}_{0kd}$ are 1s; and $\mathbf{H}_{0kj}$, $\tilde{\mathbf{H}}_{0kl}$, $\mathbf{\Sigma}_{0k\tau}$, $\mathbf{\Sigma}_{0x}$, $\mathbf{\Sigma}_{0ky}$, $\mathbf{\Sigma}_{0kd}$, and $\mathbf{V}_{0k}^{-1}$ are 10 times the identity matrices of appropriate order, $\alpha_{0kj} = \tilde{\alpha}_{0kl} = 5$, $\beta_{0kj} = \tilde{\beta}_{0kl} = 6$, and $\rho_{0k} = 13$. Based on some pilot runs, we found that the MCMC algorithm converged within 8000 iterations. After discarding 8000 burn-in iterations, an additional 10 000 observations were used to compute the modified DIC values. The modified DIC values corresponding to M_k were $\text{DIC}_{M_1} = 74\,512$, $\text{DIC}_{M_2} = 73\,035$, and $\text{DIC}_{M_3} = 78\,160$, respectively. Therefore, the two-component model M_2 was selected. To select appropriate mechanisms for missing responses and covariates, we compared M_2 with the following two-component models:

M_4 : the missing data in $\mathbf{y}$ are treated as MAR, and in $\mathbf{d}$ and $\mathbf{x}$ are treated as nonignorable;

M_5 : the missing data in $\mathbf{d}$ are treated as MAR, and in $\mathbf{y}$ and $\mathbf{x}$ are treated as nonignorable;

M_6 : the missing data in **x** are treated as MAR, and in **y** and **d** are treated as nonignorable;

M_7 : the missing data in **y**, **d**, and **x** are all treated as MAR;

M_8 : instead of using logistic regression models (7.27)–(7.29), the probit regression models are used to model the missingness mechanisms;

M_9 : the explanatory covariates in models (7.27)–(7.29) are specified as

$$\text{logit}\{p(r_{ij}^y = 1|\mathbf{y}_i, \boldsymbol{\varphi}_{ky})\} = \varphi_0^y + \varphi_j^y y_{ij},$$

$$\text{logit}\{p(r_{ij}^d = 1|\mathbf{d}_i, \boldsymbol{\varphi}_{kd})\} = \varphi_0^d + \varphi_j^d d_{ij},$$

$$\text{logit}\{p(r_{ij}^x = 1|\mathbf{x}_i, \boldsymbol{\varphi}_x)\} = \varphi_0^x + \varphi_j^x x_{ij}.$$

In the above model settings, $M_4, \ldots, M_9$ have the same number of components as the true model but have different missingness mechanisms for **y**, **d**, and **x**, respectively. The modified DIC values for $M_4, \ldots, M_9$ were $\text{DIC}_{M_4} = 73\,458$, $\text{DIC}_{M_5} = 73\,162$, $\text{DIC}_{M_6} = 73\,131$, $\text{DIC}_{M_7} = 74\,001$, $\text{DIC}_{M_8} = 73\,088$, and $\text{DIC}_{M_9} = 73, 862$. Again, M_2, with the smallest $\text{DIC}_{M_2} = 73\,035$, was selected.

On the basis of the selected model M_2, 10 000 observations collected after convergence were used to obtain the Bayesian estimates. The path diagrams of components 1 and 2 are presented in Figures 7.2 and 7.3, respectively, together with the Bayesian estimates of some

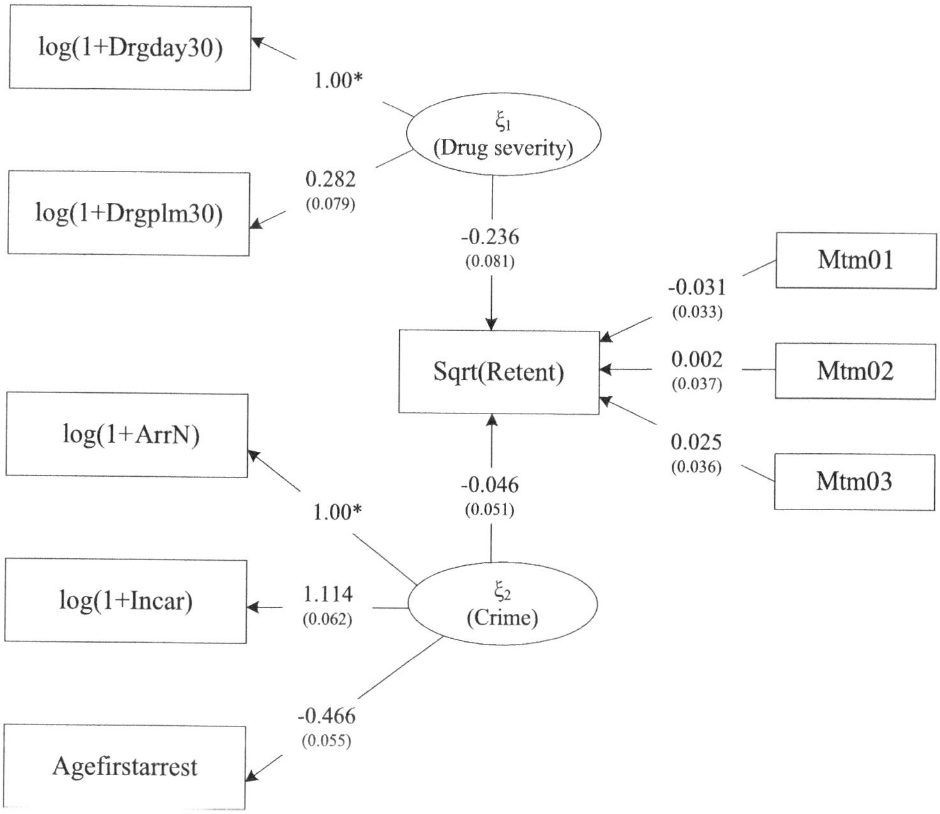

Figure 7.2 Path diagram of component 1 in the polydrug use example.

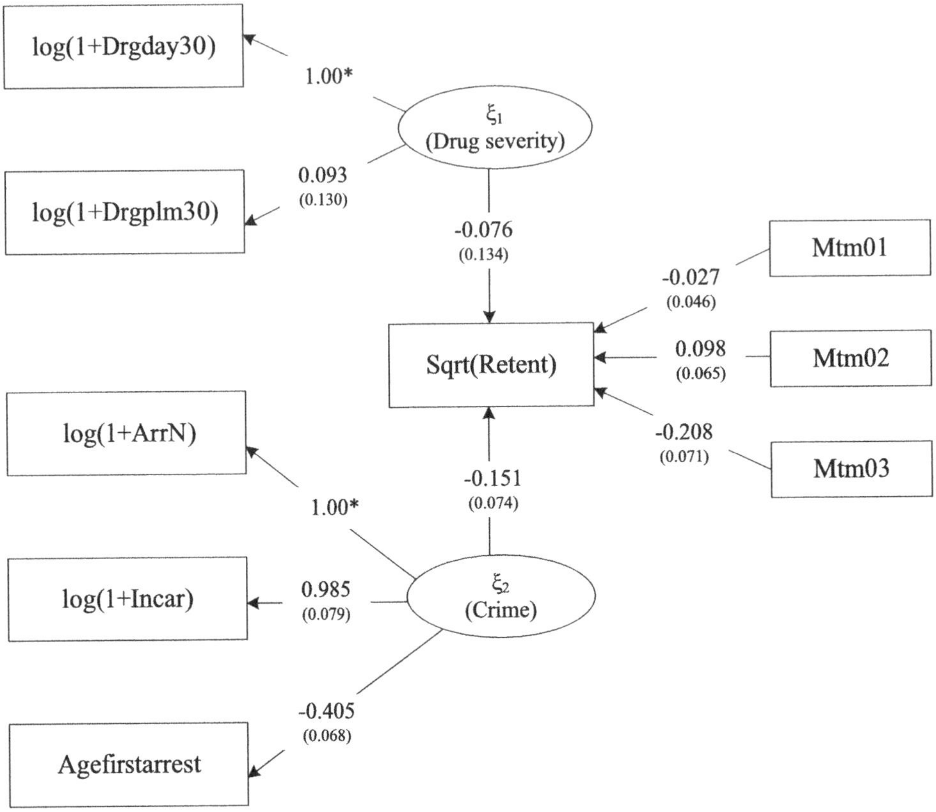

Figure 7.3 Path diagram of component 2 in the polydrug use example.

interesting component-specific parameters. The Bayesian estimates of other parameters and their corresponding standard error estimates (SE) are presented in Table 7.5. We draw the following conclusions: (i) For components 1 and 2, the influences of latent variables 'drug severity' and 'crime' on retention have different patterns. This indicates that the mixture SEM with two components is necessary. For component 1, the effect of 'drug severity' is significant ($\hat{\gamma}_{11} = -0.236$, SE = 0.081), while the effect of 'crime' is insignificant ($\hat{\gamma}_{12} = -0.046$, SE = 0.051). Hence, it seems that in this component, participants with less drug use tend to stay in the treatment longer. In contrast, for component 2, the effect of 'drug severity' is insignificant ($\hat{\gamma}_{21} = -0.076$, SE = 0.134), while the effect of 'crime' is significant ($\hat{\gamma}_{22} = -0.151$, SE = 0.074). Thus, the participants with fewer drug-related crime records tend to stay in treatment longer. Moreover, as the difference in sizes of $\hat{\gamma}_{11}$ and $\hat{\gamma}_{12}$, and $\hat{\gamma}_{21}$ and $\hat{\gamma}_{22}$ are substantial, more attention should be paid to the significant effects. (ii) For components 1 and 2, the effects of treatment motivation on retention are different. In particular, for component 1, the effect of 'Mtm03' on 'retention' is insignificant ($\hat{b}_{13} = 0.025$, SE = 0.036), while for component 2, the corresponding effect is significant ($\hat{b}_{23} = -0.208$, SE = 0.071). (iii) There are differences in other parameter estimates in the two components. For example, estimates of $\lambda_{1,32}$ and $\lambda_{2,32}$, μ_{1j} and μ_{2j} for $j = 1, \ldots, 6$, and some nuisance parameters in the logistic regression models are quite different. (iv) τ_{11} and τ_{13} are significant, indicating that both service and

Table 7.5 Bayesian estimates of the parameters in the illustrative example.

	Component 1			Component 2	
Par.	Est	SE		Est	SE
μ_1	−0.008	0.069		0.460	0.124
μ_2	−0.297	0.055		0.615	0.077
μ_3	−0.620	0.079		1.209	0.141
μ_4	−0.122	0.041		0.248	0.052
μ_5	−0.052	0.033		0.114	0.051
μ_6	0.019	0.038		−0.003	0.049
ψ_2	0.364	0.051		0.545	0.079
ψ_3	0.371	0.053		0.163	0.090
ψ_4	0.364	0.032		0.441	0.051
ψ_5	0.304	0.036		0.383	0.049
ψ_6	0.956	0.059		0.762	0.061
ϕ_{11}	0.435	0.069		0.403	0.068
ϕ_{21}	0.037	0.025		0.041	0.038
ϕ_{22}	0.537	0.047		0.655	0.074
ψ_δ	0.903	0.051		0.833	0.066
φ_0^y	−4.393	0.598		−1.892	0.516
φ_1^y	−0.309	0.083		−0.236	0.153
φ_2^y	0.228	0.086		0.107	0.110
φ_3^y	−1.787	0.477		−1.075	0.360
φ_4^y	−0.162	0.125		−0.023	0.108
φ_5^y	0.050	0.105		0.044	0.124
φ_6^y	0.040	0.073		0.185	0.110
φ_0^d	−4.001	0.841		−1.326	0.586
φ_1^d	5.715	0.344		3.117	0.402
φ_2^d	−5.589	0.184		−4.965	0.595
φ_3^d	−2.139	0.463		−0.407	0.279
τ_{10}	0.827	0.246			
τ_{11}	−0.257	0.074			
τ_{12}	0.028	0.016			
τ_{13}	0.058	0.018			
Non-component-specific parameters					
φ_0^x	−3.930	0.301	φ_2^x	−3.069	0.217
φ_1^x	1.055	0.142	φ_3^x	2.451	0.169

drug tests received by the participants are useful to predict their component probabilities. (v) Many parameter estimates in φ_y, φ_d, and φ_x are substantially different from zero, indicating the necessity of the nonignorable mechanisms in the analysis of missing data. (vi) The different estimates of φ_y and φ_d in the two components imply the existence of component-specific patterns in the missingness mechanisms for both responses and covariates. These conclusions reconfirm the above model comparison result in selecting a mixture SEM with two components.

To investigate the sensitivity of Bayesian estimation and model selection to the prior input given in (7.31) and (7.32), the above analyses were repeated with some perturbations of the current prior inputs. Bayesian estimates obtained are close to those given in Table 7.5. The DIC values consistently selected model M_2 under the different prior inputs. The computer program for conducting this analysis is written in R compiled C code, which is given in the following website:

`www.wiley.com/go/medical_behavioral_sciences`

Appendix 7.1 The permutation sampler

Let $\boldsymbol{\psi} = (\boldsymbol{\Omega}, \mathbf{W}, \boldsymbol{\theta})$. The permutation sampler for generating $\boldsymbol{\psi}$ from the posterior $p(\boldsymbol{\psi}|\mathbf{Y})$ is implemented as follows:

1. Generate $\tilde{\boldsymbol{\psi}}$ from the unconstrained posterior $p(\boldsymbol{\psi}|\mathbf{Y})$ using standard Gibbs sampling steps.

2. Select some permutation $\rho(1), \ldots, \rho(K)$ of the current labeling of the states and define $\boldsymbol{\psi} = \rho(\tilde{\boldsymbol{\psi}})$ from $\tilde{\boldsymbol{\psi}}$ by reordering the labeling through this permutation, $(\boldsymbol{\theta}_1, \ldots, \boldsymbol{\theta}_K) := (\boldsymbol{\theta}_{\rho(1)}, \ldots, \boldsymbol{\theta}_{\rho(K)})$, and $\mathbf{W} = (w_1, \ldots, w_n) := (\rho(w_1), \ldots, \rho(w_n))$.

One application of permutation sampling is the random permutation sampler, where each sweep of the MCMC chain is concluded by relabeling the states through a random permutation of $\{1, \ldots, K\}$. This method delivers a sample that explores the whole unconstrained parameter space and jumps between the various labeling subspaces in a balanced fashion. Another application of the permutation sampler is the permutation sampling under identifiability constraints. A common way to include an identifiability constraint is to use a permutation sampler, where the permutation is selected in such a way that the identifiability constraint is fulfilled.

Appendix 7.2 Searching for identifiability constraints

For $k = 1, \ldots, K$, let $\boldsymbol{\theta}_k$ denote the parameter vector corresponding to the kth component. As suggested by Frühwirth-Schnatter (2001), the MCMC output of the random permutation sampler can be explored to find a suitable identifiability constraint. It is sufficient to consider only the parameters in $\boldsymbol{\theta}_1$, because a balanced sample from the unconstrained posterior will contain the same information for all parameters in $\boldsymbol{\theta}_k$ with $k > 1$. As the random permutation sampler jumps between the various labeling subspaces, part of the values sampled for $\boldsymbol{\theta}_1$ will belong to the first state, part will belong to the second state, and so on. To differ for various states, it is most useful to consider bivariate scatter plots of θ_{1i} versus θ_{1l} for possible combinations of i and l, where θ_{1i} and θ_{1l} indicate the ith and the lth element of $\boldsymbol{\theta}_1$, respectively. Jumping between the labeling subspaces produces groups in these scatter plots that correspond to different states. By describing the difference between the various groups geometrically, identification of a unique labeling subspace through conditions on the state-specific parameters is attempted. If the values sampled for a certain component of $\boldsymbol{\theta}$ differ markedly between the groups when jumping between the labeling subspaces, then an order condition on this component could be used to separate the labeling subspaces, while if the values sampled for a certain component of $\boldsymbol{\theta}$ hardly differ between the states when jumping between the labeling subspaces, then this component will be a poor candidate for separating the labeling subspaces.

Appendix 7.3 Conditional distributions: Modified mixture SEMs

The full conditional distribution of $\mathbf{Y}_{\text{mis}}$ is given by

$$p(\mathbf{Y}_{\text{mis}}|\mathbf{R}^y, \mathbf{Y}_{\text{obs}}, \boldsymbol{\Omega}, \mathbf{Z}, \boldsymbol{\theta}_*) = \prod_{i=1}^{n} p\big(\mathbf{y}_{i,\text{mis}}|\mathbf{r}_i^y, \mathbf{y}_{i,\text{obs}}, \boldsymbol{\omega}_i, z_i = k, \boldsymbol{\theta}_*\big), \quad \text{and}$$

$$\begin{aligned} p(\mathbf{y}_{i,\text{mis}}|\mathbf{r}_i^y, \mathbf{y}_{i,\text{obs}}, \boldsymbol{\omega}_i, z_i = k, \boldsymbol{\theta}_*) &\propto p\left(\mathbf{r}_i^y|\mathbf{y}_i, z_i = k, \boldsymbol{\varphi}_{ky}\right) p(\mathbf{y}_{i,\text{mis}}|\boldsymbol{\omega}_i, z_i = k, \boldsymbol{\theta}_k) \\ &\propto \exp\Bigg[-\frac{1}{2}(\mathbf{y}_{i,\text{mis}} - \boldsymbol{\mu}_{k,\text{mis}} - \boldsymbol{\Lambda}_{k,\text{mis}}\boldsymbol{\omega}_i)^T \boldsymbol{\Psi}_{k,\text{mis}}^{-1}(\mathbf{y}_{i,\text{mis}} - \boldsymbol{\mu}_{k,\text{mis}} - \boldsymbol{\Lambda}_{k,\text{mis}}\boldsymbol{\omega}_i) \\ &\quad + \left(\sum_{j=1}^{p} r_{ij}^y\right)\left(\boldsymbol{\varphi}_{ky}^T\mathbf{u}_i^y\right) - p\log\left\{1 + \exp\left(\boldsymbol{\varphi}_{ky}^T\mathbf{u}_i^y\right)\right\}\Bigg], \end{aligned} \tag{7.A1}$$

where $\boldsymbol{\mu}_{k,\text{mis}}$ is the subvector of $\boldsymbol{\mu}_k$, $\boldsymbol{\Lambda}_{k,\text{mis}}$ and $\boldsymbol{\Psi}_{k,\text{mis}}$ are the submatrices of $\boldsymbol{\Lambda}_k$ and $\boldsymbol{\Psi}_k$ corresponding to $\mathbf{y}_{i,\text{mis}}$, respectively.

The full conditional distribution of $\mathbf{D}_{\text{mis}}$ is given by

$$p(\mathbf{D}_{\text{mis}}|\mathbf{R}^d, \mathbf{D}_{\text{obs}}, \boldsymbol{\Omega}, \mathbf{Z}, \boldsymbol{\theta}_*) = \prod_{i=1}^{n} p(\mathbf{d}_{i,\text{mis}}|\mathbf{r}_i^d, \mathbf{d}_{i,\text{obs}}, \boldsymbol{\omega}_i, z_i = k, \boldsymbol{\theta}_*), \text{ and}$$

$$\begin{aligned} &p(\mathbf{d}_{i,\text{mis}}|\mathbf{r}_i^d, \mathbf{d}_{i,\text{obs}}, \boldsymbol{\omega}_i, z_i = k, \boldsymbol{\theta}_*) \\ &\quad\propto p\left(\mathbf{r}_i^d|\mathbf{d}_i, z_i = k, \boldsymbol{\varphi}_{kd}\right) p(\boldsymbol{\eta}_i|\boldsymbol{\xi}_i, \mathbf{d}_i, z_i = k, \boldsymbol{\theta}_k) p(\mathbf{d}_{i,\text{mis}}|z_i = k, \boldsymbol{\tau}_{kd}) \\ &\quad\propto \exp\Bigg[-\frac{1}{2}(\boldsymbol{\eta}_i - \boldsymbol{\Lambda}_{\omega k}\mathbf{G}(\boldsymbol{\omega}_i))^T \boldsymbol{\Psi}_{\delta k}^{-1}(\boldsymbol{\eta}_i - \boldsymbol{\Lambda}_{\omega k}\mathbf{G}(\boldsymbol{\omega}_i)) \\ &\qquad + \left(\sum_{j=1}^{m_2} r_{ij}^d\right)\left(\boldsymbol{\varphi}_{kd}^T\mathbf{u}_i^d\right) - m_2\log\left\{1 + \exp\left(\boldsymbol{\varphi}_{kd}^T\mathbf{u}_i^d\right)\right\}\Bigg] \cdot p(\mathbf{d}_{i,\text{mis}}|\boldsymbol{\tau}_{kd}, z_i = k). \end{aligned} \tag{7.A2}$$

The full conditional distribution of $\mathbf{X}_{\text{mis}}$ is given by

$$p(\mathbf{X}_{\text{mis}}|\mathbf{R}^x, \mathbf{X}_{\text{obs}}, \mathbf{Z}, \boldsymbol{\theta}_*) = \prod_{i=1}^{n} p(\mathbf{x}_{i,\text{mis}}|\mathbf{r}_i^x, \mathbf{x}_{i,\text{obs}}, z_i, \boldsymbol{\theta}_*), \quad \text{and}$$

$$\begin{aligned} p\left(\mathbf{x}_{i,\text{mis}}|\mathbf{r}_i^x, \mathbf{x}_{i,\text{obs}}, z_i, \boldsymbol{\theta}_*\right) &\propto p(z_i|\boldsymbol{\tau}, \mathbf{x}_i) p\left(\mathbf{r}_i^x|\mathbf{x}_i, \boldsymbol{\varphi}_x\right) p(\mathbf{x}_i|\boldsymbol{\tau}_x) \\ &\propto \exp\Bigg[\boldsymbol{\tau}_{z_i}^T\mathbf{x}_i - \log\left\{\sum_{j=1}^{K}\exp\left(\boldsymbol{\tau}_j^T\mathbf{x}_i\right)\right\} + \left(\sum_{j=1}^{m_1} r_{ij}^x\right)\left(\boldsymbol{\varphi}_x^T\mathbf{u}_i^x\right) \\ &\quad - m_1\log\left\{1 + \exp\left(\boldsymbol{\varphi}_x^T\mathbf{u}_i^x\right)\right\}\Bigg] \cdot p(\mathbf{x}_i|\boldsymbol{\tau}_x). \end{aligned} \tag{7.A3}$$

The full conditional distribution of $\boldsymbol{\Omega}$ is given by

$$p(\boldsymbol{\Omega}|\mathbf{Y}, \mathbf{D}, \mathbf{Z}, \boldsymbol{\theta}_*) = \prod_{i=1}^{n} p(\boldsymbol{\omega}_i|\mathbf{y}_i, \mathbf{d}_i, z_i = k, \boldsymbol{\theta}_*), \quad \text{and}$$

$$\begin{aligned}
&p(\boldsymbol{\omega}_i|\mathbf{y}_i, \mathbf{d}_i, z_i = k, \boldsymbol{\theta}_*) \\
&\quad \propto p(\mathbf{y}_i|\boldsymbol{\omega}_i, z_i = k, \boldsymbol{\theta}_k) p(\boldsymbol{\eta}_i|\boldsymbol{\xi}_i, \mathbf{d}_i, z_i = k, \boldsymbol{\theta}_k) p(\boldsymbol{\xi}_i|z_i = k, \boldsymbol{\theta}_k) \\
&\quad \propto \exp\Big[-\frac{1}{2}(\mathbf{y}_i - \boldsymbol{\mu}_k - \boldsymbol{\Lambda}_k\boldsymbol{\omega}_i)^T \boldsymbol{\Psi}_k^{-1} (\mathbf{y}_i - \boldsymbol{\mu}_k - \boldsymbol{\Lambda}_k\boldsymbol{\omega}_i) \\
&\qquad -\frac{1}{2}(\boldsymbol{\eta}_i - \boldsymbol{\Lambda}_{\omega k}\mathbf{G}(\boldsymbol{\omega}_i))^T \boldsymbol{\Psi}_{\delta k}^{-1} (\boldsymbol{\eta}_i - \boldsymbol{\Lambda}_{\omega k}\mathbf{G}(\boldsymbol{\omega}_i)) - \frac{1}{2}\boldsymbol{\xi}_i^T \boldsymbol{\Phi}_k^{-1}\boldsymbol{\xi}_i \Big].
\end{aligned} \tag{7.A4}$$

The full conditional distribution of $\mathbf{Z}$ is given by

$$p(\mathbf{Z}|\mathbf{R}^y, \mathbf{R}^d, \mathbf{Y}, \boldsymbol{\Omega}, \mathbf{D}, \mathbf{X}, \boldsymbol{\theta}_*) = \prod_{i=1}^{n} p\left(z_i|\mathbf{r}_i^y, \mathbf{r}_i^d, \mathbf{y}_i, \boldsymbol{\omega}_i, \mathbf{d}_i, \mathbf{x}_i, \boldsymbol{\theta}_*\right), \text{ and}$$

$$p\left(z_i = k|\mathbf{r}_i^y, \mathbf{r}_i^d, \mathbf{y}_i, \boldsymbol{\omega}_i, \mathbf{d}_i, \mathbf{x}_i, \boldsymbol{\theta}_*\right) = \frac{\pi_{ik} p_k\left(\mathbf{r}_i^y, \mathbf{r}_i^d, \mathbf{y}_i, \boldsymbol{\omega}_i, \mathbf{d}_i|\boldsymbol{\theta}_k, \boldsymbol{\varphi}_{ky}, \boldsymbol{\varphi}_{kd}, \boldsymbol{\tau}_{kd}\right)}{\sum_{j=1}^{K} \pi_{ij} p_j\left(\mathbf{r}_i^y, \mathbf{r}_i^d, \mathbf{y}_i, \boldsymbol{\omega}_i, \mathbf{d}_i|\boldsymbol{\theta}_k, \boldsymbol{\varphi}_{ky}, \boldsymbol{\varphi}_{kd}, \boldsymbol{\tau}_{kd}\right)}, \tag{7.A5}$$

where π_{ik} is defined in (7.23) and $p_k(\mathbf{r}_i^y, \mathbf{r}_i^d, \mathbf{y}_i, \boldsymbol{\omega}_i, \mathbf{d}_i|\boldsymbol{\theta}_k, \boldsymbol{\varphi}_{ky}, \boldsymbol{\varphi}_{kd}, \boldsymbol{\tau}_{kd})$ is given as follows:

$$\begin{aligned}
&\log p_k(\mathbf{r}_i^y, \mathbf{r}_i^d, \mathbf{y}_i, \boldsymbol{\omega}_i, \mathbf{d}_i|\boldsymbol{\theta}_k, \boldsymbol{\varphi}_{ky}, \boldsymbol{\varphi}_{kd}, \boldsymbol{\tau}_{kd}) \\
&= \left(\sum_{j=1}^{p} r_{ij}^y\right)\left(\boldsymbol{\varphi}_{ky}^T\mathbf{u}_i^y\right) - p\log\left\{1 + \exp\left(\boldsymbol{\varphi}_{ky}^T\mathbf{u}_i^y\right)\right\} - \frac{1}{2}(\mathbf{y}_i - \boldsymbol{\mu}_k - \boldsymbol{\Lambda}_k\boldsymbol{\omega}_i)^T \boldsymbol{\Psi}_k^{-1}(\mathbf{y}_i - \boldsymbol{\mu}_k - \boldsymbol{\Lambda}_k\boldsymbol{\omega}_i) \\
&\quad -\frac{1}{2}(\boldsymbol{\eta}_i - \boldsymbol{\Lambda}_{\omega k}\mathbf{G}(\boldsymbol{\omega}_i))^T \boldsymbol{\Psi}_{\delta k}^{-1}(\boldsymbol{\eta}_i - \boldsymbol{\Lambda}_{\omega k}\mathbf{G}(\boldsymbol{\omega}_i)) - \frac{1}{2}\boldsymbol{\xi}_i^T \boldsymbol{\Phi}_k^{-1}\boldsymbol{\xi}_i \\
&\quad + \left(\sum_{j=1}^{m_2} r_{ij}^d\right)\left(\boldsymbol{\varphi}_{kd}^T\mathbf{u}_i^d\right) - m_2\log\left\{1 + \exp\left(\boldsymbol{\varphi}_{kd}^T\mathbf{u}_i^d\right)\right\} + \log p(\mathbf{d}_i|\boldsymbol{\tau}_{kd}, z_i = k) \\
&\quad -\frac{1}{2}\big\{\log|\boldsymbol{\Psi}_k| + \log|\boldsymbol{\Psi}_{\delta k}| + \log|\boldsymbol{\Phi}_k| + (p+q)\log(2\pi)\big\}.
\end{aligned}$$

The full conditional distribution of $\boldsymbol{\theta}$ is as follows. Let $\boldsymbol{\Omega}_1 = (\boldsymbol{\eta}_1, \ldots, \boldsymbol{\eta}_n)$, $\boldsymbol{\Omega}_2 = (\boldsymbol{\xi}_1, \ldots, \boldsymbol{\xi}_n)$, and $\mathbf{G} = (\mathbf{G}(\boldsymbol{\omega}_1), \ldots, \mathbf{G}(\boldsymbol{\omega}_n))$. Further, let $\mathbf{Y}_k$, $\boldsymbol{\Omega}_k$, $\boldsymbol{\Omega}_{1k}$, $\boldsymbol{\Omega}_{2k}$, and $\mathbf{G}_k$ be the submatrices of $\mathbf{Y}$, $\boldsymbol{\Omega}$, $\boldsymbol{\Omega}_1$, $\boldsymbol{\Omega}_2$, and $\mathbf{G}$ respectively such that all the ith columns with $z_i \neq k$ are deleted. Under the conjugate prior distributions in (7.31), it can be shown that the full conditional distributions of components of $\boldsymbol{\theta}_k$ are:

$$[\boldsymbol{\mu}_k|\cdot] \stackrel{D}{=} N\left[\left(\boldsymbol{\Sigma}_{0k}^{-1} + n_k\boldsymbol{\Psi}_k^{-1}\right)^{-1}\left(n_k\boldsymbol{\Psi}_k^{-1}\bar{\mathbf{Y}}_k + \boldsymbol{\Sigma}_{0k}^{-1}\boldsymbol{\mu}_{0k}\right), \left(\boldsymbol{\Sigma}_{0k}^{-1} + n_k\boldsymbol{\Psi}_k^{-1}\right)^{-1}\right],$$

$$[\boldsymbol{\Lambda}_{kj}|\cdot] \stackrel{D}{=} N\left[\tilde{\boldsymbol{\Lambda}}_{kj}^*, \psi_{kj}\mathbf{H}_{kj}^*\right], \quad \left[\psi_{kj}^{-1}|\cdot\right] \stackrel{D}{=} \text{Gamma}\left[n_k/2 + \alpha_{0kj}, \beta_{kj}^*\right],$$

$$[\boldsymbol{\Lambda}_{\omega kl}|\cdot] \stackrel{D}{=} N\left[\tilde{\boldsymbol{\Lambda}}_{\omega kl}^*, \psi_{\delta kl}\tilde{\mathbf{H}}_{kl}^*\right], \quad \left[\psi_{\delta kl}^{-1}|\cdot\right] \stackrel{D}{=} \text{Gamma}\left[n_k/2 + \tilde{\alpha}_{0kl}, \tilde{\beta}_{kl}^*\right],$$

$$[\boldsymbol{\Phi}_k|\cdot] \stackrel{D}{=} \text{IW}_{q_2}\left[\left(\boldsymbol{\Omega}_{2k}\boldsymbol{\Omega}_{2k}^T + \mathbf{V}_{0k}^{-1}\right), n_k + \rho_{0k}\right],$$

where $n_k = \sum_{i=1}^n I(z_i = k)$, in which $I(\cdot)$ is an indicator function, $\bar{\mathbf{Y}}_k = \sum_{i,z_i=k}(\mathbf{y}_i - \boldsymbol{\Lambda}_k\boldsymbol{\omega}_i)/n_k$, and

$$\tilde{\boldsymbol{\Lambda}}_{kj}^* = \mathbf{H}_{kj}^*\left[\mathbf{H}_{0kj}^{-1}\boldsymbol{\Lambda}_{0kj} + \boldsymbol{\Omega}_k\mathbf{Y}_{kj}^*\right], \quad \mathbf{H}_{kj}^* = \left(\mathbf{H}_{0kj}^{-1} + \boldsymbol{\Omega}_k\boldsymbol{\Omega}_k^T\right)^{-1},$$

$$\beta_{kj}^* = \beta_{0kj} + \left[\mathbf{Y}_{kj}^{*T}\mathbf{Y}_{kj}^* - \tilde{\boldsymbol{\Lambda}}_{kj}^{*T}\mathbf{H}_{kj}^{*-1}\tilde{\boldsymbol{\Lambda}}_{kj}^* + \boldsymbol{\Lambda}_{0kj}^T\mathbf{H}_{0kj}^{-1}\boldsymbol{\Lambda}_{0kj}\right]\Big/2,$$

$$\tilde{\boldsymbol{\Lambda}}_{\omega kl}^* = \tilde{\mathbf{H}}_{kl}^*\left[\tilde{\mathbf{H}}_{0kl}^{-1}\tilde{\boldsymbol{\Lambda}}_{0kl} + \mathbf{G}_k\boldsymbol{\Omega}_{1kl}\right], \quad \tilde{\mathbf{H}}_{kl}^* = \left(\tilde{\mathbf{H}}_{0kl}^{-1} + \mathbf{G}_k\mathbf{G}_k^T\right)^{-1},$$

$$\tilde{\beta}_{kl}^* = \tilde{\beta}_{0kl} + \left[\boldsymbol{\Omega}_{1kl}^T\boldsymbol{\Omega}_{1kl} - \tilde{\boldsymbol{\Lambda}}_{\omega kl}^{*T}\tilde{\mathbf{H}}_{kl}^{*-1}\tilde{\boldsymbol{\Lambda}}_{\omega kl}^* + \tilde{\boldsymbol{\Lambda}}_{0kl}^T\tilde{\mathbf{H}}_{0kl}^{-1}\tilde{\boldsymbol{\Lambda}}_{0kl}\right]\Big/2,$$

where $\mathbf{Y}_{kj}^{*T}$ is the jth row of $\mathbf{Y}_k^*$ which is a matrix whose columns are equal to the columns of $\mathbf{Y}_k$ minus $\boldsymbol{\mu}_k$, and $\boldsymbol{\Omega}_{1kl}^T$ is the lth row of $\boldsymbol{\Omega}_{1k}$.

The full conditional distribution of $\boldsymbol{\varphi}_y$ is given by

$$p(\boldsymbol{\varphi}_{ky}|\mathbf{R}^y, \mathbf{Y}, \mathbf{Z}) \propto \left\{\prod_{i,z_i=k} p\left(\mathbf{r}_i^y|\mathbf{y}_i, \boldsymbol{\varphi}_{ky}\right)\right\}p(\boldsymbol{\varphi}_{ky}) \propto \tag{7.A6}$$

$$\exp\left[\sum_{i,z_i=k}\left\{\left(\sum_{j=1}^p r_{ij}^y\right)\left(\boldsymbol{\varphi}_{ky}^T\mathbf{u}_i^y\right) - p\log\left(1 + \exp\left(\boldsymbol{\varphi}_{ky}^T\mathbf{u}_i^y\right)\right)\right\} - \frac{1}{2}(\boldsymbol{\varphi}_{ky} - \boldsymbol{\varphi}_{0ky})^T\boldsymbol{\Sigma}_{0ky}^{-1}(\boldsymbol{\varphi}_{ky} - \boldsymbol{\varphi}_{0ky})\right].$$

The full conditional distribution of $\boldsymbol{\varphi}_d$ is given by

$$p(\boldsymbol{\varphi}_{kd}|\mathbf{R}^d, \mathbf{D}, \mathbf{Z}) \propto \left\{\prod_{i,z_i=k} p\left(\mathbf{r}_i^d|\mathbf{d}_i, \boldsymbol{\varphi}_{kd}\right)\right\}p(\boldsymbol{\varphi}_{kd}) \propto \tag{7.A7}$$

$$\exp\left[\sum_{i,z_i=k}\left\{\left(\sum_{j=1}^{m_2} r_{ij}^d\right)\left(\boldsymbol{\varphi}_{kd}^T\mathbf{u}_i^d\right) - m_2\log\left(1 + \exp\left(\boldsymbol{\varphi}_{kd}^T\mathbf{u}_i^d\right)\right)\right\} - \frac{1}{2}(\boldsymbol{\varphi}_{kd} - \boldsymbol{\varphi}_{0kd})^T\boldsymbol{\Sigma}_{0kd}^{-1}(\boldsymbol{\varphi}_{kd} - \boldsymbol{\varphi}_{0kd})\right].$$

The full conditional distribution of $\boldsymbol{\varphi}_x$ is given by

$$p(\boldsymbol{\varphi}_x|\mathbf{R}^x, \mathbf{X}) \propto \left\{\prod_{i=1}^n p\left(\mathbf{r}_i^x|\mathbf{x}_i, \boldsymbol{\varphi}_x\right)\right\}p(\boldsymbol{\varphi}_x) \propto \tag{7.A8}$$

$$\exp\left[\sum_{i=1}^n\left\{\left(\sum_{j=1}^{m_1} r_{ij}^x\right)\left(\boldsymbol{\varphi}_x^T\mathbf{u}_i^x\right) - m_1\log(1 + \exp\left(\boldsymbol{\varphi}_x^T\mathbf{u}_i^x\right))\right\} - \frac{1}{2}(\boldsymbol{\varphi}_x - \boldsymbol{\varphi}_{0x})^T\boldsymbol{\Sigma}_{0x}^{-1}(\boldsymbol{\varphi}_x - \boldsymbol{\varphi}_{0x})\right].$$

Finally, the full conditional distribution of $\boldsymbol{\tau}$ is given by

$$p(\boldsymbol{\tau}_k|\mathbf{Z}, \mathbf{X}, \boldsymbol{\tau}_{-k}) \propto p(\mathbf{Z}|\boldsymbol{\tau}, \mathbf{X})p(\boldsymbol{\tau}_k) = \left\{\prod_{i=1}^{n} p(z_i|\boldsymbol{\tau}, \mathbf{x}_i)\right\} p(\boldsymbol{\tau}_k)$$
$$\propto \left\{\prod_{i=1}^{n} \frac{\exp\left(\boldsymbol{\tau}_{z_i}^T \mathbf{x}_i\right)}{\sum_{j=1}^{K} \exp\left(\boldsymbol{\tau}_j^T \mathbf{x}_i\right)}\right\} \exp\left\{-\frac{1}{2}(\boldsymbol{\tau}_k - \boldsymbol{\mu}_{0k\tau})^T \boldsymbol{\Sigma}_{0k\tau}^{-1}(\boldsymbol{\tau}_k - \boldsymbol{\mu}_{0k\tau})\right\}, \tag{7.A9}$$

where $\boldsymbol{\tau}_{-k}$ is $\boldsymbol{\tau}$ with $\boldsymbol{\tau}_k$ deleted.

The full conditional distributions in (7.A1)–(7.A9) are nonstandard; we will use the MH algorithm to simulate observations from them. The full conditional distributions of $\boldsymbol{\tau}_x$ and $\boldsymbol{\tau}_d$ depend on their prior distributions and the distributions of $\mathbf{x}_i$ and $\mathbf{d}_i$, respectively; they can be easily derived on a problem-by-problem basis.

References

Arminger, G., Stein, P. and Wittenberg, J. (1999) Mixtures of conditional mean- and covariance-structure models. *Psychometrika*, **64**, 475–494.

Cai, J. H., Song, X. Y. and Hser, Y. I. (2010) A Bayesian analysis of mixture structural equation models with nonignorable missing responses and covariates. *Statistics in Medicine*, **29**, 1861–1874.

Celeux, G., Forbes, F., Robert, C. P. and Titterington, D. M. (2006) Deviance information criteria for missing data models. *Bayesian Analysis*, **1**, 651–674.

Diebolt, J. and Robert, C. P. (1994) Estimation of finite mixture distributions through Bayesian sampling. *Journal of the Royal Statistical Society, Series B*, **56**, 363–375.

Dolan, C. V. and van der Maas, H. L. J. (1998) Fitting multivariage normal finite mixtures subject to structural equation modeling. *Psychometrika*, **63**, 227–253.

Elliott, M. R., Gallo, J. J., Ten Have, T. R., Bogner, H. R. and Katz, I. R. (2005) Using a Bayesian latent growth curve model to identify trajectories of positive affect and negative events following myocardial infarction, *Biostatistics*, **6**, 119–143.

Frühwirth-Schnatter, S. (2001) Markov chain Monte Carlo estimation of classical and dynamic switching and mixture models. *Journal of the American Statistical Association*, **96**, 194–209.

Geman, S. and Geman, D. (1984) Stochastic relaxation, Gibbs distributions, and the Bayesian restoration of images. *IEEE Transactions on Pattern Analysis and Machine Intelligence*, **6**, 721–741.

Guo, J., Wall, M. and Amemiya, Y. (2006) Latent class regression on latent factors. *Biostatistics*, **7**, 145–163.

Hastings, W. K. (1970) Monte Carlo sampling methods using Markov chains and their applications. *Biometrika*, **57**, 97–109.

Hathaway, R. J. (1985) A constrained formulation of maximum-likelihood estimation for normal mixture distributions. *Annals of Statistics*, **13**, 795–800.

Ibrahim, J. G., Chen, M. H. and Lipsitz, S. R. (2001) Missing responses in generalised linear mixed models when the missing data mechanism is nonignorable. *Biometrika*, **88**, 551–564.

Jedidi, K., Jagpal, H. S. and DeSarbo, W. S. (1997) STEMM: A general finite mixture structural equation model. *Journal of Classification*, **14**, 23–50.

Kass, R. E. and Raftery, A. E. (1995) Bayes factors. *Journal of the American Statistical Association*, **90**, 773–795.

Lee, S. Y. (2007a) *Structural Equation Modeling: A Bayesian Approach*. Chichester: John Wiley & Sons, Ltd.

Lee, S. Y. (2007b) Bayesian analysis of mixtures structural equation models with missing data. In S. Y. Lee (ed.), *Handbook of Latent Variable and Related Models*. Amsterdam: Elsevier.

Lee, S. Y. and Song, X. Y. (2002) Bayesian selection on the number of factors in a factor analysis model. *Behaviormetrika*, **29**, 23–39.

Lee, S. Y. and Song, X. Y. (2003) Bayesian model selection for mixtures of structural equation models with an unknown number of components. *British Journal of Mathematical and Statistical Psychology*, **56**, 145–165.

Lindley, D. V. and Smith, A. F. M. (1972) Bayes estimates for the linear model (with discussion). *Journal of the Royal Statistical Society, Series B*, **34**, 1–41.

Lindsay, B. G. and Basak, P. (1993) Multivariate normal mixtures: A fast consistent method of moments. *Journal of the American Statistical Association*, **88**, 468–476.

Metropolis, N., Rosenbluth, A. W., Rosenbluth, M. N., Teller, A. H. and Teller, E. (1953) Equation of state calculations by fast computing machines. *Journal of Chemical Physics*, **21**, 1087–1092.

Muthén, B. and Shedden, K. (1999) Finite mixture modeling with mixture outcomes using the EM algorithm. *Biometrics*, **55**, 463–469.

Pettit, L. I. and Smith, A. F. M. (1985) Outliers and influential observations in linear models. In J. M. Bernardo *et al.* (eds), *Bayesian Statistics 2*, pp. 473–494. Amsterdam: Elsevier.

Richardson, S. and Green, P. J. (1997) On Bayesian analysis of mixtures with an unknown number of components (with discussion). *Journal of the Royal Statistical Society, Series B*, **59**, 731–792.

Robert, C. P. (1996) Mixtures of distributions: Inference and estimation. In W. R. Gilks, S. Richardson and D. J. Spiegelhalter (eds), *Markov Chain Monte Carlo in Practice*, pp. 441–464. London: Chapman & Hall.

Roeder, K. and Wasserman, L. (1997) Practical Bayesian density estimation using mixtures of normals. *Journal of the American Statistical Association*, **92**, 894–902.

Song, X. Y. and Lee, S. Y. (2007) Bayesian analysis of latent variable models with non-ignorable missing outcomes from exponential family. *Statistics in Medicine*, **26**, 681–693.

Spiegelhalter, D. J., Best, N. G., Carlin, B. P. and van der Linde, A. (2002) Bayesian measures of model complexity and fit (with discussion). *Journal of the Royal Statistical Society, Series B*, **64**, 583–639.

Spiegelhalter, D. J., Thomas, A., Best, N. G. and Lunn, D. (2003) *WinBUGS User Manual. Version 1.4*. Cambridge: MRC Biostatistics Unit.

Yung, Y. F. (1997) Finite mixtures in confirmatory factor-analysis models. *Psychometrika*, **62**, 297–330.

Zhu, H. T. and Lee, S. Y. (2001) A Bayesian analysis of finite mixtures in the LISREL model. *Psychometrika*, **66**, 133–152.

8

Structural equation modeling for latent curve models

8.1 Introduction

Latent curve models (LCMs) are popular longitudinal methods in the analysis of individual differences in the patterns of change, which usually involves a random intercept and a random slope (they are grouped as a latent growth factor) with each pair forming a different trajectory over time. LCM techniques have been developed via the incorporation of many features of structural equation models; see Meredith and Tisak (1990), and Bollen and Curran (2006). For instance, the random intercept and slope are respectively considered as latent variables representing initial status and rate of change of the outcome variable. In this way, SEM techniques provide powerful tools for developing more useful LCMs for analyzing complex dynamic changes. In this chapter we introduce the basic LCM and some of its extensions, for example the LCM involving second-order latent variables (Jöreskog, 1970) with ordered categorical variables. Again, Bayesian methods that utilize data augmentation and MCMC methods are introduced to analyze the LCMs. Two real longitudinal studies are presented to illustrate the Bayesian methodologies. One is about the health-related quality of life of stroke survivors, and the other relates to a longitudinal study of cocaine use.

This chapter is organized as follows. The backgrounds of the aforementioned real studies are described in Section 8.2. Some LCMs are described in Section 8.3, using the longitudinal study of cocaine use as an illustrative example. The Bayesian approach is presented in Section 8.4. Section 8.5 provides the Bayesian analyses of the two real studies. Finally, Section 8.6 introduces some other extensions of the basic LCM.

Basic and Advanced Bayesian Structural Equation Modeling: With Applications in the Medical and Behavioral Sciences,
First Edition. Xin-Yuan Song and Sik-Yum Lee.

8.2 Background to the real studies

8.2.1 A longitudinal study of quality of life of stroke survivors

Stroke is a major health issue in the older population as it not only affects physical impairment but also leads to disability with regard to activities of daily living (ADL), social nonparticipation (handicap), and depression. Such changes have a substantial influence on health-related quality of life (HRQOL) of stroke survivors. Analyses of the dynamic changes in HRQOL of stroke survivors and the associated factors of these changes have received much attention in the field. Ahlsiö *et al.* (1984) found that even though HRQOL was associated with greater disability, it failed to improve over time even when ADL function increased. Kwok *et al.* (2006) found that the environment and social interaction domains of HRQOL decreased during the first year after a stroke, and depression had a more generalized adverse effect on HRQOL than basic functional disabilities. Moreover, they observed that ADL, including instrumental ADL, remained stable, while the occupation and orientation domains of handicap, and depression deteriorated. In order to examine the relative importance of the above mentioned interrelated factors in determining HRQOL in the first year after a stroke, we will apply a dynamic LCM to study how changes in HRQOL relate to changes in ADL, handicap, and depression. The results may help steer the development of appropriate interventions to promote the HRQOL of stroke survivors.

Data were obtained from patients with acute stroke within 2 days of admission, and at follow-up 3, 6, and 12 months after stroke. Outcome measures obtained from questionnaires included the modified Barthel Index (MBI) score (Shah *et al.*, 1989), Geriatric Depression Scale (GDS) score (Chiu *et al.*, 1994), the abbreviated Hong Kong version of World Health Organization Quality of Life measure (WHOQOL BREF (HK)) score, and the London Handicap Scale (LHS) score (Harwood *et al.*, 1994). Patients' ADL were assessed through the MBI, which is a good measurement instrument in terms of reliability and validity, and has been already applied to most studies of stroke as the measure of functional status. The MBI has 10 items on activities of daily living. A total score of up to 20 indicates full independence in ADL; a higher score represents a higher level of independence. Post-stroke depression was measured using the GDS, which has 15 items. A score of 8 or more indicates depression. The HRQOL data set comprises 24 items covering four domains: physical health (PHY), psychological health (PSY), social interaction (SO), and environment (EN). The stroke survivors are required to respond to the items on a five-point Likert scale in which the categories range from 'Not at all' (scored 1) to 'An extreme amount' (scored 5). The domain scores are converted by normogram to 100% score. Finally, handicap is defined as the disadvantage brought on by impairment and disabilities experienced by an individual, taking into account the influence of physical and psychological effects of a disease, the physical and social environment, and the effects of health service provisions. The most applied generic measure of handicap in stroke survivors is the LHS. It consists of six questions measuring the levels of handicap (scores ranging from 1 to 6) on six dimensions including mobility, independence, occupation, social integration, orientation, and economic self-sufficiency. A higher score indicates a greater handicap. The stroke survivors were requested to mark the response that best describes their situations. The total score of all six domains was used to indicate overall handicap level. Recognizing that MBI, LHS, and GDS could change over time, LCMs are used to assess how the changes in these variables influence the growth of each of the four HRQOL domains at three time points.

8.2.2 A longitudinal study of cocaine use

Cocaine use is a major social and health problem in many countries, and as such it is interesting to study the dynamic influences of various latent variables on the dynamic change in cocaine use. In the literature on cocaine use, many studies have shown that psychiatric problems have a substantial impact on cocaine use (Brown *et al.*, 1998; Hser *et al.*, 2006). Moreover, the treatment of a cocaine patient and family support are other important influences on cocaine use. To gain a better understanding of the these issues, the UCLA Center for Advancing Longitudinal Drug Abuse Research collected various measures from patients admitted in 1988–1989 to the West Los Angeles Veterans Affairs Medical Center and met the DSM III-R criteria for cocaine dependence (Kasarabada *et al.*, 1999). These patients were assessed at baseline, 1 year after treatment, 2 years after treatment, and 12 years after treatment in 2002 ($t = 1, 2, 3, 4$). Measures at each time point include the number of days of cocaine use per month (CC), times per month in formal treatment (TR), Beck Inventory (BI), depression (DEP), anxiety (AN), and family support (FS), where CC, TR, BI, DEP, and AN are continuous, while FS is ordered categorical on a three-point scale. Since some patients were confirmed to be deceased, some declined to be interviewed, and some were out of the country, there is a considerable amount of missing data. In order to efficiently analyze the data, it is necessary to take into account the following features in developing LCMs and associated statistical methods.

Firstly, we consider an LCM based on cocaine use measured at $t = 1, \ldots, 4$ with a latent variable η_1 on initial status (intercept) of cocaine use, and a latent variable η_2 on rate of change (slope) of cocaine use. Another LCM is considered on the basis of TR measured at $t = 1, \ldots, 4$ with latent variables ξ_{11} and ξ_{21} on the initial status of TR and the rate of change of TR, respectively. The effects of $\{\xi_{11}, \xi_{21}\}$ on $\{\eta_1, \eta_2\}$ can be assessed through a simple structural equation. Similarly, we consider one more LCM based on FS measured at $t = 1 \ldots, 4$, and obtain the initial status of FS (ξ_{12}) and rate of change of FS (ξ_{22}) via growth curve modeling. The effects of $\{\xi_{12}, \xi_{22}\}$ together with $\{\xi_{11}, \xi_{21}\}$ on $\{\eta_1, \eta_2\}$ are assessed by incorporating them into a structural equation. Based on the same rationale, we can first obtain latent variables (intercept, slope) based on the measures of DEP at each time point, and then assess the effects of these latent variables on $\{\eta_1, \eta_2\}$. However, with the inclusion of BI and AN, we are interested not only in DEP, but also in a latent variable 'psychiatric problems (PP)' that should be assessed by three observed variables BI, DEP, and AN. Hence, at each time point we first use a measurement equation to group BI, DEP, and AN into the latent variable PP, then construct an LCM on the basis of PP at $t = 1, \ldots, 4$ to obtain the initial status of PP (ξ_{13}) and rate of change of PP (ξ_{23}). Here, we call a latent variable obtained from several observed variables a 'first-order latent variable' (e.g. $\eta_1, \eta_2, \xi_{11}, \xi_{21}, \xi_{12}, \xi_{22}$, PP); and call a latent variable obtained from several latent variables (e.g. ξ_{13}, ξ_{23}) a 'second-order latent variable' (see Jöreskog, 1970). Hence, it is desirable to establish a comprehensive LCM that accommodates the effects of both first- and second-order latent variables on the growth factors of the outcome variables.

Secondly, as pointed out by Li *et al.* (2000), it is important to include the interaction of latent variables in assessing the joint effect of dynamic latent variables. Hence, the LCM accommodates a nonlinear structural equation which subsumes polynomials (including interaction and higher-order terms) of the first- and second-order latent variables.

Thirdly, the LCM accommodates mixed continuous and ordered categorical data, which are very common in practice.

Finally, the LCM accommodates missing data, which are very common in longitudinal studies.

8.3 Latent curve models

8.3.1 Basic latent curve models

The basic latent curve model (see Meredith and Tisak, 1990; Bollen and Curran, 2006) can be viewed as the following common factor analysis model:

$$\mathbf{y} = \boldsymbol{\Lambda}\boldsymbol{\eta} + \boldsymbol{\epsilon}_y, \tag{8.1}$$

where $\mathbf{y}$ is a $T \times 1$ vector of repeated measures, $\boldsymbol{\Lambda}$ is a $T \times m$ parameter matrix of sequential fixed values of the growth curve records, $\boldsymbol{\eta}$ is an $m \times 1$ outcome latent growth factor which contains scores on the m factors for a given individual, and $\boldsymbol{\epsilon}_y$ is a $T \times 1$ vector of residual errors. The pattern of $\boldsymbol{\Lambda}$ can be interpreted as representing a particular aspect of change in y across the T occasions. It is assumed that $\boldsymbol{\epsilon}_y$ is distributed as $N[\mathbf{0}, \boldsymbol{\Psi}_y]$, where $\boldsymbol{\Psi}_y$ is a diagonal matrix with diagonal elements ψ_{yt}, for $t = 1, \ldots, T$. When $m = 2$, equation (8.1) is expressed in the following matrix form:

$$\begin{pmatrix} y_1 \\ y_2 \\ \vdots \\ y_T \end{pmatrix} = \begin{pmatrix} 1 & t_1 \\ 1 & t_2 \\ \vdots & \vdots \\ 1 & t_T \end{pmatrix} \begin{pmatrix} \eta_1 \\ \eta_2 \end{pmatrix} + \begin{pmatrix} \epsilon_{y1} \\ \epsilon_{y2} \\ \vdots \\ \epsilon_{yT} \end{pmatrix}. \tag{8.2}$$

The first column in $\boldsymbol{\Lambda}$ can be used to define an intercept factor, which represents an initial status of change in y. The second column in $\boldsymbol{\Lambda}$ represents the known times of measurement $(t_1, \ldots, t_T)$ and constraints (the values of t should reflect the spacing between measurement occasions), and the latent growth factor $\boldsymbol{\eta}$ contains the initial status η_1 (intercept) and rate of change η_2 (slope). The two-factor linear LCM is specified in (8.2) so that the intercept factor (fixed at a constant value of 1) serves as the starting point (initial status) for any change (growth) across time and the slope factor captures the rate of change of the trajectory over time. The scaling of the slope can be specified by using either fixed value restrictions (e.g. $0, 1, \ldots, T-1$) representing a straight-line growth, or unspecified value restrictions (where $t_1 = 0$ and $t_2 = 1$ are fixed for model identification, and the remaining $t_3, \ldots, t_T$ are freely estimated) allowing estimation of an optimal pattern of change over measurement occasions (Meredith and Tisak, 1990).

The equation for the latent growth factor $\boldsymbol{\eta}$ can be simply written as

$$\boldsymbol{\eta} = \boldsymbol{\beta} + \boldsymbol{\Pi}\boldsymbol{\eta} + \boldsymbol{\delta}, \tag{8.3}$$

where $\boldsymbol{\beta}$ is an $m \times 1$ vector of the population average of the latent individual growth factors, $\boldsymbol{\Pi}$ is an $m \times m$ matrix of coefficients expressing the structural relations between the $\boldsymbol{\eta}$ variables, and $\boldsymbol{\delta}$ is an $m \times 1$ vector of random residuals.

To illustrate the model framework, we use the example in the longitudinal study of cocaine use across four measurement occasions. Let $\mathbf{y} = (y_1, y_2, y_3, y_4)^T$, and $\boldsymbol{\Pi} = \mathbf{0}$. Then equations

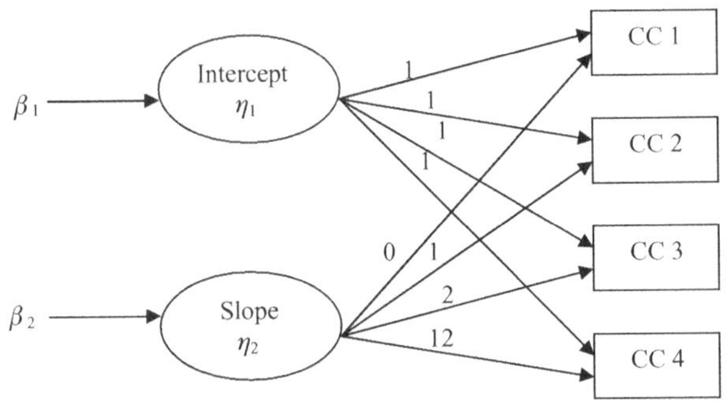

Figure 8.1 Path diagram of the model defined in (8.4) and (8.5). In all path diagrams in this chapter, error terms are omitted for brevity. Reproduced by permission of Taylor & Francis from Song, X. Y., Lee, S. Y. and Hser, Y. I. (2009). Bayesian analysis of multivariate latent curve models with nonlinear longitudinal latent effects. *Structural Equation Modeling – A Multidisciplinary Journal*, **16**, 245–266.

(8.2) and (8.3) can be expressed in the following form to represent the model in Figure 8.1:

$$\begin{pmatrix} y_1 \\ y_2 \\ y_3 \\ y_4 \end{pmatrix} = \begin{pmatrix} 1 & 0 \\ 1 & 1 \\ 1 & 2 \\ 1 & 12 \end{pmatrix} \begin{pmatrix} \eta_1 \\ \eta_2 \end{pmatrix} + \begin{pmatrix} \epsilon_{y1} \\ \epsilon_{y2} \\ \epsilon_{y3} \\ \epsilon_{y4} \end{pmatrix}, \tag{8.4}$$

$$\begin{pmatrix} \eta_1 \\ \eta_2 \end{pmatrix} = \begin{pmatrix} \beta_1 \\ \beta_2 \end{pmatrix} + \begin{pmatrix} \delta_1 \\ \delta_2 \end{pmatrix}. \tag{8.5}$$

The four measurement occasions are 1989 (baseline), 1990 (1 year after treatment), 1991 (2 years after treatment), and 2002 (12 years after treatment). Thus, the fixed times of measurement t_1, t_2, t_3, and t_4 are set to 0, 1, 2, and 12 to reflect the spacing between measurement occasions.

8.3.2 Latent curve models with explanatory latent variables

The previous model can be extended to include the following explanatory latent growth factors:

$$\begin{pmatrix} \mathbf{x}_1 \\ \mathbf{x}_2 \\ \vdots \\ \mathbf{x}_r \end{pmatrix} = \begin{pmatrix} \mathbf{\Lambda} & \mathbf{0} & \cdots & \mathbf{0} \\ \mathbf{0} & \mathbf{\Lambda} & \cdots & \mathbf{0} \\ \vdots & \vdots & \ddots & \vdots \\ \mathbf{0} & \mathbf{0} & \cdots & \mathbf{\Lambda} \end{pmatrix} \begin{pmatrix} \boldsymbol{\xi}_1 \\ \boldsymbol{\xi}_2 \\ \vdots \\ \boldsymbol{\xi}_r \end{pmatrix} + \begin{pmatrix} \boldsymbol{\epsilon}_{x1} \\ \boldsymbol{\epsilon}_{x2} \\ \vdots \\ \boldsymbol{\epsilon}_{xr} \end{pmatrix}, \tag{8.6}$$

where $\mathbf{0}$ is a $T \times m$ matrix with elements 0. For $k = 1, \ldots, r$, $\boldsymbol{\xi}_k$ is the kth latent growth factor that includes growth parameters (e.g. intercept, slope), $\mathbf{x}_k$ and $\boldsymbol{\epsilon}_{xk}$ are defined similarly to $\mathbf{y}$ and $\boldsymbol{\epsilon}_y$, and $\mathbf{\Lambda}$ is defined similarly to equation (8.1). It is assumed that $\boldsymbol{\epsilon}_{xk}$ is distributed as $N[\mathbf{0}, \mathbf{\Psi}_{xk}]$, where $\mathbf{\Psi}_{xk}$ is a diagonal matrix with diagonal elements $\psi_{x1k}, \ldots, \psi_{xTk}$. The latent growth factors $\boldsymbol{\xi}_k$ ($k = 1, \ldots, r$) are the first-order explanatory latent variables.

In the cocaine use data, the key outcome variable is 'cocaine use' (CC), and η_1 and η_2 are the latent growth parameters where η_1 (intercept) specifies the initial status of individual

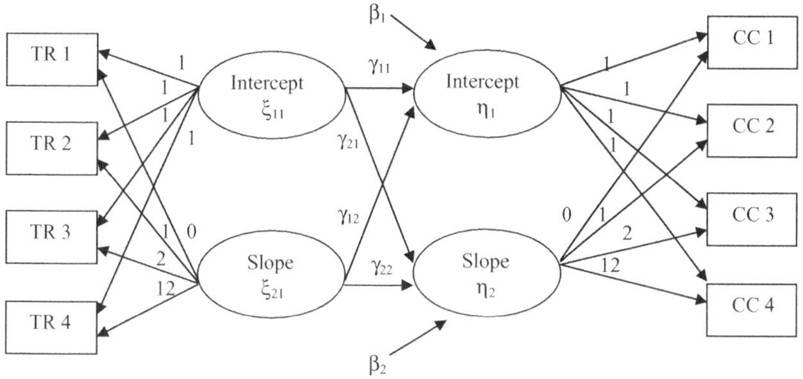

Figure 8.2 Path diagram of the model defined in (8.4), (8.7), and (8.8). Reproduced by permission of Taylor & Francis from Song, X. Y., Lee, S. Y. and Hser, Y. I. (2009). Bayesian analysis of multivariate latent curve models with nonlinear longitudinal latent effects. *Structural Equation Modeling – A Multidisciplinary Journal*, **16**, 245–266.

growth and η_2 (slope) specifies the rate of change over the four measurement time points. Let $\mathbf{x}_1 = (x_{11}, x_{21}, x_{31}, x_{41})^T$ be a vector of treatment measured at four time occasions, and $\boldsymbol{\xi}_1 = (\xi_{11}, \xi_{21})^T$ such that

$$\begin{pmatrix} x_{11} \\ x_{21} \\ x_{31} \\ x_{41} \end{pmatrix} = \begin{pmatrix} 1 & 0 \\ 1 & 1 \\ 1 & 2 \\ 1 & 12 \end{pmatrix} \begin{pmatrix} \xi_{11} \\ \xi_{21} \end{pmatrix} + \begin{pmatrix} \epsilon_{x11} \\ \epsilon_{x21} \\ \epsilon_{x31} \\ \epsilon_{x41} \end{pmatrix}. \tag{8.7}$$

The growth factor in relation to treatment, $\boldsymbol{\xi}_1$, can be regarded as an explanatory latent growth factor with intercept (ξ_{11}) and slope (ξ_{21}). The LCM with this explanatory latent growth factor can be expressed by equations (8.4), (8.7), and

$$\begin{pmatrix} \eta_1 \\ \eta_2 \end{pmatrix} = \begin{pmatrix} \beta_1 \\ \beta_2 \end{pmatrix} + \begin{pmatrix} \gamma_{11} & \gamma_{12} \\ \gamma_{21} & \gamma_{22} \end{pmatrix} \begin{pmatrix} \xi_{11} \\ \xi_{21} \end{pmatrix} + \begin{pmatrix} \delta_1 \\ \delta_2 \end{pmatrix}. \tag{8.8}$$

The path diagram of this LCM is depicted in Figure 8.2.

8.3.3 Latent curve models with longitudinal latent variables

To incorporate longitudinal latent variables, we further consider the following measurement model (Song *et al.*, 2009):

$$\mathbf{u}_t = \boldsymbol{\Lambda}_{ut}\boldsymbol{\omega}_{ut} + \boldsymbol{\epsilon}_{ut}, \quad t = 1, \ldots, T, \tag{8.9}$$

where $\mathbf{u}_t$ is a $p \times 1$ vector of measurements, $\boldsymbol{\Lambda}_{ut}$ is a $p \times q$ loading matrix, $\boldsymbol{\omega}_{ut}$ is a $q \times 1$ vector of latent variables, and $\boldsymbol{\epsilon}_{ut}$ is a $p \times 1$ vector of unique variances in $\mathbf{u}_t$. It is assumed that $\boldsymbol{\epsilon}_{ut}$ follows the distribution $N[\mathbf{0}, \boldsymbol{\Psi}_{ut}]$, where $\boldsymbol{\Psi}_{ut}$ is a diagonal matrix with diagonal elements

$\psi_{ut1}, \ldots, \psi_{utp}$. Equation (8.9) can be expressed in the following form:

$$\begin{pmatrix} u_{t1} \\ u_{t2} \\ \vdots \\ u_{tp} \end{pmatrix} = \begin{pmatrix} \lambda_{ut,11} & \lambda_{ut,12} & \cdots & \lambda_{ut,1q} \\ \lambda_{ut,21} & \lambda_{ut,22} & \cdots & \lambda_{ut,2q} \\ \vdots & \vdots & \ddots & \vdots \\ \lambda_{ut,p1} & \lambda_{ut,p2} & \cdots & \lambda_{ut,pq} \end{pmatrix} \begin{pmatrix} \omega_{ut1} \\ \omega_{ut2} \\ \vdots \\ \omega_{utq} \end{pmatrix} + \begin{pmatrix} \epsilon_{ut1} \\ \epsilon_{ut2} \\ \vdots \\ \epsilon_{utp} \end{pmatrix}, \tag{8.10}$$

where some $\lambda_{ut,ij}$ are fixed at 0 or 1 for model identification. As the latent variables ω_{utk}, $k = 1, \ldots, q$ defined in equation (8.9) or (8.10) are related to observed variables measured at multiple time points $t_1, \ldots, t_T$, they are regarded as longitudinal latent variables. Let $\boldsymbol{\omega}_k = (\omega_{u1k}, \ldots, \omega_{uTk})^T$ and $\boldsymbol{\epsilon}_{\omega k} = (\epsilon_{\omega 1k}, \ldots, \epsilon_{\omega Tk})^T$. We can use the following LCM to investigate the patterns of change in these longitudinal latent variables:

$$\boldsymbol{\omega}_k = \boldsymbol{\Lambda}\boldsymbol{\xi}_{r+k} + \boldsymbol{\epsilon}_{\omega k}, \quad k = 1, \ldots, q, \tag{8.11}$$

where $\boldsymbol{\xi}_{r+k}$ is an $m \times 1$ latent growth factor that includes growth parameters, r is specified in equation (8.6), and $\boldsymbol{\Lambda}$ is defined similarly to equation (8.1). We assume that $\boldsymbol{\epsilon}_{\omega k}$ follows the distribution $N[\mathbf{0}, \boldsymbol{\Psi}_{\omega k}]$, where $\boldsymbol{\Psi}_{\omega k}$ is a diagonal matrix with diagonal elements $\psi_{\omega tk}$, for $t = 1, \ldots, T$ and $k = 1, \ldots, q$. If $m = 2$, then $\boldsymbol{\xi}_{r+k} = (\xi_{1,r+k}, \xi_{2,r+k})^T$, and equation (8.11) has the form

$$\begin{pmatrix} \omega_{u1k} \\ \omega_{u2k} \\ \vdots \\ \omega_{uTk} \end{pmatrix} = \begin{pmatrix} 1 & t_1 \\ 1 & t_2 \\ \vdots & \vdots \\ 1 & t_T \end{pmatrix} \begin{pmatrix} \xi_{1,r+k} \\ \xi_{2,r+k} \end{pmatrix} + \begin{pmatrix} \epsilon_{\omega 1k} \\ \epsilon_{\omega 2k} \\ \vdots \\ \epsilon_{\omega Tk} \end{pmatrix}, \quad k = 1, \ldots, q, \tag{8.12}$$

where $\xi_{1,r+k}$ and $\xi_{2,r+k}$ denote the intercept and slope in latent growth factor $\boldsymbol{\xi}_{r+k}$.

In the cocaine use example, 'psychiatric problems' is a longitudinal latent variable, which is formed by three observed variables, Beck Inventory (BI), depression (DEP), and anxiety (AN), at multiple time points. The related measurement equation, which is a special case of equation (8.10), is given by

$$\begin{pmatrix} u_{t1} \\ u_{t2} \\ u_{t3} \end{pmatrix} = \begin{pmatrix} 1 \\ \lambda_{ut,21} \\ \lambda_{ut,31} \end{pmatrix} \omega_{ut1} + \begin{pmatrix} \epsilon_{ut1} \\ \epsilon_{ut2} \\ \epsilon_{ut3} \end{pmatrix}, \quad t = 1, \ldots, 4, \tag{8.13}$$

where the 1s in $\boldsymbol{\Lambda}_{ut}$ are fixed to identify the factor analysis model. The LCM (see equation (8.12)) that describes the pattern of change of the longitudinal latent variable ω_{ut1} is defined as

$$\begin{pmatrix} \omega_{u11} \\ \omega_{u21} \\ \omega_{u31} \\ \omega_{u41} \end{pmatrix} = \begin{pmatrix} 1 & 0 \\ 1 & 1 \\ 1 & 2 \\ 1 & 12 \end{pmatrix} \begin{pmatrix} \xi_{13} \\ \xi_{23} \end{pmatrix} + \begin{pmatrix} \epsilon_{\omega 11} \\ \epsilon_{\omega 21} \\ \epsilon_{\omega 31} \\ \epsilon_{\omega 41} \end{pmatrix}, \tag{8.14}$$

where ξ_{13} and ξ_{23} can be regarded as the second-order latent variables. The path diagram for equations (8.13) and (8.14) is shown in Figure 8.3.

In general, let $\boldsymbol{\xi} = (\boldsymbol{\xi}_1^T, \ldots, \boldsymbol{\xi}_r^T, \boldsymbol{\xi}_{r+1}^T, \ldots, \boldsymbol{\xi}_{r+q}^T)^T$ be the vector of explanatory latent growth factors that are either first- or second-order latent variables. To assess the linear and nonlinear effects of the explanatory latent growth factors in $\boldsymbol{\xi}$ on the latent growth factor $\boldsymbol{\eta}$, we further

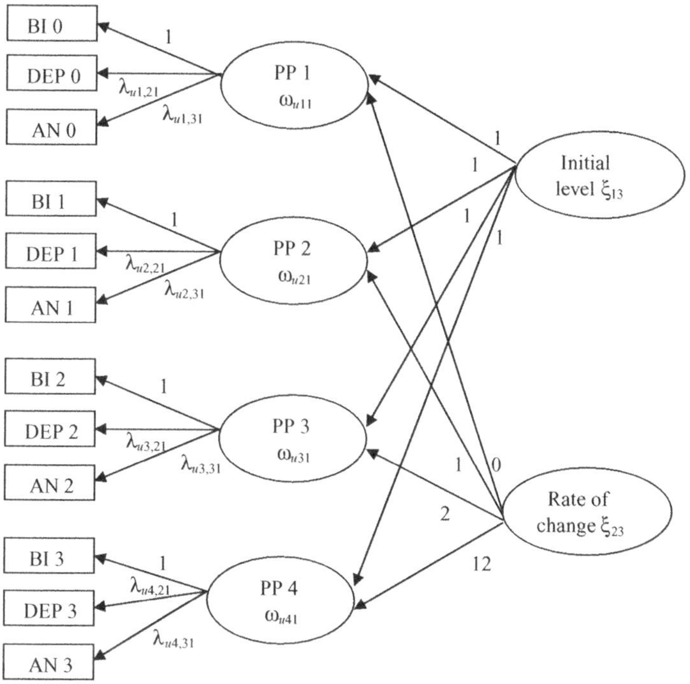

Figure 8.3 Path diagram of the model defined in (8.13) and (8.14). Reproduced by permission of Taylor & Francis from Song, X. Y., Lee, S. Y. and Hser, Y. I. (2009). Bayesian analysis of multivariate latent curve models with nonlinear longitudinal latent effects. *Structural Equation Modeling – A Multidisciplinary Journal*, **16**, 245–266.

propose the following nonlinear structural equation:

$$\boldsymbol{\eta} = \boldsymbol{\beta} + \boldsymbol{\Pi}\boldsymbol{\eta} + \boldsymbol{\Gamma}\mathbf{F}(\boldsymbol{\xi}) + \boldsymbol{\delta}, \tag{8.15}$$

where $\boldsymbol{\Gamma}$ is a matrix of unknown regression coefficients, $\mathbf{F}(\boldsymbol{\xi}) = (f_1(\boldsymbol{\xi}), \ldots, f_h(\boldsymbol{\xi}))^T$ is a vector-valued function containing nonzero differentiable functions $f_1, \ldots, f_h$, and $h \geq r + q$. Here, $\boldsymbol{\xi}$ is distributed as $N[\mathbf{0}, \boldsymbol{\Phi}]$, $\boldsymbol{\delta}$ is a vector of residuals with distribution $N[\mathbf{0}, \boldsymbol{\Psi}_\delta]$, in which $\boldsymbol{\Psi}_\delta$ is a diagonal matrix with diagonal elements $\psi_{\delta k}, k = 1, \ldots, m$, and $\boldsymbol{\xi}$ and $\boldsymbol{\delta}$ are independent. Note that $\boldsymbol{\Phi}$ contains variances and covariances of explanatory latent growth factors which describe the relationships between the aspects of change represented by various growth curve parameters for different response variables. Let $\boldsymbol{\Lambda}_\delta = (\boldsymbol{\Pi}, \boldsymbol{\Gamma})$, $\boldsymbol{\zeta} = (\boldsymbol{\eta}^T, \boldsymbol{\xi}^T)^T$, and $\mathbf{G}(\boldsymbol{\zeta}) = (\boldsymbol{\eta}^T, \mathbf{F}(\boldsymbol{\xi})^T)^T$; then equation (8.15) can be rewritten as

$$\boldsymbol{\eta} = \boldsymbol{\beta} + \boldsymbol{\Lambda}_\delta\mathbf{G}(\boldsymbol{\zeta}) + \boldsymbol{\delta}. \tag{8.16}$$

In the analysis of cocaine use data, we are interested in the longitudinal effects of treatment (TR), family support (FS), and psychiatric problems (PP) on cocaine use (CC), where 'psychiatric problems (PP)' is a latent variable. Specifically, we aim to study how the dynamic changes in the latent growth factors $\boldsymbol{\xi}_1$ (TR), $\boldsymbol{\xi}_2$ (FS), and $\boldsymbol{\xi}_3$ (PP) influence the latent growth factor $\boldsymbol{\eta}$ (CC). Here, $m = 2$, $r = 2$, $q = 1$, and each $\boldsymbol{\xi}_k = (\xi_{1k}, \xi_{2k})^T$ $(k = 1, 2, 3)$ includes the intercept and slope that represent the initial status and rate of changes in TR, FS, and PP,

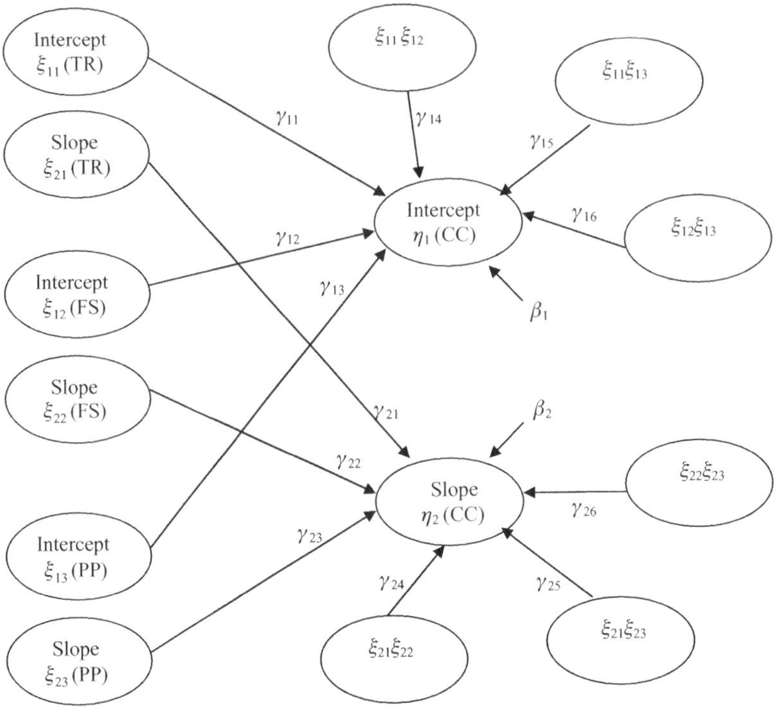

Figure 8.4 Path diagram of the model defined in (8.17) and (8.18). Reproduced by permission of Taylor & Francis from Song, X. Y., Lee, S. Y. and Hser, Y. I. (2009). Bayesian analysis of multivariate latent curve models with nonlinear longitudinal latent effects. *Structural Equation Modeling – A Multidisciplinary Journal*, **16**, 245–266.

respectively. An interesting model is described as follows and depicted in Figure 8.4:

$$\eta_1 = \beta_1 + \gamma_{11}\xi_{11} + \gamma_{12}\xi_{12} + \gamma_{13}\xi_{13} + \gamma_{14}\xi_{11}\xi_{12} + \gamma_{15}\xi_{11}\xi_{13} + \gamma_{16}\xi_{12}\xi_{13} + \delta_1, \quad (8.17)$$

$$\eta_2 = \beta_2 + \gamma_{21}\xi_{21} + \gamma_{22}\xi_{22} + \gamma_{23}\xi_{23} + \gamma_{24}\xi_{21}\xi_{22} + \gamma_{25}\xi_{21}\xi_{23} + \gamma_{26}\xi_{22}\xi_{23} + \delta_2, \quad (8.18)$$

where the regression coefficients γ_{11}, γ_{12}, and γ_{13} respectively represent the effect of initial status in treatment, family support, and psychiatric problems on the initial status in cocaine use, whereas γ_{21}, γ_{22}, and γ_{23} respectively represent the effect of rate of change in treatment, family support, and psychiatric problems on the rate of change in cocaine use. The other coefficients represent various interactive effects of explanatory growth factors on the outcome growth factor. For example, equation (8.18) can be used to examine how the impact of joint changes in TR, FS, and PP influences the change in CC. Hence, the significance of parameters γ_{24}, γ_{25}, and γ_{26} essentially answers the question: whether the simultaneous change (interaction effect) in explanatory latent growth factors in treatment, psychiatric problems, or family support influences the rate of change in the outcome growth factor in cocaine use.

So far we have focused our attention on continuous repeated measures. However, in the cocaine use study, some of the observed variables y, x, and u are ordered categorical variables. These ordered categorical variables will be treated in a familiar manner. Let z be the underlying continuous unobservable variable that corresponds to an ordered categorical variable x. Then, for $k = 1, \ldots, r$ and $t = 1, \ldots, T$,

$$x_{tk} = j, \quad \text{if } \alpha_{tk,j} \leq z_{tk} < \alpha_{tk,j+1}, \ j = 0, \ldots, h_k, \tag{8.19}$$

where $\{-\infty = \alpha_{tk,0} < \alpha_{tk,1} < \ldots < \alpha_{tk,h_k} < \alpha_{tk,h_k+1} = \infty\}$ is the set of threshold parameters that defines the $h_k + 1$ categories. For identification, as suggested by Bollen and Curran (2006), we set the first threshold $\alpha_{tk,1}$ to 0 and ψ_{xtk} to 1 for $k = 1, \ldots, r$ and $t = 1, 2, \ldots, T$. The extension to more complex situations where all y, x, and u include ordered categorical components is straightforward.

In Section 8.5, we will apply a comprehensive LCM defined by equations (8.1), (8.6), (8.9), (8.11), and (8.15) to the two sets of longitudinal data that are respectively related to the HRQOL of stroke survivors and cocaine use. Equation (8.19) will be incorporated if we encounter ordered categorical variables. Moreover, data that are missing at random can be treated using the method described in Chapter 5.

8.4 Bayesian analysis

To use the Bayesian approach to analyze the above LCM, let $\boldsymbol{\theta}$ be the vector containing the unknown free parameters of the model, and $\boldsymbol{\alpha}$ be the vector containing the unknown thresholds. In the Bayesian approach, $(\boldsymbol{\theta}, \boldsymbol{\alpha})$ is considered as random with a prior distribution $p(\boldsymbol{\theta}, \boldsymbol{\alpha})$. Let $\mathbf{D} = \{\mathbf{Y}, \mathbf{X}, \mathbf{U}\}$, where $\mathbf{Y}$, $\mathbf{X}$, and $\mathbf{U}$ include all three kinds of observed variables defined in equations (8.2), (8.6), and (8.10); $\mathbf{Z}$ includes all underlying continuous variables that correspond to ordered categorical variables in $\mathbf{D}$. Bayesian inference is based on the posterior distribution of $(\boldsymbol{\theta}, \boldsymbol{\alpha})$ given the observed data set $\mathbf{D}$ and $p(\boldsymbol{\theta}, \boldsymbol{\alpha})$.

In the context of our LCM, it is rather difficult to compute the posterior mean mainly because of the existence of a lot of first- and second-order latent variables, unobservable continuous variables, and the nonlinearity of the structural equation. To solve this difficulty, we adopt a commonly used strategy in Bayesian analysis that involves two key steps. The first step is to augment the observed data with all the latent variables to form a complete data set. Let Ξ include all latent growth factors ($\boldsymbol{\eta}$ and $\boldsymbol{\xi}$), and let $\boldsymbol{\Omega}$ include all longitudinal latent variables. The complete data set is $\{\mathbf{Z}, \Xi, \boldsymbol{\Omega}, \mathbf{D}\}$. Treating $\mathbf{Z}$, Ξ, and $\boldsymbol{\Omega}$ as random unknown quantities, the joint posterior density is $p(\boldsymbol{\theta}, \boldsymbol{\alpha}, \mathbf{Z}, \Xi, \boldsymbol{\Omega}|\mathbf{D})$. The second step is to draw a sufficiently large sample of observations from the joint posterior distribution $[\boldsymbol{\theta}, \boldsymbol{\alpha}, \mathbf{Z}, \Xi, \boldsymbol{\Omega}|\mathbf{D}]$, say $\{(\boldsymbol{\theta}^{(j)}, \boldsymbol{\alpha}^{(j)}, \mathbf{Z}^{(j)}, \Xi^{(j)}, \boldsymbol{\Omega}^{(j)}), j = 1, \ldots, J\}$. The Bayesian estimate of $(\boldsymbol{\theta}, \boldsymbol{\alpha})$ can be obtained through the sample mean, and the standard error estimates can be obtained through the sample covariance matrix. Moreover, estimates of the various latent variables can be obtained from $\Xi^{(j)}$ and $\boldsymbol{\Omega}^{(j)}$ for $j = 1, \ldots, J$, respectively. The task of simulating observations from the joint posterior distributions can be carried out with the well-known Gibbs sampler (Geman and Geman, 1984), which iteratively simulates observations from $p(\boldsymbol{\theta}|\boldsymbol{\alpha}, \mathbf{Z}, \Xi, \boldsymbol{\Omega}, \mathbf{D})$, $p(\boldsymbol{\alpha}, \mathbf{Z}|\boldsymbol{\theta}, \Xi, \boldsymbol{\Omega}, \mathbf{D})$, $p(\Xi|\boldsymbol{\theta}, \boldsymbol{\alpha}, \mathbf{Z}, \boldsymbol{\Omega}, \mathbf{D})$, and $p(\boldsymbol{\Omega}|\boldsymbol{\theta}, \boldsymbol{\alpha}, \mathbf{Z}, \Xi, \mathbf{D})$.

Recall that the selection of the appropriate prior distribution for $(\boldsymbol{\theta}, \boldsymbol{\alpha})$ is an important issue in the Bayesian approach. As before, it is natural to assume that $p(\boldsymbol{\theta}, \boldsymbol{\alpha}) = p(\boldsymbol{\theta})p(\boldsymbol{\alpha})$. To deal with the situation with little or no information about threshold parameters, the following noninformative prior distribution is used for the prior distribution $p(\boldsymbol{\alpha})$:

$$p(\alpha_{tk,2}, \ldots, \alpha_{tk,h_k}) \propto C, \quad k = 1, \ldots, r, \ t = 1, \ldots, T, \tag{8.20}$$

where C is a constant. Similarly to most Bayesian analyses of latent variable models (see previous chapters, and Lee, 2007), we use conjugate prior distributions for $p(\boldsymbol{\theta})$. More specifically, the following conjugate prior distributions are considered:

$$
\begin{aligned}
&\psi_{yt}^{-1} \stackrel{D}{=} \text{Gamma}[a_{0yt}, b_{0yt}], \quad t = 1, \ldots, T, \\
&\psi_{xtk}^{-1} \stackrel{D}{=} \text{Gamma}[a_{0xtk}, b_{0xtk}], \quad k = 1, \ldots, r,\ t = 1, \ldots, T, \\
&\psi_{\omega tk}^{-1} \stackrel{D}{=} \text{Gamma}[a_{0\omega tk}, b_{0\omega tk}], \quad k = 1, \ldots, q,\ t = 1, \ldots, T, \\
&\psi_{utk}^{-1} \stackrel{D}{=} \text{Gamma}[a_{0utk}, b_{0utk}], \quad k = 1, \ldots, p,\ t = 1, \ldots, T, \\
&[\boldsymbol{\Lambda}_{utk}|\psi_{utk}] \stackrel{D}{=} N[\boldsymbol{\Lambda}_{0utk}, \psi_{utk}\boldsymbol{\Sigma}_{0utk}], \quad k = 1, \ldots, p,\ t = 1, \ldots, T, \\
&\psi_{\delta k}^{-1} \stackrel{D}{=} \text{Gamma}[a_{0\delta k}, b_{0\delta k}],\ [\boldsymbol{\Lambda}_{\delta k}|\psi_{\delta k}] \stackrel{D}{=} N[\boldsymbol{\Lambda}_{0\delta k}, \psi_{\delta k}\boldsymbol{\Sigma}_{0\delta k}], \quad k = 1, \ldots, m, \\
&\boldsymbol{\beta} \stackrel{D}{=} N[\boldsymbol{\beta}_0, \boldsymbol{\Sigma}_0], \quad \text{and} \quad \boldsymbol{\Phi}^{-1} \stackrel{D}{=} W_{m(r+q)}[\mathbf{R}_0, \rho_0],
\end{aligned}
\tag{8.21}
$$

where ψ_{yt}, ψ_{xtk}, and $\psi_{\omega tk}$ are the tth diagonal elements of $\boldsymbol{\Psi}_y$, $\boldsymbol{\Psi}_{xk}$, and $\boldsymbol{\Psi}_{\omega k}$, and ψ_{utk} and $\psi_{\delta k}$ are the kth diagonal elements of $\boldsymbol{\Psi}_{ut}$ and $\boldsymbol{\Psi}_{\delta}$, respectively; $\boldsymbol{\Lambda}_{utk}^T$ and $\boldsymbol{\Lambda}_{\delta k}^T$ are the kth rows of $\boldsymbol{\Lambda}_{ut}$ and $\boldsymbol{\Lambda}_{\delta}$, respectively; and a_{0yt}, b_{0yt}, a_{0xtk}, b_{0xtk}, $a_{0\omega tk}$, $b_{0\omega tk}$, a_{0utk}, b_{0utk}, $a_{0\delta k}$, $b_{0\delta k}$, $\boldsymbol{\beta}_0$, $\boldsymbol{\Sigma}_0$, $\boldsymbol{\Lambda}_{0utk}$, $\boldsymbol{\Sigma}_{0utk}$, $\boldsymbol{\Lambda}_{0\delta k}$, $\boldsymbol{\Sigma}_{0\delta k}$, $\mathbf{R}_0$, and ρ_0 are the hyperparameters in the prior distributions. Under the above conjugate prior distributions, the full conditional distributions required for implementing the Gibbs sampler are presented in Appendix 8.1.

The convergence of the MCMC algorithm can be determined by examining the plots of a number (usually three) of different sequences of simulated observations with different initial values. At convergence, these sequences of observations should mix well. Suppose that the algorithm reaches convergence after the Kth iteration; a sufficient number of simulated observations, say J, after the Kth iteration are then collected to conduct statistical inference. Finally, Bayesian model comparison statistics, such as the Bayes factor, DIC, or L_ν-measure, can be calculated using the simulated observations through the methods described in previous chapters.

8.5 Applications to two longitudinal studies

8.5.1 Longitudinal study of cocaine use

The data set in this example is obtained from a longitudinal study about cocaine use conducted by the UCLA Center for Advancing Longitudinal Drug Abuse Research. Various measures were collected from 321 patients who were admitted in 1988–1989 to the West Los Angeles Veterans Affairs Medical Center and who met the DSM III-R criteria for cocaine dependence (Kasarabada *et al.*, 1999). These patients were assessed at baseline, 1 year after treatment, 2 years after treatment, and 12 years after treatment in 2002 ($t_1 = 0, t_2 = 1, t_3 = 2, t_4 = 12$). Among those patients located at the 12-year follow-up (96.9%), some were confirmed to be deceased (8.7%), some declined to be interviewed, and some were either out of the country or too ill to be interviewed after 1 year, 2 years, or 12 years after treatment. Consequently, there is a large amount of missing data in this data set. For brevity, the missing data are treated as missing at random (MAR). In this analysis, seven variables are involved. The first variable, 'days of cocaine use per month' (CC), is associated with the cocaine use of the patients. The second variable, 'times per month in formal treatment' (TR), is associated with frequencies of patient participation in treatment. The third variable, 'family support' (FS), is associated with the family support that the patients had, which is an ordered categorical variable on a three-point scale. The three variables 'Beck Inventory' (BI), 'depression' (DEP), and 'anxiety' (AN) are associated with the mental health or psychiatric problems of the patients; the latter two are measured based on the Hopkins Symptom Check List (HSCL-58: Hser *et al.*, 2006).

In this analysis, the outcome latent growth factor ($\boldsymbol{\eta}$) represents the pattern of change in CC. The first explanatory latent growth factor $\boldsymbol{\xi}_1$ represents the pattern of change in TR. The second explanatory latent growth factor $\boldsymbol{\xi}_2$ represents the pattern of change in FS. The variables BI, DEP, and AN with repeated measurements (at $t = 1, \ldots, 4$) formed a longitudinal latent variable $\boldsymbol{\omega}_{ut}$, which can be interpreted as 'psychiatric problems' (PP). Thus, the third explanatory latent growth factor $\boldsymbol{\xi}_3$ represents the patterns of change in PP. To study the possible effects of treatment, family support, and psychiatric problems of the patients on cocaine use, we propose the multivariate LCM as described in Figure 8.5. The interaction effects between the initial status or between the rates of change are assessed through the structural equations given in (8.17) and (8.18). Among the observed variables, only FS is an ordered categorical variable on a three-point scale, so we write $\alpha_{t,j}$ instead of $\alpha_{tk,j}$, and we fix $\alpha_{t,1} = 0.0$ and $\psi_{xt2} = 1.0$ to identify the model.

The Bayesian estimates of the unknown parameters were obtained using WinBUGS. In specifying the hyperparameters in the prior distributions, we use the following hierarchical prior inputs: $\boldsymbol{\beta}_0 \sim N[\mathbf{0}, 4\mathbf{I}]$, $\boldsymbol{\Lambda}_{0utk} \sim N[\mathbf{0}, 4\mathbf{I}]$, and $\boldsymbol{\Lambda}_{0\delta k} \sim N[\mathbf{0}, 4\mathbf{I}]$, where $\mathbf{I}$ is an identity matrix of appropriate dimension. The values of other hyperparameters are given by $a_{0yt} = a_{0xtk} = a_{0\omega tk} = a_{0utk} = a_{0\delta k} = 10$, $b_{0yt} = b_{0xtk} = b_{0\omega tk} = b_{0utk} = b_{0\delta k} = 4$, $\rho_0 = 6$, and $\mathbf{R}_0 = \mathbf{I}$. With three different starting values, the WinBUGS outputs showed that the sequences produced by the Gibbs sampler algorithm mixed well in less than 4000 iterations. We took a burn-in phase of 4000 iterations, and collected a further $J = 30\,000$ observations to produce the Bayesian estimates, which are reported in Table 8.1. The corresponding WinBUGS code is presented in Appendix 8.2. The estimated structural equations of (8.17) and (8.18) are given by

$$\eta_1 = \underset{(0.254)}{0.566} - \underset{(0.291)}{0.064}\xi_{11} + \underset{(0.362)}{0.383}\xi_{12} + \underset{(0.353)}{0.159}\xi_{13} - \underset{(0.293)}{0.123}\xi_{11}\xi_{12} + \underset{(0.254)}{0.016}\xi_{11}\xi_{13} - \underset{(0.173)}{0.014}\xi_{12}\xi_{13},$$

$$\eta_2 = \underset{(0.014)}{-0.060} + \underset{(0.135)}{0.006}\xi_{21} - \underset{(0.065)}{0.034}\xi_{22} + \underset{(0.219)}{0.517}\xi_{23} + \underset{(0.410)}{0.619}\xi_{21}\xi_{22} + \underset{(0.494)}{0.951}\xi_{21}\xi_{23} + \underset{(0.465)}{0.704}\xi_{22}\xi_{23}.$$

The values in parentheses provide the standard error estimates of the associated parameters.

From Table 8.1 and the above equations, we are led to the following conclusions. Firstly, all estimates of $\lambda_{ut,i1}$, $t = 1, \ldots, 4$, $i = 2, 3$, are large, indicating strong associations between observed variables and the corresponding latent variables.

Secondly, in the above estimated structural equations, $\beta_1 = 0.566$ (0.254), $\beta_2 = -0.060$ (0.014), and $\gamma_{23} = 0.517$ (0.219) are statistically significant at the 0.05 level. The value of γ_{23} represents the positive effect of rate of change in 'psychiatric problems' on the rate of change in 'cocaine use'. This positive effect shows that as a patient's rate of change in 'psychiatric problems' increases over time, his/her rate of change in cocaine use also increases. The following interesting phenomenon is also found in predicting the longitudinal change in cocaine use (η_2). Although the coefficients $\gamma_{21} = 0.006$ (0.135), $\gamma_{22} = -0.034$ (0.065) are small and nonsignificant, the coefficients of the interaction terms $\gamma_{24} = 0.619$ (0.410), $\gamma_{25} = 0.951$ (0.494), and $\gamma_{26} = 0.704$ (0.465) are relatively large. These marginally significant

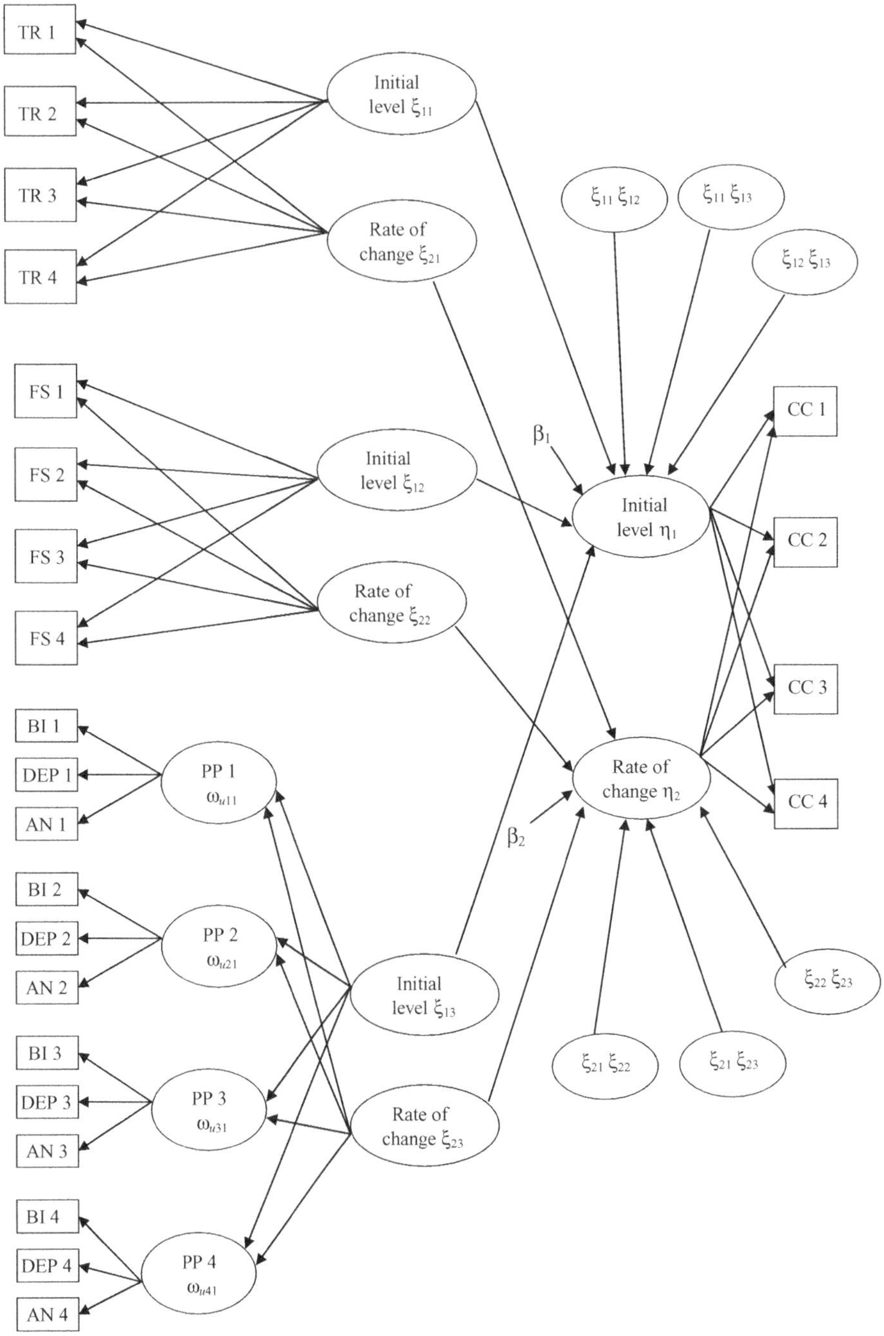

Figure 8.5 Path diagram of the LCM for the longitudinal study of cocaine use. Reproduced by permission of Taylor & Francis from Song, X. Y., Lee, S. Y. and Hser, Y. I. (2009). Bayesian analysis of multivariate latent curve models with nonlinear longitudinal latent effects. *Structural Equation Modeling – A Multidisciplinary Journal*, **16**, 245–266.

Table 8.1 Bayesian estimates and standard error estimates of the parameters in the cocaine study example.

Par	Est	Std	Par	Est	Std	Par	Est	Std
$\lambda_{u1,21}$	2.083	0.053	ψ_{y1}	1.361	0.136	ϕ_{11}	0.669	0.077
$\lambda_{u1,31}$	1.828	0.051	ψ_{y2}	0.564	0.068	ϕ_{12}	−0.052	0.009
$\lambda_{u2,21}$	2.169	0.052	ψ_{y3}	0.564	0.065	ϕ_{13}	0.528	0.109
$\lambda_{u2,31}$	2.173	0.055	ψ_{y4}	0.293	0.070	ϕ_{14}	0.014	0.021
$\lambda_{u3,21}$	2.028	0.046	ψ_{x11}	0.591	0.065	ϕ_{15}	0.708	0.091
$\lambda_{u3,31}$	2.091	0.051	ψ_{x21}	0.746	0.073	ϕ_{16}	0.002	0.006
$\lambda_{u4,21}$	1.959	0.065	ψ_{x31}	0.614	0.063	ϕ_{22}	0.015	0.001
$\lambda_{u4,31}$	1.843	0.063	ψ_{x41}	0.249	0.052	ϕ_{23}	−0.031	0.012
γ_{11}	−0.064	0.291	ψ_{u11}	0.554	0.054	ϕ_{24}	−0.007	0.002
γ_{12}	0.383	0.362	ψ_{u12}	0.203	0.034	ϕ_{25}	−0.040	0.012
γ_{13}	0.159	0.353	ψ_{u13}	0.384	0.048	ϕ_{26}	0.002	0.000
γ_{14}	−0.123	0.293	ψ_{u21}	0.608	0.056	ϕ_{33}	1.430	0.293
γ_{15}	0.016	0.254	ψ_{u22}	0.220	0.037	ϕ_{34}	0.023	0.034
γ_{16}	−0.014	0.173	ψ_{u23}	0.437	0.056	ϕ_{35}	1.596	0.209
γ_{21}	0.006	0.135	ψ_{u31}	0.547	0.051	ϕ_{36}	−0.009	0.009
γ_{22}	−0.034	0.065	ψ_{u32}	0.159	0.024	ϕ_{44}	0.053	0.014
γ_{23}	0.517	0.219	ψ_{u33}	0.344	0.043	ϕ_{45}	0.045	0.039
γ_{24}	0.619	0.410	ψ_{u41}	0.604	0.060	ϕ_{46}	−0.000	0.001
γ_{25}	0.951	0.494	ψ_{u42}	0.181	0.028	ϕ_{55}	2.064	0.190
γ_{26}	0.704	0.465	ψ_{u43}	0.277	0.035	ϕ_{56}	−0.012	0.011
β_1	0.566	0.254	$\psi_{\omega 1}$	0.175	0.025	ϕ_{66}	0.007	0.000
β_2	−0.060	0.014	$\psi_{\omega 2}$	0.128	0.017	$\alpha_{1,2}$	2.703	0.196
$\psi_{\delta 1}$	0.340	0.060	$\psi_{\omega 3}$	0.126	0.016	$\alpha_{2,2}$	3.172	0.218
$\psi_{\delta 2}$	0.038	0.003	$\psi_{\omega 4}$	0.163	0.026	$\alpha_{3,2}$	3.425	0.236
						$\alpha_{4,2}$	2.502	0.269

Reproduced by permission of Taylor & Francis from Song, X. Y., Lee, S. Y. and Hser, Y. I. (2009). Bayesian analysis of multivariate latent curve models with nonlinear longitudinal latent effects. *Structural Equation Modeling – A Multidisciplinary Journal*, **16**, 245–266.

coefficients indicate interactions between the dynamic latent growth factors (ξ_{21} and ξ_{22}, ξ_{21} and ξ_{23}, or ξ_{22} and ξ_{23}), which suggest joint effects of longitudinal changes in treatment, family support, and psychiatric problems on longitudinal change in cocaine use behavior. This finding shows that the integrated approach (combining formal medical treatment, increasing family support, and reducing psychiatric problems) is more efficient than simple medical treatment in reducing cocaine use of patients.

Thirdly, the significant variances in both the intercept and the slope, $\psi_{\delta 1} = 0.340$ (0.060) and $\psi_{\delta 2} = 0.038$ (0.003), indicate substantial individual differences in both initial level and growth of cocaine use. Similarly, the significant variances $\phi_{11} = 0.669$ (0.077), $\phi_{33} = 1.430$ (0.293), and $\phi_{55} = 2.064$ (0.190) indicate substantial individual differences in initial level of treatment, family support, and psychiatric problems. Although the variances $\phi_{22} = 0.015$ (0.001), $\phi_{44} = 0.053$ (0.014), and $\phi_{66} = 0.007$ (0.000) are small, they are also significant due to their small standard errors, indicating substantial individual differences in the rate of change in treatment, family support, and psychiatric problems.

Finally, most of the covariances in $\mathbf{\Phi}$ are small except for ϕ_{13}, ϕ_{15}, and ϕ_{35}. The large positive covariance $\phi_{13} = 0.528$ (0.109) indicates a strong positive correlation between the initial levels of treatment and family support. Similarly, $\phi_{15} = 0.708$ (0.091) indicates a strong positive correlation between the initial levels of treatment and psychiatric problems, and $\phi_{35} = 1.596$ (0.209) indicates a very strong positive correlation between the initial levels of family support and psychiatric problems. Interpretations of other less important parameters are not presented here to save space.

To cross-validate the results, different prior inputs are used to conduct the Bayesian analysis. We found that the results obtained were very close to those given in Table 8.1. This finding is consistent with the fact that the Bayesian estimates are not very sensitive to the prior inputs.

To provide more confidence in results given above, and to demonstrate the comprehensive LCM and statistical methodology, we presented a simulation study with a similar design to the longitudinal study of the cocaine use. The model is defined by equations (8.4), (8.7), (8.13), (8.14), (8.17), and (8.18) and is depicted in Figure 8.5, except that the linear time trajectories are designated as $t_1 = 1, t_2 = 2, t_3 = 3, t_4 = 4$. The sample size is 500 and the population values of the parameters are set as follows: $\lambda_{ut,21} = \lambda_{ut,31} = 0.8, t = 1, \ldots, 4$; $\gamma_{11} = \gamma_{13} = \gamma_{22} = 0.6, \gamma_{12} = \gamma_{21} = \gamma_{23} = -0.6, \gamma_{14} = \gamma_{16} = \gamma_{25} = -0.4, \gamma_{15} = \gamma_{24} = \gamma_{26} = 0.4$; $\beta_1 = 0.5, \beta_2 = -0.5$; $\psi_{yt} = \psi_{xt1} = \psi_{\omega t} = \psi_{utj} = 0.5, t = 1, \ldots, 4, j = 1, 2, 3$; $\psi_{\delta 1} = \psi_{\delta 2} = 0.36$; $\mathbf{\Phi} = (\phi_{kj})_{6\times 6}$ with $\phi_{kk} = 1.0$ and $\phi_{kj} = 0.3, \ k \neq j$. We assume that $\mathbf{x}_2$ in equation (8.6) includes ordered categorical measurements at each time point on a five-point scale. The population values of thresholds are $\alpha_{t,1} = 0.0, \alpha_{t,2} = 1.0, \alpha_{t,3} = 2.0$, and $\alpha_{t,4} = 3.0$, for $t = 1, \ldots, 4$. Here, $\alpha_{t,1}$ and ψ_{xt2} $(t = 1, \ldots, 4)$ are respectively fixed at 0 and 1 to identify the auxiliary threshold model. To accelerate the convergence of the MCMC algorithm in the simulation, $\alpha_{t,4}$ $(t = 1, \ldots, 4)$ are also fixed at their true values. About 30% of the data points are created to be missing, and they are treated as MAR in this simulation.

The Bayesian estimates of the unknown parameters based on 100 replications were found using R2WinBUGS (Sturtz *et al.*, 2005). First, a few tests performed using WinBUGS showed that the Gibbs sampler algorithm converged in less than 4000 iterations; then $J = 6000$ observations were collected after a burn-in phase of 4000 iterations to produce the Bayesian estimates in each replication. The means (Mean) and root mean squares (RMS) of the Bayesian estimates are reported in Table 8.2. We see from this table that the means of Bayesian estimates of the unknown parameters are close to the true values, and the root mean squares of the Bayesian estimates based on 100 replications are small, indicating that the Bayesian estimates are accurate.

8.5.2 Health-related quality of life for stroke survivors

In order to better understand the relationships among HRQOL and (MBI, LHS, GDS), we used the LCM to analyze the relevant longitudinal data. Ideally, a comprehensive LCM that involves all 24 items associated with HRQOL, MBI, LHS, and GDS should be considered at each of the time points. At each time point, physical health (PHY), psychological health (PSY), social interaction (SO), and environment (EN) are identified as latent variables through the measurement equation of an SEM based on the appropriate items in the HRQOL data set. Then

Table 8.2 Bayesian estimates, standard error estimates, and root mean squares of the parameters in the simulation study.

True value	Mean	RMS	True value	Mean	RMS	True value	Mean	RMS
$\lambda_{u1,21} = 0.8$	0.810	0.038	$\psi_{y1} = 0.5$	0.479	0.056	$\phi_{11} = 1.0$	0.986	0.087
$\lambda_{u1,31} = 0.8$	0.815	0.044	$\psi_{y2} = 0.5$	0.497	0.040	$\phi_{12} = 0.3$	0.310	0.058
$\lambda_{u2,21} = 0.8$	0.805	0.023	$\psi_{y3} = 0.5$	0.497	0.049	$\phi_{13} = 0.3$	0.367	0.116
$\lambda_{u2,31} = 0.8$	0.805	0.025	$\psi_{y4} = 0.5$	0.482	0.084	$\phi_{14} = 0.3$	0.332	0.078
$\lambda_{u3,21} = 0.8$	0.800	0.013	$\psi_{x11} = 0.5$	0.509	0.056	$\phi_{15} = 0.3$	0.289	0.064
$\lambda_{u3,31} = 0.8$	0.800	0.017	$\psi_{x21} = 0.5$	0.504	0.038	$\phi_{16} = 0.3$	0.303	0.063
$\lambda_{u4,21} = 0.8$	0.799	0.012	$\psi_{x31} = 0.5$	0.499	0.046	$\phi_{22} = 1.0$	1.006	0.067
$\lambda_{u4,31} = 0.8$	0.800	0.013	$\psi_{x41} = 0.5$	0.494	0.079	$\phi_{23} = 0.3$	0.378	0.117
$\gamma_{11} = 0.6$	0.621	0.070	$\psi_{u11} = 0.5$	0.506	0.049	$\phi_{24} = 0.3$	0.320	0.074
$\gamma_{12} = -0.6$	−0.567	0.085	$\psi_{u12} = 0.5$	0.502	0.045	$\phi_{25} = 0.3$	0.287	0.059
$\gamma_{13} = 0.6$	0.622	0.081	$\psi_{u13} = 0.5$	0.500	0.046	$\phi_{26} = 0.3$	0.302	0.050
$\gamma_{14} = -0.4$	−0.353	0.089	$\psi_{u21} = 0.5$	0.503	0.044	$\phi_{33} = 1.0$	1.182	0.277
$\gamma_{15} = 0.4$	0.454	0.108	$\psi_{u22} = 0.5$	0.499	0.039	$\phi_{34} = 0.3$	0.509	0.238
$\gamma_{16} = -0.4$	−0.375	0.088	$\psi_{u23} = 0.5$	0.501	0.040	$\phi_{35} = 0.3$	0.333	0.104
$\gamma_{21} = -0.6$	−0.573	0.054	$\psi_{u31} = 0.5$	0.506	0.054	$\phi_{36} = 0.3$	0.403	0.133
$\gamma_{22} = 0.6$	0.584	0.054	$\psi_{u32} = 0.5$	0.498	0.041	$\phi_{44} = 1.0$	1.132	0.210
$\gamma_{23} = -0.6$	−0.574	0.051	$\psi_{u33} = 0.5$	0.495	0.042	$\phi_{45} = 0.3$	0.345	0.087
$\gamma_{24} = 0.4$	0.390	0.057	$\psi_{u41} = 0.5$	0.491	0.048	$\phi_{46} = 0.3$	0.318	0.080
$\gamma_{25} = -0.4$	−0.392	0.055	$\psi_{u42} = 0.5$	0.500	0.042	$\phi_{55} = 1.0$	0.939	0.132
$\gamma_{26} = 0.4$	0.387	0.062	$\psi_{u43} = 0.5$	0.504	0.036	$\phi_{56} = 0.3$	0.311	0.056
$\beta_1 = 0.5$	0.464	0.070	$\psi_{\omega 1} = 0.5$	0.513	0.073	$\phi_{66} = 1.0$	1.010	0.077
$\beta_2 = -0.5$	−0.466	0.053	$\psi_{\omega 2} = 0.5$	0.503	0.062			
$\psi_{\delta 1} = 0.36$	0.388	0.062	$\psi_{\omega 3} = 0.5$	0.491	0.058			
$\psi_{\delta 2} = 0.36$	0.359	0.043	$\psi_{\omega 4} = 0.5$	0.501	0.089			
$\alpha_{1,2} = 1.0$	1.200	0.218	$\alpha_{1,3} = 2.0$	2.264	0.278			
$\alpha_{2,2} = 1.0$	1.104	0.132	$\alpha_{2,3} = 2.0$	2.211	0.173			
$\alpha_{3,2} = 1.0$	1.049	0.100	$\alpha_{3,3} = 2.0$	2.064	0.123			
$\alpha_{4,2} = 1.0$	0.967	0.096	$\alpha_{4,3} = 2.0$	1.962	0.109			

Reproduced by permission of Taylor & Francis from Song, X. Y., Lee, S. Y. and Hser, Y. I. (2009). Bayesian analysis of multivariate latent curve models with nonlinear longitudinal latent effects. *Structural Equation Modeling – A Multidisciplinary Journal*, **16**, 245–266.

the dynamic interrelationships of these latent variables and (MBI, LHS, GDS) are assessed using the comprehensive LCM by considering all the time points together. However, this comprehensive LCM would be very tedious. To save time, it may be desirable to obtain scores for the aforementioned latent variables first, and then analyze the dynamic interrelationships of each of those latent variables with (MBI, LHS, GDS) via four separate LCMs. There are at least two ways to obtain such scores. One is to use a factor analysis model to estimate the factor scores; while the other is simply to take the averages of the corresponding items. In this illustrative example, we use the latter method for simplicity. Therefore, based on three time points, four LCMs for {PHY, MBI, LHS, GDS}, {PSY, MBI, LHS, GDS}, {SO, MBI,

Table 8.3 Results of latent curve model analysis for PHY, PSY, SO, and EN domains of HRQOL.

	Initial level of ADL (ξ_1)	Initial level of handicap (ξ_3)	Initial level of depression (ξ_5)
Initial level of PHY	0.174* (0.069) [0.039, 0.307]	−0.475* (0.097) [−0.669, −0.290]	−0.310* (0.068) [−0.439, −0.177]
Initial level of PSY	0.167* (0.068) [0.034, 0.303]	−0.070 (0.095) [−0.193, 0.184]	−0.782* (0.068) [−0.910, −0.647]
Initial level of SO	0.032 (0.096) [−0.166, 0.211]	0.088 (0.135) [−0.182, 0.350]	−0.511* (0.096) [−0.698, −0.330]
Initial level of EN	0.075 (0.081) [−0.084, 0.232]	−0.191 (0.114) [−0.431, 0.025]	−0.540* (0.081) [−0.700, −0.385]
	Rate of change of ADL (ξ_2)	**Rate of change of handicap (ξ_4)**	**Rate of change of depression (ξ_6)**
Rate of change of PHY	0.280 (0.167) [−0.031, 0.617]	−0.312 (0.163) [−0.623, 0.014]	−0.328* (0.152) [−0.645, −0.042]
Rate of change of PSY	0.168 (0.166) [−0.139,0.510]	−0.179 (0.163) [−0.499, 0.139]	−0.445* (0.146) [−0.726, −0.154]
Rate of change of SO	−0.083 (0.203) [−0.478, 0.315]	−0.001 (0.201) [−0.381, 0.404]	−0.417* (0.186) [−0.771, −0.045]
Rate of change of EN	−0.128 (0.169) [−0.459, 0.202]	−0.282 (0.168) [−0.617, 0.042]	−0.539* (0.155) [−0.848, −0.242]

Note: Values are coefficient estimates, standard error estimates (given in parentheses) and 95% highest probability density (HPD) intervals (in brackets). The estimates with asterisks are statistically significant as their associated HPD intervals do not include zero.

Abbreviations: PHY, physical health; PSY, psychological health; SO, social interaction; EN, environment; ADL, activities of daily living.

Reproduced by permission of the American Heart Association from Pan, J. H., Song, X. Y., Lee, S. Y. and Kwok, T. (2008). Longitudinal analysis of quality of life for stroke survivors using latent curve models. *Stroke*, **39**, 2795–2802.

LHS, GDS}, and {EN, MBI, LHS, GDS} are established. The results of the analysis for the four HRQOL domains are shown in Table 8.3. As an example, the LCM for the physical health domain is shown in Figure 8.6, and the corresponding estimated structural equations, predicted by MBI, LHS, and GDS are as follows:

$$\eta_1 = -0.001 + 0.174\xi_1 - 0.475\xi_3 - 0.310\xi_5,$$

$$\eta_2 = -0.013 + 0.280\xi_2 - 0.312\xi_4 - 0.328\xi_6,$$

where η_1 is the initial level of the physical health domain, and η_2 is the rate of change in the physical health domain. Therefore, initial physical health was significantly associated with ADL, handicap, and depression, while the rate of change in physical health was significantly and inversely associated with rate of change in GDS only.

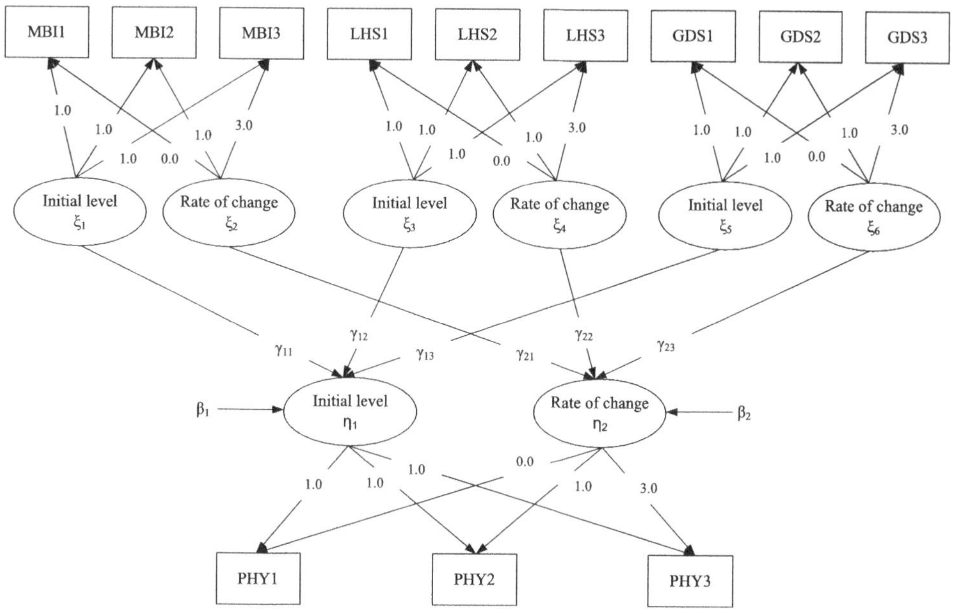

Figure 8.6 Path diagram of the LCM for HRQOL of stroke survivors. Reproduced by permission of the American Heart Association from Pan, J. H., Song, X. Y., Lee, S. Y. and Kwok, T. (2008). Longitudinal analysis of quality of life for stroke survivors using latent curve models. *Stroke*, **39**, 2795–2802.

The initial levels of the other three HRQOL domains were associated with depression only, except that psychological domain was marginally significantly associated with ADL as well. Similar to the physical health domain, the rates of change in these three HRQOL domains were associated with the rate of change in depression only.

For stroke survivors, activities of daily living, handicap, and depression are all important predictors of HRQOL. The relative importance of these interrelated variables in determining HRQOL was the subject of this study. The main finding of our analysis was that change in mood is the most significant effect on the HRQOL of stroke survivors, while changes in basic ADL and handicap had insignificant effects; see Pan *et al.* (2008) for more detailed interpretation of the results.

8.6 Other latent curve models

In previous sections, we have introduced a comprehensive LCM that accommodates the effects of dynamic changes and their interactions in explanatory variables on the dynamic changes in outcome variables. We have introduced second-order latent variables in LCMs to explore dynamic changes in longitudinal latent variables. As there has been increasing use of LCMs in various fields, we hope that modeling interactions among the first- and second-order latent variables (growth factors) will have wide applications in the analysis of longitudinal studies in various disciplines. Besides the comprehensive LCM described above, the following extensions of the basic LCM are also useful in substantive research.

8.6.1 Nonlinear latent curve models

The basic LCM can be generalized to incorporate nonlinear trajectories and effects of covariates. With this extension, a higher-order polynomial is used to describe a nonlinear pattern of dynamic change in individual characteristics. A longitudinal study of depression in multiple sclerosis (MS) by Beal *et al.* (2007) is used here to illustrate the nonlinear LCMs. This study focused on three specific research issues: (1) to reveal the patterns of change in depressive symptoms over time; (2) to identify substantial effects of covariates such as age (Age), type of MS (TMS), years since diagnosis of MS (YMS), and functional limitation (FL) on the trajectory of depression over time; (3) to examine the correlations between characteristics of change in functional limitations and depressive symptoms over the period of the study. The data were collected from 607 persons with MS over a period of 7 years, with initial recruitment in 1999, as part of an ongoing longitudinal study of quality of life (Stuifbergen *et al.*, 2006) in chronic illness. A nonlinear trajectory in depression for the sample is suggested by an examination of randomly selected empirical growth plots. A three-factor LCM is used to model the trajectories of depression for the MS sample:

$$\begin{pmatrix} y_1 \\ y_2 \\ \vdots \\ y_T \end{pmatrix} = \begin{pmatrix} 1 & t_1 & t_1^2 \\ 1 & t_2 & t_2^2 \\ \vdots & \vdots & \vdots \\ 1 & t_T & t_T^2 \end{pmatrix} \begin{pmatrix} \eta_1 \\ \eta_2 \\ \eta_3 \end{pmatrix} + \begin{pmatrix} \epsilon_{y1} \\ \epsilon_{y2} \\ \vdots \\ \epsilon_{yT} \end{pmatrix}, \tag{8.22}$$

where η_1, η_2, and η_3 represent the individual-specific random intercept, slope, and quadratic slope, respectively. As depicted in Figure 8.7, the change pattern and the correlations between

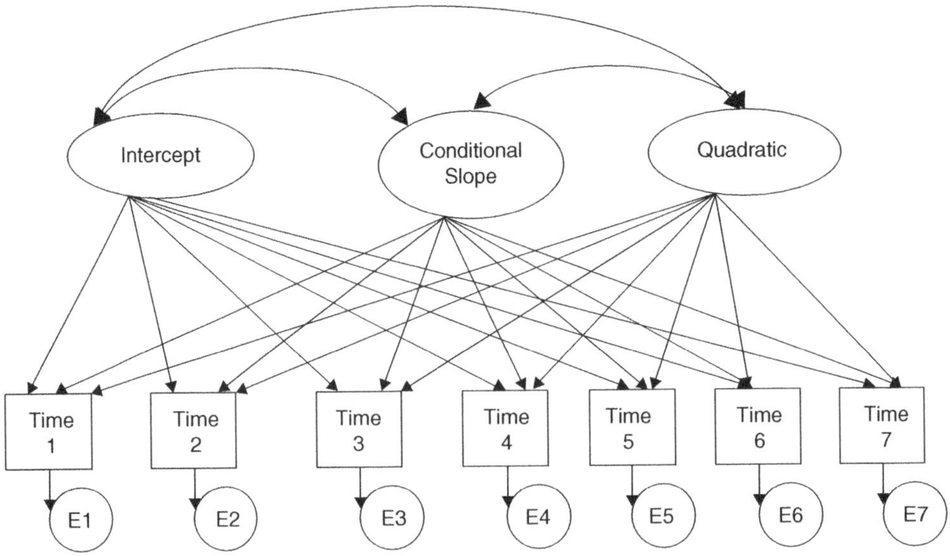

Figure 8.7 Quadratic LCM of depression across seven time points. Reprinted from Beal, C., Stuifbergen, A. K., Sands, D. V. and Brown, A. (2007). Depression in multiple sclerosis: a longitudinal analysis. *Archives of Psychiatric Nursing*, **21**, 181–191, with permission from Elsevier.

the characteristics of change in depressive symptoms are analyzed. Furthermore, predictors of change in depression are examined by regressing the intercept, slope, and quadratic slope on the covariates of interest, leading to the following equations:

$$\eta_1 = \beta_1 + \gamma_{11}(\text{Age}) + \gamma_{12}(\text{TMS}) + \gamma_{13}(\text{FL}) + \delta_1, \tag{8.23}$$

$$\eta_2 = \beta_2 + \gamma_{21}(\text{Age}) + \gamma_{22}(\text{TMS}) + \gamma_{23}(\text{FL}) + \delta_2, \tag{8.24}$$

$$\eta_3 = \beta_3 + \gamma_{31}(\text{Age}) + \gamma_{32}(\text{TMS}) + \gamma_{33}(\text{FL}) + \delta_3, \tag{8.25}$$

The findings of Beal *et al.* (2007) associated with the aforementioned three specific issues were obtained through the nonlinear LCM. First, there is no significant trend of increase or decrease in depressive symptoms, although these fluctuate over time for individuals. Second, younger age, longer time since diagnosis of MS, progressive forms of MS, and greater extent of functional limitations will result in greater depressive symptoms at time 1. Third, functional limitation shows an association with depression at all time periods, but other covariates do not. In addition, gender does not predict the changes in depressive symptoms. These results indicate that screening for depression in all persons with MS is necessary and important.

8.6.2 Multilevel latent curve models

In some circumstances, clinical trials involve a multilevel design, leading to hierarchically longitudinal data. For example, to evaluate the effects of a neighborhood walking program on quality of life (QOL) among older adults, Fisher and Li (2004) used a multilevel sampling scheme to collect a sample of neighborhoods from a large metropolitan city, from which older adult residents were randomly recruited. This two-level design results in a nested data structure in which participants are clustered within neighborhoods. The substantive interest of this study focuses on whether a 6-month neighborhood walking program improves neighborhood-level QOL for senior residents. A two-level LCM of QOL, with individual- and neighborhood-level data structures, is shown in Figure 8.8. All the measures involved are assessed at baseline, 3 months, and 6 months into the study period. Compared to the control neighborhoods, results from the two-level LCM indicate that physical, mental, and satisfaction with life aspects of QOL are significantly improved over the course of the 6-month intervention, which concludes that it is feasible and beneficial to implement a neighborhood-based walking program of low to moderate intensity in order to promote QOL among senior residents at a community level.

8.6.3 Mixture latent curve models

Heterogeneity is commonly encountered in longitudinal analysis of practical applications. For heterogeneous data, there exist some latent classes under which the characteristics of interest may present completely different change patterns. Mixture LCMs can be used to characterize the heterogeneity and to reveal specific change pattern for each distinctive latent class. Compared with the basic LCM, the additional tasks in applying mixture LCMs are to identify the number of latent classes, to detect the membership of each individual observation, and to predict the probability of each individual falling in a specific class. In order to formulate the probability of individual i belonging to latent class k, the following multinomial logistic

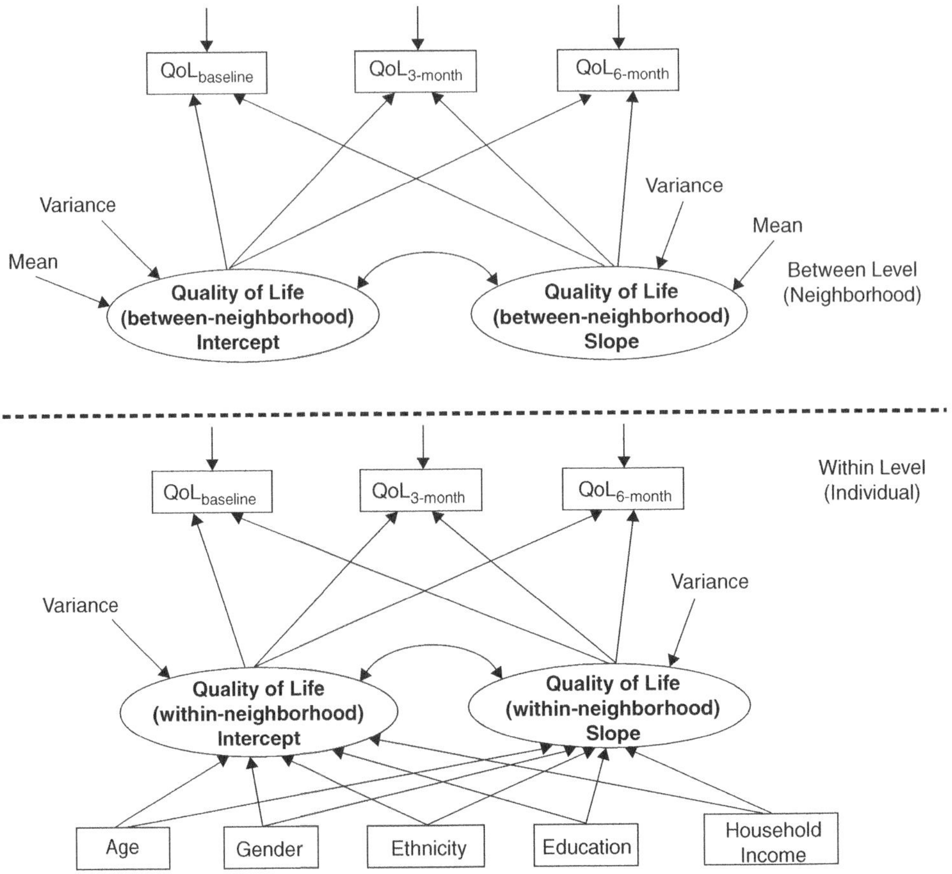

Figure 8.8 Multilevel LCM for QOL in older adults. Reproduced from Fisher, K. J. and Li, F. Z. (2004). A community-based walking trial to improve neighborhood quality of life in older adults: A multilevel analysis. *Annals of Behavioral Medicine*, **28**, 186–194, with kind permission from Springer Science and Business Media.

regression model is introduced (see also Section 7.3): for $k = 1, \ldots, K$,

$$p(C_i = k|x_{i1}, \ldots, x_{ip}) = \frac{\exp(a_{0k} + a_{1k}x_{i1} + \ldots + a_{pk}x_{ip})}{\sum_{j=1}^{K} \exp(a_{0j} + a_{1j}x_{i1} + \ldots + a_{pj}x_{ip})}, \tag{8.26}$$

where K is the number of latent classes, C_i is the class membership for individual i, $x_{i1}, \ldots, x_{ip}$ are covariates that may potentially influence the chances of individual i belonging to latent class k, and $a_{0k}, a_{1k}, \ldots, a_{pk}$ are corresponding regression coefficients that reflect the importance of potential covariates.

Hser *et al.* (2008) applied this model to examine long-term trajectories of drug use for primary heroin, cocaine, and meth users. The data include 629 primary heroin users, 694 cocaine users, and 474 meth users. The main outcome measure is the number of days using the primary drug per month. As shown in Figure 8.9, the analysis of mixture LCMs reveals five distinctive groups with different drug use trajectories over the 10-year follow-up: consistently

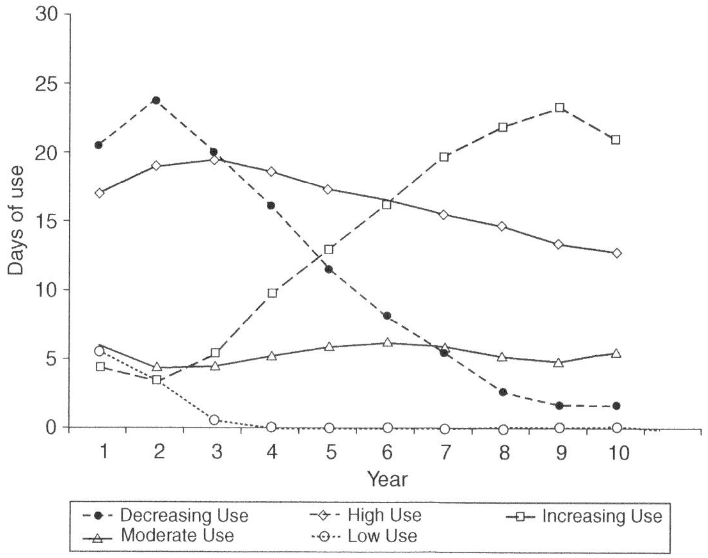

Figure 8.9 Five-group classification of drug use trajectories based on mixture LCM. Reproduced by permission of Taylor & Francis from Hser, Y. I., Huang, D., Brecht, M. L., Li, L. B. and Evans, E. (2008). Contrasting trajectories of heroin, cocaine, and methamphetamine. *Journal of Addictive Diseases*, **27**, 13–22.

high use, increasing use, decreasing use, moderate use, and low use. In addition, primary drug type is significantly associated with different trajectory patterns. Heroin users are most likely in the consistently high use group, cocaine and meth users are most likely in the moderate use group. The study also reveals that users in the high use group have earlier onsets of drug use and crime, longer incarceration durations, and fewer periods of employment than those in other groups. Compared with other existing studies of drug addiction, the use of mixture LCMs in this analysis emphasizes the heterogeneity of drug use patterns and the importance of understanding and addressing the full spectrum of drug use patterns over time.

Another application of mixture LCMs is the analysis of depression in persons with myocardial infarction (MI). Elliott *et al.* (2006) analyzed affect and event data from post-MI subjects in order to understand how mood and reactivity to negative events over time relate to diagnostic level depression. In this study, 35 patients who had experienced an MI within the past year and were currently in treatment were investigated. The affect scores and event indicators (indicating presence of positive, negative, and neutral events) of the patients were collected for up to 35 consecutive days. The analysis of mixture LCMs suggests a two-class model for the MI patients: an 'optimist' class with stable positive affect and declining perceived negative events; and a 'pessimist' class with declining positive affect and continuing perceived negative events. Depressed subjects had a 92% chance of belonging to the pessimist class, compared with 62% among nondepressed subjects. This finding uncovers some hitherto unobserved structure in the positive affect and negative event data in this sample. The key advantage of using mixture LCMs in this study is that persons who are most at risk of developing major or minor depression can be identified, which will assist in developing more specific interventions or treatments.

Appendix 8.1 Conditional distributions

Conditional Distribution $p(\boldsymbol{\alpha}, \mathbf{Z}|\cdot)$

In this appendix, we only discuss the situation where $\mathbf{z}_k$ includes the underlying unobservable continuous variables corresponding to $\mathbf{x}_k$, and $\mathbf{Z} = (\mathbf{z}_1, \ldots, \mathbf{z}_r)$ and $\mathbf{X} = (\mathbf{x}_1, \ldots, \mathbf{x}_r)$. Other situations where $\mathbf{Z}$ corresponds to $\mathbf{Y}$ and $\mathbf{U}$ are similar. Let $\boldsymbol{\alpha}_{tk} = (\alpha_{tk,2}, \ldots, \alpha_{tk,h_k})$, $\boldsymbol{\Lambda}_t^T$ be the tth row of $\boldsymbol{\Lambda}$, and z_{tk} be the tth element of $\mathbf{z}_k$. Then

$$p(\boldsymbol{\alpha}, \mathbf{Z}|\cdot) = \prod_{k=1}^{r}\prod_{t=1}^{T} p(\boldsymbol{\alpha}_{tk}, z_{tk}|\cdot) \propto \prod_{k=1}^{r}\prod_{t=1}^{T} \phi\{\psi_{xtk}^{-1/2}\left(z_{tk} - \boldsymbol{\Lambda}_t^T \boldsymbol{\xi}_k\right)\} I_{[\alpha_{tk,x_{tk}}, \alpha_{tk,x_{tk}+1})}(z_{tk}), \quad (8.A1)$$

where $\phi(\cdot)$ is the standard normal density function.

Conditional Distribution $p(\Xi|\cdot)$.

Note that once $\mathbf{Z}$ is given, Ξ is independent of $\boldsymbol{\alpha}$ and $\mathbf{X}$. Then

$$\begin{aligned} p(\boldsymbol{\zeta}|\boldsymbol{\theta}, \boldsymbol{\Omega}, \mathbf{Y}, \mathbf{Z}, \mathbf{U}) &\propto p(\boldsymbol{\Omega}, \mathbf{Y}, \mathbf{Z}, \mathbf{U}|\boldsymbol{\theta}, \boldsymbol{\zeta}) p(\boldsymbol{\zeta}|\boldsymbol{\theta}) \\ &\propto p(\mathbf{y}|\boldsymbol{\theta}, \boldsymbol{\eta}) p(\boldsymbol{\eta}|\boldsymbol{\xi}) p(\boldsymbol{\xi}|\boldsymbol{\theta}) \left[\prod_{k=1}^{r} p(\mathbf{z}_k|\boldsymbol{\theta}, \boldsymbol{\xi}_k)\right]\left[\prod_{k=1}^{q} p(\boldsymbol{\omega}_k|\boldsymbol{\theta}, \boldsymbol{\xi}_{r+k})\right]. \end{aligned}$$

It follows that $p(\boldsymbol{\zeta}|\cdot)$ is proportional to

$$\begin{aligned} \exp\Bigg[-\frac{1}{2}\Big\{ &(\mathbf{y} - \boldsymbol{\Lambda}\boldsymbol{\eta})^T \boldsymbol{\Psi}_y^{-1}(\mathbf{y} - \boldsymbol{\Lambda}\boldsymbol{\eta}) + [\boldsymbol{\eta} - \boldsymbol{\beta} - \boldsymbol{\Lambda}_\delta \mathbf{G}(\boldsymbol{\zeta})]^T \boldsymbol{\Psi}_\delta^{-1}[\boldsymbol{\eta} - \boldsymbol{\beta} - \boldsymbol{\Lambda}_\delta \mathbf{G}(\boldsymbol{\zeta})] \\ &+ \boldsymbol{\xi}^T \boldsymbol{\Phi}^{-1}\boldsymbol{\xi} + \sum_{k=1}^{r}(\mathbf{z}_k - \boldsymbol{\Lambda}\boldsymbol{\xi}_k)^T \boldsymbol{\Psi}_{xk}^{-1}(\mathbf{z}_k - \boldsymbol{\Lambda}\boldsymbol{\xi}_k) + \sum_{k=1}^{q}(\boldsymbol{\omega}_k - \boldsymbol{\Lambda}\boldsymbol{\xi}_{r+k})^T \boldsymbol{\Psi}_{\omega k}^{-1}(\boldsymbol{\omega}_k - \boldsymbol{\Lambda}\boldsymbol{\xi}_{r+k})\Big\}\Bigg]. \end{aligned} \quad (8.A2)$$

Conditional Distribution $p(\boldsymbol{\Omega}|\cdot)$.

Given Ξ, note that $\boldsymbol{\Omega}$ is independent of $\boldsymbol{\alpha}$, $\mathbf{Z}$, $\mathbf{Y}$, and $\mathbf{X}$, and $\{\boldsymbol{\omega}_k, k = 1, \ldots, q\}$ is the appropriate permutation of $\{\boldsymbol{\omega}_{ut}, t = 1, \ldots, T\}$. Thus we have

$$p(\boldsymbol{\Omega}|\cdot) = p(\boldsymbol{\Omega}|\boldsymbol{\theta}, \boldsymbol{\xi}, \mathbf{U}) \propto p(\mathbf{U}|\boldsymbol{\theta}, \boldsymbol{\Omega}) p(\boldsymbol{\Omega}|\boldsymbol{\theta}, \boldsymbol{\xi}) = \prod_{t=1}^{T} p(\mathbf{u}_t|\boldsymbol{\theta}, \boldsymbol{\omega}_{ut}) \prod_{k=1}^{q} p(\boldsymbol{\omega}_k|\boldsymbol{\theta}, \boldsymbol{\xi}_{r+k}).$$

It follows that $p(\boldsymbol{\Omega}|\cdot)$ is proportional to

$$\exp\left[-\frac{1}{2}\left\{\sum_{t=1}^{T}(\mathbf{u}_t - \boldsymbol{\Lambda}_{ut}\boldsymbol{\omega}_{ut})^T \boldsymbol{\Psi}_{ut}^{-1}(\mathbf{u}_t - \boldsymbol{\Lambda}_{ut}\boldsymbol{\omega}_{ut}) + \sum_{k=1}^{q}(\boldsymbol{\omega}_k - \boldsymbol{\Lambda}\boldsymbol{\xi}_{r+k})^T \boldsymbol{\Psi}_{\omega k}^{-1}(\boldsymbol{\omega}_k - \boldsymbol{\Lambda}\boldsymbol{\xi}_{r+k})\right\}\right], \quad (8.A3)$$

where $\boldsymbol{\omega}_{ut} = (\omega_{ut1}, \ldots, \omega_{utq})^T$ for $t = 1, \ldots, T$, and $\boldsymbol{\omega}_k = (\omega_{u1k}, \ldots, \omega_{uTk})^T$ for $k = 1, \ldots, q$.

Conditional Distribution $p(\boldsymbol{\theta}|\cdot)$.

Let $\mathbf{Z}_k = (\mathbf{z}_{k1}, \ldots, \mathbf{z}_{kn})$, $\mathbf{U}_t = (\mathbf{u}_{t1}, \ldots, \mathbf{u}_{tn})$, $\boldsymbol{\Omega}_1 = (\boldsymbol{\eta}_1, \ldots, \boldsymbol{\eta}_n)$, $\tilde{\boldsymbol{\Omega}}_1 = (\boldsymbol{\eta}_1 - \boldsymbol{\beta}, \ldots, \boldsymbol{\eta}_n - \boldsymbol{\beta})$, $\boldsymbol{\Omega}_{2k} = (\boldsymbol{\omega}_{k1}, \ldots, \boldsymbol{\omega}_{kn})$ for $k = 1, \ldots, q$, $\boldsymbol{\Omega}_{3t} = (\boldsymbol{\omega}_{ut1}, \ldots, \boldsymbol{\omega}_{utn})$ for $t = 1, \ldots, T$, $\Xi_k = (\boldsymbol{\xi}_{k1}, \ldots, \boldsymbol{\xi}_{kn})$ for $k = 1, \ldots, r + q$, $\boldsymbol{\Omega}_2 = (\Xi_1^T, \ldots, \Xi_{r+q}^T)^T$, and $\mathbf{G} = (\mathbf{G}(\boldsymbol{\zeta}_1), \ldots,$

$\mathbf{G}(\boldsymbol{\zeta}_n))$, where n is the sample size. Let $\mathbf{Y}_t^T$, $\mathbf{Z}_{tk}^T$, $\boldsymbol{\Omega}_{2tk}^T$, and $\boldsymbol{\Lambda}_t^T$ be the tth rows of $\mathbf{Y}$, $\mathbf{Z}_k$, $\boldsymbol{\Omega}_{2k}$, and $\boldsymbol{\Lambda}$, respectively, and let $\mathbf{U}_{tk}^T$, $\boldsymbol{\Omega}_{1k}^T$, $\tilde{\boldsymbol{\Omega}}_{1k}^T$, and $\boldsymbol{\Lambda}_{utk}^T$ be the kth rows of $\mathbf{U}_t$, $\boldsymbol{\Omega}_1$, $\tilde{\boldsymbol{\Omega}}_1$, and $\boldsymbol{\Lambda}_{ut}$, respectively. It can be shown (see Lee and Song, 2003) that

$$
\begin{aligned}
&\left[\psi_{yt}^{-1}|\mathbf{Y}_t, \boldsymbol{\Omega}_1, \boldsymbol{\Lambda}_t\right] \stackrel{D}{=} \text{Gamma}[n/2 + a_{0yt}, b_{yt}], \quad t = 1, \ldots, T, \\
&\left[\psi_{xtk}^{-1}|\mathbf{Z}_k, \boldsymbol{\Xi}_k, \boldsymbol{\Lambda}_t\right] \stackrel{D}{=} \text{Gamma}[n/2 + a_{0xtk}, b_{xtk}], \quad k = 1, \ldots, r,\ t = 1, \ldots, T, \\
&\left[\psi_{\omega tk}^{-1}|\boldsymbol{\Omega}_{2k}, \boldsymbol{\Xi}_{r+k}, \boldsymbol{\Lambda}_t\right] \stackrel{D}{=} \text{Gamma}[n/2 + a_{0\omega tk}, b_{\omega tk}], \quad k = 1, \ldots, q,\ t = 1, \ldots, T, \\
&[\boldsymbol{\Lambda}_{utk}|\mathbf{U}_t, \boldsymbol{\Omega}_{3t}, \psi_{utk}] \stackrel{D}{=} N[\boldsymbol{\mu}_{utk}, \psi_{utk}\boldsymbol{\Sigma}_{utk}], \quad k = 1, \ldots, p,\ t = 1, \ldots, T, \qquad (8.\text{A4}) \\
&\left[\psi_{utk}^{-1}|\mathbf{U}_t, \boldsymbol{\Omega}_{3t}\right] \stackrel{D}{=} \text{Gamma}[n/2 + a_{0utk}, b_{utk}], \quad k = 1, \ldots, p,\ t = 1, \ldots, T, \\
&[\boldsymbol{\Lambda}_{\delta k}|\tilde{\boldsymbol{\Omega}}_1, \boldsymbol{\Omega}_2, \psi_{\delta k}] \stackrel{D}{=} N[\boldsymbol{\mu}_{\delta k}, \psi_{\delta k}\boldsymbol{\Sigma}_{\delta k}], \quad k = 1, \ldots, m, \\
&\left[\psi_{\delta k}^{-1}|\tilde{\boldsymbol{\Omega}}_1, \boldsymbol{\Omega}_2\right] \stackrel{D}{=} \text{Gamma}[n/2 + a_{0\delta k}, b_{\delta k}], \quad k = 1, \ldots, m, \\
&[\boldsymbol{\beta}|\boldsymbol{\Omega}_1, \boldsymbol{\Omega}_2, \boldsymbol{\Lambda}_\delta, \boldsymbol{\Psi}_\delta] \stackrel{D}{=} N[\boldsymbol{\mu}_\beta, \boldsymbol{\Sigma}_\beta], \quad [\boldsymbol{\Phi}|\boldsymbol{\Omega}_2] \stackrel{D}{=} \text{IW}_{m(r+q)}\left[\left(\boldsymbol{\Omega}_2\boldsymbol{\Omega}_2^T + \mathbf{R}_0^{-1}\right), n + \rho_0\right],
\end{aligned}
$$

where $b_{yt} = b_{0yt} + [\mathbf{Y}_t^T\mathbf{Y}_t - 2\boldsymbol{\Lambda}_t^T\boldsymbol{\Omega}_1\mathbf{Y}_t + \boldsymbol{\Lambda}_t^T(\boldsymbol{\Omega}_1\boldsymbol{\Omega}_1^T)\boldsymbol{\Lambda}_t]/2$, $b_{xtk} = b_{0xtk} + [\mathbf{Z}_{tk}^T\mathbf{Z}_{tk} - 2\boldsymbol{\Lambda}_t^T \boldsymbol{\Xi}_k\mathbf{Z}_{tk} + \boldsymbol{\Lambda}_t^T(\boldsymbol{\Xi}_k\boldsymbol{\Xi}_k^T)\boldsymbol{\Lambda}_t]/2$, $b_{\omega tk} = b_{0\omega tk} + [\boldsymbol{\Omega}_{2tk}^T\boldsymbol{\Omega}_{2tk} - 2\boldsymbol{\Lambda}_t^T\boldsymbol{\Xi}_{r+k}\boldsymbol{\Omega}_{2tk} + \boldsymbol{\Lambda}_t^T(\boldsymbol{\Xi}_{r+k}\boldsymbol{\Xi}_{r+k}^T) \boldsymbol{\Lambda}_t]/2$, $\boldsymbol{\mu}_{utk} = \boldsymbol{\Sigma}_{utk}(\boldsymbol{\Sigma}_{0utk}^{-1}\boldsymbol{\Lambda}_{0utk} + \boldsymbol{\Omega}_{3t}\mathbf{U}_{tk})$, $\boldsymbol{\Sigma}_{utk} = (\boldsymbol{\Sigma}_{0utk}^{-1} + \boldsymbol{\Omega}_{3t}\boldsymbol{\Omega}_{3t}^T)^{-1}$, $b_{utk} = b_{0utk} + [\mathbf{U}_{tk}^T\mathbf{U}_{tk} - \boldsymbol{\mu}_{utk}^T\boldsymbol{\Sigma}_{utk}^{-1}\boldsymbol{\mu}_{utk} + \boldsymbol{\Lambda}_{0utk}^T\boldsymbol{\Sigma}_{0utk}^{-1}\boldsymbol{\Lambda}_{0utk}]/2$, $\boldsymbol{\mu}_{\delta k} = \boldsymbol{\Sigma}_{\delta k}(\boldsymbol{\Sigma}_{0\delta k}^{-1}\boldsymbol{\Lambda}_{0\delta k} + \mathbf{G}\tilde{\boldsymbol{\Omega}}_{1k})$, $\boldsymbol{\Sigma}_{\delta k} = (\boldsymbol{\Sigma}_{0\delta k}^{-1} + \mathbf{G}\mathbf{G}^T)^{-1}$, $b_{\delta k} = b_{0\delta k} + [\tilde{\boldsymbol{\Omega}}_{1k}^T\tilde{\boldsymbol{\Omega}}_{1k} - \boldsymbol{\mu}_{\delta k}^T\boldsymbol{\Sigma}_{\delta k}^{-1}\boldsymbol{\mu}_{\delta k} + \boldsymbol{\Lambda}_{0\delta k}^T\boldsymbol{\Sigma}_{0\delta k}^{-1}\boldsymbol{\Lambda}_{0\delta k}]/2$, $\boldsymbol{\mu}_\beta = \boldsymbol{\Sigma}_\beta[\boldsymbol{\Psi}_\delta^{-1}\sum_{i=1}^n(\boldsymbol{\eta}_i - \boldsymbol{\Lambda}_\delta\mathbf{G}(\boldsymbol{\zeta}_i)) + \boldsymbol{\Sigma}_0^{-1}\boldsymbol{\beta}_0]$, and $\boldsymbol{\Sigma}_\beta = (\boldsymbol{\Sigma}_0^{-1} + n\boldsymbol{\Psi}_\delta^{-1})^{-1}$.

The conditional distributions involved in (8.A3) and (8.A4) are standard, and simulating observations from them is straightforward. As the conditional distributions in (8.A1) and (8.A2) are nonstandard, the Metropolis–Hastings (Metropolis *et al.*, 1953; Hastings, 1970) algorithm will be used to simulate observations from them; see Cowles (1996), Lee and Song (2003).

Appendix 8.2 WinBUGS code for the analysis of cocaine use data

```
model{
     for(i in 1:N){
     # structural equation
     xi[i,1:6]~dmnorm(u[1:6],phi[1:6,1:6])
     for(j in 1:2){ xxi[i,j]~dnorm(nu[i,j],psd[j]) }
     nu[i,1]<-vu[1]+gam[1]*xi[i,1]+gam[2]*xi[i,3]+gam[3]*xi[i,5]
     +gam[4]*xi[i,1]*xi[i,3]+gam[5]*xi[i,1]*xi[i,5]+gam[6]*xi[i,3]*xi[i,5]
     nu[i,2]<-vu[2]+gam[7]*xi[i,2]+gam[8]*xi[i,4]+gam[9]*xi[i,6]
     +gam[10]*xi[i,2]*xi[i,4]+gam[11]*xi[i,2]*xi[i,6]+gam[12]*xi[i,4]*xi[i,6]

     # measurement models
     for(j in 1:20){ y[i,j]~dnorm(mu[i,j],psi[j]) }
         mu[i,1]<- xxi[i,1]
         mu[i,2]<- xxi[i,1]+xxi[i,2]
         mu[i,3]<- xxi[i,1]+2*xxi[i,2]
         mu[i,4]<- xxi[i,1]+12*xxi[i,2]
         mu[i,5]<- xi[i,1]
         mu[i,6]<- xi[i,1]+xi[i,2]
         mu[i,7]<- xi[i,1]+2*xi[i,2]
         mu[i,8]<- xi[i,1]+12*xi[i,2]
         mu[i,9]<- xi1[i,1]
         mu[i,10]<- lam[1]*xi1[i,1]
         mu[i,11]<- lam[2]*xi1[i,1]
         mu[i,12]<- xi1[i,2]
         mu[i,13]<- lam[3]*xi1[i,2]
         mu[i,14]<- lam[4]*xi1[i,2]
         mu[i,15]<- xi1[i,3]
         mu[i,16]<- lam[5]*xi1[i,3]
         mu[i,17]<- lam[6]*xi1[i,3]
         mu[i,18]<- xi1[i,4]
         mu[i,19]<- lam[7]*xi1[i,4]
         mu[i,20]<- lam[8]*xi1[i,4]

         xi1[i,1]<- xi[i,3]
         xi1[i,2]<- xi[i,3]+xi[i,4]
         xi1[i,3]<- xi[i,3]+2*xi[i,4]
         xi1[i,4]<- xi[i,3]+12*xi[i,4]

       for(j in 1:4){ z1[i,j]~dcat(p1[i,j,1:C1])
                      p1[i,j,1]<-Q1[i,j,1]
                      for(t in 2:C1-1){ p1[i,j,t]<- Q1[i,j,t]-Q1[i,j,t-1] }
                      p1[i,j,C1]<- 1-Q1[i,j,C1-1]
       for(t in 1:C1-1){ logit(Q1[i,j,t])<- alph1[j,t]-mu[i,20+2*j-1] } }
 #end j

       for(j in 1:4){ z2[i,j]~dcat(p2[i,j,1:C2])
                      p2[i,j,1]<-Q2[i,j,1]
                      for(t in 2:C2-1){ p2[i,j,t]<- Q2[i,j,t]-Q2[i,j,t-1] }
                      p2[i,j,C2]<- 1-Q2[i,j,C2-1]
       for(t in 1:C2-1){ logit(Q2[i,j,t])<- alph2[j,t]-mu[i,20+2*j] } }
 #end j
```

```
    mu[i,21]<- xi2[i,1]
    mu[i,22]<- lam[9]*xi2[i,1]
    mu[i,23]<- xi2[i,2]
    mu[i,24]<- lam[10]*xi2[i,2]
    mu[i,25]<- xi2[i,3]
    mu[i,26]<- lam[11]*xi2[i,3]
    mu[i,27]<- xi2[i,4]
    mu[i,28]<- lam[12]*xi2[i,4]

    xi2[i,1]<- xi[i,5]
    xi2[i,2]<- xi[i,5]+xi[i,6]
    xi2[i,3]<- xi[i,5]+2*xi[i,6]
    xi2[i,4]<- xi[i,5]+12*xi[i,6] }

   # thresholds for latent variables

  for(j in 1:4){ alph1[j,2]~ dnorm(0.0, 2.0)I(alph1[j,1],) }

  for(j in 1:4){
          alph2[j,2]~ dnorm(0.0, 2.0)I(alph2[j,1],alph2[j,3])
          alph2[j,3]~ dnorm(0.0, 2.0)I(alph2[j,2],alph2[j,4])
          alph2[j,4]~ dnorm(0.0, 2.0)I(alph2[j,3],) }

        for(j in 1:4){ alph1[j, 1]<- 0   alph2[j, 1]<- 0 }

   # priors on loadings and coefficients
   vu[1]~dnorm(0.0,4.0)      vu[2]~dnorm(0.0,4.0)
   for(j in 1:12){ lam[j]~ dnorm(1.0, 4.0) }
   for(j in 1:12){ gam[j]~ dnorm(1.0, 4.0) }

  # priors on precisions
   for(j in 1:20){ psi[j]~dgamma(10.0,4.0)
                   v[j]<-1/psi[j] }
   for(j in 1:2) { psd[j]~dgamma(10.0,4.0)
                   vd[j]<- 1/psd[j] }
   phi[1:6,1:6]~dwish(RR[1:6,1:6],6)
   phx[1:6,1:6]<- inverse(phi[1:6,1:6])

   # put all the parameters' results into bb

   for(j in 1:2){ bb[j]<- vu[j]  }
   for(j in 1:12){ bb[2+j]<- lam[j] }
   for(j in 1:12){ bb[14+j]<- gam[j] }
   for(j in 1:2){ bb[26+j]<- vd[j] }
   for(j in 1:20){ bb[28+j]<- v[j] }
   for(j in 1:6){ bb[48+j]<- phx[1,j] }
   for(j in 2:6){ bb[54+j-1]<- phx[2,j] }
   for(j in 3:6){ bb[59+j-2]<- phx[3,j] }
   for(j in 4:6){ bb[63+j-3]<- phx[4,j] }
   for(j in 5:6){ bb[66+j-4]<- phx[5,j] }
   for(j in 6:6){ bb[68+j-5]<- phx[6,j] }
   for(j in 1:4){ bb[69+j]<- alph1[j,2] }
   for(j in 1:4){ bb[73+j]<- alph2[j,2] }
   for(j in 1:4){ bb[77+j]<- alph2[j,3] }
   for(j in 1:4){ bb[81+j]<- alph2[j,4] }
}
```

```
# init 1 list(paste initial value 1)
# init 2 list(paste initial value 2)
# init 3 list(paste initial value 3)

#Data list(N=321, u=c(0,0,0,0,0,0),  C1=3, C2=5,
    RR=structure(.Data= c(1.0, 0.0, 0.0, 0.0, 0.0, 0.0,
                          0.0, 1.0, 0.0, 0.0, 0.0, 0.0,
                          0.0, 0.0, 1.0, 0.0, 0.0, 0.0,
                          0.0, 0.0, 0.0, 1.0, 0.0, 0.0,
                          0.0, 0.0, 0.0, 0.0, 1.0, 0.0,
                          0.0, 0.0, 0.0, 0.0, 0.0, 1.0), .Dim= c(6,6)),
y=structure(.Data=c(paste continuous variable), .Dim=c(321,20)),
z1=structure(.Data=c(paste the first ordinal variable), .Dim=c(321,4)),
z2=structure(.Data=c(paste the second ordinal variable), .Dim=c(321,4)))
} #end
```

References

Ahlsiö, B., Britton, M., Murray, V. and Theorell, T. (1984) Disablement and quality of life after stroke. *Stroke*, **15**, 886–890.

Beal, C. C., Stuifbergen, A. K., Sands, D. V. and Brown, A. (2007) Depression in multiple sclerosis: A longitudinal analysis. *Archives of Psychiatric Nursing*, **21**, 181–191.

Bollen, K. A. and Curran, P. J. (2006) *Latent Curve Models – A Structural Equation Perspective*. Hoboken, NJ: John Wiley & Sons, Inc.

Brown, R. A., Monti, P. M., Myers, M. G., Martin, R. A., Rivinus, T., Dubreuil, M. E. T. and Rohsenow, D. J. (1998) Depression among cocaine abusers in treatment: Relation to cocaine and alcohol use and treatment outcome. *American Journal of Psychiatry*, **155**, 220–225.

Chiu, H. F., Lee, H. C., Wing, Y. K., Kwong, P. K., Leung, C. M. and Chung, D. W. (1994) Reliability, validity and structure of the Chinese geriatric depression scale in a Hong Kong context: A preliminary report. *Singapore Medical Journal*, **35**, 477–480.

Cowles, M. K. (1996) Accelerating Monte Carlo Markov chain convergence for cumulative-link generalized linear models. *Statistics and Computing*, **6**, 101–111.

Elliott, M. R., Gallo, J. J., Ten Have, T. R., Bogner, H. R. and Katz, I. R. (2006) Using a Bayesian latent growth curve model to identify trajectories of positive affect and negative events following myocardial infarction. *Biostatistics*, **6**, 119–143.

Fisher, K. J. and Li, F. Z. (2004) A community-based walking trial to improve neighborhood quality of life in older adults: A multilevel analysis. *Annals of Behavioral Medicine*, **28**, 186–194.

Geman, S. and Geman, D. (1984) Stochastic relaxation, Gibbs distribution and the Bayesian restoration of images. *IEEE Transactions on Pattern Analysis and Machine Intelligence*, **6**, 721–741.

Harwood, R. H., Rogers, A., Dickinson, E. and Ebrahim, S. (1994) Measuring handicap: The London Handicap Scale, a new outcome measure for chronic disease. *Quality in Health Care*, **3**, 11–16.

Hastings, W. K. (1970) Monte Carlo sampling methods using Markov chains and their application. *Biometrika*, **57**, 97–109.

Hser, Y. I., Stark, M. E., Paredes, A., Huang, D., Anglin, M. D. and Rawson, R. (2006) A 12-year follow-up of a treated cocaine-dependent sample. *Journal of Substance Abuse Treatment*, **30**, 219–226.

Hser, Y. I., Huang, D., Brecht, M. L., Li, L. B. and Evans, E. (2008) Contrasting trajectories of heroin, cocaine, and methamphetamine. *Journal of Addictive Diseases*, **27**, 13–21.

Jöreskog, K. G. (1970) A general method for analysis of covariance structures. *Biometrika*, **57**, 239–251.

Kasarabada, D. N., Anglin, M. D., Khalsa-Denison, E. and Paredes, A. (1999) Differential effects of treatment modality on psychosocial functioning of cocaine-dependent men. *Journal of Clinical Psychology*, **55**, 257–274.

Kwok, T., Lo, R. S., Wong, E., Wai-Kwong, T., Mok, V. and Kai-Sing, W. (2006) Quality of life of stroke survivors: A 1-year follow-up study. *Archives of Physical Medicine and Rehabilitation*, **87**, 1177–1182.

Lee, S. Y. (2007) *Structural Equation Modeling: A Bayesian Approach*. Chichester: John Wiley & Sons, Ltd.

Lee, S. Y. and Song, X. Y. (2003) Model comparison of nonlinear structural equation models with fixed covariates. *Psychometrika*, **68**, 27–47.

Li, F. Z., Duncan, T. E. and Acock, A. (2000) Modeling interaction effects in latent growth curve models. *Structural Equation Modeling – A Multidisciplinary Journal*, **7**, 497–533.

Meredith, W. and Tisak, J. (1990) Latent curve analysis. *Psychometrika*, **55**, 107–122.

Metropolis, N., Rosenbluth, A. W., Rosenbluth, M. N., Teller, A. H. and Teller, E. (1953) Equations of state calculations by fast computing machine. *Journal of Chemical Physics*, **21**, 1087–1091.

Pan, J. H., Song, X. Y., Lee, S. Y. and Kwok, T. (2008) Longitudinal analysis of quality of life for stroke survivors using latent curve models. *Stroke*, **39**, 2795–2802.

Shah, S., Vanclay, F. and Cooper, B. (1989) Improving the sensitivity of the Barthel Index for stroke rehabilitation. *Journal of Clinical Epidemiology*, **42**, 703–709.

Song, X. Y., Lee, S. Y. and Hser, Y. I. (2009) Bayesian analysis of multivariate latent curve models with nonlinear longitudinal latent effects. *Structural Equation Modeling – A Multidisciplinary Journal*, **16**, 245–266.

Stuifbergen, A. K., Blozis, S. A., Harrison, T. C. and Becker, H. A. (2006) Exercise, functional limitations, and quality of life: A longitudinal study of persons with multiple sclerosis. *Archives of Physical Medicine and Rehabilitation*, **87**, 935–943.

Sturtz, S., Ligges, U. and Gelman, A. (2005) R2WinBUGS: A package for running WinBUGS from R. *Journal of Statistical Software*, **12**, 1–16.

9

Longitudinal structural equation models

9.1 Introduction

Analysis of longitudinal data in order to study dynamic changes of various aspects in a statistical or psychometric model has received much attention in statistics as well as medical, social, and psychological research. So far, most longitudinal models have focused on a univariate observed variable measured repeatedly over time. However, for most substantive research, interest lies mainly in the analysis of models defined with multivariate random vectors. Hence, it is necessary to develop multivariate longitudinal models to analyze multivariate data that are measured repeatedly over time. In the field of SEM, longitudinal models were developed by Jöreskog and Sörbom (1977). In their model, an SEM was defined at each time point, then a comprehensive longitudinal SEM that links all the individual SEMs at each time point was formulated. Since the work of Jöreskog and Sörbom(1977), not much further work on longitudinal SEMs has been done, although much progress has been made in statistical methods for analyzing SEMs based on multivariate data measured at a single time point (see Bollen, 1989; Lee, 2007; and previous chapters). The reason may be that the covariance matrix of the observed (and latent) variables involved at all the time points can be very complicated, and hence the classical covariance structure approach is inadequate to cope with such complicated models.

One of the main goals of this chapter is to formulate a longitudinal SEM for analyzing multivariate longitudinal data at different time points. Suppose that at each time point, we can establish an appropriate SEM which involves factor loadings in the measurement equation to relate the observed variables to the latent variables, and regression coefficients in the structural equation to assess the effects of explanatory latent variables on outcome latent variables. In order to study, first, the effects of outcome and explanatory latent variables at previous time points $1, \ldots, t-1$ and explanatory latent variables at time point t on outcome latent variables

Basic and Advanced Bayesian Structural Equation Modeling: With Applications in the Medical and Behavioral Sciences,
First Edition. Xin-Yuan Song and Sik-Yum Lee.

at time point t, and second, the dynamic changes of various aspects of the model (such as factor loadings, regression coefficients, and correlations among latent variables, etc.) over time, it is desirable to formulate a longitudinal SEM that links up the individual SEMs established at the different time points. Moreover, it is desirable to include a component to accommodate characteristics that are invariant over time.

Following on from Song *et al.* (2009, 2011), we consider a longitudinal two-level SEM to assess dynamic changes that are variant and invariant over time. More specifically, let $\mathbf{u}_{gt}$ be a random vector for the gth ($g = 1, \ldots, G$) individual measured at time point t ($t = 1, \ldots, T$). A two-level model for $\mathbf{u}_{gt}$ will be defined by $\mathbf{u}_{gt} = \mathbf{y}_g + \mathbf{v}_{gt}$, where $\mathbf{y}_g$ is the second-level random vector that is independent of t and is used to account for the invariant characteristics over time; while $\mathbf{v}_{gt}$, which depends on t, is the first-level random vector to account for characteristics that change dynamically with t. In general, any general SEMs can be used to model $\mathbf{y}_g$ and/or $\mathbf{v}_{gt}$. In this chapter, for brevity, a confirmatory factor analysis model will be used to model $\mathbf{y}_g$. A nonlinear SEM with fixed covariates will be defined for $\mathbf{v}_{gt}$, in which the latent variables at each time point are divided into outcome and explanatory latent variables, and their dynamic relationships over time are assessed by a flexible autoregressive nonlinear structural equation (see Section 9.2). To cope with the complex nature of real-world data in substantive research, the dynamic two-level nonlinear SEM also accommodates mixed continuous and ordered categorical variables, and missing data that are missing at random (MAR). Note that nonignorable missing data can be handled through the methodologies presented in Section 5.4.4.

In the literature, specific SEMs or latent variable models have been developed for analyzing longitudinal data; however, their objectives and/or formulations are quite different from the current dynamic two-level nonlinear SEMs. For example, a standard growth curve model (see Bollen and Curran, 2006; Song *et al.*, 2009; and Chapter 8) can be viewed as the confirmatory factor analysis model $\mathbf{x}_i = \boldsymbol{\Lambda}\boldsymbol{\omega}_i + \boldsymbol{\epsilon}_i$, where $\mathbf{x}_i$ is a vector of repeated measures of a univariate observed variable, $\boldsymbol{\Lambda}$ is the factor loading matrix of sequential known values of the growth curve records, $\boldsymbol{\omega}_i$ is the latent growth factor usually containing the 'initial status' (intercept) and 'rate of change' (slope), and $\boldsymbol{\epsilon}_i$ is the vector of residuals. This is a single-level SEM, in which the latent variables in $\boldsymbol{\omega}_i$ are used to assess the change in the characteristic of the univariate observed variable over time rather than the dynamic changes of the latent vectors. Hence, the formulation of a growth curve model is much less general, and the interpretation of the latent variables is very different. Dunson (2003) proposed a dynamic latent variable model, which allows mixtures of count, categorical, and continuous response variables, for analyzing multivariate longitudinal data. In this model, the latent variable $\boldsymbol{\omega}_{it}$ at time t for individual i is regressed on the linear terms of the past latent vectors $\boldsymbol{\omega}_{i1}, \ldots, \boldsymbol{\omega}_{i,t-1}$ through a regression equation with fixed covariates. It is also a single-level model, and its latent variables are not divided into explanatory and outcome latent variables. Compared with Dunson's single-level latent variable model, the current longitudinal two-level SEM includes a second-level model for assessing the individuals' characteristics that are invariant with time. Moreover, latent variables at the first level of our model are divided into explanatory and outcome latent variables; and the dynamic nonlinear effects of explanatory latent variables on outcome latent variables are assessed through a rather general autoregressive nonlinear structural equation (see equation (9.5)). Other popular longitudinal models in the statistics and/or biostatistics literature, such as the linear mixed model (Verbeke and Molenberghs, 2000) and the generalized linear mixed model (Diggle *et al.*, 2002), do not involve the latent traits and their associated structural equation. Clearly, the objectives and formulations of these models and the current longitudinal SEM are very different. Finally, as described in Section 9.2, the dynamic two-level SEM is also different from the existing multilevel SEMs.

Again Bayesian methodologies that are based on the idea of data augmentation and MCMC methods such as the Gibbs sampler and the Metropolis–Hastings algorithm are presented to estimate the unknown parameters in the model. For model comparison, as the computational burden for evaluating the Bayes factor via path sampling is heavy due to a large number of parameters and latent variables in the longitudinal SEM, we use the L_ν-measure as a model comparison statistic. Results obtained from a simulation study and an application on cocaine use are provided to illustrate the Bayesian methodologies.

9.2 A two-level SEM for analyzing multivariate longitudinal data

We consider a set of observations of a $p \times 1$ random vector $\mathbf{u}_{gt}$ for individual $g = 1, \ldots, G$, which is measured at several time points $t = 1, \ldots, T$. The collection $\mathbf{U} = \{\mathbf{u}_{gt}, g = 1, \ldots, G, t = 1, \ldots, T\}$ can be regarded as an observed sample of hierarchical observations that were measured at different time points (first level), and nested in the individuals (second level). For the gth individual measured at time points s and t, $\mathbf{u}_{gs}$ and $\mathbf{u}_{gt}$ are correlated. But $\mathbf{u}_{gt}$ and $\mathbf{u}_{ht}$ are independent for $g \neq h$. Hence, the following two-level SEM is used to model $\mathbf{u}_{gt}$:

$$\mathbf{u}_{gt} = \mathbf{y}_g + \mathbf{v}_{gt}, \tag{9.1}$$

where $\mathbf{y}_g$ and $\mathbf{v}_{gt}$ are the random vectors that respectively model the second-level effect of the gth individual, and the first-level effect with respect to the gth individual at time t. Note that the correlation between $\mathbf{u}_{gt_i}$ and $\mathbf{u}_{gt_j}$ is captured by $\mathbf{y}_g$. Moreover, as $\mathbf{y}_g$ is not dependent on t, it is invariant over time and is included in the model to assess characteristics that are invariant over time. On the other hand, $\mathbf{v}_{gt}$, which depends on t, is used to assess the characteristics that change dynamically over time. The random vectors $\mathbf{y}_g$ and $\mathbf{v}_{gt}$ could be modeled by any general SEMs. The choice of model depends on the nature of the problem and the amount of information available for the first and second levels of the model. As our main interest is in studying various characteristics that change dynamically over time, we use a rather general first-level model for $\mathbf{v}_{gt}$. Since the information available at the second level may be much less than the first level, and it may not be desirable to use a complicated model to account for the effects that are invariant over time, we use a relatively simple second-level model for $\mathbf{y}_g$.

More specifically, the second-level model for assessing characteristics of individuals that are invariant over time is defined by

$$\mathbf{y}_g = \mathbf{A}_0\mathbf{c}_{g0} + \mathbf{\Lambda}_0\boldsymbol{\omega}_{g0} + \boldsymbol{\epsilon}_{g0}, \tag{9.2}$$

where $\mathbf{c}_{g0}$ is a vector of fixed covariates, $\boldsymbol{\omega}_{g0}$ is a $q_0 \times 1$ vector of latent variables, $\boldsymbol{\epsilon}_{g0}$ is a vector of residual errors, and $\mathbf{A}_0$ and $\mathbf{\Lambda}_0$ are matrices of unknown coefficients. This is a confirmatory factor analysis model with covariates, which is formulated to study the relationships of the observed variables in $\mathbf{u}_{gt}$ and the latent variables in $\boldsymbol{\omega}_{g0}$ with respect to different individuals but common to all time points. This model is regarded as a second-level measurement equation in the multilevel SEM terminology. We assume that $\boldsymbol{\omega}_{g0}$ is independently and identically distributed (i.i.d.) as $N[\mathbf{0}, \mathbf{\Phi}_0]$, and that $\boldsymbol{\epsilon}_{g0}$ is independent of $\boldsymbol{\omega}_{g0}$, and i.i.d. as $N[\mathbf{0}, \mathbf{\Psi}_0]$, where $\mathbf{\Psi}_0$ is a diagonal matrix.

Next, we consider the following measurement model for the more important first-level random vector $\mathbf{v}_{gt}$:

$$\mathbf{v}_{gt} = \mathbf{A}_t \mathbf{c}_{gt} + \boldsymbol{\Lambda}_t \boldsymbol{\omega}_{gt} + \boldsymbol{\epsilon}_{gt}, \quad g = 1, \ldots, G, \; t = 1, \ldots, T, \tag{9.3}$$

in which the definitions of $\mathbf{A}_t$, $\mathbf{c}_{gt}$, $\boldsymbol{\Lambda}_t$, $\boldsymbol{\omega}_{gt}$, and $\boldsymbol{\epsilon}_{gt}$ are similar to those given in equation (9.2), except that here they are defined at time point t nested within the individual g, and that the distribution of $\boldsymbol{\epsilon}_{gt}$ is $N[\mathbf{0}, \boldsymbol{\Psi}_t]$, where $\boldsymbol{\Psi}_t$ is assumed to be a diagonal matrix for brevity. Hence, we assume that the random vector $\mathbf{u}_{gt}$ conditional on $\mathbf{y}_g$ has the following structure:

$$\mathbf{u}_{gt} = \mathbf{y}_g + \mathbf{A}_t \mathbf{c}_{gt} + \boldsymbol{\Lambda}_t \boldsymbol{\omega}_{gt} + \boldsymbol{\epsilon}_{gt}, \quad g = 1, \ldots, G, \; t = 1, \ldots, T. \tag{9.4}$$

Conditional on $\mathbf{y}_g$, equation (9.4) accounts for dependency among the observed variables measured for individual g at a given time point t through the fixed covariates $\mathbf{c}_{gt}$ and the shared latent vector $\boldsymbol{\omega}_{gt}$. By estimating the regression coefficients $\mathbf{A}_t$ and $\boldsymbol{\Lambda}_t$, this measurement equation is useful for studying how the relationships of the observed variables and the corresponding fixed covariates and latent variables change dynamically over time.

We consider a partition of $\boldsymbol{\omega}_{gt}$ into $(\boldsymbol{\eta}_{gt}^T, \boldsymbol{\xi}_{gt}^T)^T$, where $\boldsymbol{\eta}_{gt}$ and $\boldsymbol{\xi}_{gt}$ are q_1-dimensional outcome and q_2-dimensional explanatory random latent vectors respectively, and $q = q_1 + q_2$. Effects of the explanatory latent variables $\boldsymbol{\xi}_{gt}$ at the current time point and the latent variables at previous time points on the outcome latent variables $\boldsymbol{\eta}_{gt}$ are studied through the following autoregressive nonlinear structural equation: for $g = 1, \ldots, G$,

$$\begin{aligned} \boldsymbol{\eta}_{g1} &= \mathbf{B}_0 \mathbf{d}_{g0} + \mathbf{B}_1 \mathbf{d}_{g1} + \boldsymbol{\Gamma}_1^* \mathbf{F}_1^*(\boldsymbol{\xi}_{g1}) + \boldsymbol{\delta}_{g1}, \\ \boldsymbol{\eta}_{gt} &= \mathbf{B}_0 \mathbf{d}_{g0} + \mathbf{B}_t \mathbf{d}_{gt} + \boldsymbol{\Gamma}_t^* \mathbf{F}_t^*(\boldsymbol{\omega}_{g1}, \ldots, \boldsymbol{\omega}_{g,t-1}, \boldsymbol{\xi}_{gt}) + \boldsymbol{\delta}_{gt}, \quad t = 2, \ldots, T, \end{aligned} \tag{9.5}$$

where $\mathbf{B}_0$, $\mathbf{B}_t$, and $\boldsymbol{\Gamma}_t^*$ are matrices of unknown coefficients, $\mathbf{d}_{g0}$ is a vector of fixed covariates which is independent of t, $\mathbf{d}_{gt}$ is another vector of fixed covariates, $\boldsymbol{\delta}_{gt}$ is a vector of residual errors, and $\mathbf{F}_t^* = (f_{t1}, \ldots, f_{tr})$ is a vector-valued function in which f_{tj} is a differentiable function of the explanatory latent vector $\boldsymbol{\xi}_{gt}$ at the current time point, and the latent vectors $\boldsymbol{\omega}_{g1}, \ldots, \boldsymbol{\omega}_{g,t-1}$ at previous time points. The residual vector $\boldsymbol{\delta}_{gt}$ is independent of $\boldsymbol{\epsilon}_{gt}$, $\boldsymbol{\omega}_{g1}, \ldots, \boldsymbol{\omega}_{g,t-1}$, and $\boldsymbol{\xi}_{gt}$. Moreover, these residual errors are i.i.d. $N[\mathbf{0}, \boldsymbol{\Psi}_{\delta t}]$, where $\boldsymbol{\Psi}_{\delta t}$ is a diagonal matrix. Let $\boldsymbol{\xi}_g = (\boldsymbol{\xi}_{g1}^T, \ldots, \boldsymbol{\xi}_{gT}^T)^T$; the distribution of $\boldsymbol{\xi}_g$ is assumed to be $N[\mathbf{0}, \boldsymbol{\Phi}]$, where $\boldsymbol{\Phi}$ contains the covariance matrix $\boldsymbol{\Phi}_{tt}$ of $\boldsymbol{\xi}_{gt}$, and the covariance matrix $\boldsymbol{\Phi}_{t_i t_j}$ of $\boldsymbol{\xi}_{gt_i}$ and $\boldsymbol{\xi}_{gt_j}$ at different time points t_i and t_j.

The first and second terms of equation (9.5) allow for direct effects of observed predictors that are invariant over time ($\mathbf{d}_{g0}$) and variant over time ($\mathbf{d}_{gt}$) on the outcome latent variables. The term $\boldsymbol{\Gamma}_t^* \mathbf{F}_t^*(\cdot)$ is very important for assessing the dynamic effects of explanatory latent variables on the outcome latent vector $\boldsymbol{\eta}_{gt}$. It is very general and allows various flexible autoregressive structures for recovering different complicated dependencies (through general differentiable functions f_{tj}) of the outcome latent variables in $\boldsymbol{\eta}_{gt}$ at the current time point and across both outcome latent variables at previous time points, and explanatory latent variables at previous and current time points. For example, typical special cases are, for $t = 2, \ldots, T$,

(a) $\boldsymbol{\eta}_{gt} = \boldsymbol{\beta}_{t-1} \boldsymbol{\eta}_{g,t-1} + \boldsymbol{\Gamma}_1 \boldsymbol{\xi}_{g1} + \ldots + \boldsymbol{\Gamma}_{t-1} \boldsymbol{\xi}_{g,t-1} + \boldsymbol{\Gamma}_t \mathbf{F}_t(\boldsymbol{\xi}_{gt}) + \boldsymbol{\delta}_{gt}$,

(b) $\boldsymbol{\eta}_{gt} = \boldsymbol{\beta}_1 \boldsymbol{\eta}_{g1} + \ldots + \boldsymbol{\beta}_{t-1} \boldsymbol{\eta}_{g,t-1} + \boldsymbol{\Gamma}_t \mathbf{F}_t(\boldsymbol{\xi}_{gt}) + \boldsymbol{\delta}_{gt}$,

(c) $\boldsymbol{\eta}_{gt} = \boldsymbol{\beta}_{t-1} \boldsymbol{\eta}_{g,t-1} + \boldsymbol{\Gamma}_{t-1} \mathbf{F}_{t-1}(\boldsymbol{\xi}_{g,t-1}) + \boldsymbol{\Gamma}_t \mathbf{F}_t(\boldsymbol{\xi}_{gt}) + \boldsymbol{\delta}_{gt}$, where $\mathbf{F}_{t-1}$ and $\mathbf{F}_t$ are vectors of differentiable functions. In special case (a), $\boldsymbol{\eta}_{gt}$ is regressed on the linear explanatory latent vectors at all previous time points, the outcome latent vector at $t-1$, and finally nonlinear terms of explanatory latent variables at the current time point. The autoregressive structure (b) allows $\boldsymbol{\eta}_{gt}$ to depend on the previous outcome latent vectors $\boldsymbol{\eta}_{g1}, \ldots, \boldsymbol{\eta}_{g,t-1}$ and a general function $\mathbf{F}_t(\boldsymbol{\xi}_{gt})$ of the current explanatory latent vector $\boldsymbol{\xi}_{gt}$. By means of (c), the linear effects of the latent vector $\boldsymbol{\eta}_{g,t-1}$ at time $t-1$, and general nonlinear effects $\mathbf{F}_{t-1}(\boldsymbol{\xi}_{g,t-1})$ and $\mathbf{F}_t(\boldsymbol{\xi}_{g,t})$ of the explanatory latent vectors at previous time $t-1$ and current time t on the current outcome latent vector $\boldsymbol{\eta}_{gt}$ can be assessed. To simplify notation, let $\boldsymbol{\Lambda}_{\omega t} = (\mathbf{B}_t, \boldsymbol{\Gamma}_t^*)$ and $\mathbf{h}_{gt} = (\mathbf{d}_{gt}^T, \mathbf{F}_t^*(\boldsymbol{\omega}_{g1}, \ldots, \boldsymbol{\omega}_{g,t-1}, \boldsymbol{\xi}_{gt})^T)^T$. Then equation (9.5) can be rewritten as

$$\boldsymbol{\eta}_{gt} = \mathbf{B}_0\mathbf{d}_{g0} + \boldsymbol{\Lambda}_{\omega t}\mathbf{h}_{gt} + \boldsymbol{\delta}_{gt}. \tag{9.6}$$

Other multilevel SEMs have been developed to analyze hierarchical data collected from units that are nested within clusters; see Chapter 6 and references therein. The objectives of those multilevel SEMs are to handle the hierarchical effects rather than the dynamic changes of characteristics. Due to different objectives, the formulations of the first-level model for $\mathbf{v}_{gt}$ in those multilevel SEMs are quite different, and do not accommodate certain important features of the current dynamic model. For example, their matrices of coefficient parameters and covariance matrices of errors in the first-level model vary with the cluster g rather than t; see equations (6.1) and (6.4). Moreover, for $t \neq r$, the $\mathbf{v}_{gt}$ and $\mathbf{v}_{gr}$ in other two-level SEMs are assumed to be independent; however, $\mathbf{v}_{gt}$ and $\mathbf{v}_{gr}$ are correlated in the current two-level longitudinal SEM.

As ordered categorical data are very common in substantive research, the Bayesian methodologies for analyzing the longitudinal SEM are introduced to account for mixed continuous and categorical variables. Suppose that $\mathbf{u}_{gt}$ is composed of a subvector $\mathbf{x}_{gt}$ of observed measurements, and a subvector $\mathbf{w}_{gt}$ of unobserved measurements whose information is given by ordered categorical observations. In a generic sense, the relation of an ordered categorical variable z and its underlying continuous variable w is defined by $z = k$ if $\alpha_k \leq w < \alpha_{k+1}$, for $k = 0, 1, \ldots, m$, where $\{-\infty = \alpha_0 < \alpha_1 < \ldots < \alpha_m < \alpha_{m+1} = \infty\}$ is the set of threshold parameters that define the $m+1$ categories. Moreover, missing data that are MAR (Little and Rubin, 2002) are handled through the procedure given in Song and Lee (2002). Details are omitted here for brevity.

This two-level longitudinal SEM is not identified without imposing identification constraints. Existing methods suggested in the SEM literature can be adopted for identifying various components of the current model. For example, the identification problem associated with an ordered categorical variable can be solved by fixing the thresholds α_1 and/or α_m at some appropriate preassigned values (see Section 5.2), and the covariance structures in the first- and second-level models can be identified by fixing appropriate elements in $\boldsymbol{\Lambda}_0$, and $\boldsymbol{\Lambda}_t$ at preassigned values (see Song and Lee, 2008).

9.3 Bayesian analysis of the two-level longitudinal SEM

9.3.1 Bayesian estimation

In the Bayesian estimation of the longitudinal two-level nonlinear SEM with missing categorical data, we adopt a commonly used strategy in the Bayesian analysis of SEMs that involves two key steps. The first step is to augment the observed data with all the latent variables and the missing data to form a complete data set and then consider the resulting joint posterior distribution. The second step is to draw a sufficiently large sample of observations from the joint posterior distribution via MCMC methods such as the Gibbs sampler and the MH algorithm.

Let $\boldsymbol{\alpha}$ be the vector that contains all the unknown thresholds, and let $\boldsymbol{\theta}$ be the parameter vector that contains all the unknown distinct structural parameters in $\{\mathbf{A}_t, \boldsymbol{\Lambda}_t, \boldsymbol{\Psi}_t, t = 0, 1, \ldots, T\}$ and $\{\boldsymbol{\Lambda}_{\omega t}, \boldsymbol{\Psi}_{\delta t}, \mathbf{B}_0, \boldsymbol{\Phi}_0, \boldsymbol{\Phi}, t = 1, \ldots, T\}$, which are involved in the measurement and structural equations, respectively. Let $\mathbf{z}_{gt} = (z_{gt1}, \ldots, z_{gts})^T$ be an $s \times 1$ vector of ordered categorical observations, and $\mathbf{u}_{gt} = \{\mathbf{w}_{gt}, \mathbf{x}_{gt}\}$, where $\mathbf{x}_{gt}$ is a vector of continuous measurements and $\mathbf{w}_{gt}$ is the latent continuous measurement corresponding to $\mathbf{z}_{gt}$. Let $\mathbf{u}_g = \{\mathbf{u}_{gt}, t = 1, \ldots, T\}$, $\mathbf{Z} = \{\mathbf{z}_{gt}, g = 1, \ldots, G, t = 1, \ldots, T\}$, $\mathbf{W} = \{\mathbf{w}_{gt}, g = 1, \ldots, G, t = 1, \ldots, T\}$, and $\mathbf{X} = \{\mathbf{x}_{gt}, g = 1, \ldots, G, t = 1, \ldots, T\}$. Moreover, let $\boldsymbol{\omega}_g = (\boldsymbol{\eta}_{g1}^T, \ldots, \boldsymbol{\eta}_{gT}^T, \boldsymbol{\xi}_{g1}^T, \ldots, \boldsymbol{\xi}_{gT}^T)^T$, $\boldsymbol{\Omega}_1 = \{\boldsymbol{\omega}_g, g = 1, \ldots, G\}$, $\boldsymbol{\Omega}_0 = \{\boldsymbol{\omega}_{g0}, g = 1, \ldots, G\}$, and $\mathbf{Y} = \{\mathbf{y}_g, g = 1, \ldots, G\}$ be matrices of various kinds of latent vectors at the first and second levels. To obtain the Bayesian estimates of the unknown parameters in $\boldsymbol{\alpha}$ and $\boldsymbol{\theta}$, observations are simulated from the joint posterior distribution $[\boldsymbol{\theta}, \boldsymbol{\alpha}, \mathbf{W}, \mathbf{Y}, \boldsymbol{\Omega}_0, \boldsymbol{\Omega}_1 | \mathbf{X}, \mathbf{Z}]$ by implementing the Gibbs sampler (Geman and Geman, 1984) and the MH algorithm (Metropolis *et al.*, 1953; Hastings, 1970).

Since the joint posterior distribution depends on the prior distribution of $\boldsymbol{\theta}$ through $p(\boldsymbol{\theta})$, the selection of the appropriate prior distribution for $\boldsymbol{\theta}$ is an important issue in the Bayesian approach. As in previous chapters, we use conjugate prior distributions. Recall that the key advantage of a conjugate prior distribution is that the resulting posterior distribution will follow the same parametric form of the prior distribution (see Lee, 2007); and hence conjugacy ensures proper posterior distributions and a relatively easy derivation of the conditional distributions. More specifically, the prior distributions of the unknown parameters in $\boldsymbol{\theta}$ are given as follows. For $t = 0, 1, \ldots, T$ and $k = 1, \ldots, p$, let ψ_{tk} be the variance of ϵ_{gtk}, and $\mathbf{A}_{tk}^T$ and $\boldsymbol{\Lambda}_{tk}^T$ be the kth rows of $\mathbf{A}_t$ and $\boldsymbol{\Lambda}_t$, respectively. Moreover, for $t = 1, \ldots, T$ and $l = 1, \ldots, q_1$, let $\psi_{\delta tl}$ be the lth diagonal elements of $\boldsymbol{\Psi}_{\delta t}$, and $\boldsymbol{\Lambda}_{\omega tl}^T$ and $\mathbf{B}_{0l}^T$ be the lth rows of $\boldsymbol{\Lambda}_{\omega t}$ and $\mathbf{B}_0$, respectively. The following common conjugate prior distributions in Bayesian analysis of SEMs are used:

$$\begin{aligned}
&\psi_{0k}^{-1} \stackrel{D}{=} \text{Gamma}[\alpha_{0k}, \beta_{0k}], \quad [\boldsymbol{\Lambda}_{0k}|\psi_{0k}] \stackrel{D}{=} N[\tilde{\boldsymbol{\Lambda}}_{0k}, \psi_{0k}\mathbf{H}_{0k}],\\
&\mathbf{A}_{0k} \stackrel{D}{=} N[\tilde{\mathbf{A}}_{0k}, \mathbf{H}_{0ak}],\\
&\mathbf{B}_{0l} \stackrel{D}{=} N[\mathbf{b}_{0l}, \mathbf{H}_{0bl}], \quad \boldsymbol{\Phi}_0^{-1} \stackrel{D}{=} W_{q_0}[\mathbf{R}_0, \rho_0], \quad \boldsymbol{\Phi}^{-1} \stackrel{D}{=} W_{q_2 \times T}[\mathbf{R}_w, \rho_w],
\end{aligned} \tag{9.7}$$

and for $t = 1, \ldots, T$,

$$\begin{aligned}
&\psi_{tk}^{-1} \stackrel{D}{=} \text{Gamma}[\alpha_{0tk}, \beta_{0tk}], \quad [\boldsymbol{\Lambda}_{tk}|\psi_{tk}] \stackrel{D}{=} N[\boldsymbol{\Lambda}_{0tk}, \psi_{tk}\mathbf{H}_{0tk}],\\
&\mathbf{A}_{tk} \stackrel{D}{=} N[\mathbf{A}_{0tk}, \mathbf{H}_{0atk}],\\
&\psi_{\delta tl}^{-1} \stackrel{D}{=} \text{Gamma}[\tilde{\alpha}_{0tl}, \tilde{\beta}_{0tl}], \quad [\boldsymbol{\Lambda}_{\omega tl}|\psi_{\delta tl}] \stackrel{D}{=} N[\tilde{\boldsymbol{\Lambda}}_{0tl}, \psi_{\delta tl}\tilde{\mathbf{H}}_{0tl}],
\end{aligned} \tag{9.8}$$

where $\alpha_{0k}, \beta_{0k}, \alpha_{0tk}, \beta_{0tk}, \tilde{\alpha}_{0tl}, \tilde{\beta}_{0tl}, \tilde{\boldsymbol{\Lambda}}_{0k}, \tilde{\mathbf{A}}_{0k}, \mathbf{b}_{0l}, \boldsymbol{\Lambda}_{0tk}, \mathbf{A}_{0tk}, \tilde{\boldsymbol{\Lambda}}_{0tl}, \rho_0, \rho_w$, and the positive definite matrices $\mathbf{H}_{0k}, \mathbf{H}_{0ak}, \mathbf{H}_{0bl}, \mathbf{H}_{0tk}, \mathbf{H}_{0atk}, \tilde{\mathbf{H}}_{0tl}, \mathbf{R}_0, \mathbf{R}_w$ are hyperparameters whose values are assumed to be preassigned based on the prior information. Moreover, we use the common noninformative prior distributions for the unknown thresholds in $\boldsymbol{\alpha}$ (see Chapter 5). Under the above prior distributions, the full conditional distributions required in implementing the

Gibbs sampler are presented in Appendix 9.1, together with a brief discussion on the MH algorithm for simulating observations from some nonstandard conditional distributions.

As before, the convergence of the algorithm can be determined by examining the plots of a number (usually three) of different sequences of simulated observations with different initial values. At convergence, these sequences should mix well together. Suppose that the algorithm converges after the Kth iteration; a sufficient number of simulated observations, say J, after the Kth iteration are then collected. Statistical inference for the model can be conducted on the basis of a sample of observations, $\{(\boldsymbol{\theta}^{(j)}, \boldsymbol{\alpha}^{(j)}, \mathbf{W}^{(j)}, \mathbf{Y}^{(j)}, \boldsymbol{\Omega}_0^{(j)}, \boldsymbol{\Omega}_1^{(j)}), j = 1, \ldots, J\}$, simulated via the Gibbs sampler from the joint posterior distribution. The Bayesian estimate of $(\boldsymbol{\theta}, \boldsymbol{\alpha})$ and their standard error estimates can be obtained from the sample means and sample covariance matrices of $\{(\boldsymbol{\theta}^{(j)}, \boldsymbol{\alpha}^{(j)}), j = 1, \ldots, J\}$, respectively. Moreover, Bayesian estimates of the latent variables can be obtained similarly.

9.3.2 Model comparison via the L_ν-measure

We now consider the important issue of model comparison. Due to the high dimensionality and the complexity of the longitudinal two-level nonlinear SEM with categorical data, the commonly used Bayesian model comparison statistics, such as the Bayes factor, require considerable computational effort to obtain. Hence, we use the L_ν-measure as the Bayesian statistic for model comparison; see Section 4.3.3.

To compute the L_ν-measure for the two-level longitudinal SEM with ordered categorical variables, we first dichotomize the ordered categorical responses as follows (see Chen *et al.*, 2004): for $t = 1, \ldots, T$, $j = 1, \ldots, s$, and $g = 1, \ldots, G$,

$$z_{gtj,k} = \begin{cases} 1 & \text{if } k = z_{gtj}, \\ 0 & \text{if } k \neq z_{gtj}. \end{cases}$$

Let $\mathbf{z}^*_{gtj} = (z_{gtj,0}, \ldots, z_{gtj,m_j})^T$, where $m_j + 1$ is the number of categories for z_{gtj}; and let $(\mathbf{z}^{*\text{rep}T}_{gt1}, \ldots, \mathbf{z}^{*\text{rep}T}_{gts})^T$ and $\mathbf{x}^{\text{rep}}_{gt}$ be the future dichotomized vector of an ordered categorical response $\mathbf{z}_{gt}$ and the future vector of continuous response $\mathbf{x}_{gt}$ of an imaginary replicated experiment, respectively. For some $0 \leq \nu \leq 1$, we consider the following multivariate version of the L_ν-measure (see Song *et al.*, 2011):

$$L_\nu(\mathbf{X}, \mathbf{Z}) = \sum_{g=1}^{G} \sum_{t=1}^{T} \left[\text{tr}\{\text{Cov}(\mathbf{x}^{\text{rep}}_{gt} | \mathbf{X}, \mathbf{Z})\} + \nu (E(\mathbf{x}^{\text{rep}}_{gt} | \mathbf{X}, \mathbf{Z}) - \mathbf{x}_{gt})^T (E(\mathbf{x}^{\text{rep}}_{gt} | \mathbf{X}, \mathbf{Z}) - \mathbf{x}_{gt}) \right]$$

$$+ \sum_{g=1}^{G} \sum_{t=1}^{T} \sum_{j=1}^{s} \left[\text{tr}\{\text{Cov}(\mathbf{z}^{*\text{rep}}_{gtj} | \mathbf{X}, \mathbf{Z})\} + \nu (E(\mathbf{z}^{*\text{rep}}_{gtj} | \mathbf{X}, \mathbf{Z}) - \mathbf{z}^*_{gtj})^T (E(\mathbf{z}^{*\text{rep}}_{gtj} | \mathbf{X}, \mathbf{Z}) - \mathbf{z}^*_{gtj}) \right], \quad (9.9)$$

where the expectation is taken with respect to the posterior predictive distribution of $p(\mathbf{x}^{\text{rep}}_{gt}, \mathbf{z}^{*\text{rep}}_{gtj} | \mathbf{X}, \mathbf{Z})$. It can be seen from equation (9.9) that both the first and the second terms of $L_\nu(\mathbf{X}, \mathbf{Z})$ are a sum of two components. The first component is related to the variability of the prediction, whereas the second component is related to the discrepancy between the prediction and the observed data. Hence, small values of the L_ν-measure indicate predictions close to the observed values with low variability. Naturally, the model with the smallest L_ν-measure is selected from a collection of competing models. Note that using $\nu = 1$ gives equal weight to the squared bias and the variance component. However, allowing ν to vary provides more flexibility in the tradeoff between bias and variance. As suggested by Ibrahim *et al.* (2001), we take $v = 0.5$ in the real example presented in Section 9.5. Details for approximating the covariances and expectations with MCMC samples are given in Appendix 9.2.

9.4 Simulation study

Results obtained in the following simulation study are reported here to empirically evaluate the performance of the Bayesian approach for estimation. A special case of the longitudinal two-level SEM defined in equations (9.1)–(9.3) and (9.5) with $p = 9$ and $G = 800$ at four time points is considered. We used a two-factor confirmatory factor analysis model for the second-level model associated with individuals, where the true population values of the parameters are given as follows: $\mathbf{A}_0 = \mathbf{0}$,

$$\mathbf{\Lambda}_0^T = \begin{bmatrix} 0.6 & 1 & 0.6 & 0 & 0 & 0 & 0 & 0 & 0 \\ 0 & 0 & 0 & 0.6 & 1 & 0.6 & 0.6 & 0.6 & 0.6 \end{bmatrix}, \quad \mathbf{\Psi}_0 = \text{diag}(0.2, \ldots, 0.2),$$

and the elements in $\mathbf{\Phi}_0$ are taken as $\phi_{0,11} = 1.0, \phi_{0,12} = 0.3$, and $\phi_{0,22} = 1.0$. For the measurement equations of the first-level model associated with $t = 1, \ldots, 4$ (see equation (9.3)), the covariates are all equal to 1.0. Hence, $\mathbf{A}_t$ is a vector of intercepts, whose true values are all equal to 0.5. The true values of parameters in $\mathbf{\Psi}_t$ and $\mathbf{\Lambda}_t$ are $\mathbf{\Psi}_t = \text{diag}(0.5, 0.5, 1, 0.5, 0.5, 1, 0.5, 0.5, 1)$ and

$$\mathbf{\Lambda}_t^T = \begin{bmatrix} 1 & 0.8 & 0.8 & 0 & 0 & 0 & 0 & 0 & 0 \\ 0 & 0 & 0 & 1 & 0.8 & 0.8 & 0 & 0 & 0 \\ 0 & 0 & 0 & 0 & 0 & 0 & 1 & 0.8 & 0.8 \end{bmatrix}.$$

The 1s and 0s in $\mathbf{\Lambda}_0$, $\mathbf{\Lambda}_t$, and $\mathbf{\Psi}_t$ are fixed to identify the model. The latent variables in $\boldsymbol{\omega}_{gt} = (\eta_{gt}, \xi_{1gt}, \xi_{2gt})^T$ are modeled through the following structural equation: for $g = 1, \ldots, 800$ and $t = 1, \ldots, 4$,

$$\eta_{gt} = b_{10}d_{1g0} + b_t d_{gt} + \beta_{t-1}\eta_{g,t-1} + \gamma_{t1}\xi_{1gt} + \gamma_{t2}\xi_{2gt} + \delta_{gt}, \tag{9.10}$$

where the fixed covariates d_{1g0} are independently generated from the standard normal distribution, and the fixed covariates d_{gt} are generated from a Bernoulli distribution with probability of success 0.6. The true values of the parameters involved in equation (9.10) are: $b_{10} = 0.5$, and, for all $t = 1, \ldots, 4$, $b_t = 0.7$, $\gamma_{t1} = \gamma_{t2} = 0.6$, $\psi_{\delta t} = 0.36$, $(\phi_{t,11}, \phi_{t,12}, \phi_{t,22})$ in $\mathbf{\Phi}_{tt}$ equal to $(1.0, 0.3, 1.0)$, and covariances of ξ_{igt_j} and ξ_{kgt_l} are all 0.3. For $t = 2, 3, 4$, $\beta_{t-1} = 0.6$. Based on the above specifications of the model and the true parameter values, continuous observations of $\mathbf{u}_{gt}$ can be generated. To consider the model with ordered categorical data, the 1st, 2nd, 4th, 5th, 7th, and 8th entries in every $\mathbf{u}_{gt}$ were transformed to ordered categorical using the thresholds $(-1.2, -0.6, 0.6, 1.2)$; while the 3rd, 6th, and 9th entries were transformed to dichotomous variables with the threshold 0.0. Moreover, missing data are considered by randomly deleting some entries in $\mathbf{u}_{gt}$. About 80% of the observations in the data set are fully observed. The total number of parameters in this longitudinal two-level SEM is 201. Using the conjugate prior distributions with reasonably accurate prior inputs, it is observed from a few test runs that the MCMC algorithm converged within 6000 iterations. Hence, for each of the 100 replications, a total of 14 000 observations were collected after discarding 6000 burn-in iterations to obtain the Bayesian results. The bias (Bias) and the root mean squares (RMS) between the estimates and the true population values of the parameters were computed as follows:

$$\text{Bias of } \hat{\theta}(h) = 100^{-1} \sum_{r=1}^{100} [\hat{\theta}_r(h) - \theta_0(h)],$$

$$\text{RMS of } \hat{\theta}(h) = \left\{ 100^{-1} \sum_{r=1}^{100} [\hat{\theta}_r(h) - \theta_0(h)]^2 \right\}^{1/2},$$

where $\theta_0(h)$ is the hth element of the true parameter vector, and $\hat{\theta}_r(h)$ is its Bayesian estimate at the rth replication. Simulation results obtained on the basis of 100 replications are presented in Tables 9.1 and 9.2. We observe from these tables that the bias and RMS are rather small. These results indicate that the empirical performance of the Bayesian estimates obtained using the Bayesian approach is satisfactory. To save space, results associated with the nuisance threshold parameters are omitted.

9.5 Application: Longitudinal study of cocaine use

We illustrate the Bayesian methodology through a longitudinal data set on cocaine use and related phenomena; see Song *et al.* (2009). Cocaine use is a major social and health problem in many countries. In the United States, cocaine is consistently detected in the urine specimens from approximately one-third of arrestees tested across the nation each year, and it is the illegal drug mentioned most often in emergency department records. There are various latent traits that influence cocaine use. Specifically, many studies have shown substantial impact of psychiatric problems on cocaine-dependent patients (see Carroll *et al.*, 1993; Patkar *et al.*, 2004), and social support is another key latent trait (see Weisner *et al.*, 2003; Hser, 2007). Although treatment for cocaine use has received considerable attention in recent years, the longitudinal pattern of cocaine use in relation to psychiatric problems and social support has not yet been adequately explicated. To illustrate the Bayesian methodology, the data set, obtained from a longitudinal study of cocaine use conducted at the UCLA Center for Advancing Longitudinal Drug Abuse Research, is analyzed. In this data set, observations were obtained from cocaine-dependent patients at intake, 1 year, 2 years, and 12 years after treatment (Hser *et al.*, 2006). The longitudinal two-level SEM is applied to assess the dynamic effects of the latent traits (psychiatric problems and social support) on cocaine use.

Various measures were collected from patients admitted to the West Los Angeles Veterans Affairs Medical Center in 1988–1989 who met the DSM III-R criteria for cocaine dependence (Kasarabada *et al.*, 1999). Data obtained from these patients were obtained at baseline, 1 year after treatment, 2 years after treatment, and 12 years after treatment ($t = t_1, t_2, t_3, t_4$) in 2002–2003. Among those patients located at the 12-year follow-up, some were confirmed to be deceased, some declined to be interviewed, and some were either out of the country or too ill to be interviewed. As a result, there is a considerable amount of missing data. The following observed variables at each time t are involved in the current analysis: (i) cocaine use (CC), an ordered categorical variable coded 0 to 4 to denote fewer than 2 days of cocaine use per month, 2–7 days, 8–14 days, 15–25 days, and more than 25 days, respectively; (ii) Beck Inventory (BI), an ordered categorical variable coded 0 to 4 to denote scores that are less than 3.0, between 3.0 and 8.0, between 9.0 and 20.0, between 21 and 30, and larger than 30; (iii) depression (DEP), an ordered categorical variable based on the Hopkins Symptom

Table 9.1 Bias and root mean squares of parameter estimates in the first-level model.

Measurement model						Structural equation					
Par	Bias	RMS	Par	Bias	RMS	Par	Bias	RMS	Par	Bias	RMS
$\lambda_{1,21}$	0.001	0.044	$a_{1,1}$	0.001	0.067	b_{10}	−0.006	0.030	ϕ_{11}	−0.047	0.132
$\lambda_{1,31}$	0.002	0.078	$a_{1,2}$	−0.003	0.077	b_1	0.003	0.074	ϕ_{12}	−0.031	0.078
$\lambda_{1,52}$	0.038	0.080	$a_{1,3}$	0.005	0.082	b_2	−0.029	0.101	ϕ_{13}	−0.023	0.084
$\lambda_{1,62}$	0.059	0.113	$a_{1,4}$	−0.001	0.053	b_3	0.001	0.099	ϕ_{14}	−0.019	0.074
$\lambda_{1,83}$	0.046	0.077	$a_{1,5}$	0.004	0.061	b_4	−0.030	0.095	ϕ_{15}	−0.033	0.074
$\lambda_{1,93}$	0.045	0.113	$a_{1,6}$	0.021	0.088	β_1	0.012	0.060	ϕ_{16}	−0.019	0.073
$\lambda_{2,21}$	−0.012	0.035	$a_{1,7}$	−0.019	0.058	β_2	0.009	0.046	ϕ_{17}	−0.024	0.071
$\lambda_{2,31}$	0.002	0.066	$a_{1,8}$	−0.004	0.048	β_3	0.008	0.048	ϕ_{18}	−0.017	0.055
$\lambda_{2,52}$	0.029	0.080	$a_{1,9}$	0.006	0.065	γ_{11}	0.009	0.076	ϕ_{22}	−0.076	0.141
$\lambda_{2,62}$	0.021	0.099	$a_{2,1}$	0.013	0.100	γ_{12}	0.033	0.078	ϕ_{23}	−0.018	0.069
$\lambda_{2,83}$	0.024	0.074	$a_{2,2}$	0.008	0.085	γ_{21}	0.009	0.079	ϕ_{24}	−0.032	0.069
$\lambda_{2,93}$	0.022	0.092	$a_{2,3}$	0.033	0.108	γ_{22}	0.011	0.074	ϕ_{25}	−0.027	0.061
$\lambda_{3,21}$	0.005	0.046	$a_{2,4}$	0.002	0.048	γ_{31}	0.020	0.069	ϕ_{26}	−0.034	0.067
$\lambda_{3,31}$	0.025	0.094	$a_{2,5}$	−0.001	0.053	γ_{32}	0.001	0.070	ϕ_{27}	−0.024	0.069
$\lambda_{3,52}$	0.043	0.080	$a_{2,6}$	0.011	0.071	γ_{41}	0.008	0.090	ϕ_{28}	−0.027	0.061
$\lambda_{3,62}$	0.030	0.101	$a_{2,7}$	−0.006	0.052	γ_{42}	0.020	0.063	ϕ_{33}	−0.049	0.139
$\lambda_{3,83}$	0.030	0.074	$a_{2,8}$	−0.012	0.042	ϕ_{47}	−0.023	0.061	ϕ_{34}	−0.023	0.070
$\lambda_{3,93}$	0.036	0.090	$a_{2,9}$	−0.007	0.080	ϕ_{48}	−0.029	0.062	ϕ_{35}	−0.029	0.077
$\lambda_{4,21}$	0.004	0.040	$a_{3,1}$	−0.012	0.123	ϕ_{55}	−0.069	0.142	ϕ_{36}	−0.018	0.074
$\lambda_{4,31}$	0.041	0.099	$a_{3,2}$	−0.010	0.108	ϕ_{56}	−0.020	0.059	ϕ_{37}	−0.029	0.076
$\lambda_{4,52}$	0.039	0.082	$a_{3,3}$	0.005	0.115	ϕ_{57}	−0.036	0.078	ϕ_{38}	−0.020	0.062
$\lambda_{4,62}$	0.039	0.120	$a_{3,4}$	−0.010	0.056	ϕ_{58}	−0.017	0.060	ϕ_{44}	−0.048	0.141
$\lambda_{4,83}$	0.022	0.067	$a_{3,5}$	−0.012	0.058	ϕ_{66}	−0.048	0.106	ϕ_{45}	−0.025	0.064
$\lambda_{4,93}$	0.035	0.107	$a_{3,6}$	−0.012	0.065	ϕ_{67}	−0.022	0.068	ϕ_{46}	−0.031	0.065
$a_{3,7}$	−0.001	0.058	$a_{4,4}$	0.002	0.054	ϕ_{68}	−0.024	0.062	ϕ_{77}	−0.060	0.144
$a_{3,8}$	0.004	0.059	$a_{4,5}$	0.001	0.058	ϕ_{78}	−0.014	0.062	ϕ_{88}	−0.049	0.111
$a_{3,9}$	0.014	0.065	$a_{4,6}$	−0.007	0.062						
$a_{4,1}$	0.004	0.116	$a_{4,7}$	−0.005	0.053						
$a_{4,2}$	0.000	0.103	$a_{4,8}$	−0.005	0.049						
$a_{4,3}$	0.010	0.118	$a_{4,9}$	0.004	0.063						

Table 9.2 Bias and root mean squares of parameter estimates in the second-level model.

Par	Bias	RMS	Par	Bias	RMS	Par	Bias	RMS
$\lambda_{0,11}$	0.030	0.071	$\lambda_{0,72}$	0.004	0.041	$\phi_{0,11}$	−0.084	0.163
$\lambda_{0,31}$	0.034	0.075	$\lambda_{0,82}$	0.008	0.042	$\phi_{0,12}$	−0.009	0.080
$\lambda_{0,42}$	0.012	0.036	$\lambda_{0,92}$	0.014	0.053	$\phi_{0,22}$	−0.033	0.088
$\lambda_{0,62}$	0.016	0.059						

Checklist-58 scores, coded 0 to 4 to denote scores that are less than 1.1, between 1.1 and 1.4, between 1.4 and 1.8, between 1.8 and 2.5, and larger than 2.5; (iv) number of friends (NF), an ordered categorical variable coded 0 to 4 to denote no friend, 1 friend, 2–4 friends, 5–8 friends, more than 9 friends; (v) 'have someone to talk to about problem (TP)'; (vi) 'currently employed (EMP)'; and (vii) 'alcohol dependence (AD) at baseline'. The last three variables are dichotomous variables with {0, 1} for {no, yes}. The sample size is 227, and the frequencies of all variables at different time points are given in Table 9.3.

In the Bayesian analysis, we consider observed variables (CC, BI, DEP, NF, TP) and two fixed covariates (EMP, AD) for each individual who was measured at the four time points.

Table 9.3 Frequencies of the ordered categorical variables at different time points in the cocaine use example.

		Categories							
Variables		0	1	2	3	4	No = 0	Yes = 1	Total
	CC	13	24	38	37	115			227
	BI	14	45	66	27	11			163
	DEP	15	29	31	58	26			159
$t = 1$	NF	28	30	65	27	8			158
	TP						30	174	204
	EMP						90	137	227
	AD						121	106	227
	CC	92	46	23	22	44			227
	BI	30	59	67	22	9			187
	DEP	39	47	41	49	17			193
$t = 2$	NF	26	28	92	21	18			185
	TP						15	182	197
	EMP						72	155	227
	AD						121	106	227
	CC	108	31	25	16	47			227
	BI	37	54	74	20	9			194
	DEP	48	41	46	41	13			189
$t = 3$	NF	22	22	96	29	23			192
	TP						9	205	214
	EMP						82	145	227
	AD						121	106	227
	CC	174	15	14	8	15			226
	BI	58	73	68	10	16			225
	DEP	64	54	43	46	20			227
$t = 4$	NF	21	38	113	27	25			224
	TP						22	202	224
	EMP						86	141	227
	AD						121	106	227

The longitudinal two-level SEM (see equations (9.1)–(9.3) and (9.5)) is applied to analyze this data set. The following second-level model, which is a two-factor confirmatory factor analysis model, is used to assess invariant effects over time:

$$\mathbf{y}_g = \mathbf{\Lambda}_0 \boldsymbol{\omega}_{g0} + \boldsymbol{\epsilon}_{g0}, \quad g = 1, \ldots, 227, \tag{9.11}$$

where $\mathbf{y}_g$ includes the observed variables (CC, BI, DEP, NF, TP) for the gth individual, $\boldsymbol{\omega}_{g0} = (\omega_{g01}, \omega_{g02})^T$, $\mathbf{\Psi}_0 = \text{diag}(0, \psi_{02}, \psi_{03}, \psi_{04}, \psi_{05})$,

$$\mathbf{\Lambda}_0^T = \begin{bmatrix} 1 & 0 & 0 & 0 & 0 \\ 0 & \lambda_{0,22} & 1 & \lambda_{0,42} & \lambda_{0,52} \end{bmatrix}, \text{ and } \mathbf{\Phi}_0 = \begin{bmatrix} \phi_{0,11} & \\ \phi_{0,21} & \phi_{0,22} \end{bmatrix},$$

where the 0s and 1s in $\mathbf{\Lambda}_0$ and $\mathbf{\Psi}_0$ are fixed to identify the model. As y_{g1} is fully defined by CC, $\lambda_{0,11}$ and ψ_{01} are respectively fixed at 1 and 0 in line with the common SEM practice (Bollen, 1989; Lee, 2007). In this second-level model, ω_{g01} can be interpreted as the invariant portion of cocaine use and ω_{g02} can be interpreted as a general latent factor that is invariant over time. The covariance of ω_{g01} and ω_{g02} is assessed by $\phi_{0,21}$. We now consider the first-level model for assessing various dynamic effects that change over time. Based on the meaning of the observed variables, the measurement equation of the first-level model is defined by

$$\mathbf{v}_{gt} = \mathbf{A}_t \mathbf{c}_{gt} + \mathbf{\Lambda}_t \boldsymbol{\omega}_{gt} + \boldsymbol{\epsilon}_{gt}, \quad g = 1, \ldots, 227, \; t = t_1, \ldots, t_4, \tag{9.12}$$

where $\mathbf{c}_{gt} = 1$, $\mathbf{A}_t$ is a vector of intercepts, $\boldsymbol{\omega}_{gt} = (\eta_{gt}, \xi_{1gt}, \xi_{2gt})^T$, and

$$\mathbf{\Lambda}_t^T = \begin{bmatrix} 1 & 0 & 0 & 0 & 0 \\ 0 & 1 & \lambda_{t,32} & 0 & 0 \\ 0 & 0 & 0 & 1 & \lambda_{t,53} \end{bmatrix},$$

in which the 1s and 0s are fixed parameters. The non-overlapping structure of $\mathbf{\Lambda}_t$ is used to obtain a clear interpretation of the latent variables. Based on the structure of $\mathbf{\Lambda}_t$ and the meaning of the observed variables, the latent variables η_{gt}, ξ_{1gt}, and ξ_{2gt} can be clearly interpreted as 'cocaine use' (CC), 'psychiatric problems', and 'social support'. In the structural equation of this first-level model, cocaine use is treated as the outcome latent variable (η_{gt}), and it is regressed on various explanatory latent variables, and fixed covariates EMP (d_{gt}) and AD (d_{g0}) that are variant and invariant over time, respectively. We applied the L_ν-measure to compare several models. Here, we only report the results obtained in comparing the following two competing models, which have the same second-level model and the same measurement equation in the first-level model. However, two different structural equations in the first-level model were considered:

$$M_1 : \eta_{g1} = b_0 d_{g0} + b_1 d_{g1} + \gamma_{11}\xi_{1g1} + \gamma_{21}\xi_{2g1} + \gamma_{31}\xi_{1g1}\xi_{2g1} + \delta_{g1}, \quad \text{for } t = t_1,$$

$$\eta_{gt} = b_0 d_{g0} + b_t d_{gt} + \beta_{t-1}\eta_{g,t-1} + \gamma_{1t}\xi_{1gt} + \gamma_{2t}\xi_{2gt} + \gamma_{3t}\xi_{1gt}\xi_{2gt} + \delta_{gt}, \quad \text{for } t = t_2, t_3, t_4;$$

$$M_2 : \eta_{g1} = b_0 d_{g0} + b_1 d_{g1} + \gamma_{11}\xi_{1g1} + \gamma_{21}\xi_{2g1} + \delta_{g1}, \quad \text{for } t = t_1,$$

$$\eta_{gt} = b_0 d_{g0} + b_t d_{gt} + \beta_{t-1}\eta_{g,t-1} + \gamma_{1t}\xi_{1gt} + \gamma_{2t}\xi_{2gt} + \delta_{gt}, \quad \text{for } t = t_2, t_3, t_4.$$

Of these competing models, M_1 is more general than M_2, which does not involve any interactions. Each of them involves a large number (more than 90) of unknown parameters. To reduce the total number of unknown parameters, the nuisance threshold parameters associated with the categorical variables were not treated as unknown but fixed at $\alpha_{jh} = \Phi^{*-1}(\rho_{jh})$, where $\Phi^*(\cdot)$ is the distribution function of $N[0, 1]$, and ρ_{jh} are the observed cumulative marginal proportions of the categories with $z_j < h$. Bayesian results were obtained using 10 000 observations simulated after 40 000 burn-in iterations from the joint posterior distribution via the Gibbs sampler together with the MH algorithm.

The L_ν-measures associated with M_1 and M_2 are equal to 3891.4 and 3886.1, respectively. Hence, the simpler model M_2 with no interaction term is selected. The PP p-value (see Gelman *et al.*, 1996) associated with M_2 is 0.618, which indicates that the selected model M_2 fits the sample data. The Bayesian estimates of some parameters in the first-level and second-level models are respectively presented in the path diagrams displayed in Figures 9.1 and 9.2, together with their standard error estimates. Bayesian estimates of the parameters in $\mathbf{\Phi}$ are presented in Table 9.4.

The longitudinal patterns of the more important parameters in the first-level model are presented in Figures 9.3 and 9.4. Based on Figures 9.1, 9.3, and 9.4, the following phenomena are observed. (i) At all time points ($t = t_1, \ldots, t_4$), $\hat{\lambda}_{32}$ is close to 1.0. This indicates that BI and DEP give equal constant loadings over time on the latent variable 'psychiatric problems, ξ_{1gt}'; and that the association between 'psychiatric problems' and {BI, DEP} is very stable over time (they both measure depression symptoms). (ii) The effect of fixed covariate AD on CC is minor. (iii) The fixed covariate EMP has a negative effect on CC at all time points (see the line labeled 'b' in Figure 9.3), which reveals that having a job reduces cocaine use. (iv) The positive effect of the latent variable 'social support' on cocaine use at baseline changes quickly to negative effects at 2 years after intake, as well as years after treatment (see the line labeled 'γ_2'). This shows that social support has a substantial impact of reducing cocaine use during the past-treatment period. (v) We note that $\hat{\gamma}_1$ decreases from baseline to 1 or 2 years after intake, but rebounds during the long-term follow-up period. This indicates that the impact of psychiatric problems is still strong for a long period of time after treatment, although it may be reduced during treatment or shortly after. (vi) It is interesting to find that estimates of the variances $\hat{\phi}_{11}$, $\hat{\phi}_{22}$, and $\hat{\phi}_{12}$ are basically constant over time (see Figure 9.4). (vii) The changes in $\hat{\lambda}_{53}$, $\hat{\gamma}_1$, and $\hat{\gamma}_2$ are substantial from baseline to 1 or 2 years after intake, but less substantial in the subsequent years (see Figure 9.3). (viii) The effects of cocaine use from $t = t_1$ to $t = t_2$, and from $t = t_2$ to $t = t_3$ are -0.009 $(=\hat{\beta}_1)$ and 0.578 $(=\hat{\beta}_2)$, respectively. After a time difference of 10 years, the corresponding effect from $t = t_3$ to $t = t_4$ is reduced to 0.033 $(=\hat{\beta}_3)$ (see Figure 9.1). These findings are consistent with the previous literature that shows a strong stability of cocaine use over time. The present modeling results also demonstrate a positive association of psychiatric problems with cocaine use at the baseline and the long-term follow-up period. The increasingly negative association of social support with cocaine use is obvious at the later follow-up points, which suggests that the social support becomes a stronger factor influencing cocaine use when the treatment effects dissipate at the longer follow-up point, and future studies are needed to further this investigation. To save space, the straightforward interpretation of the second-level model is not discussed.

9.6 Discussion

This chapter introduces a general longitudinal two-level nonlinear SEM with covariates for analyzing longitudinal data that involve mixed continuous and ordered categorical observations, as well as missing data. Various characteristics that are variant and invariant over time can be assessed through the two-level structure of the model. We wish to point out that the structural

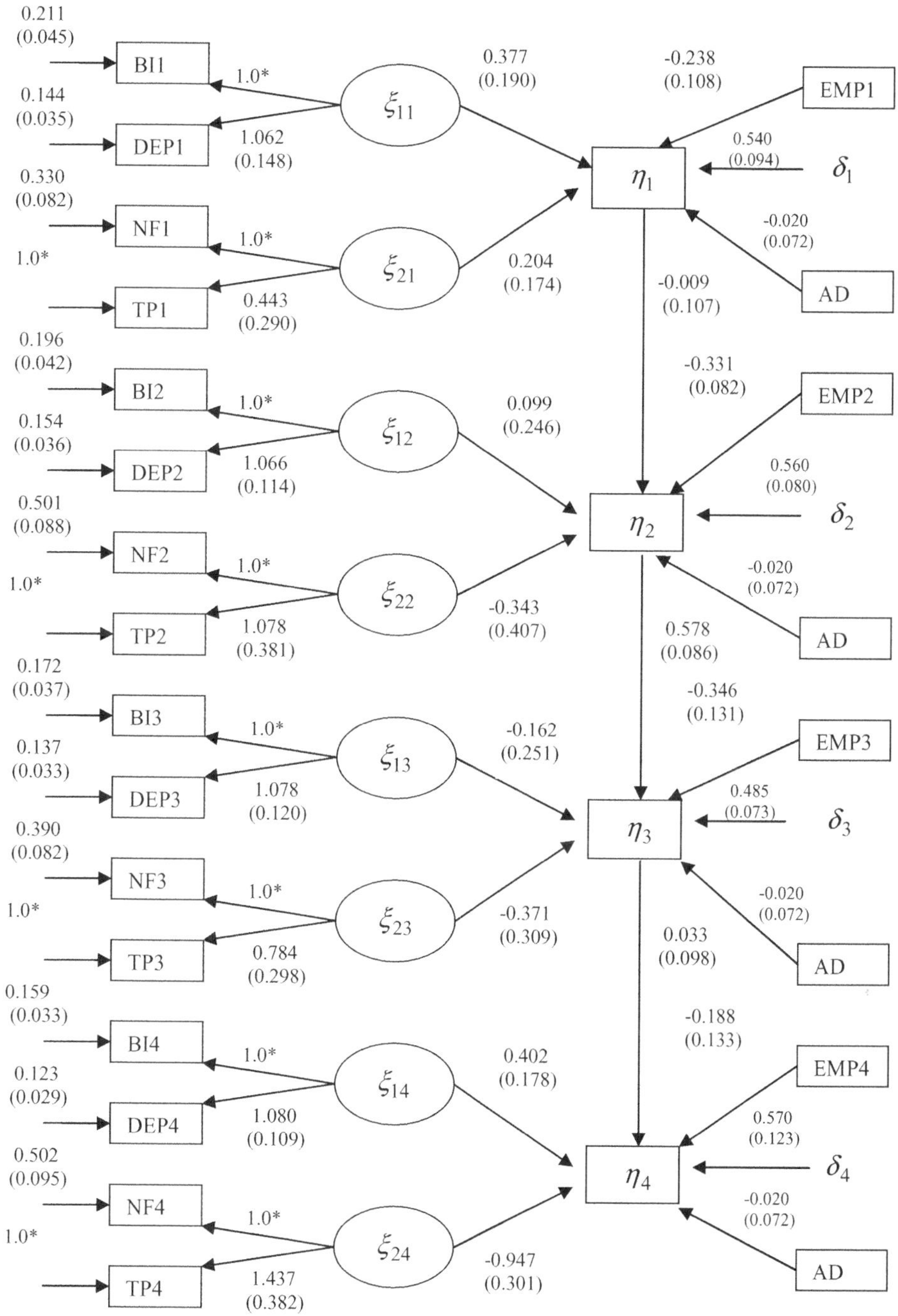

Figure 9.1 Path diagram and estimates of parameters of the first-level model in the selected model, where observed variables are represented by rectangles, latent variables are represented by ellipses, and standard error estimates are in parentheses. Here, η_t, ξ_{1t}, and ξ_{2t} respectively denote cocaine use (CC), psychiatric problems, and social support at $t = 1, \ldots, 4$.

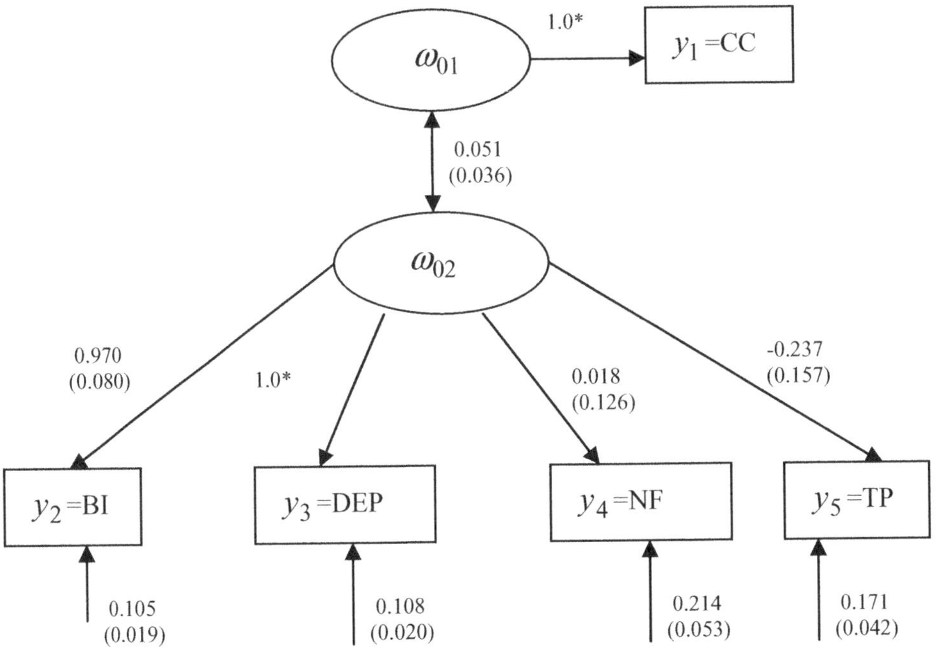

Figure 9.2 Path diagram and estimates of parameters of the second-level model in the selected model.

Table 9.4 Bayesian estimates and their standard error estimates (in parentheses) of $\mathbf{\Phi} = [\mathbf{\Phi}_{t_i t_j}]$ in the cocaine use example.

$t = 1$	0.340							
	(0.080)							
	−0.187	0.374						
	(0.060)	(0.125)						
$t = 2$	0.086	−0.085	0.436					
	(0.049)	(0.065)	(0.083)			symmetric		
	−0.073	0.177	−0.240	0.267				
	(0.048)	(0.088)	(0.084)	(0.112)				
$t = 3$	0.089	−0.272	0.221	−0.213	0.439			
	(0.056)	(0.078)	(0.073)	(0.077)	(0.108)			
	−0.035	0.256	−0.213	0.203	−0.305	0.357		
	(0.047)	(0.084)	(0.071)	(0.084)	(0.065)	(0.094)		
$t = 4$	−0.079	−0.034	−0.091	−0.030	0.033	−0.019	0.393	
	(0.053)	(0.057)	(0.049)	(0.061)	(0.056)	(0.057)	(0.078)	
	0.092	0.039	−0.101	0.128	−0.142	0.098	−0.171	0.287
	(0.051)	(0.063)	(0.056)	(0.067)	(0.068)	(0.061)	(0.050)	(0.083)

Reproduced by permission of Taylor & Francis from Song, X. Y., Lu, Z. H., Hser, Y. I. and Lee, S. Y. (2011). A Bayesian approach for analyzing longitudinal structural equation models. *Structural Equation Modeling - A multidisciplinary Journal*, **18**, 183–194.

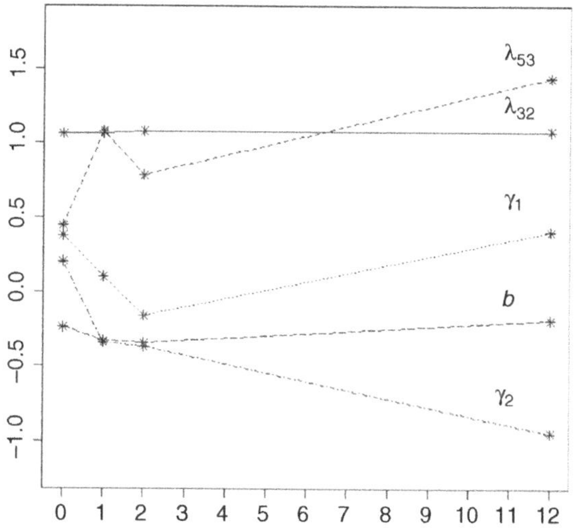

Figure 9.3 Plots of Bayesian estimates of λ_{32}, λ_{53}, b, γ_1, and γ_2 at $t = t_1, \ldots, t_4$.

equation (see equation (9.5)) of the first-level model is very general. Various autoregressive relationships among latent variables at different time points can be analyzed. Clearly, the classical covariance structure approach cannot be applied to analyze the current complicated SEM. Hence, we utilize Bayesian methodologies for estimation and model comparison, and show that they are effective in the analysis of the longitudinal SEM. This is a typical example to illustrate that data augmentation coupled with MCMC methods can be applied to efficiently analyze complicated SEMs.

Like many SEMs, the current longitudinal two-level SEM was considered under the crucial assumption that the distributions of latent variables and residual errors are normal.

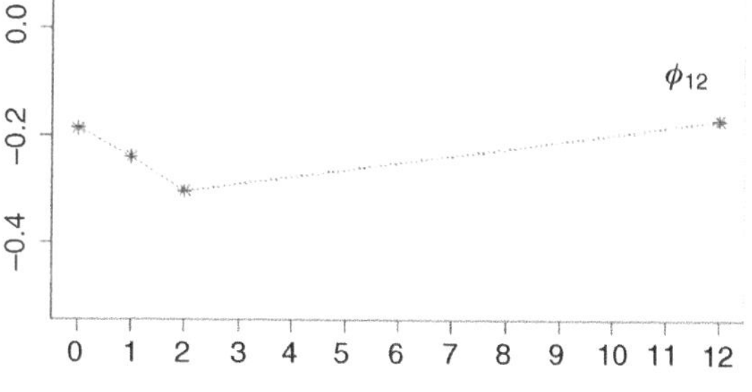

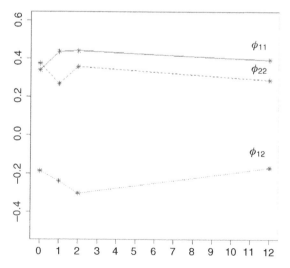

Figure 9.4 Plots of Bayesian estimates of ϕ_{11}, ϕ_{12}, and ϕ_{22} at $t = t_1, \ldots, t_4$.

As this assumption may not be true in substantive research, development of robust methods for analyzing nonnormal longitudinal data is important. Hence, a natural extension of the current model is to assume that the distributions of the latent variables or residual errors in both first- and second-level models are unknown, and to model these unknown distributions through Bayesian semiparametric modeling based on a truncated Dirichlet process with stick-breaking priors; see details in Chapter 10 and Song *et al.* (2011).

Appendix 9.1 Full conditional distributions for implementing the Gibbs sampler

Recall that $\mathbf{u}_{gt} = \{\mathbf{w}_{gt}, \mathbf{x}_{gt}\}$ for $g = 1, \ldots, G$ and $t = 1, \ldots, T$. Let $\mathbf{U} = \{\mathbf{u}_{gt}, \; g = 1, \ldots, G, t = 1, \ldots, T\}$; then $\mathbf{U} = (\mathbf{W}, \mathbf{X})$. Hence, the conditional distributions of $\mathbf{Y}$, $\mathbf{\Omega}_0$, $\mathbf{\Omega}_1$, and $\boldsymbol{\theta}$ given $\mathbf{U}$ are independent of $\mathbf{Z}$ and $\boldsymbol{\alpha}$.

Sampling from $[\mathbf{Y}|\mathbf{\Omega}_0, \mathbf{\Omega}_1, \mathbf{U}, \boldsymbol{\theta}]$, $[\mathbf{\Omega}_0|\mathbf{Y}, \mathbf{\Omega}_1, \mathbf{U}, \boldsymbol{\theta}]$, *and* $[\mathbf{\Omega}_1|\mathbf{Y}, \mathbf{\Omega}_0, \mathbf{U}, \boldsymbol{\theta}]$

Based on the definition and properties of the current model, it can be shown that

$$p(\mathbf{Y}|\mathbf{\Omega}_0, \mathbf{\Omega}_1, \mathbf{U}, \boldsymbol{\theta}) = \prod_{g=1}^{G} p(\mathbf{y}_g|\boldsymbol{\omega}_{g0}, \boldsymbol{\omega}_g, \mathbf{u}_g, \boldsymbol{\theta}),$$

where

$$p(\mathbf{y}_g|\boldsymbol{\omega}_{g0}, \boldsymbol{\omega}_g, \mathbf{u}_g, \boldsymbol{\theta}) \stackrel{D}{=} N\Bigg[\mathbf{\Sigma}_v\Bigg\{\sum_{t=1}^{T} \mathbf{\Psi}_t^{-1}(\mathbf{u}_{gt} - \mathbf{A}_t\mathbf{c}_{gt} - \mathbf{\Lambda}_t\boldsymbol{\omega}_{gt})$$

$$+ \mathbf{\Psi}_0^{-1}(\mathbf{A}_0\mathbf{c}_{g0} + \mathbf{\Lambda}_0\boldsymbol{\omega}_{g0})\Bigg\}, \mathbf{\Sigma}_v\Bigg], \quad \text{with } \mathbf{\Sigma}_v = \left(\sum_{t=1}^{T} \mathbf{\Psi}_t^{-1} + \mathbf{\Psi}_0^{-1}\right)^{-1}; \tag{9.A1}$$

$$p(\mathbf{\Omega}_0|\mathbf{Y}, \mathbf{\Omega}_1, \mathbf{U}, \boldsymbol{\theta}) = \prod_{g=1}^{G} p(\boldsymbol{\omega}_{g0}|\mathbf{y}_g, \boldsymbol{\theta}),$$

where

$$p(\boldsymbol{\omega}_{g0}|\mathbf{y}_g, \boldsymbol{\theta}) \stackrel{D}{=} N[\mathbf{m}_{g0}, \mathbf{\Sigma}_{g0}],$$

$$\text{with } \mathbf{m}_{g0} = \mathbf{\Sigma}_{g0}\mathbf{\Lambda}_0^T\mathbf{\Psi}_0^{-1}(\mathbf{y}_g - \mathbf{A}_0\mathbf{c}_{g0}), \quad \mathbf{\Sigma}_{g0} = \left(\mathbf{\Phi}_0^{-1} + \mathbf{\Lambda}_0^T\mathbf{\Psi}_0^{-1}\mathbf{\Lambda}_0\right)^{-1}; \tag{9.A2}$$

and

$$p(\mathbf{\Omega}_1|\mathbf{Y}, \mathbf{\Omega}_0, \mathbf{U}, \boldsymbol{\theta}) = \prod_{g=1}^{G} p(\boldsymbol{\omega}_g|\mathbf{y}_g, \mathbf{u}_g, \boldsymbol{\theta}),$$

where

$$p(\boldsymbol{\omega}_g|\mathbf{y}_g, \mathbf{u}_g, \boldsymbol{\theta}) \propto$$

$$\exp\Bigg[-\frac{1}{2}\Bigg\{\boldsymbol{\xi}_g^T\mathbf{\Phi}^{-1}\boldsymbol{\xi}_g + \sum_{t=1}^{T}(\mathbf{u}_{gt} - \mathbf{y}_g - \mathbf{A}_t\mathbf{c}_{gt} - \mathbf{\Lambda}_t\boldsymbol{\omega}_{gt})^T\mathbf{\Psi}_t^{-1}(\mathbf{u}_{gt} - \mathbf{y}_g - \mathbf{A}_t\mathbf{c}_{gt} - \mathbf{\Lambda}_t\boldsymbol{\omega}_{gt})$$

$$+ \sum_{t=1}^{T}(\boldsymbol{\eta}_{gt} - \mathbf{B}_0\mathbf{d}_{g0} - \mathbf{\Lambda}_{\omega t}\mathbf{h}_{gt})^T\mathbf{\Psi}_{\delta t}^{-1}(\boldsymbol{\eta}_{gt} - \mathbf{B}_0\mathbf{d}_{g0} - \mathbf{\Lambda}_{\omega t}\mathbf{h}_{gt})\Bigg\}\Bigg]. \tag{9.A3}$$

Sampling from $[\boldsymbol{\theta}, \boldsymbol{\alpha}, \mathbf{W}|\mathbf{Y}, \mathbf{\Omega}_0, \mathbf{\Omega}_1, \mathbf{X}, \mathbf{Z}]$

Observations can be simulated from $[\boldsymbol{\theta}, \boldsymbol{\alpha}, \mathbf{W}|\mathbf{Y}, \mathbf{\Omega}_0, \mathbf{\Omega}_1, \mathbf{X}, \mathbf{Z}]$ by completing the following updates in each cycle of the Gibbs sampler.

(i) Sampling from $[\mathbf{\Lambda}_t, \mathbf{A}_t, \psi_{tk}|\mathbf{Y}, \mathbf{\Omega}_1, \mathbf{U}]$. Let $\mathbf{\Omega}_{1t} = (\boldsymbol{\omega}_{1t}, \ldots, \boldsymbol{\omega}_{Gt})$, $\mathbf{C}_t = (\mathbf{c}_{1t}, \ldots, \mathbf{c}_{Gt})$, $\tilde{\mathbf{u}}_{gt} = \mathbf{u}_{gt} - \mathbf{y}_g - \mathbf{A}_t\mathbf{c}_{gt}$, $\tilde{\mathbf{u}}^*_{gt} = \mathbf{u}_{gt} - \mathbf{y}_g - \mathbf{\Lambda}_t\boldsymbol{\omega}_{gt}$, $\tilde{\mathbf{U}}_t = (\tilde{\mathbf{u}}_{1t}, \ldots, \tilde{\mathbf{u}}_{Gt})$, $\tilde{\mathbf{U}}^*_t = (\tilde{\mathbf{u}}^*_{1t}, \ldots, \tilde{\mathbf{u}}^*_{Gt})$, and $\tilde{\mathbf{U}}^T_{tk}$ and $\tilde{\mathbf{U}}^{*^T}_{tk}$ be the kth rows of $\tilde{\mathbf{U}}_t$ and $\tilde{\mathbf{U}}^*_t$, respectively. Moreover, let $\mathbf{H}_{\epsilon tk} = (\mathbf{H}^{-1}_{0tk} + \mathbf{\Omega}_{1t}\mathbf{\Omega}^T_{1t})^{-1}$, $\mathbf{\Lambda}_{\epsilon tk} = \mathbf{H}_{\epsilon tk}(\mathbf{H}^{-1}_{0tk}\mathbf{\Lambda}_{0tk} + \mathbf{\Omega}_{1t}\tilde{\mathbf{U}}_{tk})$, $\beta_{\epsilon tk} = \beta_{0tk} + (\tilde{\mathbf{U}}^T_{tk}\tilde{\mathbf{U}}_{tk} - \mathbf{\Lambda}^T_{\epsilon tk}\mathbf{H}^{-1}_{\epsilon tk}\mathbf{\Lambda}_{\epsilon tk} + \mathbf{\Lambda}^T_{0tk}\mathbf{H}^{-1}_{0tk}\mathbf{\Lambda}_{0tk})/2$, $\mathbf{H}_{atk} = (\mathbf{H}^{-1}_{0atk} + \psi^{-1}_{tk}\mathbf{C}_t\mathbf{C}^T_t)^{-1}$, and $\mathbf{A}_{atk} = \mathbf{H}_{atk}(\mathbf{H}^{-1}_{0atk}\mathbf{A}_{0atk} + \psi^{-1}_{tk}\mathbf{C}_t\tilde{\mathbf{U}}^*_{tk})$. It can be shown that, for $k = 1, \ldots, p$ and $t = 1, \ldots, T$,

$$[\psi^{-1}_{tk}|\mathbf{Y}, \mathbf{\Omega}_1, \mathbf{U}, \mathbf{A}_t] \stackrel{D}{=} \text{Gamma}[G/2 + \alpha_{0tk}, \beta_{\epsilon tk}],$$

$$[\mathbf{\Lambda}_{tk}|\mathbf{Y}, \mathbf{\Omega}_1, \mathbf{U}, \mathbf{A}_t, \psi_{tk}] \stackrel{D}{=} N[\mathbf{\Lambda}_{\epsilon tk}, \psi_{tk}\mathbf{H}_{\epsilon tk}], \text{ and}$$

$$[\mathbf{A}_{tk}|\mathbf{Y}, \mathbf{\Omega}_1, \mathbf{U}, \mathbf{\Lambda}_t, \psi_{tk}] \stackrel{D}{=} N[\mathbf{A}_{atk}, \mathbf{H}_{atk}].$$

(ii) Sampling from $[\mathbf{\Lambda}_0, \mathbf{A}_0, \psi_{0k}|\mathbf{Y}, \mathbf{\Omega}_0]$. Let $\mathbf{C}_0 = (\mathbf{c}_{10}, \ldots, \mathbf{c}_{G0})$, $\tilde{\mathbf{y}}_g = \mathbf{y}_g - \mathbf{A}_0\mathbf{c}_{g0}$, $\tilde{\mathbf{y}}^*_g = \mathbf{y}_g - \mathbf{\Lambda}_0\boldsymbol{\omega}_{g0}$, $\tilde{\mathbf{Y}} = (\tilde{\mathbf{y}}_1, \ldots, \tilde{\mathbf{y}}_G)$, $\tilde{\mathbf{Y}}^* = (\tilde{\mathbf{y}}^*_1, \ldots, \tilde{\mathbf{y}}^*_G)$, and $\tilde{\mathbf{Y}}^T_k$ and $\tilde{\mathbf{Y}}^{*^T}_k$ be the kth rows of $\tilde{\mathbf{Y}}$ and $\tilde{\mathbf{Y}}^*$, respectively. Moreover, let $\mathbf{H}_{\epsilon k} = (\mathbf{H}^{-1}_{0k} + \mathbf{\Omega}_0\mathbf{\Omega}^T_0)^{-1}$, $\mathbf{\Lambda}_{\epsilon k} = \mathbf{H}_{\epsilon k}(\mathbf{H}^{-1}_{0k}\tilde{\mathbf{\Lambda}}_{0k} + \mathbf{\Omega}_0\tilde{\mathbf{Y}}_k)$, $\beta_{\epsilon k} = \beta_{0k} + (\tilde{\mathbf{Y}}^T_k\tilde{\mathbf{Y}}_k - \mathbf{\Lambda}^T_{\epsilon k}\mathbf{H}^{-1}_{\epsilon k}\mathbf{\Lambda}_{\epsilon k} + \tilde{\mathbf{\Lambda}}^T_{0k}\mathbf{H}^{-1}_{0k}\tilde{\mathbf{\Lambda}}_{0k})/2$, $\mathbf{H}_{ak} = (\mathbf{H}^{-1}_{0ak} + \psi^{-1}_{0k}\mathbf{C}_0\mathbf{C}^T_0)^{-1}$, and $\mathbf{A}_{\epsilon k} = \mathbf{H}_{ak}(\mathbf{H}^{-1}_{0ak}\tilde{\mathbf{A}}_{0k} + \psi^{-1}_{0k}\mathbf{C}_0\tilde{\mathbf{Y}}^*_k)$. It can be shown that, for $k = 1, \ldots, p$,

$$[\psi^{-1}_{0k}|\mathbf{Y}, \mathbf{\Omega}_0, \mathbf{A}_0] \stackrel{D}{=} \text{Gamma}[G/2 + \alpha_{0k}, \beta_{\epsilon k}],$$

$$[\mathbf{\Lambda}_{0k}|\mathbf{Y}, \mathbf{\Omega}_0, \mathbf{A}_0, \psi_{0k}] \stackrel{D}{=} N[\mathbf{\Lambda}_{\epsilon k}, \psi_{0k}\mathbf{H}_{\epsilon k}], \text{ and}$$

$$[\mathbf{A}_{0k}|\mathbf{Y}, \mathbf{\Omega}_0, \mathbf{\Lambda}_0, \psi_{0k}] \stackrel{D}{=} N[\mathbf{A}_{\epsilon k}, \mathbf{H}_{ak}].$$

(iii) Sampling from $[\mathbf{B}_0, \mathbf{\Phi}, \mathbf{\Lambda}_{\omega t}, \mathbf{\Psi}_{\delta t}|\mathbf{\Omega}_1]$. Let $\mathbf{D}_0 = (\mathbf{d}_{10}, \ldots, \mathbf{d}_{G0})$, $\mathbf{F}_{gt} = \mathbf{F}^*_t(\boldsymbol{\omega}_{g1}, \ldots, \boldsymbol{\omega}_{g,t-1}, \boldsymbol{\xi}_{gt})$, $\tilde{\mathbf{F}}_t = (\mathbf{h}_{1t}, \ldots, \mathbf{h}_{Gt})$, $\tilde{\boldsymbol{\eta}}_{gt} = \boldsymbol{\eta}_{gt} - \mathbf{B}_0\mathbf{d}_{g0}$, $\tilde{\boldsymbol{\eta}}^*_{gt} = \boldsymbol{\eta}_{gt} - \mathbf{\Lambda}_{\omega t}\mathbf{h}_{gt}$, $\tilde{\mathbf{E}}_t = (\tilde{\boldsymbol{\eta}}_{1t}, \ldots, \tilde{\boldsymbol{\eta}}_{Gt})$, $\tilde{\mathbf{E}}^T_{tl}$ be the lth row of $\tilde{\mathbf{E}}_t$, and $\mathbf{\Omega}_\xi = (\boldsymbol{\xi}_1, \ldots, \boldsymbol{\xi}_G)$. Moreover, let $\tilde{\mathbf{H}}_{\omega tl} = (\tilde{\mathbf{H}}^{-1}_{0tl} + \tilde{\mathbf{F}}_t\tilde{\mathbf{F}}^T_t)^{-1}$, $\tilde{\mathbf{\Lambda}}_{\omega tl} = \tilde{\mathbf{H}}_{\omega tl}(\tilde{\mathbf{H}}^{-1}_{0tl}\tilde{\mathbf{\Lambda}}_{0tl} + \tilde{\mathbf{F}}_t\tilde{\mathbf{E}}_{tl})$, $\tilde{\beta}_{\delta tl} = \tilde{\beta}_{0tl} + (\tilde{\mathbf{E}}^T_{tl}\tilde{\mathbf{E}}_{tl} - \tilde{\mathbf{\Lambda}}^T_{\omega tl}\tilde{\mathbf{H}}^{-1}_{\omega tl}\tilde{\mathbf{\Lambda}}_{\omega tl} + \tilde{\mathbf{\Lambda}}^T_{0tl}\tilde{\mathbf{H}}^{-1}_{0tl}\tilde{\mathbf{\Lambda}}_{0tl})/2$, $\mathbf{H}_l = [\mathbf{H}^{-1}_{0bl} + (\sum_{t=1}^T \psi^{-1}_{\delta tl})\mathbf{D}_0\mathbf{D}^T_0]^{-1}$, and $\mathbf{b}_l = \mathbf{H}_l[\mathbf{H}^{-1}_{0bl}\mathbf{b}_{0l} + \sum_{g=1}^G(\sum_{t=1}^T \tilde{\eta}^*_{gtl}/\psi_{\delta tl})\mathbf{d}_{g0}]$, where $\tilde{\eta}^*_{gtl}$ is the lth element of $\tilde{\boldsymbol{\eta}}^*_{gt}$. Then, for $l = 1, \ldots, q_1$ and $t = 1, \ldots, T$,

$$[\psi^{-1}_{\delta tl}|\mathbf{\Omega}_1, \mathbf{B}_0, \mathbf{\Lambda}_{\omega tl}] \stackrel{D}{=} \text{Gamma}[G/2 + \tilde{\alpha}_{0tl}, \tilde{\beta}_{\delta tl}],$$

$$[\mathbf{\Lambda}_{\omega tl}|\mathbf{\Omega}_1, \mathbf{B}_0, \psi_{\delta tl}] \stackrel{D}{=} N[\tilde{\mathbf{\Lambda}}_{\omega tl}, \psi_{\delta tl}\tilde{\mathbf{H}}_{\omega tl}],$$

$$[\mathbf{B}_{0l}|\mathbf{\Omega}_1, \mathbf{\Lambda}_{\omega 1l}, \ldots, \mathbf{\Lambda}_{\omega tl}, \psi_{\delta 1l}, \ldots, \psi_{\delta Tl}] \stackrel{D}{=} N[\mathbf{b}_l, \mathbf{H}_l], \text{ and}$$

$$[\mathbf{\Phi}|\mathbf{\Omega}_1] \stackrel{D}{=} \text{IW}_{q_2 \times T}\left[\left(\mathbf{\Omega}_\xi\mathbf{\Omega}^T_\xi + \mathbf{R}^{-1}_w\right), G + \rho_w\right].$$

(iv) Sampling from $[\mathbf{\Phi}_0|\mathbf{\Omega}_0]$. It can be shown that

$$[\mathbf{\Phi}_0|\mathbf{\Omega}_0] \stackrel{D}{=} \text{IW}_{q_0}\left[\left(\mathbf{\Omega}_0\mathbf{\Omega}^T_0 + \mathbf{R}^{-1}_0\right), G + \rho_0\right].$$

(v) Sampling from $[\boldsymbol{\alpha}, \mathbf{W}|\mathbf{Y}, \mathbf{\Omega}_1, \mathbf{Z}, \boldsymbol{\theta}]$. For $k = 1, \ldots, s$ and $t = 1, \ldots, T$, let $\boldsymbol{\alpha}_{tk}$ be the parameter vector of the unknown thresholds corresponding to z_{gtk}, $\mathbf{W}_t = (\mathbf{w}_{1t}, \ldots, \mathbf{w}_{Gt})$,

$\mathbf{Z}_t = (\mathbf{z}_{1t}, \ldots, \mathbf{z}_{Gt})$, $\mathbf{W}_{tk}$ and $\mathbf{Z}_{tk}$ be the kth rows of $\mathbf{W}_t$ and $\mathbf{Z}_t$, respectively. Assume $z_{gtk} = 0, \ldots, b_{tk}$. It is natural to use the following noninformative prior distribution for the unknown thresholds in $\boldsymbol{\alpha}_{tk}$: $\pi(\alpha_{tk,2}, \ldots, \alpha_{tk,b_{tk}-1}) \propto c$ for $\alpha_{tk,2} < \ldots < \alpha_{tk,b_{tk}-1}$, where c is a constant. Given $\mathbf{Y}$ and $\boldsymbol{\Omega}_1$, the ordered categorical data $\mathbf{Z}$ and the thresholds corresponding to different rows are conditionally independent, and

$$p(\boldsymbol{\alpha}_{tk}, \mathbf{W}_{tk}|\mathbf{Y}, \boldsymbol{\Omega}_1, \mathbf{Z}_{tk}, \boldsymbol{\theta}) = p(\boldsymbol{\alpha}_{tk}|\mathbf{Y}, \boldsymbol{\Omega}_1, \mathbf{Z}_{tk}, \boldsymbol{\theta})p(\mathbf{W}_{tk}|\boldsymbol{\alpha}_{tk}, \mathbf{Y}, \boldsymbol{\Omega}_1, \mathbf{Z}_{tk}, \boldsymbol{\theta}), \quad (9.A4)$$

with

$$p(\boldsymbol{\alpha}_{tk}|\mathbf{Y}, \boldsymbol{\Omega}_1, \mathbf{Z}_{tk}, \boldsymbol{\theta}) \propto \prod_{g=1}^{G} \Big\{ \Phi^*[\psi_{tk}^{-1/2}(\alpha_{tk,z_{gtk}+1} - y_{gk} - \mathbf{A}_{tk}^T\mathbf{c}_{gt} - \boldsymbol{\Lambda}_{tk}^T\boldsymbol{\omega}_{gt})]$$

$$-\Phi^*\big[\psi_{tk}^{-1/2}\big(\alpha_{tk,z_{gtk}} - y_{gk} - \mathbf{A}_{tk}^T\mathbf{c}_{gt} - \boldsymbol{\Lambda}_{tk}^T\boldsymbol{\omega}_{gt}\big)\big]\Big\}, \quad (9.A5)$$

and $p(\mathbf{W}_{tk}|\boldsymbol{\alpha}_{tk}, \mathbf{Y}, \boldsymbol{\Omega}_1, \mathbf{Z}_{tk}, \boldsymbol{\theta})$ is a product of $p(w_{gtk}|\boldsymbol{\alpha}_{tk}, \mathbf{Y}, \boldsymbol{\Omega}_1, \mathbf{Z}_{tk}, \boldsymbol{\theta})$, where

$$p(w_{gtk}|\boldsymbol{\alpha}_{tk}, \mathbf{Y}, \boldsymbol{\Omega}_1, \mathbf{Z}_{tk}, \boldsymbol{\theta}) \overset{D}{=} N\left(y_{gk} + \mathbf{A}_{tk}^T\mathbf{c}_{gt} + \boldsymbol{\Lambda}_{tk}^T\boldsymbol{\omega}_{gt}, \psi_{tk}\right) I_{(\alpha_{tk,z_{gtk}}, \alpha_{tk,z_{gtk}+1}]}(w_{gtk}), \quad (9.A6)$$

in which y_{gk} and w_{gtk} are the kth elements of $\mathbf{y}_g$ and $\mathbf{w}_{gt}$, respectively, $I_A(w)$ is an indicator function which takes 1 if $w \in A$ and 0 otherwise, and $\Phi^*(\cdot)$ denotes the standard normal cumulative distribution function.

We consider an MH algorithm for generating observations from the target distribution $p(\boldsymbol{\alpha}_{tk}, \mathbf{W}_{tk}|\mathbf{Y}, \boldsymbol{\Omega}_1, \mathbf{Z}_{tk}, \boldsymbol{\theta})$. The joint target density of $\boldsymbol{\alpha}_{tk}$ and $\mathbf{W}_{tk}$ in the MH algorithm is given by (9.A4). However, in the proposal distribution, $\boldsymbol{\alpha}_{tk}$ is not simulated from equation (9.A5). Instead, at the lth MH iteration, a vector of thresholds $(\alpha_{tk,2}, \ldots, \alpha_{tk,b_{tk}-1})$ is generated from the univariate truncated normal distribution $\alpha_{tk,z} \sim N(\alpha_{tk,z}^{(l)}, \sigma_{\alpha_{tk}}^2)I_{(\alpha_{tk,z-1}, \alpha_{tk,z+1}^{(l)}]}(\alpha_{tk,z})$ for $z = 2, \ldots, b_{tk} - 1$, where $\alpha_{tk,z}^{(l)}$ is the current value of $\alpha_{tk,z}$ at the lth iteration of the Gibbs sampler, and $\sigma_{\alpha_{tk}}^2$ is a preassigned constant. The acceptance probability for $(\boldsymbol{\alpha}_{tk}, \mathbf{W}_{tk})$ as a new observation is $\min(1, R_{tk})$, where

$$R_{tk} = \frac{p(\boldsymbol{\alpha}_{tk}, \mathbf{W}_{tk}|\mathbf{Y}, \boldsymbol{\Omega}_1, \mathbf{Z}_{tk}, \boldsymbol{\theta})p\big(\boldsymbol{\alpha}_{tk}^{(l)}, \mathbf{W}_{tk}^{(l)}|\boldsymbol{\alpha}_{tk}, \mathbf{W}_{tk}, \mathbf{Y}, \boldsymbol{\Omega}_1, \mathbf{Z}_{tk}, \boldsymbol{\theta}\big)}{p\big(\boldsymbol{\alpha}_{tk}^{(l)}, \mathbf{W}_{tk}^{(l)}|\mathbf{Y}, \boldsymbol{\Omega}_1, \mathbf{Z}_{tk}, \boldsymbol{\theta}\big)p\big(\boldsymbol{\alpha}_{tk}, \mathbf{W}_{tk}|\boldsymbol{\alpha}_{tk}^{(l)}, \mathbf{W}_{tk}^{(l)}, \mathbf{Y}, \boldsymbol{\Omega}_1, \mathbf{Z}_{tk}, \boldsymbol{\theta}\big)}.$$

Let $\tilde{w}_{gtk} = y_{gk} + \mathbf{A}_{tk}^T\mathbf{c}_{gt} + \boldsymbol{\Lambda}_{tk}^T\boldsymbol{\omega}_{gt}$; it can be shown that

$$R_{tk} = \prod_{z=2}^{b_{tk}-1} \frac{\Phi^*\big[\big(\alpha_{tk,z+1}^{(l)} - \alpha_{tk,z}^{(l)}\big)/\sigma_{\alpha_{tk}}\big] - \Phi^*\big[\big(\alpha_{tk,z-1} - \alpha_{tk,z}^{(l)}\big)/\sigma_{\alpha_{tk}}\big]}{\Phi^*\big[\big(\alpha_{tk,z+1} - \alpha_{tk,z}\big)/\sigma_{\alpha_{tk}}\big] - \Phi^*\big[\big(\alpha_{tk,z-1}^{(l)} - \alpha_{tk,z}\big)/\sigma_{\alpha_{tk}}\big]}$$

$$\times \prod_{g=1}^{G} \frac{\Phi^*\big[\psi_{tk}^{-1/2}\big(\alpha_{tk,z_{gtk}+1} - \tilde{w}_{gtk}\big)\big] - \Phi^*\big[\psi_{tk}^{-1/2}\big(\alpha_{tk,z_{gtk}} - \tilde{w}_{gtk}\big)\big]}{\Phi^*\big[\psi_{tk}^{-1/2}\big(\alpha_{tk,z_{gtk}+1}^{(l)} - \tilde{w}_{gtk}\big)\big] - \Phi^*\big[\psi_{tk}^{-1/2}\big(\alpha_{tk,z_{gtk}}^{(l)} - \tilde{w}_{gtk}\big)\big]}.$$

As R_{tk} does not depend on $\mathbf{W}_{tk}$, it is unnecessary to generate a new $\mathbf{W}_{tk}$ in any iteration in which the new value of $\boldsymbol{\alpha}_{tk}$ is not accepted. For an accepted $\boldsymbol{\alpha}_{tk}$, a new $\mathbf{W}_{tk}$ is simulated from equation (9.A6).

Appendix 9.2 Approximation of the L_ν-measure in equation (9.9) via MCMC samples

We denote the parameters at the mth iteration with an additional superscript (m). First, we note that

$$\text{Cov}\left(\mathbf{x}_{gt}^{\text{rep}}|\mathbf{X},\mathbf{Z}\right) = E\left(\mathbf{x}_{gt}^{\text{rep}}\mathbf{x}_{gt}^{\text{rep}T}|\mathbf{X},\mathbf{Z}\right) - E\left(\mathbf{x}_{gt}^{\text{rep}}|\mathbf{X},\mathbf{Z}\right)E\left(\mathbf{x}_{gt}^{\text{rep}T}|\mathbf{X},\mathbf{Z}\right),$$

where $E(\mathbf{x}_{gt}^{\text{rep}}\mathbf{x}_{gt}^{\text{rep}T}|\mathbf{X},\mathbf{Z})$ and $E(\mathbf{x}_{gt}^{\text{rep}}|\mathbf{X},\mathbf{Z})$ can be approximated by MCMC samples as follows:

$$\begin{aligned}
&E\left(\mathbf{x}_{gt}^{\text{rep}}\mathbf{x}_{gt}^{\text{rep}T}|\mathbf{X},\mathbf{Z}\right)\\
&= E\left(E(\mathbf{x}_{gt}^{\text{rep}}\mathbf{x}_{gt}^{\text{rep}T}|\boldsymbol{\theta},\mathbf{Y},\boldsymbol{\Omega}_1)|\mathbf{X},\mathbf{Z}\right)\\
&= E\left(\text{Cov}\left(\mathbf{x}_{gt}^{\text{rep}}|\boldsymbol{\theta},\mathbf{Y},\boldsymbol{\Omega}_1\right) + E\left(\mathbf{x}_{gt}^{\text{rep}}|\boldsymbol{\theta},\mathbf{Y},\boldsymbol{\Omega}_1\right)E\left(\mathbf{x}_{gt}^{\text{rep}T}|\boldsymbol{\theta},\mathbf{Y},\boldsymbol{\Omega}_1\right)|\mathbf{X},\mathbf{Z}\right)\\
&\approx \frac{1}{M}\sum_{m=1}^{M}\left[\text{Cov}\left(\mathbf{x}_{gt}^{\text{rep}}|\boldsymbol{\theta}^{(m)},\mathbf{Y}^{(m)},\boldsymbol{\Omega}_1^{(m)}\right) + E\left(\mathbf{x}_{gt}^{\text{rep}}|\boldsymbol{\theta}^{(m)},\mathbf{Y}^{(m)},\boldsymbol{\Omega}_1^{(m)}\right)E\left(\mathbf{x}_{gt}^{\text{rep}T}|\boldsymbol{\theta}^{(m)},\mathbf{Y}^{(m)},\boldsymbol{\Omega}_1^{(m)}\right)\right]\\
&= \frac{1}{M}\sum_{m=1}^{M}\left[\boldsymbol{\Psi}_{tx}^{(m)} + \left(\mathbf{y}_{gx}^{(m)} + \mathbf{A}_{tx}^{(m)}\mathbf{c}_{gt} + \boldsymbol{\Lambda}_{tx}^{(m)}\boldsymbol{\omega}_{gt}^{(m)}\right)\left(\mathbf{y}_{gx}^{(m)} + \mathbf{A}_{tx}^{(m)}\mathbf{c}_{gt} + \boldsymbol{\Lambda}_{tx}^{(m)}\boldsymbol{\omega}_{gt}^{(m)}\right)^T\right]
\end{aligned}$$

and

$$E\left(\mathbf{x}_{gt}^{\text{rep}}|\mathbf{X},\mathbf{Z}\right) = E\left(E(\mathbf{x}_{gt}^{\text{rep}}|\boldsymbol{\theta},\mathbf{Y},\boldsymbol{\Omega}_1)|\mathbf{X},\mathbf{Z}\right) \approx \frac{1}{M}\sum_{m=1}^{M}\left(\mathbf{y}_{gx}^{(m)} + \mathbf{A}_{tx}^{(m)}\mathbf{c}_{gt} + \boldsymbol{\Lambda}_{tx}^{(m)}\boldsymbol{\omega}_{gt}^{(m)}\right),$$

where $\boldsymbol{\Psi}_{tx}^{(m)}$ is the covariance matrix of $\boldsymbol{\epsilon}_{gt}$ corresponding to the continuous measurements $\mathbf{x}_{gt}$, and $\mathbf{y}_{gx}^{(m)}$, $\mathbf{A}_{tx}^{(m)}$, and $\boldsymbol{\Lambda}_{tx}^{(m)}$ consist of rows of $\mathbf{y}_{g}^{(m)}$, $\mathbf{A}_{t}^{(m)}$, and $\boldsymbol{\Lambda}_{t}^{(m)}$ that correspond to $\mathbf{x}_{gt}$, respectively.

For $k = 0, 1\ldots, m_j$, as $z_{gtj,k}$ is a binary random variable, we have $\text{Var}(z_{gtj,k}^{\text{rep}}|\mathbf{X},\mathbf{Z}) = E(z_{gtj,k}^{\text{rep}}|\mathbf{X},\mathbf{Z}) \times (1 - E(z_{gtj,k}^{\text{rep}}|\mathbf{X},\mathbf{Z}))$. Because $\text{tr}\{\text{Cov}(\mathbf{z}_{gtj}^{*\text{rep}}|\mathbf{X},\mathbf{Z})\} = \sum_{k=0}^{m_j}\text{Var}(z_{gtj,k}^{\text{rep}}|\mathbf{X},\mathbf{Z})$, we only need to calculate $E(z_{gtj,k}^{\text{rep}}|\mathbf{X},\mathbf{Z})$ to obtain the second summation in (9.9). Let z_{gtj}^{rep} be the future replicate of the ordered categorical variable z_{gtj} corresponding to $\mathbf{z}_{gtj}^{*\text{rep}}$; we have

$$\begin{aligned}
E\left(z_{gtj,k}^{\text{rep}}|\mathbf{X},\mathbf{Z}\right) &= E\left(E\left(z_{gtj,k}^{\text{rep}}|\boldsymbol{\alpha},\boldsymbol{\theta},\mathbf{Y},\boldsymbol{\Omega}_1\right)|\mathbf{X},\mathbf{Z}\right)\\
&= E\left(P\left(z_{gtj}^{\text{rep}} = k|\boldsymbol{\alpha},\boldsymbol{\theta},\mathbf{Y},\boldsymbol{\Omega}_1\right)|\mathbf{X},\mathbf{Z}\right)\\
&\approx \frac{1}{M}\sum_{m=1}^{M}P\left(z_{gtj}^{\text{rep}} = k|\boldsymbol{\alpha}^{(m)},\boldsymbol{\theta}^{(m)},\mathbf{Y}^{(m)},\boldsymbol{\Omega}_1^{(m)}\right)\\
&= \frac{1}{M}\sum_{m=1}^{M}\left\{\Phi^*\left(\frac{\alpha_{tj,k+1}^{(m)} - \left(y_{gj}^{(m)} + \mathbf{A}_{tj}^{(m)}c_{gt} + \boldsymbol{\Lambda}_{tj}^{(m)^T}\boldsymbol{\omega}_{gt}^{(m)}\right)}{\psi_{tk}^{(m)}}\right)\right.\\
&\qquad\left. -\Phi^*\left(\frac{\alpha_{tj,k}^{(m)} - \left(y_{gj}^{(m)} + \mathbf{A}_{tj}^{(m)}c_{gt} + \boldsymbol{\Lambda}_{tj}^{(m)^T}\boldsymbol{\omega}_{gt}^{(m)}\right)}{\psi_{tk}^{(m)}}\right)\right\}.
\end{aligned}$$

References

Bollen, K. A. (1989) *Structural Equations with Latent Variables*. New York: John Wiley & Sons, Inc.

Bollen, K. A. and Curran, P. J. (2006) *Latent Curve Models – A Structural Equation Perspective*. Hoboken, NJ: John Wiley & Sons, Inc.

Carroll, K. M., Power, M. E., Bryant, K. and Rounsaville, B. J. (1993) One-year follow-up status of treatment-seeking cocaine abusers. Psychopathology and dependence severity as predictors of outcome. *Journal of Nervous and Mental Disease*, **181**, 71–79.

Chen, M. H., Dey, D. K. and Ibrahim, J. G. (2004) Bayesian criterion based model assessment for categorical data. *Biometrika*, **91**, 45–63.

Diggle, P. J., Heagerty, P. J., Liang, K. Y. and Zeger, S. L. (2002) *Analysis of Longitudinal Data* (2nd edn). Oxford: Oxford University Press.

Dunson, D. B. (2003) Dynamic latent trait models for multidimensional longitudinal data. *Journal of the American Statistical Association*, **98**, 555–563.

Gelman, A., Meng, X. L. and Stern, H. (1996) Posterior predictive assessment of model fitness via realized discrepancies. *Statistica Sinica*, **6**, 733–760.

Geman, S. and Geman, D. (1984) Stochastic relaxation, Gibbs distributions and the Bayesian restoration of images. *IEEE Transactions on Pattern Analysis and Machine Intelligence*, **6**, 721–741.

Hastings, W. K. (1970) Monte Carlo sampling methods using Markov chains and their applications. *Biometrika*, **57**, 97–109.

Hser, Y. (2007) Predicting long-term stable recovery from heroin addiction: Findings from a 33-year follow-up study. *Journal of Addictive Diseases*, **26**, 51–60.

Hser, Y., Stark, M. E., Paredes, A., Huang, D., Anglin, M. D. and Rawson, R. (2006) A 12-year follow-up of a treated cocaine-dependent sample. *Journal of Substance Abuse Treatment*, **30**, 219–226.

Ibrahim, J. G., Chen, M. H. and Sinha, D. (2001) Criterion-based methods for Bayesian model assessment. *Statistica Sinica*, **11**, 419–443.

Jöreskog, K. G. and Sörbom, D. (1977) Statistical models and methods for analysis of longitudinal data. In D. J. Aigner and A. S. Goldberger (eds), *Latent Variables in Socio-economic Models*, pp. 285–325. Amsterdam: North-Holland.

Kasarabada, N. D., Anglin, M. D., Khalsa-Denison, E. and Paredes, A. (1999) Differential effects of treatment modality on psychosocial functioning of cocaine-dependent men. *Journal of Clinical Psychology*, **55**, 257–274.

Lee, S. Y. (2007) *Structural Equation Modeling: A Bayesian Approach*. Chichester: John Wiley & Sons, Ltd.

Little, R. J. A. and Rubin, D. B. (2002) *Statistical Analysis with Missing Data* (2nd edn). Hoboken, NJ: John Wiley & Sons, Inc.

Metropolis, N., Rosenbluth, A. W., Rosenbluth, M. N., Teller, A. H. and Teller, E. (1953) Equation of state calculations by fast computing machines. *Journal of Chemical Physics*, **21**, 1087–1092.

Patkar, A. A., Thornton, C. C., Mannelli, P., Hill, K. P., Gottheil, E., Vergare, M. J. and Weinstein, S. P. (2004) Comparison of pretreatment characteristics and treatment outcomes for alcohol-, cocaine-, and multisubstance-dependent patients. *Journal of Addictive Diseases*, **23**, 93–109.

Song, X. Y. and Lee, S. Y. (2002) Analysis of structural equation model with ignorable missing continuous and polytomous data. *Psychometrika*, **67**, 261–288.

Song, X. Y. and Lee, S. Y. (2008) A Bayesian approach for analyzing hierarchical data with missing outcomes through structural equation models. *Structural Equation Modeling – A Multidisciplinary Journal*, **15**, 272–300.

Song, X. Y., Lee, S. Y. and Hser, Y. I. (2009) Bayesian analysis of multivariate latent curve models with nonlinear longitudinal latent effects. *Structural Equation Modeling – A Multidisciplinary Journal*, **16**, 245–266.

Song, X. Y., Lu, Z. H., Hser, Y. I. and Lee, S. Y. (2011) A Bayesian approach for analyzing longitudinal structural equation models. *Structural Equation Modeling – A Multidisciplinary Journal*, **18**, 183–194.

Verbeke, G. and Molenberghs, G. (2000) *Linear Mixed Models for Longitudinal Data*. New York: Springer-Verlag.

Weisner, C., Ray, G. T., Mertens, J. R., Satre, D. D. and Moore, C. (2003) Short-term alcohol and drug treatment outcomes predict long-term outcome. *Drug and Alcohol Dependence*, **71**, 281–294.

10

Semiparametric structural equation models with continuous variables

10.1 Introduction

In previous chapters, we have presented Bayesian methods for analyzing various SEMs and data structures. In those situations, we have relaxed the normal assumption of observed variables in order to take into account the complicated relationships among latent variables (for example, the nonlinear terms of explanatory latent variables in the structural equation) and the complex structures of data (e.g. heterogeneous data). However, the distributions of explanatory latent variables were assumed to be normal and Bayesian methodologies were developed under this assumption. In practice, this parametric assumption may not be always true in behavioral, medical, social, and psychological research. For a rigorous analysis, it is necessary to make sure that this assumption is not violated. However, based on the given data set and the methodologies presented in previous chapters, it is impossible to test the normal assumption for latent variables. As an example, we consider a study on kidney disease in which the effects of the explanatory latent variables 'lipid control', 'glycemic control', and 'obesity' on the outcome latent variable 'kidney disease' are examined through a structural equation. In the standard parametric Bayesian analysis, the joint distribution of 'lipid control', 'glycemic control', and 'obesity' was assumed to be multivariate normal. However, as 'lipid control', 'glycemic control', and 'obesity' are latent variables rather than observed variables, we have no information from the observed data to test their distributional assumption. One may argue that the estimates of these latent variables obtained from MCMC methods can be used. Unfortunately, these MCMC methods depend on the normal assumption of the latent variables and hence the estimates of the latent variables produced cannot be used.

Basic and Advanced Bayesian Structural Equation Modeling: With Applications in the Medical and Behavioral Sciences,
First Edition. Xin-Yuan Song and Sik-Yum Lee.

One may ask the related question: are the Bayesian results obtained using the previously presented methodologies robust to the normal assumption of the latent variables? So far, very limited simulation studies have been conducted to address this issue. However, it is expected that at least the estimates of latent variables, which are directly affected by this assumption, are not robust. Note that a primary focus of SEMs is on latent variables, which play the most important role in both the measurement and structural equations. In practice, it is of interest to consider a nonparametric or semiparametric estimation of latent variables and learn more about their true distributions.

Another motivation for introducing semiparametric methods is to handle general nonnormal data. In the SEM literature, the results of some simulation studies (e.g. Hu *et al.*, 1992; West *et al.*, 1995) have shown that statistical results obtained from the classical ML approach are not robust to the normal assumption. In fact, problems related to the normal assumption have received a great deal of attention in the field. Robust methods that are developed with the multivariate t-distribution through the classical covariance structure approach have been used for handling nonnormal data with symmetrical heavy tails (Shapiro and Browne, 1987; Kano *et al.*, 1993). Lee and Xia (2006) proposed a more general robust model that involves random weights with the t-distribution, and obtained ML results through a Monte Carlo EM algorithm. Recently, Lee and Xia (2008) developed Bayesian methods for a robust nonlinear SEM with normal/independent distributions which subsume the multivariate t-distribution, multivariate contaminated distribution, and multivariate slash distribution as special cases. However, the above statistical models and methods are still parametric. In many situations, restricting statistical inference to a parametric form may limit the scope and type of inferences. For instance, because the t-distribution is symmetric, robust methods developed based on this distribution are not effective in coping with skewed distributions or mixture distributions.

In this chapter we introduce a Bayesian semiparametric approach to analyze SEMs. It has been shown by Song *et al.* (2010) that an SEM becomes nonidentifiable when the distributions of latent variables and residual errors are unknown. To learn more about the true distribution of the explanatory latent variables, we introduce the basic Bayesian semiparametric/nonparametric approach for an SEM with semiparametric modeling for the explanatory latent variables, while the distributions of the residual errors are assumed to be normal. Theoretically, the general nonparametric approach requires the definition of random probability measures. Practically, Ferguson (1973) introduced the Dirichlet process as a random probability measure that has the following desirable properties: (i) its support is sufficiently large, and (ii) the posterior inference is analytically manageable. This Dirichlet process has been widely used in semiparametric Bayesian analyses of statistical models (e.g. West *et al.*, 1994; Müller *et al.*, 1996). To promote rapid mixing of MCMC chains and take advantage of the block coordinate update, Ishwaran and Zarepour (2000) proposed the truncation approximation of the Dirichlet process in semiparametric Bayesian inference. Ishwaran and James (2001) proposed the stick-breaking prior and the blocked Gibbs sampler for obtaining the Bayesian estimates. For model comparison, it is very difficult to apply the Bayes factor because path sampling cannot give accurate results in computing the Bayes factor for semiparametric SEMs. The main reason is that when ultilizing the path sampling procedure, one needs to assume that it is legitimate to interchange integration and differentiation (see Lee, 2007, p. 132). However, for semiparametric SEMs with the truncated Dirichlet process, the dimension of the integration related to the latent variables is extremely high (approaching infinite), and hence interchanging integration and differentiation would lead to huge errors. Therefore, we will apply the L_ν-measure for model comparison.

In the next section we present the basic Bayesian semiparametric approach in the context of a linear SEM with semiparametric modeling for the explanatory latent variables in the model. Based on the stick-breaking prior and the blocked Gibbs sampler, Bayesian methods are presented in Section 10.3 for fitting such a semiparametric SEM in which the explanatory latent variables are modeled with a truncated Dirichlet process, whilst the distributions of residual errors are assumed to be normal. Results obtained from an analysis of the kidney disease data set are provided in Section 10.4. In Section 10.5 results obtained from simulation studies related to estimation and model comparison, as well as an application of WinBUGS to model comparison, are presented. Finally, a discussion is given in Section 10.6.

10.2 Bayesian semiparametric hierarchical modeling of SEMs with covariates

For the ith individual, let $\mathbf{y}_i = (y_{i1}, \ldots, y_{ip})^T$ be a $p \times 1$ observed random vector that satisfies the measurement model

$$\mathbf{y}_i = \mathbf{A}\mathbf{c}_i + \boldsymbol{\Lambda}\boldsymbol{\omega}_i + \boldsymbol{\epsilon}_i, \quad i = 1, \ldots, n, \tag{10.1}$$

where $\mathbf{A}(p \times r_1)$ and $\boldsymbol{\Lambda}(p \times q)$ are unknown parameter matrices, $\mathbf{c}_i(r_1 \times 1)$ is a vector of fixed covariates, $\boldsymbol{\omega}_i(q \times 1)$ is a random vector of latent factors with $q < p$, and $\boldsymbol{\epsilon}_i(p \times 1)$ is a random vector of error terms. To assess the interrelationships among latent variables, we partition $\boldsymbol{\omega}_i$ into two parts $(\boldsymbol{\eta}_i^T, \boldsymbol{\xi}_i^T)^T$, where $\boldsymbol{\eta}_i(q_1 \times 1)$ and $\boldsymbol{\xi}_i(q_2 \times 1)$ represent outcome and explanatory latent variables, respectively. The interrelationships among latent variables are assessed via the structural equation

$$\boldsymbol{\eta}_i = \mathbf{B}\mathbf{d}_i + \boldsymbol{\Pi}\boldsymbol{\eta}_i + \boldsymbol{\Gamma}\boldsymbol{\xi}_i + \boldsymbol{\delta}_i, \tag{10.2}$$

where $\mathbf{B}(q_1 \times r_2)$, $\boldsymbol{\Pi}(q_1 \times q_1)$, and $\boldsymbol{\Gamma}(q_1 \times q_2)$ are unknown parameter matrices, $\mathbf{d}_i(r_2 \times 1)$ is a vector of fixed covariates, and $\boldsymbol{\delta}_i(q_1 \times 1)$ is a vector of random error terms independent of $\boldsymbol{\xi}_i$. For convenience, it is assumed that $\boldsymbol{\Pi}_0 = \mathbf{I}_{q_1} - \boldsymbol{\Pi}$ is nonsingular, and $|\boldsymbol{\Pi}_0|$ is independent of elements of $\boldsymbol{\Pi}$. As before, the fixed covariates $\mathbf{c}_i$ and $\mathbf{d}_i$ can be discrete, ordered categorical, or continuous measurements.

For the SEMs discussed in previous chapters, $\boldsymbol{\xi}_i$ is assumed to follow a multivariate normal distribution, which implies that $\mathbf{y}_i$ also follows a multivariate normal distribution. This assumption may not be true for many latent constructs in behavioral and/or biomedical research. Given the important role of latent variables in both the measurement and structural equations, applications of the standard parametric SEMs, which violate this basic crucial assumption, would lead to biased statistical results (Hu *et al.*, 1992; West *et al.*, 1995). Hence, it is desirable to consider a semiparametric approach to modeling $\boldsymbol{\xi}_i$, relaxing the basic normal assumption, and to give a more general and correct inference for the distribution of $\boldsymbol{\xi}_i$, such as detection of skewness and multimodality.

In this section we focus on the nonparametric modeling of the latent vector $\boldsymbol{\xi}_i$ in the model. As in the semiparametric Bayesian development of the random effects model (Kleinman and Ibrahim, 1998), we assume here that the random error terms $\boldsymbol{\epsilon}_i$ in (10.1) and $\boldsymbol{\delta}_i$ in (10.2) are independently distributed as $N[\mathbf{0}, \boldsymbol{\Psi}_\epsilon]$ and $N[\mathbf{0}, \boldsymbol{\Psi}_\delta]$ respectively, where $\boldsymbol{\Psi}_\epsilon$ and $\boldsymbol{\Psi}_\delta$ are diagonal matrices.

Our approach employs a Bayesian nonparametric technique of modeling the distribution of $\boldsymbol{\xi}_i$ using a random probability measure P with a nonparametric prior $\mathcal{P}$. Let $\boldsymbol{\theta}_y$ contain all the unknown parameters in $\mathbf{A}$, $\mathbf{\Lambda}$, and $\mathbf{\Psi}_\epsilon$, let $\boldsymbol{\theta}_\omega$ contain all the unknown parameters in $\mathbf{B}$, $\mathbf{\Pi}$, $\mathbf{\Gamma}$, and $\mathbf{\Psi}_\delta$, and let $\boldsymbol{\theta} = (\boldsymbol{\theta}_y, \boldsymbol{\theta}_\omega)$. The method is conceptualized by reformatting (10.1) and (10.2) through the following model (Lee *et al.*, 2008):

$$[\mathbf{y}_i|\boldsymbol{\eta}_i, \boldsymbol{\xi}_i, \boldsymbol{\theta}_y] \stackrel{D}{=} N[\mathbf{A}\mathbf{c}_i + \mathbf{\Lambda}\boldsymbol{\omega}_i, \mathbf{\Psi}_\epsilon], \tag{10.3a}$$

$$[\boldsymbol{\eta}_i|\boldsymbol{\xi}_i, \boldsymbol{\theta}_\omega] \stackrel{D}{=} N\left[\mathbf{\Pi}_0^{-1}(\mathbf{B}\mathbf{d}_i + \mathbf{\Gamma}\boldsymbol{\xi}_i), \mathbf{\Pi}_0^{-1}\mathbf{\Psi}_\delta\mathbf{\Pi}_0^{-T}\right], \tag{10.3b}$$

$$\boldsymbol{\theta} \stackrel{D}{=} g(\boldsymbol{\theta}), \tag{10.3c}$$

$$[\boldsymbol{\xi}_i|P] \stackrel{D}{=} P, \quad P \stackrel{D}{=} \mathcal{P}, \tag{10.3d}$$

where $g(\boldsymbol{\theta})$ is the prior distribution of $\boldsymbol{\theta}$, and $\mathcal{P}(\cdot)$ is a random probability measure. In general, $\mathcal{P}$ can be chosen to be the Dirichlet process (Ferguson, 1973). However, to achieve a posterior which can be efficiently fitted via the blocked Gibbs sampler (Ishwaran and James, 2001) to promote rapid mixing of Markov chains, we consider the truncation approximation Dirichlet process with stick-breaking priors. More specifically, the random probability measure in (10.3d) is defined by

$$\mathcal{P}(\cdot) = \mathcal{P}_G(\cdot) = \sum_{k=1}^{G} \pi_k \delta_{\mathbf{Z}_k}(\cdot), \quad 1 \leq G < \infty, \tag{10.4}$$

where $\delta_{\mathbf{Z}_k}(\cdot)$ denotes a discrete probability measure concentrated at $\mathbf{Z}_k$, the π_k are random variables (called random weights) chosen to be independent of $\mathbf{Z}_k$, such that $0 \leq \pi_k \leq 1$, and $\sum_{k=1}^{G} \pi_k = 1$. It is assumed that $\mathbf{Z}_k$ are independently and identically distributed random elements with a nonatomic distribution H. The random weights π_k are defined through the following stick-breaking procedure:

$$\pi_1 = \nu_1, \quad \text{and} \quad \pi_k = \nu_k \prod_{j=1}^{k-1}(1 - \nu_j), \ k = 2, \ldots, G, \tag{10.5}$$

where ν_k are independent Beta$[a_k, b_k]$ random variables for $a_k, b_k > 0$, and $\nu_G = 1$ to ensure that the sum of π_k is equal to 1. The construction of the stick-breaking priors can be informally viewed as a stick-breaking procedure, where at each stage one independently and randomly breaks what is left of a stick of unit length and assigns the length of the current break to π_k. Based on the useful result that any random probability distribution generated by a Dirichlet process can be represented by Beta$[1, \alpha]$ (Sethuraman, 1994), we consider

$$\nu_j \stackrel{D}{=} \text{Beta}[1, \alpha], \quad j = 1, \ldots, G - 1, \tag{10.6}$$

in constructing the random weights in (10.5), where α is a hyperparameter. We need to make sure that the choice of G in the truncation leads to an adequate approximation of the Dirichlet process. According to Theorem 2 in Ishwaran and James (2001), a moderate truncation leads to a very good approximation to the Dirichlet process, even for huge sample sizes. Furthermore, Ishwaran and Zarepour (2000) pointed out that the accuracy of the truncated Dirichlet process increases exponentially in terms of G, and provided additional theoretical results. Based on our practical experience in the analysis of complex semiparametric SEMs, a truncation level of $G = 300$ appears to be more than adequate.

Similar to the analysis of mixture SEMs for achieving efficient sampling, we reformulate the above model in terms of some random variables. Let $\mathbf{L} = (L_1, \ldots, L_n)^T$, where L_i are conditionally independent classification variables that identify the $\mathbf{Z}_k$ associated with $\boldsymbol{\xi}_i$ such that $\boldsymbol{\xi}_i = \mathbf{Z}_{L_i}$. Let $\boldsymbol{\pi} = (\pi_1, \ldots, \pi_G)$, and $\mathbf{Z} = (\mathbf{Z}_1, \ldots, \mathbf{Z}_G)$. The semiparametric hierarchical model defined in (10.3d) and (10.4) can be reformulated as

$$[L_i|\boldsymbol{\pi}] \stackrel{D}{=} \sum_{k=1}^{G} \pi_k \delta_k(\cdot), \quad \text{and} \quad (\boldsymbol{\pi}, \mathbf{Z}) \stackrel{D}{=} g_1(\boldsymbol{\pi}) g_2(\mathbf{Z}), \tag{10.7}$$

where $g_1(\boldsymbol{\pi})$ is given by the stick-breaking prior as defined by (10.5) and (10.6). The prior distribution involved in $g_2(\mathbf{Z})$ is taken as

$$[\mathbf{Z}_k|\boldsymbol{\mu}, \boldsymbol{\Psi}_z] \stackrel{D}{=} N[\boldsymbol{\mu}, \boldsymbol{\Psi}_z], \quad k = 1, \ldots, G, \tag{10.8}$$

where $\boldsymbol{\mu} = (\mu_1, \ldots, \mu_{q_2})^T$, and $\boldsymbol{\Psi}_z$ is a diagonal matrix with diagonal elements ψ_{zj}, $j = 1, \ldots, q_2$. The prior distributions of the hyperparameters in (10.8), and the α in the stick-breaking prior (10.6) are given, for $j = 1, \ldots, q_2$, by

$$\mu_j \stackrel{D}{=} N[0, \sigma_\mu], \quad \psi_{zj}^{-1} \stackrel{D}{=} \text{Gamma}[\rho_1, \rho_2], \quad \alpha \stackrel{D}{=} \text{Gamma}[\tau_1, \tau_2], \tag{10.9}$$

where σ_μ, ρ_1, ρ_2, τ_1, and τ_2 are preassigned given values. The values of τ_1 and τ_2 should be selected with care because they directly influence the value of α which controls the clustering behavior of $\boldsymbol{\xi}_i$. As suggested by Ishwaran (2000), we select $\tau_1 = \tau_2 = 2$ to encourage both small and large values for α. Roughly speaking, it can be seen from (10.7), (10.8), and $\boldsymbol{\xi}_i = \mathbf{Z}_{L_i}$ that we use a mixture of normals with G endpoints to approximate the general distribution of $\boldsymbol{\xi}_i$; see Roeder and Wasserman (1997) for more technical details.

The prior distribution $g(\boldsymbol{\theta})$ for $\boldsymbol{\theta}$ is given as follows. Let $\boldsymbol{\Lambda}_y = (\mathbf{A}, \boldsymbol{\Lambda})$, $\boldsymbol{\Lambda}_\omega = (\mathbf{B}, \boldsymbol{\Pi}, \boldsymbol{\Gamma})$, $\psi_{\epsilon k}$ be the kth diagonal element of $\boldsymbol{\Psi}_\epsilon$, $\boldsymbol{\Lambda}_{yk}^T$ be the kth row of $\boldsymbol{\Lambda}_y$ for $k = 1, \ldots, p$, $\psi_{\delta l}$ be the lth diagonal element of $\boldsymbol{\Psi}_\delta$, and $\boldsymbol{\Lambda}_{\omega l}^T$ be the lth row of $\boldsymbol{\Lambda}_\omega$ for $l = 1, \ldots, q_1$. The following common conjugate prior distributions in Bayesian SEM analyses are used (see Lee, 2007):

$$\begin{aligned} \psi_{\epsilon k}^{-1} &\stackrel{D}{=} \text{Gamma}[\alpha_{0\epsilon k}, \beta_{0\epsilon k}], \quad [\boldsymbol{\Lambda}_{yk}|\psi_{\epsilon k}] \stackrel{D}{=} N[\boldsymbol{\Lambda}_{0yk}, \psi_{\epsilon k}\mathbf{H}_{0yk}], \\ \psi_{\delta l}^{-1} &\stackrel{D}{=} \text{Gamma}[\alpha_{0\delta l}, \beta_{0\delta l}], \quad [\boldsymbol{\Lambda}_{\omega l}|\psi_{\delta l}] \stackrel{D}{=} N[\boldsymbol{\Lambda}_{0\omega l}, \psi_{\delta l}\mathbf{H}_{0\omega l}], \end{aligned} \tag{10.10}$$

where $\alpha_{0\epsilon k}$, $\beta_{0\epsilon k}$, $\alpha_{0\delta l}$, $\beta_{0\delta l}$, $\boldsymbol{\Lambda}_{0yk}$, $\boldsymbol{\Lambda}_{0\omega l}$, and the positive definite matrices $\mathbf{H}_{0yk}$ and $\mathbf{H}_{0\omega l}$ are hyperparameters whose values are assumed to be given from the prior information of previous studies or other sources. As we will see from the results of the simulation study presented in Section 10.5, Bayesian estimation is not very sensitive to the prior inputs of these hyperparameters for reasonably large sample sizes.

10.3 Bayesian estimation and model comparison

Let $\mathbf{Y} = (\mathbf{y}_1, \ldots, \mathbf{y}_n)$ and $\boldsymbol{\Omega}_1 = (\boldsymbol{\eta}_1, \ldots, \boldsymbol{\eta}_n)$. The blocked Gibbs sampler (Ishwaran and James, 2001) will be used to simulate a sequence of random observations from the joint posterior distribution $[\boldsymbol{\theta}, \boldsymbol{\Omega}_1, \boldsymbol{\pi}, \mathbf{Z}, \mathbf{L}, \boldsymbol{\mu}, \boldsymbol{\Psi}_z, \alpha|\mathbf{Y}]$. As before, the Bayesian estimate of $\boldsymbol{\theta}$ is taken to be the sample mean of the observations simulated from the joint posterior distribution.

The full conditional distributions in relation to $\boldsymbol{\theta}$ and $\boldsymbol{\Omega}_1$ in the parametric component are presented in Appendix 10.1. These conditional distributions can be obtained through reasoning similar to that presented in Chapter 3.

The main idea of efficient sampling for $\mathcal{P}_G(\cdot)$ is to recast the definition of $\boldsymbol{\xi}_i$ in terms of a latent variable L_i which records its cluster membership: $\boldsymbol{\xi}_i = \mathbf{Z}_{L_i}$. To explore the posterior in relation to the nonparametric component, we need to sample $(\boldsymbol{\pi}, \mathbf{Z}, \mathbf{L}, \boldsymbol{\mu}, \boldsymbol{\Psi}_z, \alpha|\boldsymbol{\theta}, \boldsymbol{\Omega}_1, \mathbf{Y})$ using the blocked Gibbs sampler. Based on the nature of these random variables, this is equivalent to sampling from the following full conditional distributions:

$$(\boldsymbol{\pi}, \mathbf{Z}|\mathbf{L}, \boldsymbol{\mu}, \boldsymbol{\Psi}_z, \alpha, \boldsymbol{\theta}, \boldsymbol{\Omega}_1, \mathbf{Y}), \quad (\mathbf{L}|\boldsymbol{\pi}, \mathbf{Z}, \boldsymbol{\theta}, \boldsymbol{\Omega}_1, \mathbf{Y}), \quad (\boldsymbol{\mu}|\mathbf{Z}, \boldsymbol{\Psi}_z), \quad (\boldsymbol{\Psi}_z|\mathbf{Z}, \boldsymbol{\mu}), \quad (\alpha|\boldsymbol{\pi}).$$

The draws of the nonparametric parameters $\boldsymbol{\pi}$, $\mathbf{Z}$, and $\mathbf{L}$ are blocked, with each step simultaneously completed in a multivariate draw to encourage mixing of Markov chains. The related conditional distributions in sampling $(\boldsymbol{\pi}, \mathbf{Z}, \mathbf{L}, \boldsymbol{\mu}, \boldsymbol{\Psi}_z, \alpha|\boldsymbol{\theta}, \boldsymbol{\Omega}_1, \mathbf{Y})$ are presented in Appendix 10.2.

Below, we consider the issue of model comparison in relation to Bayesian semiparametric SEMs. Due to complex modeling of the latent variables, path sampling is unable to provide an accurate solution for computing the Bayes factor (or the marginal likelihood). In contrast, the application of the L_ν-measure (see Section 4.3.3) is relatively easy. Let $\mathbf{Y}^{\text{rep}} = \{\mathbf{y}_1^{\text{rep}}, \ldots, \mathbf{y}_n^{\text{rep}}\}$ be future responses that have the same density as $p(\mathbf{Y}|\boldsymbol{\theta})$. Based on the identities $E(\mathbf{y}_i^{\text{rep}}|\mathbf{Y}) = E\left\{E(\mathbf{y}_i^{\text{rep}}|\mathbf{Z}, \mathbf{L}, \boldsymbol{\theta})|\mathbf{Y}\right\}$ and $E\left\{\mathbf{y}_i^{\text{rep}}(\mathbf{y}_i^{\text{rep}})^T|\mathbf{Y}\right\} = E[E\left\{\mathbf{y}_i^{\text{rep}}(\mathbf{y}_i^{\text{rep}})^T|\mathbf{Z}, \mathbf{L}, \boldsymbol{\theta}\right\}|\mathbf{Y}]$, a consistent estimate of L_ν can be obtained via ergodic averaging of an MCMC sample $\{(\boldsymbol{\theta}^{(t)}, \boldsymbol{\Omega}_1^{(t)}, \boldsymbol{\pi}^{(t)}, \mathbf{Z}^{(t)}, \mathbf{L}^{(t)}, \boldsymbol{\mu}^{(t)}, \boldsymbol{\Psi}_z^{(t)}, \alpha^{(t)}),\ t = 1, \ldots, T\}$ obtained via the blocked Gibbs sampler in the estimation. More specifically, it follows from equation (4.19) that

$$\hat{L}_\nu(\mathbf{Y}) = \sum_{i=1}^n \text{tr}\left\{\frac{1}{T}\sum_{t=1}^T\left[\boldsymbol{\Psi}_\epsilon^{(t)} + \left(\boldsymbol{\Lambda}_\eta^{(t)}\left(\boldsymbol{\Pi}_0^{(t)}\right)^{-1}\right)\boldsymbol{\Psi}_\delta^{(t)}\left(\boldsymbol{\Lambda}_\eta^{(t)}\left(\boldsymbol{\Pi}_0^{(t)}\right)^{-1}\right)^T\right] + \frac{1}{T}\sum_{t=1}^T \mathbf{m}_i^{(t)}\mathbf{m}_i^{(t)T}\right.$$
$$\left. - \left[\frac{1}{T}\sum_{t=1}^T \mathbf{m}_i^{(t)}\right]\left[\frac{1}{T}\sum_{t=1}^T \mathbf{m}_i^{(t)}\right]^T\right\} + \nu\sum_{i=1}^n \text{tr}\left\{\left[\frac{1}{T}\sum_{t=1}^T \mathbf{m}_i^{(t)} - \mathbf{y}_i\right]\left[\frac{1}{T}\sum_{t=1}^T \mathbf{m}_i^{(t)} - \mathbf{y}_i\right]^T\right\},$$

where $\mathbf{m}_i^{(t)} = \mathbf{A}^{(t)}\mathbf{c}_i + \boldsymbol{\Lambda}_\xi^{(t)}\mathbf{Z}_{L_i}^{(t)} + \boldsymbol{\Lambda}_\eta^{(t)}(\boldsymbol{\Pi}_0^{(t)})^{-1}(\mathbf{B}^{(t)}\mathbf{d}_i + \boldsymbol{\Gamma}^{(t)}\mathbf{Z}_{L_i}^{(t)})$, and $\boldsymbol{\Lambda}^{(t)} = (\boldsymbol{\Lambda}_\eta^{(t)}, \boldsymbol{\Lambda}_\xi^{(t)})$ is a partition of $\boldsymbol{\Lambda}^{(t)}$ into $\boldsymbol{\Lambda}_\eta^{(t)}$ associated with $\boldsymbol{\eta}_i$ and $\boldsymbol{\Lambda}_\xi^{(t)}$ associated with $\boldsymbol{\xi}_i$. As the MCMC sample is available in the estimation, the additional computational burden is light.

10.4 Application: Kidney disease study

The semiparametric Bayesian methodology is illustrated through an application to the study of diabetic kidney disease as described in Chapter 2. The data set in this application was obtained from patients who participated in a medical program which aims to examine the clinical and molecular epidemiology of type 2 diabetes in Hong Kong Chinese, with particular emphasis on diabetic nephropathy. The SEM will be formulated with two fixed covariates, 'smoking' and 'age', and the following observed variables: log urinary albumin creatinine ratio (lnACR), log plasma creatinine (lnPCr), high-density lipoprotein cholesterol (HDL), low-density lipoprotein cholesterol (LDL), log triglyceride (lnTG), glycemic control (HbA1c), fasting blood glucose (FBG), body mass index (BMI), hip index (HIP), and waist index (WST). As the distributions of the observed variables ACR, PCr, and TG are nonnormal (even after log transformation), we expect the latent variables to be nonnormal and the usual distributional assumption would be violated. Hence, the semiparametric Bayesian approach is useful for analyzing this data set.

In this chapter the SEM defined in (10.1) and (10.2) is applied to analyze the observed random vector $\mathbf{y}$, which consists of $p = 10$ observed variables (lnACR, lnPCr, HDL, LDL, lnTG, HbA1c, FBG, BMI, HIP, WST). After removing observations with missing entries, the sample size of the data set is 615.

From medical knowledge of the observed variables, it is clear that lnACR and lnPCr provide key information about kidney disease severity; hence, they are grouped together to form a latent variable that can be interpreted as 'kidney disease severity'. Furthermore, {HDL, LDL, lnTG} are taken to be the observed variables of a latent variable that can be interpreted as 'lipid control'. Also {HbAlc, FBG} are grouped together into a latent variable that can be interpreted as 'glycemic control', and {BMI, HIP, WST} are grouped together into a latent variable that can be interpreted as 'obesity'. As a result, it is natural for the model to have $q = 4$ latent variables. The above considerations also suggest the following non-overlapping structure for $\mathbf{\Lambda}$ to model the relationships among the observed variables and their corresponding latent variables, and to provide clear interpretations of the aforementioned latent variables:

$$\mathbf{\Lambda}^T = \begin{bmatrix} 1 & \lambda_{21} & 0 & 0 & 0 & 0 & 0 & 0 & 0 & 0 \\ 0 & 0 & 1 & \lambda_{42} & \lambda_{52} & 0 & 0 & 0 & 0 & 0 \\ 0 & 0 & 0 & 0 & 0 & 1 & \lambda_{73} & 0 & 0 & 0 \\ 0 & 0 & 0 & 0 & 0 & 0 & 0 & 1 & \lambda_{94} & \lambda_{10,4} \end{bmatrix}, \tag{10.11}$$

where the 1s and 0s are treated as fixed parameters. These fixed parameters in the non-overlapping structure ensure that the underlying model is identified. In line with standard practice in factor analysis, the fixed value 1 is also used to introduce a scale to the corresponding latent variable. Based on the objective of the study, we consider 'kidney disease severity' as the single outcome latent variable η, and 'lipid control', 'glycemic control', and 'obesity' as the explanatory latent variables ξ_1, ξ_2, and ξ_3, respectively.

Based on the reasoning given above, the measurement model is taken to be $\mathbf{y}_i = \mathbf{A}c_i + \mathbf{\Lambda}\boldsymbol{\omega}_i + \boldsymbol{\epsilon}_i$, in which the covariate c_i represents the 'age' of patients and $\mathbf{\Lambda}$ is given by (10.11). To unify the scale, the observed variables and the fixed covariate are standardized. The structural equation is given by

$$\eta_i = bd_i + \gamma_1\xi_{i1} + \gamma_2\xi_{i2} + \gamma_3\xi_{i3} + \delta_i, \tag{10.12}$$

where d_i is a binary fixed covariate concerning the 'smoking status' of patients (0 = smoker, 1 = nonsmoker). We respectively use 'age' and 'smoking status' of patients as covariates in the measurement and structural equations because we suspect that 'age' and 'smoking status' may have substantial effects on the observed variables and the outcome latent variable, respectively. Hence, we wish to assess the significance of these effects. Moreover, including these covariates provides an illustration of the model with covariates. In this example, $p = 10, r_1 = 1, r_2 = 1, q = 4, q_1 = 1$, and $q_2 = 3$.

In the analysis, the hyperparameter values in the nonparametric component are taken as $\sigma_\mu = 100$, $\rho_1 = \rho_2 = 0.01$, and $\tau_1 = \tau_2 = 2$. In defining $(L_i|\boldsymbol{\pi})$ in (10.7), the truncation level of $G = 300$ was used. We use the following *ad hoc* hyperparameter values in the conjugate prior distributions corresponding to the parametric component: the values in $\mathbf{\Lambda}_{0yk}$ corresponding to unknown parameters in $\mathbf{A}$ and $\mathbf{\Lambda}$ are taken to be 1.0; the values of $\mathbf{\Lambda}_{0\omega l}$ corresponding to b, γ_1, γ_2, and γ_3 are taken to be 0.0, and $\alpha_{0\epsilon k} = \alpha_{0\delta l} = 4$, $\beta_{0\epsilon k} = \beta_{0\delta l} = 2$, $\mathbf{H}_{0yk}$ and $\mathbf{H}_{0\omega l}$ are diagonal matrices with diagonal elements 1.0. We will check the sensitivity of the Bayesian

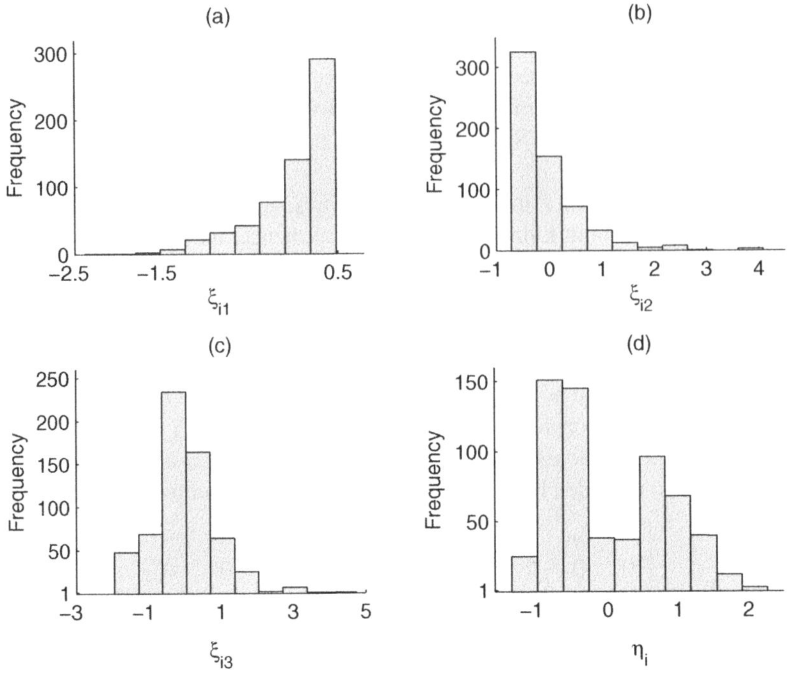

Figure 10.1 Histograms of the Bayesian estimates of latent variables (a) ξ_{i1}, (b) ξ_{i2}, (c) ξ_{i3}, and (d) η_i in the kidney disease study.

results to prior inputs. The EPSR values (Gelman, 1996) are used to diagnose convergence of the MCMC algorithm. After convergence, a total of 10 000 observations were collected to produce the Bayesian estimates of the structural parameters and their standard error estimates, as well as the estimates of the latent variables. Based on the observations $\{\mathbf{\Omega}_1^{(j)}, j = 1, \ldots, 10\,000\}$ generated using the blocked Gibbs sampler, we obtained an estimate $\hat{\eta}_i$ of η_i as the average of $\{\eta_i^{(j)}, j = 1, \ldots, 10\,000\}$, and estimates $\hat{\xi}_{ik}$ of ξ_{ik} as the average of $\{\xi_{ik}^{(j)}, j = 1, \ldots, 10\,000\}$ for $k = 1, 2, 3$. Histograms of $\{\hat{\xi}_{ik}, i = 1, \ldots, n\}$ and $\{\hat{\eta}_i, i = 1, \ldots, n\}$ are displayed in Figure 10.1, which indicates the empirical distributions of the latent variable estimates. We observe that the distributions of the latent variables are nonnormal; hence, the normal assumption on the latent variables in the parametric analysis is violated and the semiparametric approach is useful for analyzing this data set. The estimated residuals, $\hat{\boldsymbol{\epsilon}}_i = \mathbf{y}_i - \hat{\mathbf{A}}c_i - \hat{\mathbf{\Lambda}}\hat{\boldsymbol{\omega}}_i$ and $\hat{\delta}_i = \hat{\eta}_i - \hat{b}d_i - \hat{\gamma}_1\hat{\xi}_{i1} - \hat{\gamma}_2\hat{\xi}_{i2} - \hat{\gamma}_3\hat{\xi}_{i3}$, are used to reveal the adequacy of the measurement model and structural equation used to fit the data. Let ϵ_{i1} be the first element of $\boldsymbol{\epsilon}_i$; plots of the estimated residual $\hat{\epsilon}_{i1}$ versus $\hat{\xi}_{i1}$, $\hat{\xi}_{i2}$, $\hat{\xi}_{i3}$, and $\hat{\eta}_i$, and plots of $\hat{\delta}_i$ versus $\hat{\xi}_{i1}$, $\hat{\xi}_{i2}$, and $\hat{\xi}_{i3}$ are presented in Figures 10.2 and 10.3, respectively. These plots lie within two parallel horizontal lines that are centered at zero, and no linear or quadratic trends are detected. This roughly indicates that the measurement model and the structural equation are adequate in fitting the data.

Note that the parameter vector $\boldsymbol{\theta}$ does not contain the covariance matrix of $\boldsymbol{\xi}_i$, $\mathbf{\Phi} = (\phi_{kh})_{3\times3}$. To obtain an estimate of $\mathbf{\Phi}$, we denote by $\{\boldsymbol{\xi}_i^{(j)}, i = 1, \ldots, n\}$ the observations simulated

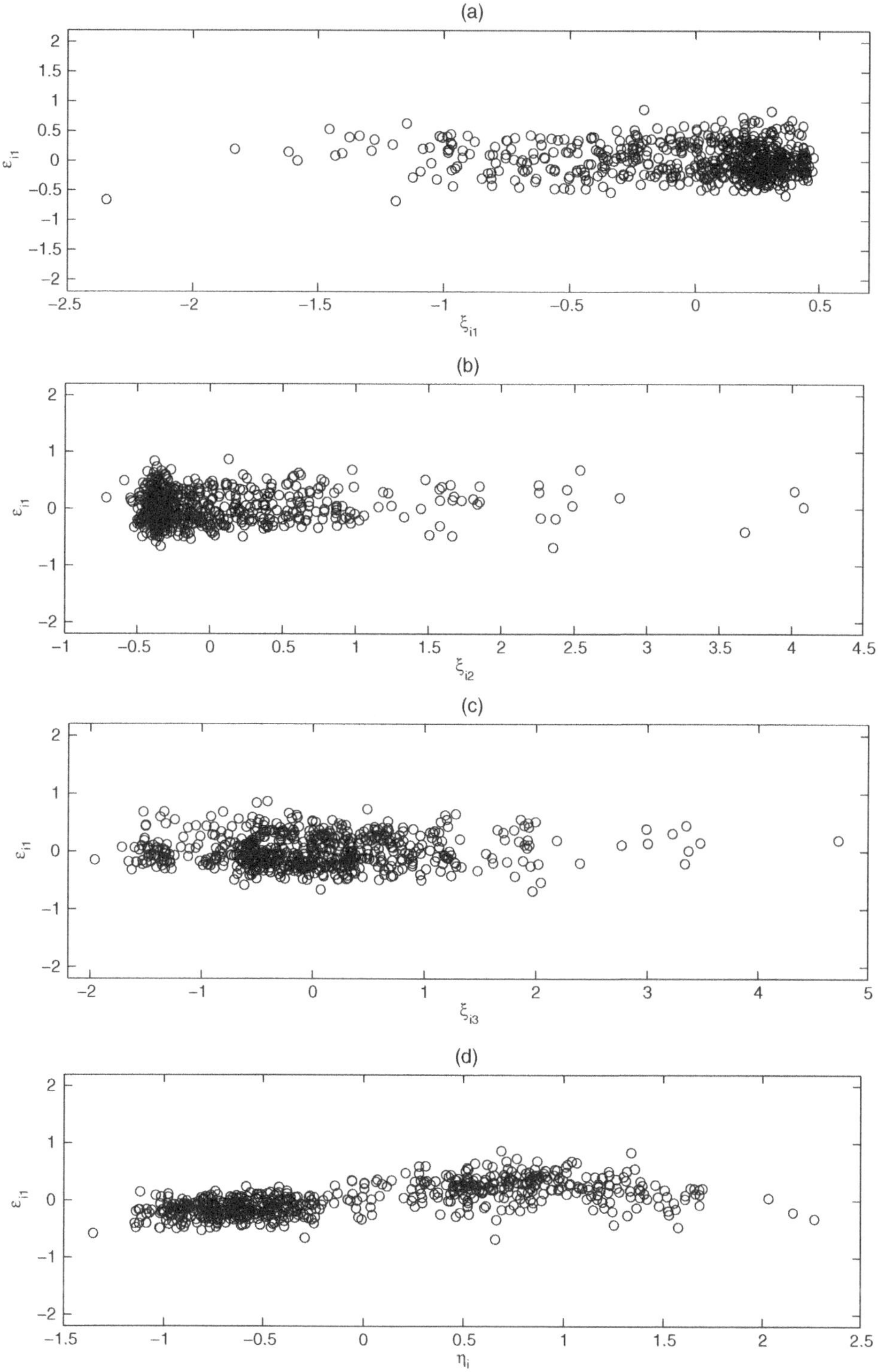

Figure 10.2 Plot of $\hat{\epsilon}_{i1}$ versus (a) $\hat{\xi}_{i1}$, (b) $\hat{\xi}_{i2}$, (c) $\hat{\xi}_{i3}$, (d) $\hat{\eta}_i$.

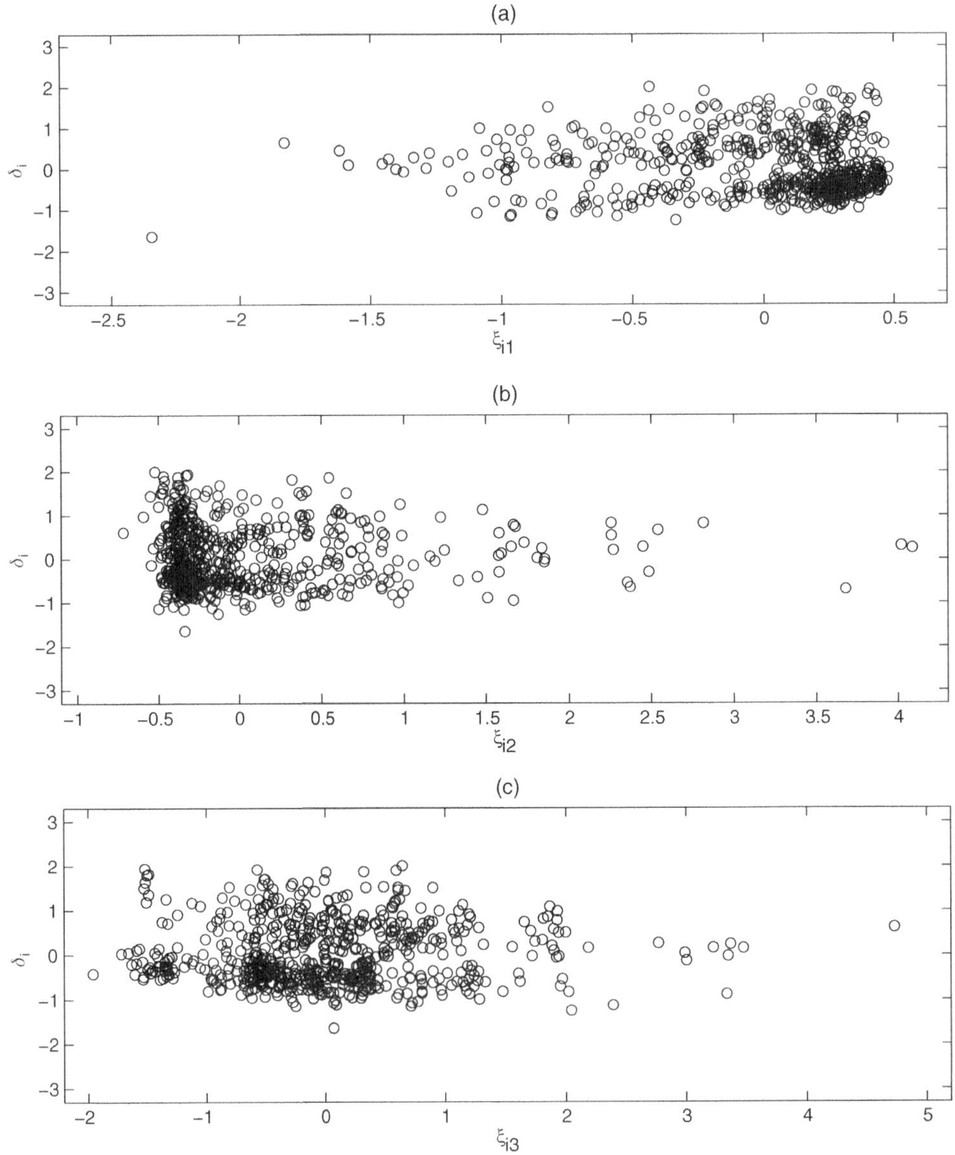

Figure 10.3 Plot of $\hat{\delta}_i$ versus (a) $\hat{\xi}_{i1}$, (b) $\hat{\xi}_{i2}$, (c) $\hat{\xi}_{i3}$.

from the posterior distribution in the *j*th Gibbs sampler iteration, and denote by $\mathbf{\Phi}^{(j)}$ the corresponding sample covariance matrix. An estimate of $\mathbf{\Phi}$ can be taken as the mean of $\mathbf{\Phi}^{(j)}$, averaging over all the Gibbs sampler iterations after the burn-in iterations. Estimates of ϕ_{kh} in $\mathbf{\Phi}$, together with Bayesian estimates of other parameters and their corresponding highest posterior density (HPD) intervals (Chen *et al.*, 2000), are presented in Table 10.1. We note that most of the HPD intervals are short. The magnitudes of the λ estimates indicate strong associations between the latent variables and most of the corresponding observed variables.

Table 10.1 Bayesian estimates of parameters and their HPD intervals: analysis of the kidney disease data.

	Semiparametric approach		Parametric approach	
Par	EST	HPD interval	EST	HPD interval
a_{11}	0.168	[0.131, 0.214]	0.145	[0.022, 0.256]
a_{21}	0.271	[0.230, 0.312]	0.253	[0.137, 0.360]
a_{31}	−0.017	[−0.061, 0.026]	0.019	[−0.101, 0.132]
a_{41}	0.069	[0.029, 0.119]	0.059	[−0.052, 0.170]
a_{51}	0.013	[−0.027, 0.035]	−0.053	[−0.170, 0.060]
a_{61}	−0.047	[−0.088, −0.010]	−0.084	[−0.189, −0.028]
a_{71}	−0.029	[−0.069, 0.001]	−0.071	[−0.183, 0.037]
a_{81}	−0.164	[−0.189, −0.126]	−0.198	[−0.314, −0.085]
a_{91}	0.020	[−0.006, 0.059]	−0.014	[−0.130, 0.105]
$a_{10,1}$	−0.090	[−0.117, −0.049]	−0.122	[−0.239, −0.007]
λ_{21}	0.761	[0.701, 0.820]	0.811	[0.667, 0.983]
λ_{42}	0.306	[0.189, 0.401]	0.327	[0.101, 0.590]
λ_{52}	1.871	[1.707, 1.966]	1.150	[0.833, 1.513]
λ_{73}	1.175	[1.075, 1.242]	0.977	[0.739, 1.228]
λ_{94}	0.987	[0.956, 1.016]	0.989	[0.918, 1.065]
$\lambda_{10,4}$	0.929	[0.895, 0.958]	0.931	[0.856, 1.010]
b	−0.028	[−0.050, −0.004]	0.013	[−0.037, 0.060]
γ_1	0.593	[0.468, 0.682]	0.720	[0.456, 1.046]
γ_2	0.108	[0.026, 0.171]	−0.034	[−0.197, 0.123]
γ_3	0.148	[0.094, 0.197]	0.049	[−0.087, 0.180]
$\psi_{\epsilon 1}$	0.213	[0.166, 0.259]	0.262	[0.162, 0.384]
$\psi_{\epsilon 2}$	0.492	[0.449, 0.536]	0.462	[0.350, 0.570]
$\psi_{\epsilon 3}$	0.811	[0.752, 0.865]	0.638	[0.487, 0.797]
$\psi_{\epsilon 4}$	0.972	[0.906, 1.037]	0.944	[0.799, 1.102]
$\psi_{\epsilon 5}$	0.209	[0.167, 0.224]	0.498	[0.323, 0.658]
$\psi_{\epsilon 6}$	0.523	[0.466, 0.556]	0.378	[0.231, 0.527]
$\psi_{\epsilon 7}$	0.340	[0.303, 0.375]	0.410	[0.261, 0.565]
$\psi_{\epsilon 8}$	0.132	[0.119, 0.145]	0.128	[0.096, 0.166]
$\psi_{\epsilon 9}$	0.190	[0.175, 0.206]	0.186	[0.147, 0.231]
$\psi_{\epsilon 10}$	0.265	[0.246, 0.289]	0.261	[0.214, 0.320]
ψ_{δ}	0.635	[0.565, 0.690]	0.515	[0.369, 0.681]
α	9.132	[7.701, 11.207]	–	–
ϕ_{11}	0.228	[0.175, 0.280]	0.387	[0.250, 0.567]
ϕ_{21}	0.083	[0.062, 0.103]	0.118	[0.039, 0.204]
ϕ_{31}	0.114	[0.093, 0.135]	0.183	[0.092, 0.287]
ϕ_{22}	0.478	[0.397, 0.551]	0.625	[0.436, 0.835]
ϕ_{32}	−0.022	[−0.050, 0.007]	0.033	[−0.133, 0.064]
ϕ_{33}	0.834	[0.790, 0.882]	0.844	[0.699, 1.008]

The estimated structural equation is $\eta_i = -0.028d_i + 0.593\xi_{i1} + 0.108\xi_{i2} + 0.148\xi_{i3}$. The interpretation of this equation is similar to the regression model, considering η as an outcome variable. It seems that the 'smoking' effect is not significant, but 'lipid control', 'glycemic control', and 'obesity' have significantly positive effects on kidney disease severity, while the impact of 'lipid control' is strongest.

To assess the sensitivity of Bayesian results to the prior inputs of the hyperparameters in prior distributions corresponding to the parametric component, the data set was reanalyzed with some perturbations of the above *ad hoc* prior inputs. We obtain close Bayesian estimates, very similar histograms of the latent variables, and very similar estimated residual plots to those given above. Moreover, we observe that the results obtained are not very sensitive to G and J (the number of iterations taken to compute the results). For example, taking $G = 100$ and $J = 4000$ gives very similar results.

We use the following competing models to illustrate the model comparison procedure via the L_ν-measure:

$$
\begin{aligned}
M_1 &: \mathbf{y}_i = \mathbf{A}\mathbf{c}_i + \mathbf{\Lambda}\boldsymbol{\omega}_i + \boldsymbol{\epsilon}_i, \quad \eta_i = bd_i + \gamma_1\xi_{i1} + \gamma_2\xi_{i2} + \gamma_3\xi_{i3} + \delta_i, \\
M_2 &: \mathbf{y}_i = \mathbf{A}\mathbf{c}_i + \mathbf{\Lambda}\boldsymbol{\omega}_i + \boldsymbol{\epsilon}_i, \quad \eta_i = \gamma_1\xi_{i1} + \gamma_2\xi_{i2} + \gamma_3\xi_{i3} + \delta_i, \\
M_3 &: \mathbf{y}_i = \mathbf{\Lambda}\boldsymbol{\omega}_i + \boldsymbol{\epsilon}_i, \quad \eta_i = bd_i + \gamma_1\xi_{i1} + \gamma_2\xi_{i2} + \gamma_3\xi_{i3} + \delta_i, \\
M_4 &: \mathbf{y}_i = \mathbf{\Lambda}\boldsymbol{\omega}_i + \boldsymbol{\epsilon}_i, \quad \eta_i = \gamma_1\xi_{i1} + \gamma_2\xi_{i2} + \gamma_3\xi_{i3} + \delta_i.
\end{aligned}
\tag{10.13}
$$

The same hyperparameter values in the prior distributions of the parameters in the parametric and nonparametric components are taken as before. The truncation level G is equal to 100. A total of 4000 observations were collected after convergence to compute the $L_{0.5}$-measures. The $L_{0.5}$-measures corresponding to $\{M_1, \ldots, M_4\}$ are $\{4947, 4952, 5067, 5070\}$, respectively. Hence, M_1 is selected. We further consider a parametric model M_5, which has the same measurement and structural equation as in M_1, but the distribution of its latent vector $\boldsymbol{\xi}_i$ is assumed to be $N[\mathbf{0}, \mathbf{\Phi}]$. Taking the prior distribution of $\mathbf{\Phi}$ to be an inverted Wishart distribution with 20 degrees of freedom and a covariance matrix $\mathbf{I}_3$, we find that the $L_{0.5}$-measure is equal to 4993. This does not change our selection of M_1.

For completeness, estimates obtained via the parametric approach are also presented in Table 10.1. We observe that some of the parameter estimates (e.g. $\hat{\lambda}_{52}, \hat{\psi}_{\epsilon 3}, \hat{\psi}_{\epsilon 5}, \hat{\psi}_{\epsilon 6}, \hat{\gamma}_1, \hat{\gamma}_2, \hat{\gamma}_3, \hat{\phi}_{11}$, and $\hat{\phi}_{22}$) are quite different from those that are obtained from the semiparametric approach; and the HPD intervals corresponding to the parametric approach are much longer.

In the real application concerning kidney disease of diabetes patients, we extend the model comparison by including the two competing semiparametric nonlinear SEMs with the following structural equations:

$$
\begin{aligned}
M_6 &: \mathbf{y}_i = \mathbf{A}\mathbf{c}_i + \mathbf{\Lambda}\boldsymbol{\omega}_i + \boldsymbol{\epsilon}_i, \\
&\quad \eta_i = bd_i + \gamma_1\xi_{i1} + \gamma_2\xi_{i2} + \gamma_3\xi_{i3} + \gamma_{12}\xi_{i1}\xi_{i2} + \gamma_{13}\xi_{i1}\xi_{i3} + \gamma_{23}\xi_{i2}\xi_{i3} + \delta_i, \\
M_7 &: \mathbf{y}_i = \mathbf{A}\mathbf{c}_i + \mathbf{\Lambda}\boldsymbol{\omega}_i + \boldsymbol{\epsilon}_i, \\
&\quad \eta_i = \gamma_1\xi_{i1} + \gamma_2\xi_{i2} + \gamma_3\xi_{i3} + \gamma_{12}\xi_{i1}\xi_{i2} + \gamma_{13}\xi_{i1}\xi_{i3} + \gamma_{23}\xi_{i2}\xi_{i3} + \delta_i.
\end{aligned}
\tag{10.14}
$$

The $L_{0.5}$-measures corresponding to M_6 and M_7 are 5007 and 5000, respectively. These values again do not affect our decision to select model M_1.

10.5 Simulation studies

10.5.1 Simulation study of estimation

The main objective of this simulation study is to investigate the empirical performance of the semiparametric approach in estimation. The data sets are simulated on the basis of an SEM similar to that in the kidney disease application with $p = 10, q = 4, r_1 = 1, r_2 = 1, q_1 = 1, q_2 = 3$, and the structure of $\mathbf{\Lambda}$ given in (10.11). The measurement model and the structural equation are defined as $\mathbf{y}_i = \mathbf{A}c_i + \mathbf{\Lambda}\boldsymbol{\omega}_i + \boldsymbol{\epsilon}_i$ and $\eta_i = bd_i + \gamma_1\xi_{i1} + \gamma_2\xi_{i2} + \gamma_3\xi_{i3} + \delta_i$, respectively. The fixed covariates c_i and d_i are drawn from $N[0, 1]$ and a Bernoulli distribution with probability of success 0.7, respectively. The true population values are taken as $\mathbf{A} = \{0.5, 0.6, 0.0, 0.0, 0.0, 0.0, 0.0, -0.5, 0.0, -0.3\}$, $b = -0.5$, $\lambda_{42} = 0.6$, $\lambda_{52} = \lambda_{73} = 1.0$, $\lambda_{21} = \lambda_{94} = \lambda_{10,4} = 0.8$, $\psi_{\epsilon 1} = \psi_{\epsilon 3} = \psi_{\epsilon 5} = \psi_{\epsilon 6} = \psi_{\epsilon 7} = \psi_{\epsilon 8} = 0.33$, $\psi_{\epsilon 2} = \psi_{\epsilon 9} = \psi_{\epsilon 10} = 0.57$, $\psi_{\epsilon 4} = 0.76$, $\gamma_1 = 0.6$, $\gamma_2 = 0.1$, $\gamma_3 = 0.2$, and $\psi_\delta = 0.395$. The explanatory latent variables ξ_{i1}, ξ_{i2}, and ξ_{i3} are independently drawn from Gamma(6, 3) to give a skewed nonnormal situation. The true covariance matrix of $\boldsymbol{\xi}_i$ is diagonal, with diagonal elements equal to 0.667. Sample sizes $n = 150$, 300, and 615 are considered, and the simulation results are obtained on the basis of 100 replications.

In each replication, the simulated data were analyzed using the semiparametric Bayesian approach with the following prior inputs for the hyperparameters in the prior distributions relating to the nonparametric component: $\sigma_\mu = 100$, $\rho_1 = \rho_2 = 0.01$, and $\tau_1 = \tau_2 = 2$. For the prior distributions relating to the parametric component, the following sets of prior inputs are considered for both approaches:

BAY1. Conjugate distributions in which $\{\mathbf{\Lambda}_{0yk}, \mathbf{\Lambda}_{0\omega l}\}$ are fixed at the true values; $\alpha_{0\epsilon k} = \alpha_{0\delta l} = 9$, $\beta_{0\epsilon k} = \beta_{0\delta l} = 4$, $\mathbf{H}_{0yk}$ and $\mathbf{H}_{0\omega l}$ are diagonal matrices with diagonal elements 0.25.

BAY2. All elements in $\mathbf{\Lambda}_{0yk}$ are taken to be 2.0, all elements in $\mathbf{\Lambda}_{0\omega l}$ are taken to be zero, $\alpha_{0\epsilon k} = \alpha_{0\delta l} = 12$, $\beta_{0\epsilon k} = \beta_{0\delta l} = 8$, $\mathbf{H}_{0yk}$ and $\mathbf{H}_{0\omega l}$ are identity matrices.

Under BAY1 and BAY2, the truncation level of the Dirichlet process is $G = 300$.

Based on the EPSR values (Gelman, 1996), the algorithm converged within 4000 iterations in a number of test runs. To be conservative, the simulation results were obtained from 5000 observations after 7000 burn-in iterations. The mean (Mean) value, and the root mean squares (RMS) between the estimates and the true values based on the 100 replications were computed. Results obtained from the Bayesian semiparametric approach with BAY1 and BAY2 prior inputs are reported in Tables 10.2 and 10.3, respectively. We observe that the mean values are close to the true values and all RMS values are small. As expected, the overall empirical performance of the Bayesian semiparametric approach is satisfactory, large sample sizes give better estimates, and the impact of prior inputs decreases with larger sample sizes. To reveal the behavior of the latent variable estimates, we randomly selected a replication, and constructed the histograms on the basis of the latent variable estimates as in the kidney disease application.

Table 10.2 Performance of the semiparametric Bayesian estimates with prior input BAY1.

	$n = 150$		$n = 300$		$n = 615$	
Par	Mean	RMS	Mean	RMS	Mean	RMS
$a_{11} = 0.5$	0.50	0.082	0.49	0.065	0.50	0.038
$a_{21} = 0.6$	0.61	0.079	0.59	0.060	0.60	0.035
$a_{31} = 0.0$	0.01	0.085	0.00	0.067	−0.01	0.041
$a_{41} = 0.0$	0.00	0.081	0.00	0.063	−0.00	0.041
$a_{51} = 0.0$	0.01	0.085	−0.01	0.058	−0.01	0.036
$a_{61} = 0.0$	−0.01	0.082	0.01	0.070	0.00	0.042
$a_{71} = 0.0$	−0.01	0.082	0.01	0.076	0.00	0.040
$a_{81} = -0.5$	−0.49	0.093	−0.50	0.063	−0.50	0.038
$a_{91} = 0.0$	0.00	0.096	−0.00	0.058	−0.01	0.045
$a_{10,1} = -0.3$	−0.30	0.082	−0.30	0.061	−0.30	0.041
$\lambda_{21} = 0.8$	0.81	0.046	0.80	0.034	0.80	0.021
$\lambda_{42} = 0.6$	0.60	0.040	0.60	0.023	0.60	0.018
$\lambda_{52} = 1.0$	1.01	0.036	1.01	0.024	1.00	0.016
$\lambda_{73} = 1.0$	1.00	0.028	1.00	0.025	1.00	0.016
$\lambda_{94} = 0.8$	0.81	0.033	0.80	0.025	0.80	0.018
$\lambda_{10,4} = 0.8$	0.81	0.036	0.80	0.024	0.80	0.016
$\psi_{\epsilon 1} = 0.33$	0.38	0.074	0.37	0.059	0.35	0.039
$\psi_{\epsilon 2} = 0.57$	0.54	0.077	0.56	0.056	0.56	0.040
$\psi_{\epsilon 3} = 0.33$	0.40	0.093	0.38	0.063	0.36	0.043
$\psi_{\epsilon 4} = 0.76$	0.72	0.103	0.74	0.070	0.75	0.043
$\psi_{\epsilon 5} = 0.33$	0.34	0.048	0.35	0.043	0.34	0.033
$\psi_{\epsilon 6} = 0.33$	0.41	0.099	0.38	0.058	0.37	0.049
$\psi_{\epsilon 7} = 0.33$	0.35	0.073	0.34	0.050	0.35	0.034
$\psi_{\epsilon 8} = 0.33$	0.42	0.103	0.41	0.091	0.38	0.059
$\psi_{\epsilon 9} = 0.57$	0.56	0.072	0.56	0.053	0.57	0.037
$\psi_{\epsilon 10} = 0.57$	0.55	0.076	0.57	0.060	0.57	0.037
$b = -0.5$	−0.52	0.101	−0.51	0.086	−0.51	0.069
$\gamma_1 = 0.6$	0.61	0.086	0.61	0.053	0.61	0.040
$\gamma_2 = 0.1$	0.10	0.086	0.10	0.060	0.10	0.040
$\gamma_3 = 0.2$	0.20	0.071	0.19	0.048	0.20	0.037
$\psi_\delta = 0.395$	0.38	0.058	0.38	0.047	0.39	0.039
$\phi_{11} = 0.67$	0.60	0.138	0.63	0.085	0.63	0.071
$\phi_{21} = 0.00$	0.01	0.059	−0.01	0.047	0.00	0.033
$\phi_{31} = 0.00$	0.00	0.062	0.00	0.047	−0.00	0.033
$\phi_{22} = 0.67$	0.62	0.132	0.64	0.087	0.64	0.062
$\phi_{32} = 0.00$	0.01	0.059	0.00	0.046	−0.00	0.034
$\phi_{33} = 0.67$	0.61	0.129	0.62	0.092	0.64	0.061

Table 10.3 Performance of the semiparametric Bayesian estimates with prior input BAY2.

	$n = 150$		$n = 300$		$n = 615$	
Par	Mean	RMS	Mean	RMS	Mean	RMS
$a_{11} = 0.5$	0.50	0.081	0.48	0.066	0.49	0.039
$a_{21} = 0.6$	0.60	0.079	0.58	0.061	0.60	0.035
$a_{31} = 0.0$	0.00	0.083	−0.00	0.067	−0.01	0.042
$a_{41} = 0.0$	0.00	0.081	0.00	0.064	−0.00	0.040
$a_{51} = 0.0$	0.00	0.085	−0.01	0.059	−0.01	0.037
$a_{61} = 0.0$	−0.00	0.084	0.01	0.072	0.00	0.042
$a_{71} = 0.0$	−0.01	0.083	0.00	0.077	0.00	0.040
$a_{81} = -0.5$	−0.48	0.094	−0.49	0.063	−0.50	0.038
$a_{91} = 0.0$	0.01	0.097	−0.00	0.059	−0.00	0.043
$a_{10,1} = -0.3$	−0.29	0.083	−0.30	0.061	−0.30	0.040
$\lambda_{21} = 0.8$	0.82	0.051	0.81	0.035	0.81	0.021
$\lambda_{42} = 0.6$	0.62	0.047	0.61	0.025	0.61	0.019
$\lambda_{52} = 1.0$	1.04	0.055	1.02	0.029	1.01	0.018
$\lambda_{73} = 1.0$	1.03	0.041	1.01	0.030	1.01	0.018
$\lambda_{94} = 0.8$	0.83	0.045	0.81	0.029	0.81	0.020
$\lambda_{10,4} = 0.8$	0.83	0.048	0.81	0.029	0.81	0.018
$\psi_{\epsilon 1} = 0.33$	0.44	0.117	0.40	0.077	0.36	0.046
$\psi_{\epsilon 2} = 0.57$	0.61	0.072	0.59	0.055	0.57	0.038
$\psi_{\epsilon 3} = 0.33$	0.46	0.144	0.41	0.092	0.38	0.059
$\psi_{\epsilon 4} = 0.76$	0.70	0.112	0.72	0.074	0.75	0.045
$\psi_{\epsilon 5} = 0.33$	0.29	0.058	0.32	0.041	0.33	0.029
$\psi_{\epsilon 6} = 0.33$	0.47	0.147	0.42	0.093	0.39	0.070
$\psi_{\epsilon 7} = 0.33$	0.30	0.066	0.32	0.051	0.33	0.028
$\psi_{\epsilon 8} = 0.33$	0.48	0.162	0.45	0.125	0.40	0.080
$\psi_{\epsilon 9} = 0.57$	0.53	0.084	0.55	0.057	0.56	0.038
$\psi_{\epsilon 10} = 0.57$	0.51	0.085	0.55	0.063	0.56	0.039
$b = -0.5$	−0.40	0.140	−0.45	0.101	−0.48	0.071
$\gamma_1 = 0.6$	0.56	0.092	0.59	0.051	0.60	0.038
$\gamma_2 = 0.1$	0.11	0.082	0.11	0.058	0.11	0.040
$\gamma_3 = 0.2$	0.20	0.068	0.19	0.046	0.20	0.037
$\psi_\delta = 0.395$	0.47	0.090	0.43	0.051	0.42	0.041
$\phi_{11} = 0.67$	0.59	0.136	0.63	0.085	0.63	0.070
$\phi_{21} = 0.00$	0.01	0.059	−0.00	0.046	0.00	0.033
$\phi_{31} = 0.00$	0.01	0.059	0.00	0.047	−0.00	0.033
$\phi_{22} = 0.67$	0.62	0.122	0.63	0.088	0.63	0.064
$\phi_{32} = 0.00$	0.01	0.056	0.00	0.045	−0.00	0.033
$\phi_{33} = 0.67$	0.59	0.141	0.61	0.096	0.64	0.063

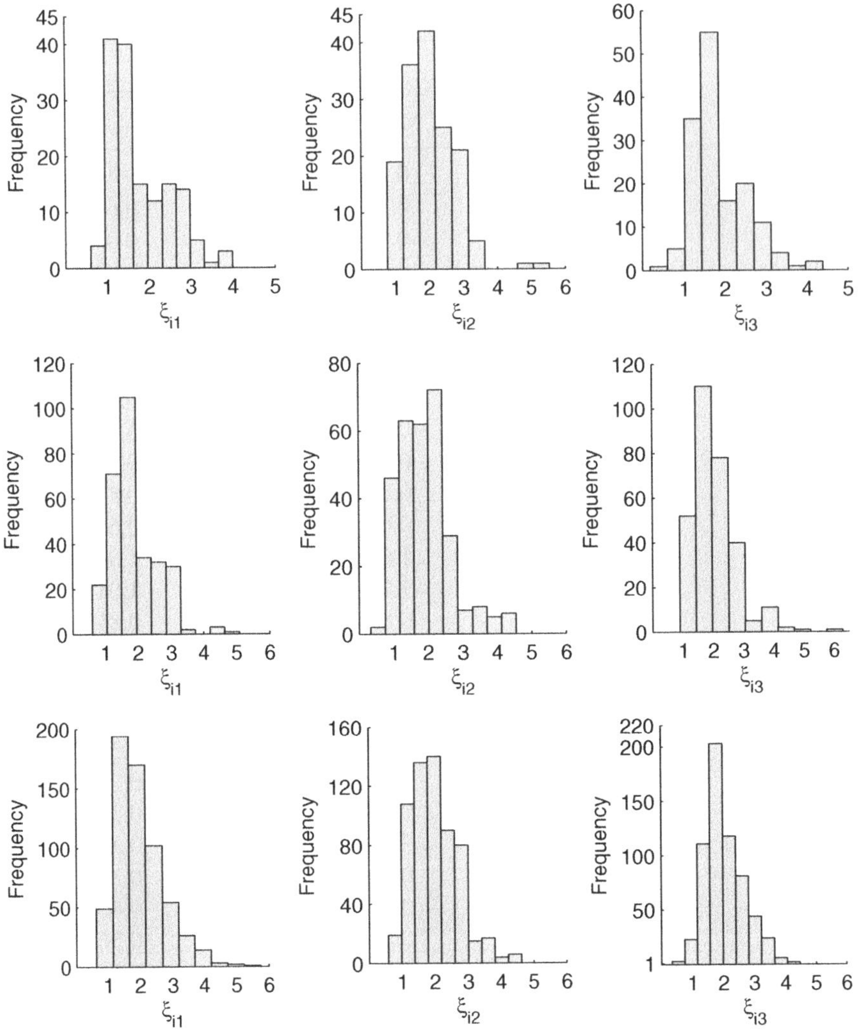

Figure 10.4 Histograms of the Bayesian estimates of the latent variables ξ_{i1}, ξ_{i2}, and ξ_{i3} in the simulation study: first row, $n = 150$; second row, $n = 300$; third row, $n = 615$.

The histograms of $\hat{\xi}_{i1}$, $\hat{\xi}_{i2}$, and $\hat{\xi}_{i3}$ for $n = 150$, 300, and 615 are presented in Figure 10.4. We observe that the empirical distributions are close to the true gamma distribution.

10.5.2 Simulation study of model comparison

The main objective of this simulation study is to evaluate the performance of the L_ν-measure in model comparison of the Bayesian semiparametric linear SEM with covariates. To save computing effort, we consider the following simple true linear SEMs. The covariates c_{ij}, $j = 1, 2$, in the measurement equation are generated from the standard normal distribution. The specifications of $\mathbf{A}$ and $\mathbf{\Lambda}$, and the true values of their parameters are given by

$$\mathbf{A}^T = \begin{bmatrix} 1.0 & 1.0 & 1.0 & 1.0 & 1.0 & 1.0 & 1.0 & 1.0 & 1.0 \\ 0.7 & 0.7 & 0.7 & 0.7 & 0.7 & 0.7 & 0.7 & 0.7 & 0.7 \end{bmatrix},$$

$$\mathbf{\Lambda}^T = \begin{bmatrix} 1 & 1.5 & 1.5 & 0 & 0 & 0 & 0 & 0 & 0 \\ 0 & 0 & 0 & 1 & 1.5 & 1.5 & 0 & 0 & 0 \\ 0 & 0 & 0 & 0 & 0 & 0 & 1 & 1.5 & 1.5 \end{bmatrix}, \tag{10.15}$$

in which 1s and 0s in $\mathbf{\Lambda}$ are treated as fixed in order to identify the model. The true value of $\psi_{\epsilon j}$ in $\mathbf{\Psi}_\epsilon$ is 0.5, $j = 1, \ldots, 9$. Let $\boldsymbol{\omega}_i = (\eta_i, \xi_{i1}, \xi_{i2})^T$. The structural equation of the true model is

$$\eta_i = bd_i + \gamma_1\xi_{i1} + \gamma_2\xi_{i2} + \delta_i, \tag{10.16}$$

where the covariate d_i is sampled from a Bernoulli distribution that takes value 1 with probability 0.7 and 0 with probability 0.3. The true values of the parameters are given by $b = 1.0$, $(\gamma_1, \gamma_2) = (0.2, 0.7)$, and $\psi_\delta = 0.5$. In this simulation study, with regard to the nonparametric component, we consider the following hyperparameter values in the prior distributions: $\sigma_\mu = 100$, $\rho_1 = \rho_2 = 0.01$, and $\tau_1 = \tau_2 = 2.0$. With regard to the parametric component, we consider the following hyperparameter values in the prior distributions: $\{\mathbf{\Lambda}_{0yk}, \mathbf{\Lambda}_{0\omega l}\}$ are fixed at the true values, $\alpha_{0\epsilon k} = \alpha_{0\delta l} = 9$, $\beta_{0\epsilon k} = \beta_{0\delta l} = 8$, and $\mathbf{H}_{0yk}$ and $\mathbf{H}_{0\omega l}$ are diagonal matrices with the diagonal elements 1.0.

Two true distributions for $\boldsymbol{\xi}_i$ are considered: (i) $\boldsymbol{\xi}_i$ is simulated from the mixture of normal distributions, $0.5N[\boldsymbol{\mu}_1, \mathbf{\Phi}_1] + 0.5N[\boldsymbol{\mu}_2, \mathbf{\Phi}_2]$, where $\boldsymbol{\mu}_1 = (-1.0, 2.0)^T$, $\boldsymbol{\mu}_2 = (1.0, -2.0)^T$, and $\mathbf{\Phi}_1 = \mathbf{\Phi}_2 = \mathbf{I}_2$; and (ii) ξ_{ij} are independently drawn from Gamma(4.0, 2.0) for $j = 1, 2$. Thus, the true distribution of $\boldsymbol{\xi}_i$ is either bimodal or skewed. Based on these specifications, data sets were obtained from random samples $\{\mathbf{y}_i, i = 1, \ldots, n\}$ with $n = 300$.

We consider the following linear SEMs:

$$\begin{aligned} M_1 &: \mathbf{y}_i = \mathbf{A}\mathbf{c}_i + \mathbf{\Lambda}\boldsymbol{\omega}_i + \boldsymbol{\epsilon}_i, & \eta_i &= bd_i + \gamma_1\xi_{i1} + \gamma_2\xi_{i2} + \delta_i, \\ M_2 &: \mathbf{y}_i = \mathbf{A}\mathbf{c}_i + \mathbf{\Lambda}\boldsymbol{\omega}_i + \boldsymbol{\epsilon}_i, & \eta_i &= \gamma_1\xi_{i1} + \gamma_2\xi_{i2} + \delta_i, \\ M_3 &: \mathbf{y}_i = \mathbf{\Lambda}\boldsymbol{\omega}_i + \boldsymbol{\epsilon}_i, & \eta_i &= bd_i + \gamma_1\xi_{i1} + \gamma_2\xi_{i2} + \delta_i, \\ M_4 &: \mathbf{y}_i = \mathbf{\Lambda}\boldsymbol{\omega}_i + \boldsymbol{\epsilon}_i, & \eta_i &= \gamma_1\xi_{i1} + \gamma_2\xi_{i2} + \delta_i, \end{aligned} \tag{10.17}$$

where M_1 represents the true model. We take $G = 100$ in the semiparametric modeling of $\boldsymbol{\xi}_i$ and the implementation of the blocked Gibbs sampler. Based on results obtained from a few test runs to investigate the convergence of the algorithm, 2000 observations were collected after 2000 burn-in iterations to obtain the Bayesian estimates and to compute the L_ν-measure. In each of the 100 replications, $L_{0.5}$-measures for $M_1, \ldots, M_4$ are computed. Recall that the $L_{0.5}$-measure selects the true model if its value for M_1 is the smallest. The $L_{0.5}$-measures correctly selected M_1 in all replications under both nonnormal distributions of $\boldsymbol{\xi}_i$. The mean and standard deviation of $L_{0.5}$-measures obtained from the 100 replications are presented in Table 10.4. Based on the simulation results, we see that the performance of this model comparison statistic is satisfactory.

Table 10.4 Mean and standard deviation (SD) of $L_{0.5}$-measures: simulation with linear SEMs.

		$L_{0.5}$	
	Fitting model	Mean	SD
ξ_i from mixture of normal	M_1	3702	117.29
	M_2	4774	200.53
	M_3	3796	134.47
	M_4	4941	205.26
ξ_i from gamma	M_1	3632	137.32
	M_2	4256	178.37
	M_3	3989	139.28
	M_4	4478	151.88

Reproduced by permission of Taylor & Francis from Song, X. Y., Xia, Y. M., Pan, J. H. and Lee, S. Y. (2011). Model comparison of Bayesian semiparametric and parametric structural equation models. *Structural Equation Modeling – A Multidisciplinary Journal*, **18**, 55–73.

10.5.3 Obtaining the L_ν-measure via WinBUGS and R2WinBUGS

The WinBUGS software(Spiegelhalter *et al.*, 2003), which is mainly based on MCMC techniques, can provide simulated samples from the joint posterior distribution of the unknown quantities. Bayesian estimates of the unknown parameters in the model and their standard error estimates can be obtained from these samples for conducting statistical inferences. As already mentioned, one of the most useful new features in WinBUGS 1.4 is the ability to call WinBUGS from within other programs, such as the R2WinBUGS package (Sturtz *et al.*, 2005) in R. Using this package, we can input a data file and a script in R, then call WinBUGS from R and run the script in WinBUGS. Finally, we can save the MCMC samples which are simulated from the posterior distribution through WinBUGS in R to calculate the L_ν-measure.

To illustrate the use of WinBUGS in conducting model comparison for Bayesian semiparametric linear SEMs with covariates, we consider the true model M_1 based on the same settings as given above. After reformulating the model, it can be transformed into the text-based BUGS language. Consider the following measurement equations: for $i = 1, 2, \ldots, 300$,

$$\begin{aligned} y_{ij} &= a_{j1}c_{i1} + a_{j2}c_{i2} + \lambda_{j1}\eta_i + \lambda_{j3}\xi_{i2} + \epsilon_{ij}, \quad j = 1, 2, 3, \\ y_{ij} &= a_{j1}c_{i1} + a_{j2}c_{i2} + \lambda_{j2}\xi_{i1} + \epsilon_{ij}, \quad j = 4, 5, 6, \\ y_{ij} &= a_{j1}c_{i1} + a_{j2}c_{i2} + \lambda_{j3}\xi_{i2} + \epsilon_{ij}, \quad j = 7, 8, 9, \end{aligned} \tag{10.18}$$

where $\epsilon_{ij} \stackrel{D}{=} N[0, \psi_{\epsilon j}]$, $j = 1, 2, \ldots, 9$. In applying WinBUGS, we reformulate the above equations as follows: for $i = 1, 2, \ldots, 300$ and $j = 1, 2, \ldots, 9$,

$$y_{ij} \stackrel{D}{=} N[\vartheta_{ij}, \psi_{\epsilon j}],$$

where

$$\begin{aligned}
\vartheta_{ij} &= a_{j1}c_{i1} + a_{j2}c_{i2} + \lambda_{j1}\eta_i + \lambda_{j3}\xi_{i2}, \quad j = 1, 2, 3, \\
\vartheta_{ij} &= a_{j1}c_{i1} + a_{j2}c_{i2} + \lambda_{j2}\xi_{i1}, \quad j = 4, 5, 6, \\
\vartheta_{ij} &= a_{j1}c_{i1} + a_{j2}c_{i2} + \lambda_{j3}\xi_{i2}, \quad j = 7, 8, 9.
\end{aligned} \tag{10.19}$$

The structural equation in this simulation study is

$$\eta_i \stackrel{D}{=} N[\mu_i, \psi_\delta], \tag{10.20}$$

where $\mu_i = bd_i + \gamma_1\xi_{i1} + \gamma_2\xi_{i2}$. The prior distribution of $(\xi_{i1}, \xi_{i2})^T$ is formulated with the truncated Dirichlet process distribution with stick-breaking priors. By using the R2WinBUGS package, we can save the observations simulated from the posterior distribution through WinBUGS in R, and they can then be used to obtain the L_ν-measure. The R2WinBUGS code related to this illustration is presented in the following website:

`www.wiley.com/go/medical_behavioral_sciences`

Refer to Sturtz *et al.* (2005) for more details on how to use R2WinBUGS package to call WinBUGS from R and to save the simulated observations in R. The $L_{0.5}$-measures obtained via WinBUGS are generally a bit larger than those obtained using our tailor-made C program. However, these $L_{0.5}$-measures also correctly selected M_1 in all 100 replications under both nonnormal distributions of $\boldsymbol{\xi}_i$. To save space, details are omitted.

10.6 Discussion

Latent variables play the most crucial role in SEMs. It is important to examine various properties of latent variables, including the interrelationships among themselves and the observed variables, as well as their true distributions. Most existing methods in SEMs are based on an assumption that the distribution of latent variables is normal. This assumption, which is impossible to test on the observed data, may not be realistic for data in behavioral, biological, and medical sciences. In this chapter, we apply a semiparametric Bayesian approach to relax this assumption in the analysis of SEMs with fixed covariates and continuous variables. This approach not only produces accurate estimates when dealing with nonnormal data but also can recover the true distribution of the important latent variables. Our methods include the formulation of a nonparametric prior for the distribution of the crucial explanatory latent variables in the model with a truncation approximation Dirichlet process, application of a blocked Gibbs sampler to obtaining estimates of the parameters and latent variables, and computation of the L_ν-measure for model comparison. As the full conditional distributions involved are the standard normal, gamma, and beta distributions, the blocked Gibbs sampler is efficient, and its implementation is straightforward. In the illustrative example, the Bayesian methodology is applied to study the effects of the explanatory latent variables, 'lipid control', 'glycemic control', and 'obesity', on the outcome latent variable 'kidney disease severity'. It is clear from both theoretical and methodological points of view that the semiparametric Bayesian approach is more general than a parametric approach with the normal assumption. Results obtained from the illustrative example and the simulation studies also indicate that the semiparametric Bayesian approach is better in many aspects.

Based on the rationale as given in this chapter, it is also desirable to develop semiparametric methods for analyzing other types of SEMs. In fact, the key ideas in formulating the Bayesian semiparametric modeling, implementing the blocked Gibbs sampler, and applying the L_ν-measure can be used similarly in other SEMs. In Section 11.3, we will discuss the Bayesian semiparametric SEM with continuous and unordered categorical analysis. Moreover, key ideas presented in this chapter can be applied to develop semiparametric SEMs in which the residual errors are modeled via a semiparametric approach; see Song *et al.* (2010).

Appendix 10.1 Conditional distributions for parametric components

Similar to the reasoning given in Lee and Song (2003), the conditional distributions for the parametric component are as follows. Let $\mathbf{u}_i = (\mathbf{c}_i^T, \boldsymbol{\omega}_i^T)^T$, $\mathbf{U} = (\mathbf{u}_1, \ldots, \mathbf{u}_n)$, $\boldsymbol{\Omega} = (\boldsymbol{\omega}_1, \ldots, \boldsymbol{\omega}_n)$, and $\mathbf{Y}_k^T$ be the kth row of $\mathbf{Y}$ with general elements y_{ik},for $i = 1, \ldots, n$ and $k = 1, \ldots, p$. It can be shown that

$$\left[\psi_{\epsilon k}^{-1}|\mathbf{Y}, \boldsymbol{\Omega}\right] \stackrel{D}{=} \text{Gamma}[n/2 + \alpha_{0\epsilon k}, \beta_{\epsilon k}] \quad \text{and} \quad [\boldsymbol{\Lambda}_{yk}|\psi_{\epsilon k}, \mathbf{Y}, \boldsymbol{\Omega}] \stackrel{D}{=} N[\boldsymbol{\mu}_{yk}, \psi_{\epsilon k}\boldsymbol{\Sigma}_{yk}],$$

where $\boldsymbol{\Sigma}_{yk} = (\mathbf{H}_{0yk}^{-1} + \mathbf{U}\mathbf{U}^T)^{-1}$, $\boldsymbol{\mu}_{yk} = \boldsymbol{\Sigma}_{yk}(\mathbf{H}_{0yk}^{-1}\boldsymbol{\Lambda}_{0yk} + \mathbf{U}\mathbf{Y}_k)$, and $\beta_{\epsilon k} = \beta_{0\epsilon k} + (\mathbf{Y}_k^T\mathbf{Y}_k - \boldsymbol{\mu}_{yk}^T\boldsymbol{\Sigma}_{yk}^{-1}\boldsymbol{\mu}_{yk} + \boldsymbol{\Lambda}_{0yk}^T\mathbf{H}_{0yk}^{-1}\boldsymbol{\Lambda}_{0yk})/2$. This gives the full conditional distributions of $\boldsymbol{\theta}_y$.

For the conditional distribution of $\boldsymbol{\theta}_\omega$, we let $\mathbf{v}_i = (\mathbf{d}_i^T, \boldsymbol{\omega}_i^T)^T$, $\mathbf{V} = (\mathbf{v}_1, \ldots, \mathbf{v}_n)$, and $\boldsymbol{\Omega}_{1k}^T$ be the kth row of $\boldsymbol{\Omega}_1$, $k = 1, \ldots, q_1$. It can be shown that

$$\left[\psi_{\delta k}^{-1}|\boldsymbol{\Omega}\right] \stackrel{D}{=} \text{Gamma}[n/2 + \alpha_{0\delta k}, \beta_{\delta k}] \quad \text{and} \quad [\boldsymbol{\Lambda}_{\omega k}|\psi_{\delta k}, \boldsymbol{\Omega}] \stackrel{D}{=} N[\boldsymbol{\mu}_{\omega k}, \psi_{\delta k}\boldsymbol{\Sigma}_{\omega k}],$$

where $\boldsymbol{\Sigma}_{\omega k} = (\mathbf{H}_{0\omega k}^{-1} + \mathbf{V}\mathbf{V}^T)^{-1}$, $\boldsymbol{\mu}_{\omega k} = \boldsymbol{\Sigma}_{\omega k}(\mathbf{H}_{0\omega k}^{-1}\boldsymbol{\Lambda}_{0\omega k} + \mathbf{V}\boldsymbol{\Omega}_{1k})$, and $\beta_{\delta k} = \beta_{0\delta k} + (\boldsymbol{\Omega}_{1k}^T\boldsymbol{\Omega}_{1k} - \boldsymbol{\mu}_{\omega k}^T\boldsymbol{\Sigma}_{\omega k}^{-1}\boldsymbol{\mu}_{\omega k} + \boldsymbol{\Lambda}_{0\omega k}^T\mathbf{H}_{0\omega k}^{-1}\boldsymbol{\Lambda}_{0\omega k})/2$.

Finally, let $\boldsymbol{\Lambda}_\eta$ and $\boldsymbol{\Lambda}_\xi$ be the submatrices of $\boldsymbol{\Lambda}$ which contain q_1 and q_2 rows of $\boldsymbol{\Lambda}$ corresponding to $\boldsymbol{\eta}_i$ and $\boldsymbol{\xi}_i$, respectively. For $i = 1, \ldots, n$, it can be shown that

$$[\boldsymbol{\eta}_i|\mathbf{y}_i, \boldsymbol{\xi}_i, \boldsymbol{\theta}_y, \boldsymbol{\theta}_\omega] \stackrel{D}{=} N[\boldsymbol{\mu}_{\eta_i}, \boldsymbol{\Sigma}_\eta],$$

where $\boldsymbol{\Sigma}_\eta = (\boldsymbol{\Pi}_0^T\boldsymbol{\Psi}_\delta^{-1}\boldsymbol{\Pi}_0 + \boldsymbol{\Lambda}_\eta^T\boldsymbol{\Psi}_\epsilon^{-1}\boldsymbol{\Lambda}_\eta)^{-1}$ and $\boldsymbol{\mu}_{\eta_i} = \boldsymbol{\Sigma}_\eta\left\{(\mathbf{B}\mathbf{d}_i + \boldsymbol{\Gamma}\boldsymbol{\xi}_i)^T\boldsymbol{\Psi}_\delta^{-1}\boldsymbol{\Pi}_0 + (\mathbf{y}_i - \mathbf{A}\mathbf{c}_i - \boldsymbol{\Lambda}_\xi\boldsymbol{\xi}_i)^T\boldsymbol{\Psi}_\epsilon^{-1}\boldsymbol{\Lambda}_\eta\right\}^T$.

Simulating observations from these conditional distributions, which are the normal and gamma distributions, is straightforward and fast.

Appendix 10.2 Conditional distributions for nonparametric components

Conditional distributions for the nonparametric component for sampling $(\boldsymbol{\pi}, \mathbf{Z}, \mathbf{L}, \boldsymbol{\mu}, \boldsymbol{\Psi}_z, \alpha|\boldsymbol{\theta}, \boldsymbol{\Omega}_1, \mathbf{Y})$ are presented here. First, consider the conditional distribution $(\boldsymbol{\pi}, \mathbf{Z}|\mathbf{L}, \boldsymbol{\mu}, \boldsymbol{\Psi}_z, \alpha, \boldsymbol{\theta}, \boldsymbol{\Omega}_1, \mathbf{Y})$. As $\boldsymbol{\pi}$ and α are independent of $\mathbf{Z}$, $\boldsymbol{\theta}$, $\boldsymbol{\Omega}_1$, and $\mathbf{Y}$, we have

$$p(\boldsymbol{\pi}, \mathbf{Z}|\mathbf{L}, \boldsymbol{\mu}, \boldsymbol{\Psi}_z, \alpha, \boldsymbol{\theta}, \boldsymbol{\Omega}_1, \mathbf{Y}) \propto p(\boldsymbol{\pi}|\mathbf{L}, \alpha)p(\mathbf{Z}|\mathbf{L}, \boldsymbol{\mu}, \boldsymbol{\Psi}_z, \boldsymbol{\theta}, \boldsymbol{\Omega}_1, \mathbf{Y}). \qquad (10.\text{A1})$$

Hence, this conditional distribution can be decomposed into two separate parts. It can be shown that the conditional distribution $(\boldsymbol{\pi}|\mathbf{L}, \alpha)$ is a generalized Dirichlet distribution, $\mathcal{G}(a_1^*, \ldots, a_{G-1}^*, b_1^*, \ldots, b_{G-1}^*)$, where $a_k^* = 1 + m_k$, $b_k^* = \alpha + \sum_{j=k+1}^{G} m_j$, $k = 1, \ldots, G-1$, and m_k is the number of L_i whose value equals k. Hence, observations can be effectively sampled through

$$\begin{aligned} \pi_1 &= \nu_1^*, \\ \pi_k &= (1-\nu_1^*)(1-\nu_2^*)\ldots(1-\nu_{k-1}^*)\nu_k^*, \quad k = 2, \ldots, G-1, \\ \pi_G &= (1-\nu_1^*)\ldots(1-\nu_{G-1}^*), \end{aligned} \qquad (10.\text{A2})$$

where $\nu_k^* \stackrel{D}{=} \text{Beta}[a_k^*, b_k^*]$, $k = 1, \ldots, G-1$. For the second part of (10.A1), let $\{L_1^*, \ldots, L_m^*\}$ be the unique set of L_i values, $\mathbf{Z}^L = (\mathbf{Z}_{L_1^*}, \ldots, \mathbf{Z}_{L_m^*})$, with $\mathbf{Z}^{[L]}$ corresponding to those values in $\mathbf{Z} = (\mathbf{Z}_1, \ldots, \mathbf{Z}_G)$ which exclude $\mathbf{Z}^L$. Then

$$p(\mathbf{Z}|\mathbf{L}, \boldsymbol{\mu}, \boldsymbol{\Psi}_z, \boldsymbol{\theta}, \boldsymbol{\Omega}_1, \mathbf{Y}) = p(\mathbf{Z}^{[L]}|\boldsymbol{\mu}, \boldsymbol{\Psi}_z)p(\mathbf{Z}^L|\mathbf{L}, \boldsymbol{\mu}, \boldsymbol{\Psi}_z, \boldsymbol{\theta}, \boldsymbol{\Omega}_1, \mathbf{Y}). \qquad (10.\text{A3})$$

The components of $(\mathbf{Z}^{[L]}|\boldsymbol{\mu}, \boldsymbol{\Psi}_z)$ are independently and identically distributed as $N[\boldsymbol{\mu}, \boldsymbol{\Psi}_z]$, and are easy to sample. Clearly,

$$p(\mathbf{Z}^L|\mathbf{L}, \boldsymbol{\mu}, \boldsymbol{\Psi}_z, \boldsymbol{\theta}, \boldsymbol{\Omega}_1, \mathbf{Y}) = \prod_{k=1}^{m} p(\mathbf{Z}_{L_k^*}|\mathbf{L}, \boldsymbol{\mu}, \boldsymbol{\Psi}_z, \boldsymbol{\theta}, \boldsymbol{\Omega}_1, \mathbf{Y}).$$

It can be shown that

$$\left[\mathbf{Z}_{L_k^*}|\mathbf{L}, \boldsymbol{\mu}, \boldsymbol{\Psi}_z, \boldsymbol{\theta}, \boldsymbol{\Omega}_1, \mathbf{Y}\right] \stackrel{D}{=} N[\boldsymbol{\mu}_k^*, \boldsymbol{\Sigma}_k^*], \qquad (10.\text{A4})$$

where $\boldsymbol{\Sigma}_k^* = \left\{\boldsymbol{\Psi}_z^{-1} + m_k^*(\boldsymbol{\Lambda}_\xi^T\boldsymbol{\Psi}_\epsilon^{-1}\boldsymbol{\Lambda}_\xi + \boldsymbol{\Gamma}^T\boldsymbol{\Psi}_\delta^{-1}\boldsymbol{\Gamma})\right\}^{-1}$ and

$$\boldsymbol{\mu}_k^* = \boldsymbol{\Sigma}_k^*\Big\{\boldsymbol{\Psi}_z^{-1}\boldsymbol{\mu} + \sum_{\{i:L_i=L_k^*\}} \left(\boldsymbol{\Lambda}_\xi^T\boldsymbol{\Psi}_\epsilon^{-1}\mathbf{R}_i + \boldsymbol{\Gamma}^T\boldsymbol{\Psi}_\delta^{-1}(\boldsymbol{\Pi}_0\boldsymbol{\eta}_i - \mathbf{B}\mathbf{d}_i)\right)\Big\},$$

in which $\mathbf{R}_i = \mathbf{y}_i - \mathbf{A}\mathbf{c}_i - \boldsymbol{\Lambda}_\eta\boldsymbol{\eta}_i$, $\boldsymbol{\Lambda}_\eta$ and $\boldsymbol{\Lambda}_\xi$ are the corresponding partitions of $\boldsymbol{\Lambda}$ with respect to $\boldsymbol{\eta}_i$ and $\boldsymbol{\xi}_i$, and $m_k^* = \#\left\{i : L_i = L_k^*\right\}$ is the number of i such that $L_i = L_k^*$.

Moreover, it can be shown that

$$[L_i|\boldsymbol{\pi}, \mathbf{Z}, \boldsymbol{\theta}, \boldsymbol{\Omega}_1, \mathbf{Y}] \stackrel{D}{=} \sum_{k=1}^{G} \pi_{ik}^*\delta_k(\cdot), \qquad (10.\text{A5})$$

where $(\pi_{i1}^*, \ldots, \pi_{iG}^*) \propto (\pi_1 p(\mathbf{y}_i|\mathbf{Z}_1, \boldsymbol{\eta}_i, \boldsymbol{\theta}_y)p(\boldsymbol{\eta}_i|\mathbf{Z}_1, \boldsymbol{\theta}_\omega), \ldots, \pi_G p(\mathbf{y}_i|\mathbf{Z}_G, \boldsymbol{\eta}_i, \boldsymbol{\theta}_y)p(\boldsymbol{\eta}_i|\mathbf{Z}_G, \boldsymbol{\theta}_\omega))$;

$$[\boldsymbol{\mu}|\mathbf{Z}, \boldsymbol{\Psi}_z] \stackrel{D}{=} N\left[\boldsymbol{\Sigma}_\mu \boldsymbol{\Psi}_z^{-1} \sum_{k=1}^{G} \mathbf{Z}_k, \boldsymbol{\Sigma}_\mu\right], \tag{10.A6}$$

where $\boldsymbol{\Sigma}_\mu = (G\boldsymbol{\Psi}_z^{-1} + \sigma_\mu^{-1}\mathbf{I}_{q_2})^{-1}$;

$$\left[\psi_{zj}^{-1}|\boldsymbol{\mu}, \mathbf{Z}\right] \stackrel{D}{=} \text{Gamma}\left[\frac{G}{2} + \rho_1, \rho_2 + \sum_{k=1}^{G}(Z_{kj} - \mu_j)^2/2\right], \tag{10.A7}$$

where Z_{kj} is the jth element of $\mathbf{Z}_k$; and

$$[\alpha|\boldsymbol{\pi}] \stackrel{D}{=} \text{Gamma}\left[G - 1 + \tau_1, \tau_2 - \sum_{k=1}^{G-1} \log(1 - \nu_k^*)\right], \tag{10.A8}$$

where ν_k^* is defined in (10.A2).

Simulating observations from the conditional distributions in (10.A2), (10.A4), and (10.A5)–(10.A8) is straightforward and fast.

References

Chen, M. H., Shao, Q. M. and Ibrahim, J. G. (2000) *Monte Carlo Methods in Bayesian Computation.* New York: Springer-Verlag.

Ferguson, T. S. (1973) A Bayesian analysis of some nonparametric problems. *Annals of Statistics*, **1**, 209–230.

Gelman, A. (1996) Inference and monitoring convergence. In W. R. Gilks, S. Richardson and D. J. Spiegelhalter (eds), *Markov Chain Monte Carlo in Practice*, pp. 131–144. London: Chapman & Hall.

Hu, L., Bentler, P. M. and Kano, Y. (1992) Can test statistics in covariance structure analysis be trusted? *Psychological Bulletin*, **112**, 351–362.

Ishwaran, H. (2000) Inference for the random effects in Bayesian generalized linear mixed models. In *ASA Proceedings of the Bayesian Statistical Science Section*, 1–10.

Ishwaran, H. and James, L. F. (2001) Gibbs sampling methods for stick-breaking priors. *Journal of the American Statistical Association*, **96**, 161–173.

Ishwaran, H. and Zarepour, M. (2000) Markov chain Monte Carlo in approximate Dirichlet and beta two-parameter process hierarchical models. *Biometrika*, **87**, 371–390.

Kano, Y., Berkane, M. and Bentler, P. M. (1993) Statistical inference based on pseudo-maximum likelihood estimators in elliptical populations. *Journal of the American Statistical Association*, **88**, 135–143.

Kleinman, K. and Ibrahim, J. (1998) A semiparametric Bayesian approach to the random effects model. *Biometrics*, **54**, 921–938.

Lee, S. Y. (2007) *Structural Equation Modeling: A Bayesian Approach.* Chichester: John Wiley & Sons, Ltd.

Lee, S. Y. and Song, X. Y. (2003) Model comparison of nonlinear structural equation models with fixed covariates. *Psychometrika*, **68**, 27–47.

Lee, S. Y. and Xia, Y. M. (2006) Maximum likelihood methods in treating outliers and symmetrically heavy-tailed distributions for nonlinear structural equation models with missing data. *Psychometrika*, **71**, 565–585.

Lee, S. Y. and Xia, Y. M. (2008) A robust Bayesian approach for structural equation models with missing data. *Psychometrika*, **73**, 343–364.

Lee, S. Y., Lu, B. and Song, X. Y. (2008) Semiparametric Bayesian analysis of structural equation models with fixed covariates. *Statistics in Medicine*, **27**, 2341–2360.

Müller, P., Erkanli, A. and West, M. (1996) Bayesian curve fitting using multivariate normal mixtures. *Biometrika*, **83**, 67–79.

Roeder, K. and Wasserman, L. (1997) Practical Bayesian density estimation using mixtures of normals. *Journal of the American Statistical Association*, **92**, 894–902.

Sethuraman, J. (1994) A constructive definition of Dirichlet priors. *Statistica Sinica*, **4**, 639–650.

Shapiro, A. and Browne, M. W. (1987) Analysis of covariance structures under elliptical distributions. *Journal of the American Statistical Association*, **82**, 1092–1097.

Song, X. Y., Pan, J. H., Kwok, T., Vandenput, L., Ohlsson, C. and Leung, P. C. (2010). A semiparametric Bayesian approach for structural equation models. *Biometrical Journal*, **52**, 314–332.

Song, X. Y., Xia, Y. M., Pan, J. H. and Lee, S. Y. (2011) Model comparison of Bayesian semiparametric and parametric structural equation models. *Structural Equation Modeling – A Multidisciplinary Journal*, **18**, 55–73.

Spiegelhalter, D. J., Thomas, A., Best, N. G. and Lunn, D. (2003) *WinBUGS User Manual, Version 1.4*, Cambridge: MRC Biostatistics Unit.

Sturtz, S., Ligges, U. and Gelman, A. (2005) R2WinBUGS: A package for running WinBUGS from R. *Journal of Statistical Software*, **12**, 1–16.

West, M., Müller, P. and Escobar, M. (1994) Hierarchical priors and mixture models with applications in regression and density estimation. In A. Smith and P. Freeman (eds), *Aspects of Uncertainty: A Tribute to D. V. Lindley*, pp. 363–386. Chichester: John Wiley & Sons, Ltd.

West, S. G., Finch, J. F. and Curran, P. J. (1995) Structural equation models with nonnormal variables: Problems and remedies. In R. H. Hoyle (ed), *Structural Equation Modeling: Concepts, Issues and Applications*, pp. 56–75. Newbary Park, CA: Sage.

11

Structural equation models with mixed continuous and unordered categorical variables

11.1 Introduction

In Chapter 5 we presented the Bayesian methodologies for analyzing SEMs with continuous and ordered categorical variables. In substantive research it is also common to encounter categorical variables in which the categories are unordered. For instance, there are different products in business and economics, and different races in sociological studies. An important model for analyzing such unordered categorical variables with a multivariate multinomial distribution is the choice model (multinomial probit model), originally developed in econometrics (McCulloch and Rossi, 1994; Imai and van Dyk, 2005). Our main motivation for introducing SEMs with unordered categorical variables is to analyze genotype variables, which have unordered carries, in medical research.

Epidemiological and family-based cohort analyses have demonstrated that diseases with complex traits such as diabetes have both genetic and environmental determinants (Seaquist *et al.*, 1989). Indeed, the importance of gene–gene and gene–environment interactions is now being recognized in the study of pathogenesis of complex diseases (Chen *et al.*, 1999). In general, given the complexity of the pathogenetic pathways in relation to the genetic and environmental determinant of various diseases, it is necessary to develop an efficient statistical method to investigate the effects of the linear and interaction terms of explanatory phenotype and genotype variables on the outcome variables. Although most observed phenotype variables are continuous, the observed genotype variables are unordered categorical with a multinomial distribution, say with possible genotype carriers $\{AA, Aa, aa\}$. Thus, the observed random vector is composed of mixed correlated continuous and multinomial variables. As our main

Basic and Advanced Bayesian Structural Equation Modeling: With Applications in the Medical and Behavioral Sciences, First Edition. Xin-Yuan Song and Sik-Yum Lee.

interest is in latent variables, it is necessary to formulate genotype latent variables through the genotype observed variables with a correlated multinomial distribution. It is well known that the analysis of correlated multinomial variables is nontrivial. SEMs may be used to assess the interrelationships among explanatory and outcome genotype and/or phenotype latent variables. Although the multinomial probit model (see McCulloch and Rossi, 1994; Imai and van Dyk, 2005) has been developed to predict multinomial variables through fixed covariates with a regression equation, no latent variables are involved in this method and thus it cannot be applied to solve the problem previously described.

In this chapter, SEMs with mixed continuous and multinomial variables are introduced to analyze the interrelationships among phenotype and genotype latent variables. The SEM is composed of two components. The first component is a confirmatory factor analysis (CFA) model in which the mean vector and the factor loading matrix are defined for modeling the multinomial variables. This component relates the latent variables with all their corresponding observed variables, and takes the measurement errors into account. The second component is a regression type structural equation, which regresses outcome latent variables on the linear and nonlinear terms of explanatory latent variables. In general applications, outcome latent variables can be related to phenotype or genotype observed variables. First, we introduce parametric SEMs with the assumption that the distribution of the explanatory latent variables is multivariate normal. The Bayes factor computed through path sampling is used for model comparison. We then discuss semiparametric SEMs without the normal assumption on the explanatory latent variables. A modification of the semiparametric Bayesian methods as presented in Chapter 10 is described to handle SEMs with unordered categorical variables. An L_ν-measure is adopted to address the issue of model comparison. Real applications related to kidney disease in diabetic patients are presented to illustrate the parametric and semiparametric SEMs.

11.2 Parametric SEMs with continuous and unordered categorical variables

11.2.1 The model

The main objective of this section is to develop a nonlinear SEM with mixed continuous and unordered categorical variables to study the interrelationships of the latent variables formed by those observed variables. Basically, we introduce a model for a $p \times 1$ observed random vector $\mathbf{y}_i$ which is composed of r continuous variables and $s = p - r$ unordered categorical variables. For notational simplicity, we assume that $\mathbf{y}_i = (x_{i1}, x_{i2}, \ldots, x_{ir}, u_{i,r+1}, u_{i,r+2}, \ldots, u_{ip})^T$. Suppose that each u_{ij} is an observed unordered categorical (multinomial) variable which takes one and only one of the possible values, $\{0, 1, \ldots, K_j - 1\}$. In a genetic application, u_{ij} denotes the $K_j = 3$ possible genotype carriers, say {AA, Aa, aa}. Following the approach of Dunson (2000) and Imai and van Dyk (2005), u_{ij} is modeled in terms of an unobserved continuous random vector $\mathbf{v}_{ij} = (v_{ij,1}, \ldots, v_{ij,K_j-1})^T$ that is related to a multivariate normal distribution such that

$$u_{ij}(\mathbf{v}_{ij}) = \begin{cases} 0, & \text{if } \max(\mathbf{v}_{ij}) < 0, \\ k, & \text{if } \max(\mathbf{v}_{ij}) = v_{ij,k} > 0, \end{cases} \quad \text{for} \quad j = r+1, \ldots, p, \tag{11.1}$$

where $\max(\mathbf{v}_{ij})$ is the largest element in the vector $\mathbf{v}_{ij}$. For an observed genotype variable u_{ij} with three outcomes, we have $\mathbf{v}_{ij} = (v_{ij,1}, v_{ij,2})^T$; $u_{ij}(\mathbf{v}_{ij}) = 0$ if both $v_{ij,1}$ and $v_{ij,2}$ are less than zero; $u_{ij}(\mathbf{v}_{ij}) = 1$ if $v_{ij,1} > v_{ij,2}$ and $v_{ij,1} > 0$; and $u_{ij}(\mathbf{v}_{ij}) = 2$ if $v_{ij,2} > v_{ij,1}$ and $v_{ij,2} > 0$.

Motivated by the development of SEMs for ordered categorical variables, we develop an SEM for the observed continuous variables in $\mathbf{y}_i$ and unobserved continuous variables in $\mathbf{v}_{ij}$. To group the observed unordered categorical variables into latent variables according to their functions, we consider the following measurement equation in modeling $\mathbf{v}_{ij}$:

$$\mathbf{v}_{ij} = \mathbf{1}_{K_j-1}\mu_j + \mathbf{1}_{K_j-1}\mathbf{\Lambda}_j^T\boldsymbol{\omega}_i + \boldsymbol{\epsilon}_{ij}, \tag{11.2}$$

where μ_j is an intercept, $\mathbf{1}_{K_j-1}$ is a $(K_j - 1) \times 1$ vector of 1s, $\mathbf{\Lambda}_j$ is a $q \times 1$ vector of parameters, $\boldsymbol{\omega}_i = (\omega_{i1}, \ldots, \omega_{iq})^T$ is a vector of correlated latent variables, and $\boldsymbol{\epsilon}_{ij}$ is a vector of random error terms. We assume that $\boldsymbol{\epsilon}_{ij} \stackrel{D}{=} N[\mathbf{0}, \mathbf{\Psi}_{\epsilon j}]$, where $\mathbf{\Psi}_{\epsilon j}$ is a diagonal matrix. The probability mass function of u_{ij} is

$$p(u_{ij} = k|\boldsymbol{\omega}_i, \mu_j, \mathbf{\Lambda}_j, \mathbf{\Psi}_{\epsilon j}) = \int_{\mathfrak{R}_{ik}} \phi_{K_j-1}(\mathbf{v}_{ij}|\mathbf{1}_{K_j-1}\mu_j + \mathbf{1}_{K_j-1}\mathbf{\Lambda}_j^T\boldsymbol{\omega}_i, \mathbf{\Psi}_{\epsilon j})d\mathbf{v}_{ij},$$

where $\phi_{K_j-1}(\cdot)$ is the density function of the $(K_j - 1)$-variate normal distribution, and

$$\mathfrak{R}_{ik} = \begin{cases} \{\mathbf{v}_{ij} : \max(\mathbf{v}_{ij}) < 0\}, & k = 0, \\ \{\mathbf{v}_{ij} : \max(\mathbf{v}_{ij}) = v_{ij,k} > 0\}, & 0 < k \leq K_j - 1, \end{cases} \tag{11.3}$$

Hence, $\mathbf{v}_{ij}$ is related to the truncated multivariate normal distribution

$$[\mathbf{v}_{ij}|u_{ij} = k, \boldsymbol{\omega}_i, \mu_j, \mathbf{\Lambda}_j, \mathbf{\Psi}_{\epsilon j}] \stackrel{D}{=} N\left[\mathbf{1}_{K_j-1}\mu_j + \mathbf{1}_{K_j-1}\mathbf{\Lambda}_j^T\boldsymbol{\omega}_i, \mathbf{\Psi}_{\epsilon j}\right] I(\mathfrak{R}_{ik}),$$

where $I(\cdot)$ is an indicator function which takes value 1 if $\mathbf{v}_{ij} \in \mathfrak{R}_{ik}$ and 0 otherwise. Note that this approach is similar to the threshold approach for modeling discrete outcomes via unobserved normal continuous variables, which has been used in the full-information item factor model (Meng and Schilling, 1996) for analyzing dichotomous variables, in the binary probit model (Albert and Chib, 1993) for analyzing binary variables, and in SEMs (Lee and Song, 2004; Lee, 2007; see also Section 5.2 above) for analyzing ordered categorical variables.

Let $\mathbf{x}_i = (x_{i1}, \ldots, x_{ir})^T$, $\mathbf{u}_i = (u_{i,r+1}, \ldots, u_{ip})^T$ corresponding to $(\mathbf{v}_{i,r+1}, \ldots, \mathbf{v}_{ip})$, and let $\mathbf{y}_i^* = (\mathbf{x}_i^T, \mathbf{v}_{i,r+1}^T, \ldots, \mathbf{v}_{ip}^T)^T$ be the $[r + \sum_{j=r+1}^p (K_j - 1)] \times 1$ vector of observed and unobserved continuous variables corresponding to $\mathbf{y}_i$. Based on equation (11.2), we use the variables in $\mathbf{y}_i^*$ as indicators to establish q latent variables $\boldsymbol{\omega}_i = (\omega_{i1}, \ldots, \omega_{iq})^T$ through the following measurement model:

$$\mathbf{y}_i^* = \begin{bmatrix} x_{i1} \\ \vdots \\ x_{ir} \\ \mathbf{v}_{i,r+1} \\ \vdots \\ \mathbf{v}_{ip} \end{bmatrix} = \begin{bmatrix} \mu_1 \\ \vdots \\ \mu_r \\ \mathbf{1}_{K_{r+1}-1}\mu_{r+1} \\ \vdots \\ \mathbf{1}_{K_p-1}\mu_p \end{bmatrix} + \begin{bmatrix} \mathbf{\Lambda}_1^T \\ \vdots \\ \mathbf{\Lambda}_r^T \\ \mathbf{1}_{K_{r+1}-1}\mathbf{\Lambda}_{r+1}^T \\ \vdots \\ \mathbf{1}_{K_p-1}\mathbf{\Lambda}_p^T \end{bmatrix} \boldsymbol{\omega}_i + \begin{bmatrix} \epsilon_{i1} \\ \vdots \\ \epsilon_{ir} \\ \boldsymbol{\epsilon}_{i,r+1} \\ \vdots \\ \boldsymbol{\epsilon}_{ip} \end{bmatrix}, \tag{11.4}$$

where the definitions of μ_j and $\mathbf{\Lambda}_j$ are the same as in (11.2), and $\epsilon_{i1}, \ldots, \epsilon_{ir}, \boldsymbol{\epsilon}_{i,r+1}, \ldots, \boldsymbol{\epsilon}_{ip}$ are independent random error terms. Let $\boldsymbol{\epsilon}_{ix} = (\epsilon_{i1}, \ldots, \epsilon_{ir})^T$; we assume that $\boldsymbol{\epsilon}_{ix} \stackrel{D}{=} N[\mathbf{0}, \mathbf{\Psi}_{\epsilon x}]$, where $\mathbf{\Psi}_{\epsilon x}$ is diagonal, and $\boldsymbol{\omega}_i$ and the $\boldsymbol{\epsilon}$s are independent. Let $\boldsymbol{\epsilon}_i = (\boldsymbol{\epsilon}_{ix}^T, \boldsymbol{\epsilon}_{i,r+1}^T, \ldots, \boldsymbol{\epsilon}_{ip}^T)^T$, $\boldsymbol{\mu} = (\mu_1, \ldots, \mu_r, \boldsymbol{\mu}_{r+1}, \ldots, \boldsymbol{\mu}_p)^T$,

$$\mathbf{E} = \begin{bmatrix} \mathbf{I}_r & \mathbf{0} & \cdots & \mathbf{0} \\ \mathbf{0} & \mathbf{1}_{K_{r+1}-1} & \cdots & \mathbf{0} \\ \vdots & \vdots & \ddots & \vdots \\ \mathbf{0} & \mathbf{0} & \cdots & \mathbf{1}_{K_p-1} \end{bmatrix}, \quad \text{and} \quad \mathbf{\Lambda} = \begin{bmatrix} \mathbf{\Lambda}_1 & \cdots & \mathbf{\Lambda}_r & \mathbf{\Lambda}_{r+1} & \cdots & \mathbf{\Lambda}_p \end{bmatrix}^T.$$

Then equation (11.4) can be rewritten as

$$\mathbf{y}_i^* = \mathbf{E}\boldsymbol{\mu} + \mathbf{E}\mathbf{\Lambda}\boldsymbol{\omega}_i + \boldsymbol{\epsilon}_i. \tag{11.5}$$

The model defined in (11.1) and (11.5) is not identified. The first model indeterminacy is due to the unordered categorical variables. It can be seen that multiplying each $v_{ij,k}$ by an arbitrary positive constant does not change the value of u_{ij} in (11.1). This indeterminacy can be solved by a method similar to that used in Meng and Schilling (1996), Dunson (2000), Shi and Lee (2000), and Lee and Song (2003): fixing $\mathbf{\Psi}_{\epsilon j} = \mathbf{I}_{K_j-1}$, an identity matrix of order $K_j - 1$, for $j = r+1, \ldots, p$. The second model indeterminacy is associated with the measurement equation defined by (11.5). This problem can be solved by the common method of fixing appropriate elements in $\mathbf{\Lambda}_j$ at preassigned values.

Let $\boldsymbol{\omega}_i = (\boldsymbol{\eta}_i^T, \boldsymbol{\xi}_i^T)^T$ be a partition of $\boldsymbol{\omega}_i$ into outcome latent variables in $\boldsymbol{\eta}_i(q_1 \times 1)$ and explanatory latent variables in $\boldsymbol{\xi}_i(q_2 \times 1)$. To assess the linear effects of some variables in $\boldsymbol{\eta}_i$ on other variables in $\boldsymbol{\eta}_i$, and the nonlinear effects of variables in $\boldsymbol{\xi}_i$ on $\boldsymbol{\eta}_i$, the SEM is defined by (11.5), together with the nonlinear structural equation

$$\boldsymbol{\eta}_i = \mathbf{\Pi}\boldsymbol{\eta}_i + \mathbf{\Gamma}\mathbf{F}(\boldsymbol{\xi}_i) + \boldsymbol{\delta}_i, \tag{11.6}$$

where $\mathbf{\Pi}$ and $\mathbf{\Gamma}$ are unknown $q_1 \times q_1$ and $q_1 \times m$ parameter matrices; $\boldsymbol{\xi}_i$ and the vector of error terms $\boldsymbol{\delta}_i$ are independently distributed as $N(\mathbf{0}, \mathbf{\Phi})$ and $N(\mathbf{0}, \mathbf{\Psi}_\delta)$, respectively; and $\mathbf{F}(\boldsymbol{\xi}_i) = (f_1(\boldsymbol{\xi}_i), \ldots, f_m(\boldsymbol{\xi}_i))^T$ is a vector-valued function with differentiable functions $f_1, \ldots, f_m$ with $m \geq q_2$. In general, $\boldsymbol{\eta}_i$ may contain latent variables which are related to observed variables in $\mathbf{x}_i$ or $\mathbf{u}_i$. Hence, we may use it for phenotype or genotype latent variables. Like other SEMs, we assume that $\mathbf{\Psi}_\delta$ is diagonal with elements $\psi_{\delta j}$, $j = 1, \ldots, q_1$. Let $\mathbf{\Lambda}_\omega = (\mathbf{\Pi}, \mathbf{\Gamma})$ and $\mathbf{G}(\boldsymbol{\omega}_i) = (\boldsymbol{\eta}_i^T, \mathbf{F}(\boldsymbol{\xi}_i)^T)^T$. Then equation (11.6) can be rewritten as

$$\boldsymbol{\eta}_i = \mathbf{\Lambda}_\omega \mathbf{G}(\boldsymbol{\omega}_i) + \boldsymbol{\delta}_i.$$

Let $\boldsymbol{\theta}$ be the parameter vector that includes all unknown structural parameters in $\boldsymbol{\mu} = (\mu_1, \ldots, \boldsymbol{\mu}_p)^T$, $\mathbf{\Lambda} = [\mathbf{\Lambda}_1, \ldots, \mathbf{\Lambda}_p]^T$, $\mathbf{\Phi}$, $\mathbf{\Lambda}_\omega$, $\mathbf{\Psi}_\delta$, and $\mathbf{\Psi}_{\epsilon x}$.

11.2.2 Application to diabetic kidney disease

The data in this application are obtained from an applied genomics program which aims to examine the clinical and molecular epidemiology of type 2 diabetes in Hong Kong Chinese, with particular emphasis on diabetic nephropathy. In the search for genetic markers for diabetic nephropathy, a panel of 65 biallelic single nucleotide polymorphisms (SNPs) in 36 genes from biochemical pathways implicated in the development and progression of cardiovascular disease were examined (Cheng *et al.*, 1999). Using this multilocus genotyping assay, SNPs in a case–control cohort consisting of type 2 diabetic patients with and without nephropathy were assessed. In this application, we are interested in incorporating multiple genetic and phenotypic pathways to study diabetic kidney disease. The outcome variable of diabetic kidney disease severity was treated as a latent variable reflected by two observed variables of urinary albumin creatinine ratio (ACR) and plasma creatinine (PCr). Based on some preliminary data analysis, and motivated by medical findings in the literature (see Song *et al.*, 2007; and the references therein), we are interested in investigating the influences of a number of continuous phenotype variables and unordered categorical genotype variables on the severity of kidney disease. The continuous phenotype variables are: fasting plasma glucose (FPG), glycated hemoglobin (HbA1c), non-high-density lipoprotein cholesterol (non-HDL-C), lower-density lipoprotein cholesterol (LDL-C), and plasma triglyceride (TG). The unordered categorical genotype variables are: beta-3 adrenergic receptor (ADRβ3), beta-2 adrenergic receptor SNP1 (ADRβ21), beta-2 adrenergic receptor SNP2 (ADRβ22), angiotensin converting enzyme (DCP1 intro 16 del/ins (DCP1)), and angiotensin II receptor type 1 AgtR1 A1166C (AGTR1). The SEM introduced in Section 11.2.1 is useful for investigating the possible linear and nonlinear effects of these phenotype and genotype variables on kidney disease.

In most medical applications, an observed variable usually only serves as an indicator for a single latent variable, and hence the corresponding $\mathbf{\Lambda}_j$ only contains a nonzero loading parameter at the appropriate position, and the remaining elements are zero. In this application, the observed random vector $\mathbf{y}_i$ has 12 variables. The first seven are the following continuous phenotype variables (xs): ACR, PCr, HbAlc, FPG, TG, non-HDL-C, and LDL-C. The remaining five unordered categorical genotype variables (us) are: ADRβ3, ADRβ21, ADRβ22, DCP1, and AGTR1. To apply the model and Bayesian methods to the analysis of these phenotype and genotype variables, the following $\mathbf{\Lambda}_1, \ldots, \mathbf{\Lambda}_{12}$ are used in the measurement model defined in equation (11.4) or (11.5):

$$[\mathbf{\Lambda}_1, \ldots, \mathbf{\Lambda}_{12}] = \begin{bmatrix} 1 & \lambda_{21} & 0 & 0 & 0 & 0 & 0 & 0 & 0 & 0 & 0 & 0 \\ 0 & 0 & 1 & \lambda_{42} & 0 & 0 & 0 & 0 & 0 & 0 & 0 & 0 \\ 0 & 0 & 0 & 0 & 1 & \lambda_{63} & \lambda_{73} & 0 & 0 & 0 & 0 & 0 \\ 0 & 0 & 0 & 0 & 0 & 0 & 0 & 1 & \lambda_{94} & \lambda_{10,4} & 0 & 0 \\ 0 & 0 & 0 & 0 & 0 & 0 & 0 & 0 & 0 & 0 & 1 & \lambda_{12,5} \end{bmatrix}, \quad (11.7)$$

where the 1s and 0s are fixed in order to give an identified model, and the λs are unknown factor loading parameters. The non-overlapping structure of $[\mathbf{\Lambda}_1, \ldots, \mathbf{\Lambda}_{12}]$ corresponds to the following five latent variables via their corresponding indicators in $\mathbf{y}_i^*$: 'kidney disease' (ω_1), with observed variables ACR and PCr; 'glycemic control' (ω_2), with observed variables HbAlc and FPG; 'lipid control' (ω_3), with observed variables TG, non-HDL-C, and LDL-C; 'β adrenergic receptor activity' (ω_4), with observed variables ADRβ3, ADRβ21, and ADRβ22; and 'angiotensin converting enzyme' (ω_5), with observed variables DCP1 and AGTR1.

In the nonlinear structural equation, we consider kidney disease severity as the outcome latent variable (η), and the explanatory latent variables are glycemic control (ξ_1), lipid control (ξ_2), β adrenergic receptor activity (ξ_3), and angiotensin converting enzyme (ξ_4). Then η is regressed on $\xi_1, \ldots, \xi_4$ through equation (11.6), with $\mathbf{\Pi} = \mathbf{0}$. As the functions $f_1, \ldots, f_m$ in $\mathbf{F}(\boldsymbol{\xi})$ can be any differentiable function, linear and nonlinear terms of $\xi_1, \ldots, \xi_4$ can be considered. An example is $\eta = \gamma_1\xi_1 + \gamma_2\xi_2 + \gamma_3\xi_3 + \gamma_4\xi_4 + \gamma_5\xi_1\xi_2 + \gamma_6\xi_1\xi_3 + \gamma_7\xi_3\xi_4 + \delta$, with $\mathbf{\Gamma} = (\gamma_1, \gamma_2, \gamma_3, \gamma_4, \gamma_5, \gamma_6, \gamma_7)$, and $\mathbf{F}(\boldsymbol{\xi}_i) = (\xi_1, \xi_2, \xi_3, \xi_4, \xi_1\xi_2, \xi_1\xi_3, \xi_3\xi_4)^T$. In this example,

$\xi_1\xi_2$ represents the phenotype interaction of ξ_1 and ξ_2, $\xi_1\xi_3$ represents a phenotype–genotype interaction of ξ_1 and ξ_3, and $\xi_3\xi_4$ represents the genotype interaction of ξ_3 and ξ_4. The existence of the interaction effects on kidney disease severity (η) is assessed via parameters γ_5, γ_6, and γ_7. Other phenotype–genotype interactions can be assessed via $\xi_1\xi_4$, $\xi_2\xi_3$, and/or $\xi_2\xi_4$.

11.2.3 Bayesian estimation and model comparison

Let $\mathbf{x}_i$ be a continuous observation and $\mathbf{u}_i = (u_{i,r+1}, \ldots, u_{ip})^T$ be an unordered categorical observation of an individual i within a random sample of size n, and let $\mathbf{V}_i = (\mathbf{v}_{i,r+1}^T, \ldots, \mathbf{v}_{ip}^T)^T$ be an unobserved continuous vector that relates to $\mathbf{u}_i$. To accommodate missing data, we let $\mathbf{x}_i = \{\mathbf{x}_{i,\text{obs}}, \mathbf{x}_{i,\text{mis}}\}$ and $\mathbf{u}_i = \{\mathbf{u}_{i,\text{obs}}, \mathbf{u}_{i,\text{mis}}\}$, where $\mathbf{x}_{i,\text{obs}}$ and $\mathbf{u}_{i,\text{obs}}$ represent the observed data, and $\mathbf{x}_{i,\text{mis}}$ and $\mathbf{u}_{i,\text{mis}}$ represent the missing data, respectively. We assume that the missing data are missing at random (Little and Rubin, 2002). Let $\mathbf{V}_i = \{\mathbf{V}_{i,\text{obs}}, \mathbf{V}_{i,\text{mis}}\}$ represent the unobserved continuous measurements, where $\mathbf{V}_{i,\text{obs}}$ and $\mathbf{V}_{i,\text{mis}}$ correspond to $\mathbf{u}_{i,\text{obs}}$ and $\mathbf{u}_{i,\text{mis}}$, respectively. Let $\mathbf{y}_{i,\text{obs}}^* = \{\mathbf{x}_{i,\text{obs}}, \mathbf{V}_{i,\text{obs}}\}$, $\mathbf{y}_{i,\text{mis}}^* = \{\mathbf{x}_{i,\text{mis}}, \mathbf{V}_{i,\text{mis}}\}$, and $\mathbf{y}_i^* = \{\mathbf{y}_{i,\text{obs}}^*, \mathbf{y}_{i,\text{mis}}^*\}$.

Let $p(\boldsymbol{\theta})$ be the prior density of $\boldsymbol{\theta}$, and let $\mathbf{X}_{\text{obs}} = \{\mathbf{x}_{i,\text{obs}}, i = 1, \ldots, n\}$ and $\mathbf{U}_{\text{obs}} = \{\mathbf{u}_{i,\text{obs}}, i = 1, \ldots, n\}$ be observed continuous and unordered categorical data, respectively. The posterior density of $\boldsymbol{\theta}$ given $\mathbf{X}_{\text{obs}}$ and $\mathbf{U}_{\text{obs}}$ is $p(\boldsymbol{\theta}|\mathbf{X}_{\text{obs}}, \mathbf{U}_{\text{obs}})$. Again the notion of data augmentation is used in the posterior analysis. Let $\mathbf{X}_{\text{mis}} = \{\mathbf{x}_{i,\text{mis}}, i = 1, \ldots, n\}$, $\mathbf{V}_{\text{obs}} = \{\mathbf{V}_{i,\text{obs}}, i = 1, \ldots, n\}$, and $\mathbf{V}_{\text{mis}} = \{\mathbf{V}_{i,\text{mis}}, i = 1, \ldots, n\}$ be the latent data; and $\boldsymbol{\Omega} = \{\boldsymbol{\omega}_i, i = 1, \ldots, n\}$ be the collection of latent variables in the model. The observed data $\{\mathbf{X}_{\text{obs}}, \mathbf{U}_{\text{obs}}\}$ are augmented with missing quantities $\{\mathbf{X}_{\text{mis}}, \mathbf{V}_{\text{obs}}, \mathbf{V}_{\text{mis}}, \boldsymbol{\Omega}\}$. A sequence of random observations will be generated from the joint posterior distribution $[\mathbf{X}_{\text{mis}}, \mathbf{V}_{\text{obs}}, \mathbf{V}_{\text{mis}}, \boldsymbol{\Omega}, \boldsymbol{\theta}|\mathbf{X}_{\text{obs}}, \mathbf{U}_{\text{obs}}]$. As before, the Gibbs sampler (Geman and Geman, 1984) and the Metropolis–Hastings (MH) algorithm (Metropolis *et al.*, 1953; Hastings, 1970) are used to simulate observations for Bayesian estimation. The simulating algorithm is implemented as follows. At the hth iteration with current values $\mathbf{X}_{\text{mis}}^{(h)}$, $\mathbf{V}_{\text{obs}}^{(h)}$, $\mathbf{V}_{\text{mis}}^{(h)}$, $\boldsymbol{\Omega}^{(h)}$, and $\boldsymbol{\theta}^{(h)}$:

(a) generate $\mathbf{X}_{\text{mis}}^{(h+1)}$ from $p\big(\mathbf{X}_{\text{mis}}|\mathbf{X}_{\text{obs}}, \mathbf{U}_{\text{obs}}, \mathbf{V}_{\text{obs}}^{(h)}, \mathbf{V}_{\text{mis}}^{(h)}, \boldsymbol{\Omega}^{(h)}, \boldsymbol{\theta}^{(h)}\big)$;

(b) generate $\mathbf{V}_{\text{obs}}^{(h+1)}$ from $p\big(\mathbf{V}_{\text{obs}}|\mathbf{X}_{\text{obs}}, \mathbf{U}_{\text{obs}}, \mathbf{X}_{\text{mis}}^{(h+1)}, \mathbf{V}_{\text{mis}}^{(h)}, \boldsymbol{\Omega}^{(h)}, \boldsymbol{\theta}^{(h)}\big)$;

(c) generate $\mathbf{V}_{\text{mis}}^{(h+1)}$ from $p\big(\mathbf{V}_{\text{mis}}|\mathbf{X}_{\text{obs}}, \mathbf{U}_{\text{obs}}, \mathbf{X}_{\text{mis}}^{(h+1)}, \mathbf{V}_{\text{obs}}^{(h+1)}, \boldsymbol{\Omega}^{(h)}, \boldsymbol{\theta}^{(h)}\big)$;

(d) generate $\boldsymbol{\Omega}^{(h+1)}$ from $p\big(\boldsymbol{\Omega}|\mathbf{X}_{\text{obs}}, \mathbf{U}_{\text{obs}}, \mathbf{X}_{\text{mis}}^{(h+1)}, \mathbf{V}_{\text{obs}}^{(h+1)}, \mathbf{V}_{\text{mis}}^{(h+1)}, \boldsymbol{\theta}^{(h)}\big)$;

(e) generate $\boldsymbol{\theta}^{(h+1)}$ from $p\big(\boldsymbol{\theta}|\mathbf{X}_{\text{obs}}, \mathbf{U}_{\text{obs}}, \mathbf{X}_{\text{mis}}^{(h+1)}, \mathbf{V}_{\text{obs}}^{(h+1)}, \mathbf{V}_{\text{mis}}^{(h+1)}, \boldsymbol{\Omega}^{(h+1)}\big)$.

The above full conditional distributions are given in Appendix 11.1.

Another important issue in the analysis of SEMs is model comparison. Here, we consider the Bayes factor (Kass and Raftery, 1995) as a statistic for model comparison. Suppose that the observed data $\mathbf{D}_{\text{obs}} = (\mathbf{X}_{\text{obs}}, \mathbf{U}_{\text{obs}})$ arose from one of two competing nonlinear SEMs, M_0 and M_1. For $l = 0, 1$, let $p(\mathbf{D}_{\text{obs}}|M_l)$ be the probability density of $\mathbf{D}_{\text{obs}}$ given M_l. The Bayes factor is defined by

$$B_{10} = \frac{p(\mathbf{D}_{\text{obs}}|M_1)}{p(\mathbf{D}_{\text{obs}}|M_0)}, \tag{11.8}$$

where

$$p(\mathbf{D}_{\text{obs}}|M_l) = \int p(\mathbf{D}_{\text{obs}}|\boldsymbol{\theta}_l, M_l)p(\boldsymbol{\theta}_l|M_l)d\boldsymbol{\theta}_l, \quad l = 0, 1,$$

in which $\boldsymbol{\theta}_l$ is the parameter vector in M_l, $p(\boldsymbol{\theta}_l|M_l)$ is its prior density, and $p(\mathbf{D}_{\text{obs}}|\boldsymbol{\theta}_l, M_l)$ is the probability density of $\mathbf{D}_{\text{obs}}$ given $\boldsymbol{\theta}_l$. Again, a path sampling procedure is applied to compute the Bayes factor for model comparison. For completeness, a brief description of this computing tool is presented in the Appendix 11.2.

11.2.4 Application to the diabetic kidney disease data

The methodologies introduced are used to analyze the diabetes data set in relation to kidney disease severity of high-risk diabetic patients as described in Section 10.2.2. Twelve phenotype and genotype observed variables, ACR, PCr, HbA1c, FPG, TG, non-HDL-C, LDL-C, ARRβ3, ARRβ21, ARRβ22, DCP1, and AGTR1, as mentioned in Section 10.2.2, were considered. Based on some preliminary analysis, we know that ACR, PCr, and TG are highly skewed. Thus, these variables are transformed via the logarithm function to lnACR, lnPCr, and lnTG. The sample size is 352. The numbers of missing entries corresponding to these variables are $\{26, 5, 0, 1, 0, 0, 36, 8, 14, 3, 1, 1\}$. To roughly unify the scale, the continuous variables are standardized using the fully observed data points. The genotype variables are coded $\{0, 1, 2\}$; these values are *ad hoc* and treated as unordered. The frequencies of these values in ADRβ3, ADRβ21, ADRβ22, DCP1, and AGTR1 are $\{264, 79, 1\}$, $\{126, 162, 56\}$, $\{306, 42, 1\}$, $\{157, 153, 41\}$, and $\{318, 33, 0\}$, respectively.

Based on the nature of the observed variables, the SEM defined by equations (11.1), (11.4), and (11.6) with the structure of $\mathbf{\Lambda}_j$ was used to fit the data set involving continuous phenotype data and the unordered categorical genotype data. Note that the measurement model defined by equation (11.4) is identified with these $\mathbf{\Lambda}_j$; and recall that the unordered categorical variables are identified by fixing the covariance matrices corresponding to $\boldsymbol{\epsilon}_{ij}$, $j = 8, \ldots, 12$ as identity matrices. The latent variables can be roughly interpreted as 'kidney disease severity' (η), 'glycemic control' (ξ_1), 'lipid control' (ξ_2), 'β adrenergic receptor activity' (ξ_3), and 'angiotensin converting enzyme' (ξ_4). We first consider the selection of an appropriate structural equation, by computing the Bayes factors through the path sampling procedure.

To obtain prior inputs for the hyperparameters in the conjugate prior distributions of $\boldsymbol{\theta}$, an auxiliary Bayesian estimation based on an encompassing model and a sample of 'control' observations among a sample size of 414 was conducted with noninformative prior distributions. Then the actual Bayesian analyses were based on the following hyperparameter values: $\alpha_{0j} = \alpha_{0\delta j} = 15$, $\beta_{0j} = \beta_{0\delta j} = 5$, $\rho_0 = 8$, $\mathbf{R}_0^{-1} = 2\mathbf{I}$, $\mathbf{\Sigma}_0$, $\mathbf{H}_{0j}$, $\mathbf{H}_{0\omega j}$ are fixed at identity matrices with appropriate dimensions, $\boldsymbol{\mu}_0 = \boldsymbol{\mu}_0^*$, $\mathbf{\Lambda}_{0j} = \mathbf{\Lambda}_j^*$, and $\mathbf{\Lambda}_{0\omega j} = \mathbf{\Lambda}_{\omega j}^*$, where $\boldsymbol{\mu}_0^*$, $\mathbf{\Lambda}_j^*$, and $\mathbf{\Lambda}_{\omega j}^*$ are estimates obtained from the auxiliary estimation. In the posterior simulation, the σ^2 in the proposal distribution of the MH algorithm was equal to 0.81, giving an approximate average acceptance rate of 0.34. In the path sampling procedure for computing the Bayes factor, the number of grids S is 20, and for each grid $L = 3000$ observations were taken after 500 burn-in iterations.

We consider competing models with the same measurement model and the following different structural equations:

$$
\begin{aligned}
M_0 &: \eta = \gamma_1\xi_1 + \gamma_2\xi_2 + \gamma_3\xi_3 + \gamma_4\xi_4 + \gamma_5\xi_1\xi_3 + \gamma_6\xi_2\xi_4 + \delta, \\
M_1 &: \eta = \gamma_1\xi_1 + \gamma_2\xi_2 + \gamma_3\xi_3 + \gamma_4\xi_4 + \gamma_5\xi_1\xi_2 + \gamma_6\xi_3\xi_4 + \delta, \\
M_2 &: \eta = \gamma_1\xi_1 + \gamma_2\xi_2 + \gamma_3\xi_3 + \gamma_4\xi_4 + \gamma_5\xi_1\xi_2 + \delta, \\
M_3 &: \eta = \gamma_1\xi_1 + \gamma_2\xi_2 + \gamma_3\xi_3 + \gamma_4\xi_4 + \gamma_5\xi_3\xi_4 + \delta, \\
M_4 &: \eta = \gamma_1\xi_1 + \gamma_2\xi_2 + \gamma_3\xi_3 + \gamma_4\xi_4 + \delta.
\end{aligned}
\tag{11.9}
$$

Note that, M_4 is nested in M_0, but M_1, M_2, and M_3 are not nested. To check the convergence of the Gibbs sampler, several parallel sequences generated with different starting values were examined and found to mix well within 7000 iterations. Hence, observations were collected after 7000 burn-in iterations. It is easy to construct a path to link the competing models in the path sampling procedure. For instance, the linked model for M_0 and M_1 is

$$M_t : \eta = \gamma_1\xi_1 + \gamma_2\xi_2 + \gamma_3\xi_3 + \gamma_4\xi_4 + t\gamma_5\xi_1\xi_2 + t\gamma_6\xi_3\xi_4 + (1-t)\gamma_7\xi_1\xi_3 + (1-t)\gamma_8\xi_2\xi_4 + \delta.$$

Clearly, when $t = 0, M_t = M_0$; and when $t = 1, M_t = M_1$. The computed log Bayes factors are $\widehat{\log B_{01}} = 1.05$, $\widehat{\log B_{02}} = 1.74$, $\widehat{\log B_{03}} = 1.32$, and $\widehat{\log B_{04}} = 1.70$. Based on the Bayes factor criterion, M_0 is selected. The posterior predictive p-value (Gelman *et al.*, 1996) for testing the goodness of fit of M_0 is 0.53, indicating that the selected model fits the data well. The nonlinear structural equation of the selected model M_0 contains all linear terms of the phenotype and genotype latent variables, and two phenotype–genotype interaction terms ($\xi_1\xi_3$, $\xi_2\xi_4$). The model comparison results between M_0 and the other models imply that M_0 is better than: (i) M_1, which contains a phenotype–phenotype interaction and a genotype–genotype interaction; (ii) M_2, which contains a phenotype–phenotype interaction; (iii) M_3, which contains a genotype–genotype interaction; and (iv) M_4, which contains no interaction. Based on M_0, we conclude that the linear effects of latent variables are inadequate in accounting for their associations with kidney disease; and phenotype–genotype interactions of glycemic control with β adrenergic receptor activity ($\xi_1\xi_3$), and lipid control with angiotensin converting enzyme ($\xi_2\xi_4$) have to be included. We have shown that these two phenotype–genotype interactions are more appropriate than the phenotype–phenotype and/or genotype–genotype interactions. The model comparison results have been cross-validated using different values of S and L in the path sampling procedure for computing the Bayes factor. We obtained similar values of $\widehat{\log B_{ij}}$ and the same conclusion as above.

A path diagram of the selected model M_0 is presented in Figure 11.1, together with the Bayesian estimates of the important parameters. These estimates were obtained from 10 000 simulated observations after 7000 burn-in iterations. We observe that the magnitudes of the λ estimates indicate strong associations between the latent variables and their corresponding indicators. The estimated structural equation is

$$\eta = -0.122\xi_1 + 0.465\xi_2 + 0.714\xi_3 + 0.619\xi_4 - 0.288\xi_1\xi_3 - 0.405\xi_2\xi_4.$$

The interpretation of this equation is similar to that of the regression model, considering η as an outcome variable and $\xi_1, \ldots, \xi_4$ as the explanatory variables. Because of the presence of the phenotype–genotype interactions, the corresponding phenotype and genotype effects should be interpreted together with the interaction effects. For example, $\partial\eta/\partial\xi_1 = -0.122 - 0.288\xi_3$

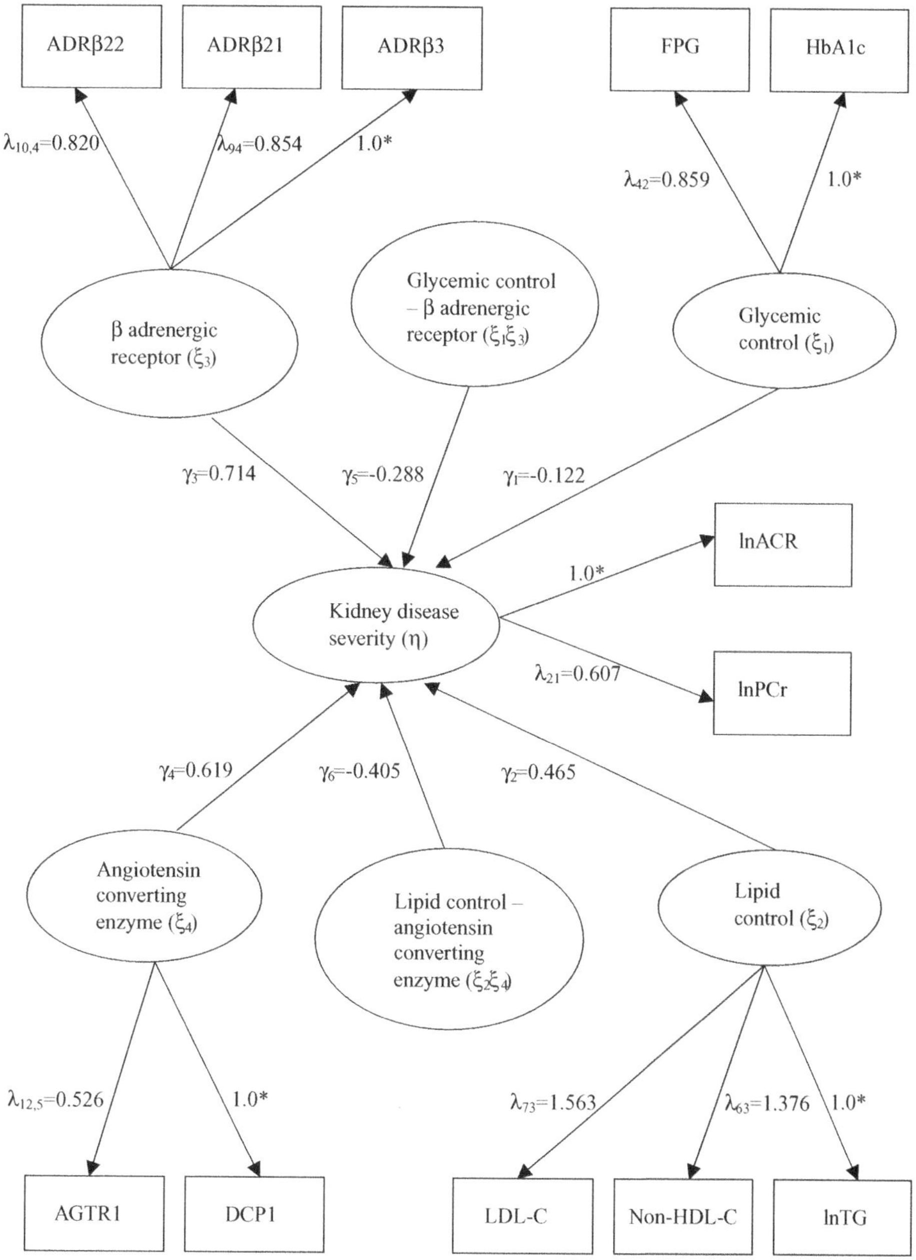

Figure 11.1 Path diagram of M_0, where latent variables and their interactions are represented by ellipses, 1.0* denotes a fixed parameter value, and λs and γs denote Bayesian estimates.

gives the change of η for a one-unit increase in ξ_1 at fixed ξ_3, and $\partial\eta/\partial\xi_3 = 0.714 - 0.288\xi_1$ gives the change of η for a one-unit increase in ξ_3 at fixed ξ_1. Bayesian estimates of $\boldsymbol{\mu}$, $\boldsymbol{\Psi}_{\epsilon x}$, and ψ_δ are respectively $\{0.023, 0.006, 0.001, -0.002, -0.006, -0.002, 0.108, -1.217, -0.315, -1.591, -0.432, -1.669\}$, $\{0.372, 0.737, 0.299, 0.468, 1.145, 0.139, 0.175\}$, and 0.360. The Bayesian estimates of the variances of the latent variables $\{\phi_{11}, \phi_{22}, \phi_{33}, \phi_{44}\}$ and their correlations $\{\phi_{12}, \phi_{13}, \phi_{14}, \phi_{23}, \phi_{24}, \phi_{34}\}$ are respectively $\{0.705, 0.459, 0.137, 0.154\}$, and $\{0.126, -0.050, 0.006, -0.041, 0.041, 0.012\}$. From the $\hat{\phi}_{ij}$, we observe that the correlations of the phenotype and genotype latent variables are small.

The Bayesian approach also produces the Bayesian estimates of the latent variables, $\hat{\boldsymbol{\omega}}_i = (\hat{\eta}_i, \hat{\xi}_{i1}, \ldots, \hat{\xi}_{i4})^T$, for $i = 1, \ldots, n$. The following estimated residuals can be obtained: $\hat{\delta}_i = \hat{\eta}_i - \hat{\gamma}_1\hat{\xi}_{i1} - \hat{\gamma}_2\hat{\xi}_{i2} - \hat{\gamma}_3\hat{\xi}_{i3} - \hat{\gamma}_4\hat{\xi}_{i4} - \hat{\gamma}_5\hat{\xi}_{i1}\hat{\xi}_{i3} - \hat{\gamma}_6\hat{\xi}_{i2}\hat{\xi}_{i4}$ and $\hat{\epsilon}_{ij} = x_{ij} - \hat{\mu}_j - \hat{\boldsymbol{\Lambda}}_j^T\hat{\boldsymbol{\omega}}_i$, for $j = 1, \ldots, 7$. Plots of $\hat{\delta}_i$ versus the phenotype latent variable $\hat{\xi}_{i1}$ and genotype latent variable $\hat{\xi}_{i3}$, and plots of $\hat{\epsilon}_{i1}$ versus $\hat{\eta}_i$, $\hat{\xi}_{i1}$, and $\hat{\xi}_{i3}$ are presented in Figure 11.2. Residual plots that correspond to other ϵ components are similar. These plots lie within two parallel horizontal lines that are centered at zero, and no linear or quadratic trends are detected. This reconfirms that the model fits the data adequately.

11.3 Bayesian semiparametric SEM with continuous and unordered categorical variables

As discussed in Chapter 10, the idea behind the development of a Bayesian semiparametric approach is to address a major concern over the crucial normal assumption for latent variables in SEMs. We recognize that even for standard SEMs with continuous variables, violation of the normal assumption (which is impossible to check) would lead to deleterious effects on statistical inference. In this section, we introduce a Bayesian semiparametric approach for analyzing SEMs with mixed continuous and unordered categorical variables, with the explanatory latent variables being modeled through an appropriate truncated Dirichlet process (DP). To gain more flexibility, fixed covariates are also accommodated in the measurement and structural equations of the model. Bayesian semiparametric approaches based on the Dirichlet process have been widely applied to various statistical models and complex data; see, for example, Müller and Rosner (1997) and Kleinman and Ibrahim (1998). In particular, Lee *et al.* (2008) utilized an approximate truncated Dirichlet process to analyze Bayesian semiparametric SEMs with continuous variables; see also Chapter 10. Although this approach works well for continuous variables, it is not suitable for modeling latent variables formed by unordered categorical variables; see Section 11.3.1 below. Here, we introduce a modified version of the truncated Dirichlet process with appropriate priors for modeling the distributions of the explanatory latent variables in the model.

We also consider the important issue of model selection. The Bayes factor is a well-known Bayesian model selection statistic, and has been applied to many parametric SEMs. However, by the same reasoning as in Chapter 10, this statistic may not be a good choice for the current semiparametric model due to some computational difficulties. First, because of the complexity induced by the semiparametric formulation of the model and the unordered categorical variables, the computational burden of the Bayes factor is extremely heavy. Moreover, path sampling, which is effective in computing Bayes factors for parametric SEMs, cannot give satisfactory results for semiparametric SEMs. Hence, as in Chapter 10, we use the L_ν-measure

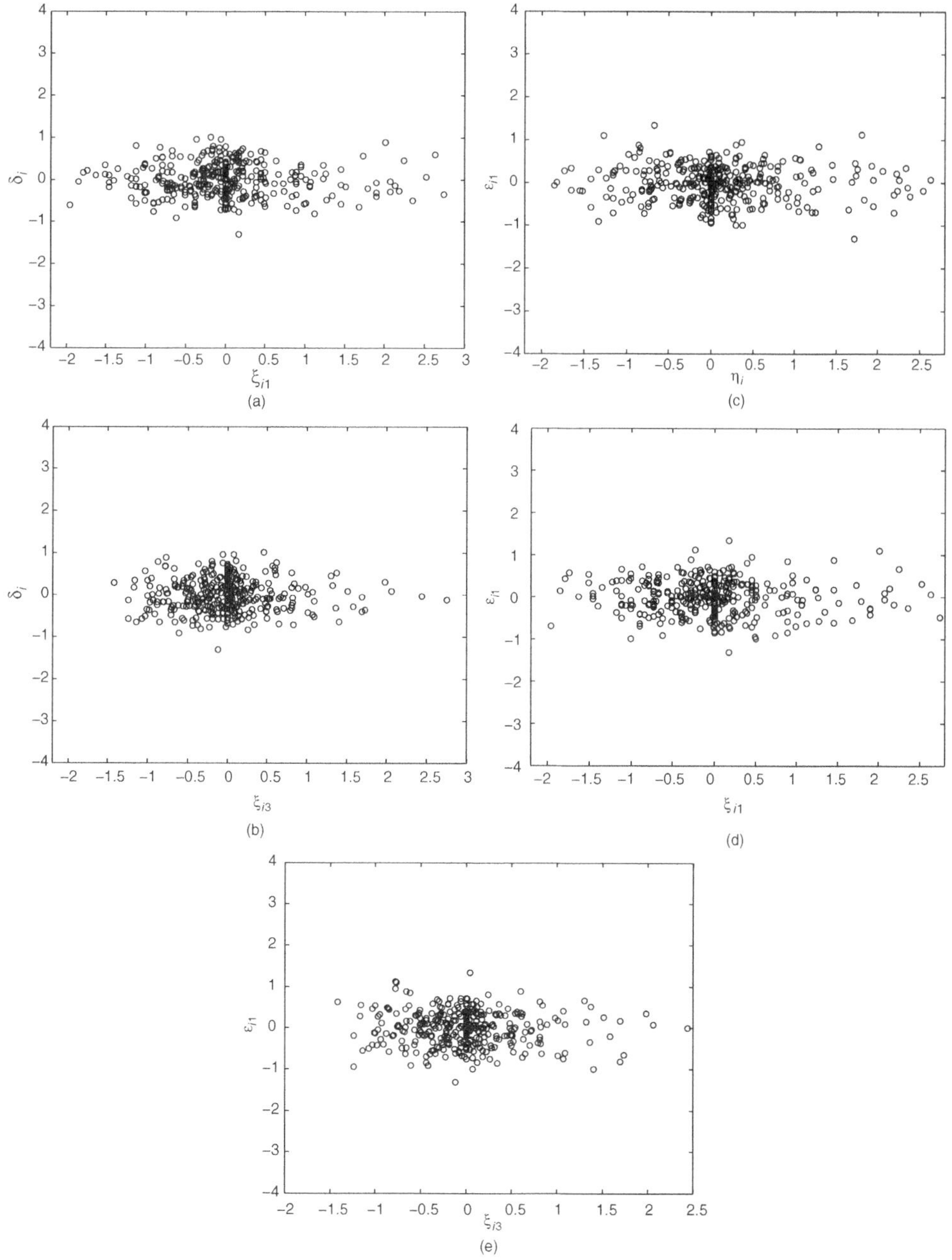

Figure 11.2 Plots of residuals $\hat{\delta}_i$ versus latent variables $\hat{\xi}_{i1}$ and $\hat{\xi}_{i3}$; and $\hat{\epsilon}_{i1}$ versus $\hat{\eta}_i$, $\hat{\xi}_{i1}$, and $\hat{\xi}_{i3}$.

as the model comparison statistic for the current semiparametric SEMs with unordered categorical variables. As this statistic can be obtained from the available outputs in the estimation, its computational burden is light.

11.3.1 Formulation of the semiparametric SEM

For completeness, we give a full description of the model. Consider a $p \times 1$ observed random vector $\mathbf{y}_i = (\mathbf{x}_i^T, \mathbf{u}_i^T)^T = (x_{i1}, \ldots, x_{ir}, u_{i,r+1}, \ldots, u_{ip})^T$, in which $\mathbf{x}_i$ contains continuous variables, and $\mathbf{u}_i$ contains unordered categorical variables. The observed continuous variables in $\mathbf{x}_i$ are related to a vector of correlated latent variables $\boldsymbol{\omega}_i^*$ and a vector of covariates $\mathbf{c}_i$ through the following confirmatory factor analysis model:

$$x_{ij} = \mathbf{A}_j^T \mathbf{c}_i + \boldsymbol{\Lambda}_j^T \boldsymbol{\omega}_i^* + \epsilon_{ij}, \quad j = 1, \ldots, r. \tag{11.10}$$

For $j = r+1, \ldots, p$, we also assume that u_{ij} is an observed unordered categorical variable which takes one and only one of the possible values $\{0, 1, \ldots, K_j - 1\}$. As before, u_{ij} is modeled through the $(K_j - 1) \times 1$ latent vector $\mathbf{v}_{ij} = (v_{ij,1}, \ldots, v_{ij,K_j-1})^T$ given by equation (11.1); and $\mathbf{v}_{ij}$ is modeled as

$$\mathbf{v}_{ij} = \mathbf{1}_{K_j-1} \mathbf{A}_j^T \mathbf{c}_i + \mathbf{1}_{K_j-1} \boldsymbol{\Lambda}_j^T \boldsymbol{\omega}_i^+ + \boldsymbol{\epsilon}_{ij}, \quad j = r+1, \ldots, p, \tag{11.11}$$

where $\mathbf{c}_i$ is a vector of covariates, $\mathbf{A}_j$ and $\boldsymbol{\Lambda}_j$ are vectors of parameters, $\boldsymbol{\omega}_i^+$ is a vector of the latent variables that are formed by unordered categorical observed variables, and $\boldsymbol{\epsilon}_{ij}$ is a vector of residual errors, which is distributed as $N[\mathbf{0}, \boldsymbol{\Psi}_j]$ and is independent of $\boldsymbol{\omega}_i^+$. To identify the unordered categorical variables, $\boldsymbol{\Psi}_j$ is fixed at $\mathbf{I}_{K_j-1}$. Define $\mathfrak{R}_{ik}$ as in (11.3). Then, for $i = 1, \ldots, n$ and $j = r+1, \ldots, p$,

$$\begin{aligned} p(u_{ij} = k|\mathbf{A}_j, \boldsymbol{\Lambda}_j, \boldsymbol{\omega}_i^+) &= p(\mathbf{v}_{ij} \in \mathfrak{R}_{ik}|\mathbf{A}_j, \boldsymbol{\Lambda}_j, \boldsymbol{\omega}_i^+) \\ &= \int_{\mathfrak{R}_{ik}} \phi_{K_j-1}\big(\mathbf{v}_{ij}|\mathbf{1}_{K_j-1}(\mathbf{A}_j^T \mathbf{c}_i + \boldsymbol{\Lambda}_j^T \boldsymbol{\omega}_i^+), \mathbf{I}_{K_j-1}\big) d\mathbf{v}_{ij} \\ &= \begin{cases} \left\{1 - \left[1 - \Phi^*(\mathbf{A}_j^T \mathbf{c}_i + \boldsymbol{\Lambda}_j^T \boldsymbol{\omega}_i^+)\right]^{K_j-1}\right\} / (K_j - 1) & \text{if } k \neq 0, \\ \left\{1 - \Phi^*(\mathbf{A}_j^T \mathbf{c}_i + \boldsymbol{\Lambda}_j^T \boldsymbol{\omega}_i^+)\right\}^{K_j-1} & \text{if } k = 0, \end{cases} \end{aligned} \tag{11.12}$$

where $\phi_{K_j-1}(\cdot)$ is the density function of the $(K_j - 1)$-variate normal distribution, and $\Phi^*(\cdot)$ is the distribution function of $N[0, 1]$.

Let $\mathbf{y}_i^* = (\mathbf{x}_i^T, \mathbf{v}_{i,r+1}^T, \ldots, \mathbf{v}_{ip}^T)^T$ be the vector of observed and unobserved continuous variables corresponding to $\mathbf{y}_i$. It follows from equations (11.10) and (11.11) that the measurement equation can be writen as

$$\mathbf{y}_i^* = \mathbf{E}\mathbf{A}\mathbf{c}_i + \mathbf{E}\boldsymbol{\Lambda}\boldsymbol{\omega}_i + \boldsymbol{\epsilon}_i, \tag{11.13}$$

where $\mathbf{E}$ and $\boldsymbol{\epsilon}_i$ are as defined in Section 11.2.1, $\boldsymbol{\omega}_i = (\boldsymbol{\omega}_i^{*T}, \boldsymbol{\omega}_i^{+T})^T$ is a $q \times 1$ vector of latent variables, and

$$\mathbf{A} = \begin{bmatrix} \mathbf{A}_1 & \cdots & \mathbf{A}_p \end{bmatrix}^T, \quad \boldsymbol{\Lambda} = \begin{bmatrix} \boldsymbol{\Lambda}_1 & \cdots & \boldsymbol{\Lambda}_r & \mathbf{0} & \cdots & \mathbf{0} \\ \mathbf{0} & \cdots & \mathbf{0} & \boldsymbol{\Lambda}_{r+1} & \cdots & \boldsymbol{\Lambda}_p \end{bmatrix}^T.$$

Let $\boldsymbol{\omega}_i = (\boldsymbol{\eta}_i^T, \boldsymbol{\xi}_i^T)^T$ be a partition of $\boldsymbol{\omega}_i$ with a vector $\boldsymbol{\eta}_i$ $(q_1 \times 1)$ of outcome latent variables and a vector $\boldsymbol{\xi}_i (q_2 \times 1)$ of explanatory latent variables. Note that $\boldsymbol{\eta}_i$ or $\boldsymbol{\xi}_i$ may involve latent variables in $\boldsymbol{\omega}_i^*$ and/or $\boldsymbol{\omega}_i^+$. The SEM introduced is defined by equation (11.13) and the structural equation

$$\boldsymbol{\eta}_i = \mathbf{B}\mathbf{d}_i + \boldsymbol{\Pi}\boldsymbol{\eta}_i + \boldsymbol{\Gamma}\boldsymbol{\xi}_i + \boldsymbol{\delta}_i, \tag{11.14}$$

where $\mathbf{B}$, $\boldsymbol{\Pi}$, and $\boldsymbol{\Gamma}$ are $q_1 \times m$, $q_1 \times q_1$, and $q_1 \times q_2$ matrices of unknown parameters; $\mathbf{d}_i(m \times 1)$ is a vector of covariates, and $\boldsymbol{\delta}_i(q_1 \times 1)$ is vector of errors that is independent of $\boldsymbol{\omega}_i$ and $\boldsymbol{\epsilon}_i$. Similarly to Chapter 10, we assume that $\boldsymbol{\epsilon}_{ix} = (\epsilon_{i1}, \ldots, \epsilon_{ir})^T$ and $\boldsymbol{\delta}_i$ are distributed as $N[\mathbf{0}, \boldsymbol{\Psi}_{\epsilon x}]$ and $N[\mathbf{0}, \boldsymbol{\Psi}_\delta]$, respectively. Hence, the covariance matrix of $\boldsymbol{\epsilon}_i$, $\boldsymbol{\Psi}_\epsilon$, is a diagonal block matrix, with the diagonal blocks equal to $\boldsymbol{\Psi}_{\epsilon x}$ and $\boldsymbol{\Psi}_j(=\mathbf{I}_{K_j-1})$, respectively. For convenience, we also assume that $\boldsymbol{\Psi}_{\epsilon x}$ and $\boldsymbol{\Psi}_\delta$ are diagonal, and $\boldsymbol{\Pi}_0 = \mathbf{I} - \boldsymbol{\Pi}$ is nonsingular with determinant independent of the elements of $\boldsymbol{\Pi}$.

11.3.2 Semiparametric hierarchical modeling via the Dirichlet process

In classical structural equation modeling, it is assumed that $\boldsymbol{\xi}_i$ follows a multivariate normal distribution. As mentioned in Chapter 10, applications of the standard parametric SEM where this assumption is violated would lead to biased results. For unordered categorical data, the problem could be more serious. Hence, it is desirable to consider a semiparametric approach to relax the basic normal assumption of $\boldsymbol{\xi}_i$.

Let $\boldsymbol{\theta}$ be the vector of unknown parameters involved in equations (11.13) and (11.14). The Bayesian semiparametric model can be reformulated as follows (Song *et al.*, 2009): for $i = 1, \ldots, n$,

$$\begin{aligned}
&[\mathbf{y}_i^*|\boldsymbol{\eta}_i, \boldsymbol{\xi}_i, \boldsymbol{\theta}] \stackrel{D}{=} N[\mathbf{E}\mathbf{A}\mathbf{c}_i + \mathbf{E}\boldsymbol{\Lambda}\boldsymbol{\omega}_i, \boldsymbol{\Psi}_\epsilon],\\
&[\boldsymbol{\eta}_i|\boldsymbol{\xi}_i, \boldsymbol{\theta}] \stackrel{D}{=} N[\boldsymbol{\Pi}_0^{-1}(\mathbf{B}\mathbf{d}_i + \boldsymbol{\Gamma}\boldsymbol{\xi}_i), \boldsymbol{\Pi}_0^{-1}\boldsymbol{\Psi}_\delta\boldsymbol{\Pi}_0^{-T}],\\
&\boldsymbol{\theta} \stackrel{D}{=} p(\boldsymbol{\theta}), \quad [\boldsymbol{\xi}_i|P] \stackrel{D}{=} P, \quad P \stackrel{D}{=} \mathcal{P}(\cdot),
\end{aligned} \tag{11.15}$$

where $p(\boldsymbol{\theta})$ is the prior distribution of $\boldsymbol{\theta}$, and $\mathcal{P}(\cdot)$ is a random probability measure. An important issue is the specification of the prior of P. Among various random probability measures that approximate the general DP, Ishwaran and James (2001) proposed the following truncated DP with stick-breaking priors (see also Chapter 10):

$$[\boldsymbol{\xi}_i|P] \stackrel{D}{=} P, \quad P \stackrel{D}{=} \mathcal{P}_G(\cdot) = \sum_{k=1}^{G} \pi_k \delta_{\mathbf{Z}_k}(\cdot), \tag{11.16}$$

where $\delta_{\mathbf{Z}_k}(\cdot)$ denotes a discrete probability measure concentrated at $\mathbf{Z}_k$, $\boldsymbol{\pi} = \{\pi_k, \ k = 1, \ldots, G\}$ is a random vector chosen to be independent of $\mathbf{Z}_k$, and

$$\begin{aligned}
\pi_1 &= V_1,\\
\pi_k &= (1 - V_1)\ldots(1 - V_{k-1})V_k, \quad k = 2, \ldots, G-1,\\
\pi_G &= (1 - V_1)\ldots(1 - V_{G-1}),
\end{aligned} \tag{11.17}$$

such that $0 \le \pi_k \le 1$ and $\sum_{k=1}^G \pi_k = 1$. Following Sethuraman (1994), V_k can be taken as independent Beta$[1, \alpha]$, where $\alpha > 0$ is a hyperparameter. Moreover, the $\mathbf{Z}_k$ are assumed to be i.i.d. $N[\boldsymbol{\mu}_z, \boldsymbol{\Sigma}_z]$. Although the above truncated DP with stick-breaking priors works well for Bayesian semiparametric SEMs with continuous variables, it cannot be directly applied to our model with unordered categorical variable because the location of P will affect the probability of the unordered categorical variables (see below).

Let $\boldsymbol{\Lambda}_\eta$ and $\boldsymbol{\Lambda}_\xi$ be the submatrices of $\boldsymbol{\Lambda}$ which contain q_1 and q_2 columns of $\boldsymbol{\Lambda}$ corresponding to $\boldsymbol{\eta}_i$ and $\boldsymbol{\xi}_i$, respectively. It follows from equations (11.13) and (11.14) that

$$p(\mathbf{y}_i^*|\boldsymbol{\theta}, P) = \int p(\mathbf{y}_i^*|\boldsymbol{\eta}_i, \boldsymbol{\xi}_i, \boldsymbol{\theta})p(\boldsymbol{\eta}_i|\boldsymbol{\xi}_i, \boldsymbol{\theta})P(d\boldsymbol{\xi}_i)d\boldsymbol{\eta}_i, \tag{11.18}$$

and its mean vector is given by

$$\boldsymbol{\mu}_{\mathbf{y}_i^*|\theta,P} = \mathbf{EAc}_i + \mathbf{E}\boldsymbol{\Lambda}_\eta\boldsymbol{\Pi}_0^{-1}\mathbf{Bd}_i + (\mathbf{E}\boldsymbol{\Lambda}_\eta\boldsymbol{\Pi}_0^{-1}\boldsymbol{\Gamma} + \mathbf{E}\boldsymbol{\Lambda}_\xi)\int \boldsymbol{\xi}_i P(d\boldsymbol{\xi}_i).$$

Based on (11.3) and (11.12), in modeling the unordered categorical variable u_{ij} through $\mathbf{v}_{ij}$ in $\mathbf{y}_i^*$, we require $\boldsymbol{\mu}_P = \int \boldsymbol{\xi}_i P(d\boldsymbol{\xi}_i) = \mathbf{0}$ with probability 1. That is, the random probability measure P in relation to semiparametric modeling of $\boldsymbol{\xi}_i$ is not arbitrary, and it is necessary to construct an appropriate P whose location is centered at zero. However, the truncated DP with stick-breaking priors in (11.16) and (11.17) is defined on an arbitrary P. Hence, it is not appropriate because the location of the random probability measure is not centered at zero. To solve this problem, a modified approach is given below.

In line with the reasoning provided in Appendix 11.3, we use the following modified truncated DP for modeling $\boldsymbol{\xi}_i$:

$$\xi_{il}|P_l \stackrel{D}{=} P_l, \quad l = 1, \ldots, q_2,$$
$$P_l \stackrel{D}{=} \frac{1}{2}\sum_{k=1}^{G} \pi_{kl}\delta_{Z_{kl}}(\cdot) + \frac{1}{2}\sum_{k=G+1}^{2G} \pi_{kl}\delta_{Z_{kl}}(\cdot), \tag{11.19}$$

in which $\mathbf{Z}_l^- = (Z_{1l}, \ldots, Z_{Gl})^T$ and $\mathbf{Z}_l^+ = (Z_{G+1,l}, \ldots, Z_{2G,l})^T$ are independent of the following distributions:

$$Z_{kl} \stackrel{D}{=} N[\mu_{zl}, \sigma_{zl}]I(Z_{kl} \leq 0), \quad k = 1, \ldots, G,$$
$$Z_{kl} \stackrel{D}{=} N[\mu_{zl}, \sigma_{zl}]I(Z_{kl} > 0), \quad k = G+1, \ldots, 2G, \tag{11.20}$$

in which $I(\cdot)$ denotes the indicator function. The random weights $\boldsymbol{\pi}_l^- = (\pi_{1l}, \ldots, \pi_{Gl})^T$ and $\boldsymbol{\pi}_l^+ = (\pi_{G+1,l}, \ldots, \pi_{2G,l})^T$ are independent, and both are constructed with a slight modification of the stick-breaking priors in (11.17). That is, for $\boldsymbol{\pi}_l^-$,

$$\pi_{1l} = V_{1l},$$
$$\pi_{kl} = (1 - V_{1l}) \ldots (1 - V_{k-1,l})V_{kl}, \quad k = 2, \ldots, G-1,$$
$$\pi_{Gl} = (1 - V_{1l}) \ldots (1 - V_{G-1,l}), \tag{11.21}$$

where V_{kl} are independently distributed as Beta$(1, \alpha_l M_l^-)$ with $\alpha_l > 0$ and $M_l^- = 1 - \Phi^*(\mu_{zl} / \sqrt{\sigma_{zl}})$; for $\boldsymbol{\pi}_l^+$,

$$\pi_{G+1,l} = U_{1l},$$
$$\pi_{G+k,l} = (1 - U_{1l}) \ldots (1 - U_{k-1,l})U_{kl}, \quad k = 2, \ldots, G-1,$$
$$\pi_{2G,l} = (1 - U_{1l}) \ldots (1 - U_{G-1,l}), \tag{11.22}$$

where U_{kl} are independent Beta$(1, \alpha_l M_l^+)$ random variables with $M_l^+ = \Phi^*(\mu_{zl}/\sqrt{\sigma_{zl}})$.

The theoretical justification for using above modified truncated DP and sticking-breaking priors in modeling $\boldsymbol{\xi}_i$ is given in Appendix 11.3. The empirical performance is examined by the simulation study in Section 11.3.4.

11.3.3 Estimation and model comparison

Let $\mathbf{Z}_l = (Z_{1l}, \ldots, Z_{2G,l})^T$, $\mathbf{Z} = (\mathbf{Z}_1, \ldots, \mathbf{Z}_{q_2})$, $\boldsymbol{\pi}_l = (\pi_{1l}, \ldots, \pi_{2G,l})^T$, and $\boldsymbol{\pi} = (\boldsymbol{\pi}_1, \ldots, \boldsymbol{\pi}_{q_2})$. The key character of the blocked Gibbs sampler is to recast the model completely by introducing cluster variables. Let $\mathbf{L} = (\mathbf{L}^1, \ldots, \mathbf{L}^{q_2})$ with $\mathbf{L}^l = (L_1^l, \ldots, L_n^l)^T$, such that $\xi_{il} = Z_{L_i^l,l}$; then (11.15) and (11.19) can be rewritten as

$$[\mathbf{y}_i^* | \boldsymbol{\eta}_i, \mathbf{Z}, \mathbf{L}, \boldsymbol{\theta}] \stackrel{D}{=} N[\mathbf{E}\mathbf{A}\mathbf{c}_i + \mathbf{E}\boldsymbol{\Lambda}\boldsymbol{\omega}_i, \boldsymbol{\Psi}_\epsilon],$$

$$[\boldsymbol{\eta}_i | \mathbf{Z}, \mathbf{L}, \boldsymbol{\theta}] \stackrel{D}{=} N[\boldsymbol{\Pi}_0^{-1}\mathbf{B}\mathbf{d}_i + \boldsymbol{\Pi}_0^{-1}\boldsymbol{\Gamma}\boldsymbol{\xi}_i, \boldsymbol{\Pi}_0^{-1}\boldsymbol{\Psi}_\delta\boldsymbol{\Pi}_0^{-T}],$$

$$[L_i^l | \boldsymbol{\pi}] \stackrel{D}{=} \frac{1}{2}\sum_{k=1}^{G} \pi_{kl}\delta_k(\cdot) + \frac{1}{2}\sum_{k=G+1}^{2G} \pi_{kl}\delta_k(\cdot), \quad l = 1, \ldots, q_2,$$

$$(\boldsymbol{\pi}, \mathbf{Z}) \stackrel{D}{=} p(\boldsymbol{\pi})p(\mathbf{Z}), \quad \text{and} \quad \boldsymbol{\theta} \stackrel{D}{=} p(\boldsymbol{\theta}), \tag{11.23}$$

where $\boldsymbol{\omega}_i = (\boldsymbol{\eta}_i^T, \boldsymbol{\xi}_i^T)^T$ with $\xi_{il} = Z_{L_i^l,l}$, and $p(\boldsymbol{\pi})$ and $p(\mathbf{Z})$ are prior densities of $\boldsymbol{\pi}$ and $\mathbf{Z}$, respectively. Let $\boldsymbol{\Lambda}_y = (\mathbf{A}, \boldsymbol{\Lambda})$, $\boldsymbol{\Lambda}_\omega = (\mathbf{B}, \boldsymbol{\Pi}, \boldsymbol{\Gamma})$, $\boldsymbol{\Psi}_{\epsilon x} = \text{diag}(\psi_{\epsilon x1}, \ldots, \psi_{\epsilon xr})$, and $\boldsymbol{\Psi}_\delta = \text{diag}(\psi_{\delta 1}, \ldots, \psi_{\delta q_1})$. Let $\boldsymbol{\Lambda}_{yj}^T$ and $\boldsymbol{\Lambda}_{\omega j}^T$ be the jth rows of $\boldsymbol{\Lambda}_y$ and $\boldsymbol{\Lambda}_\omega$, respectively. For convenience, we assume that $p(\boldsymbol{\Lambda}_y, \boldsymbol{\Psi}_\epsilon) = \{\prod_{j=1}^r p(\boldsymbol{\Lambda}_{yj}|\psi_{\epsilon xj})p(\psi_{\epsilon xj})\}\prod_{j=r+1}^p p(\boldsymbol{\Lambda}_{yj})$ and $p(\boldsymbol{\Lambda}_\omega, \boldsymbol{\Psi}_\delta) = \prod_{j=1}^{q_1} p(\boldsymbol{\Lambda}_{\omega j}|\psi_{\delta j})p(\psi_{\delta j})$. The following conjugate type prior distributions for the components of $\boldsymbol{\theta}$ are used:

$$\boldsymbol{\Lambda}_{yj} \stackrel{D}{=} N[\boldsymbol{\Lambda}_{0yj}, \mathbf{H}_{0yj}], \quad j = r+1, \ldots, p,$$

$$[\boldsymbol{\Lambda}_{yj}|\psi_{\epsilon xj}] \stackrel{D}{=} N[\boldsymbol{\Lambda}_{0yj}, \psi_{\epsilon xj}\mathbf{H}_{0yj}], \ \psi_{\epsilon xj}^{-1} \stackrel{D}{=} \text{Gamma}[\alpha_{0\epsilon j}, \beta_{0\epsilon j}], \quad j = 1, \ldots, r,$$

$$[\boldsymbol{\Lambda}_{\omega j}|\psi_{\delta j}] \stackrel{D}{=} N[\boldsymbol{\Lambda}_{0\omega j}, \psi_{\delta j}\mathbf{H}_{0\omega j}], \ \psi_{\delta j}^{-1} \stackrel{D}{=} \text{Gamma}[\alpha_{0\delta j}, \beta_{0\delta j}], \quad j = 1, \ldots, q_1. \tag{11.24}$$

where $\boldsymbol{\Lambda}_{0yj}$, $\alpha_{0\epsilon j}$, $\beta_{0\epsilon j}$, $\boldsymbol{\Lambda}_{0\omega j}$, $\alpha_{0\delta j}$, $\beta_{0\delta j}$, and the positive definite matrices $\mathbf{H}_{0yj}$ and $\mathbf{H}_{0\omega j}$ are hyperparameters. Let $\boldsymbol{\mu}_z = (\mu_{z1}, \ldots, \mu_{zq_2})^T$, $\boldsymbol{\Sigma}_z = \text{diag}\{\sigma_{z1}, \ldots, \sigma_{zq_2}\}$, $\boldsymbol{\alpha} = (\alpha_1, \ldots, \alpha_{q_2})^T$, and $\boldsymbol{\beta} = (\boldsymbol{\alpha}, \boldsymbol{\mu}_z, \boldsymbol{\Sigma}_z)$. Here, the parameters in $\boldsymbol{\beta}$ are involved in the nonparametric component. The following conjugate prior distributions for these parameters are used: for $l = 1, \ldots, q_2$,

$$[\mu_{zl}|\sigma_M] \stackrel{D}{=} N[0, \sigma_M], \quad [\sigma_{zl}^{-1}|\rho_1, \rho_2] \stackrel{D}{=} \text{Gamma}[\rho_1, \rho_2],$$

$$[\alpha_l|\tau_1, \tau_2] \stackrel{D}{=} \text{Gamma}[\tau_1, \tau_2], \tag{11.25}$$

where σ_M, ρ_1, ρ_2, τ_1, and τ_2 are hyperparameters.

To accommodate missing data, we let $\mathbf{x}_i = (\mathbf{x}_{i,\text{obs}}, \mathbf{x}_{i,\text{mis}})$ and $\mathbf{u}_i = (\mathbf{u}_{i,\text{obs}}, \mathbf{u}_{i,\text{mis}})$, where $\mathbf{x}_{i,\text{obs}}$ and $\mathbf{u}_{i,\text{obs}}$ are observed, while $\mathbf{x}_{i,\text{mis}}$ and $\mathbf{u}_{i,\text{mis}}$ are missing. For brevity, we assume that the missing data are missing at random. Let $\mathbf{X}_{\text{obs}} = \{\mathbf{x}_{1,\text{obs}}, \ldots, \mathbf{x}_{n,\text{obs}}\}$, $\mathbf{X}_{\text{mis}} = \{\mathbf{x}_{1,\text{mis}}, \ldots, \mathbf{x}_{n,\text{mis}}\}$, $\mathbf{U}_{\text{obs}} = \{\mathbf{u}_{1,\text{obs}}, \ldots, \mathbf{u}_{n,\text{obs}}\}$, $\mathbf{U}_{\text{mis}} = \{\mathbf{u}_{1,\text{mis}}, \ldots, \mathbf{u}_{n,\text{mis}}\}$, $\boldsymbol{\Omega} = \{\boldsymbol{\omega}_1, \ldots, \boldsymbol{\omega}_n\}$, and $\boldsymbol{\Omega}_1 = \{\boldsymbol{\eta}_1, \ldots, \boldsymbol{\eta}_n\}$. Further, let $\mathbf{V}_{\text{obs}}$ and $\mathbf{V}_{\text{mis}}$ include the $\mathbf{v}_{ij}$ that correspond to $\mathbf{U}_{\text{obs}}$ and $\mathbf{U}_{\text{mis}}$, respectively. The observed data $\{\mathbf{X}_{\text{obs}}, \mathbf{U}_{\text{obs}}\}$ are augmented with the missing quantities $\{\mathbf{X}_{\text{mis}}, \mathbf{V}_{\text{obs}}, \mathbf{V}_{\text{mis}}, \boldsymbol{\Omega}_1, \boldsymbol{\pi}, \mathbf{Z}, \mathbf{L}\}$ in the posterior analysis. A sequence of random observations will be generated from the joint posterior distribution $p(\mathbf{X}_{\text{mis}}, \mathbf{V}_{\text{obs}}, \mathbf{V}_{\text{mis}}, \boldsymbol{\Omega}_1, \boldsymbol{\theta}, \boldsymbol{\pi}, \mathbf{Z}, \mathbf{L}, \boldsymbol{\beta}|\mathbf{X}_{\text{obs}}, \mathbf{U}_{\text{obs}})$ through the blocked Gibbs sampler (Ishwaran and James, 2001) coupled with the MH algorithm. Some new conditional distributions involved in the blocked Gibbs sampler, together with implementation of the MH algorithm, are provided in Appendix 11.4.

Similar to the application relating to semiparametric SEM (see Chapter 10), the computation of the Bayes factor with path sampling involves an approximation of a huge-dimensional integral over $\boldsymbol{\Omega}$. Hence, path sampling cannot give accurate results for the current model. Inspired by the predictive approach for model selection and its applications to various data structures (Ibrahim *et al.*, 2001), we consider the L_ν-measure (see also Section 4.3.3), which is based on the future values of a replicate experiment and the idea that good models should give good predictions close to what has been observed. Let $\mathbf{Y}_{\text{obs}}^{\text{rep}} = (\mathbf{y}_{1,\text{obs}}^{\text{rep}}, \ldots, \mathbf{y}_{n,\text{obs}}^{\text{rep}})$ be a future response vector of a replicate experiment with the same sampling density as $p(\mathbf{Y}_{\text{obs}}|\boldsymbol{\theta})$ with $\mathbf{Y}_{\text{obs}} = \{\mathbf{X}_{\text{obs}}, \mathbf{U}_{\text{obs}}\}$. We first consider, for some $\delta \geq 0$,

$$L_1(\mathbf{Y}_{\text{obs}}, \mathbf{B}_{\text{obs}}, \delta) = E\big[\text{tr}\big(\mathbf{Y}_{\text{obs}}^{\text{rep}} - \mathbf{B}_{\text{obs}}\big)^T\big(\mathbf{Y}_{\text{obs}}^{\text{rep}} - \mathbf{B}_{\text{obs}}\big)\big] + \delta\text{tr}(\mathbf{Y}_{\text{obs}} - \mathbf{B}_{\text{obs}}), \tag{11.26}$$

where the expectation is taken with respect to the posterior predictive distribution of $p(\mathbf{Y}_{\text{obs}}^{\text{rep}}|\mathbf{Y}_{\text{obs}})$. Note that this statistic can be regarded as a multivariate version of the model assessment criterion considered by Ibrahim *et al.* (2001) for analyzing generalized linear models and survival models. By selecting $\mathbf{B}_{\text{obs}}$ as the minimizer of (11.26), it can be shown that, for some $0 \leq \nu < 1$, we have the following multivariate version of the L_ν-measure:

$$L_\nu(\mathbf{Y}_{\text{obs}}) = \sum_{i=1}^{n} \text{tr}\big\{\text{Cov}\big(\mathbf{y}_{i,\text{obs}}^{\text{rep}}|\mathbf{Y}_{\text{obs}}\big)\big\} + \nu \sum_{i=1}^{n} \text{tr}\big[\big\{E\big(\mathbf{y}_{i,\text{obs}}^{\text{rep}}|\mathbf{Y}_{\text{obs}}\big) - \mathbf{y}_{i,\text{obs}}\big\}$$
$$\big\{E\big(\mathbf{y}_{i,\text{obs}}^{\text{rep}}|\mathbf{Y}_{\text{obs}}\big) - \mathbf{y}_{i,\text{obs}}\big\}^T\big], \tag{11.27}$$

where $\nu = \delta/(\delta + 1)$. This statistic is a sum of two components. The first component relates to the variability of the prediction, while the second component measures how close its predictions are to the observed data. Clearly, a small value of the L_ν-measure indicates that the corresponding model gives predictions close to the observed values, and that the variability of the predictions is low. Hence, the model with the smallest L_ν-measure is selected from a collection of competing models. In our empirical illustrations, we choose the common value $\nu = 0.5$.

In applying the L_ν-measure for model assessment and model selection for the semiparametric SEM, we have to evaluate $\text{Cov}(\mathbf{y}_{i,\text{obs}}^{\text{rep}}|\mathbf{Y}_{\text{obs}})$ and $E(\mathbf{y}_{i,\text{obs}}^{\text{rep}}|\mathbf{Y}_{\text{obs}})$, which involve intractable multiple integrals. These integrals can be approximated by the corresponding ergodic averages of MCMC samples, $\{\mathbf{X}_{\text{mis}}^{(t)}, \mathbf{V}_{\text{obs}}^{(t)}, \mathbf{V}_{\text{mis}}^{(t)}, \boldsymbol{\Omega}_1^{(t)}, \boldsymbol{\theta}^{(t)}, \boldsymbol{\pi}^{(t)}, \mathbf{Z}^{(t)}, \mathbf{L}^{(t)}, \boldsymbol{\beta}^{(t)}, t = 1, \ldots, T\}$, which are generated using the blocked Gibbs sampler coupled with the MH algorithm in the estimation. Hence, the computational burden of $L_\nu(\mathbf{Y}_{\text{obs}})$ is light.

11.3.4 Simulation study

We conducted a simulation study to roughly reveal the performance of the Bayesian semiparametric approach in estimation and model selection, and to compare it with the parametric approach. We consider a situation with six continuous variables and three unordered categorical variables which take one and only one value in {0, 1, 2}. The measurement equation of the true model is given by

$$x_{ij} = a_j c_i + \mathbf{\Lambda}_j^T \boldsymbol{\omega}_i^* + \epsilon_{ij}, \quad j = 1, \ldots, 6,$$

$$v_{ij,l} = a_j c_i + \mathbf{\Lambda}_j^T \boldsymbol{\omega}_i^+ + \epsilon_{ij,l}, \quad j = 7, 8, 9, \; l = 1, 2. \tag{11.28}$$

The covariate c_i is generated from the standard normal distribution. The specifications of $\mathbf{A}$ and $\mathbf{\Lambda}$ in equation (11.13) and their true parameter values are given by:

$$\mathbf{A}^T = \begin{bmatrix} 0.7 & 0.7 & 0.7 & 0.7 & 0.7 & 0.7 & 0.7 & 0.7 & 0.7 \end{bmatrix},$$

$$\mathbf{\Lambda}^T = \begin{bmatrix} 1 & 0.8 & 0.8 & 0 & 0 & 0 & 0 & 0 & 0 \\ 0 & 0 & 0 & 1 & 0.8 & 0.8 & 0 & 0 & 0 \\ 0 & 0 & 0 & 0 & 0 & 0 & 1 & 0.8 & 0.8 \end{bmatrix},$$

where the 1s and 0s in $\mathbf{\Lambda}$ are treated as fixed in order to identify the model. For $j = 1, \ldots, 6$, the true value of $\psi_{\epsilon xj}$ is 1.0. Let $\boldsymbol{\omega}_i = (\eta_i, \xi_{i1}, \xi_{i2})^T$. The structural equation of the true model is

$$\eta_i = bd_i + \gamma_1 \xi_{i1} + \gamma_2 \xi_{i2} + \delta_i, \tag{11.29}$$

where the covariate d_i is generated from a Bernoulli distribution that takes 1 with probability 0.7 and 0 with probability 0.3. The true values of the parameters involved in equation (11.28) are $b = 1.0$, $(\gamma_1, \gamma_2) = (0.5, 0.7)$, and $\psi_\delta = 1.0$.

A simulation study with various nonnormal distributions of $\boldsymbol{\xi}_i$ was conducted. As the results are similar, we only present details obtained under the following two true distributions of $\boldsymbol{\xi}_i$: (I) $\boldsymbol{\xi}_i$ is drawn from the mixture of normal distributions $0.5N[\boldsymbol{\mu}_1, \mathbf{\Phi}_1] + 0.5N[\boldsymbol{\mu}_2, \mathbf{\Phi}_2]$, where $\boldsymbol{\mu}_1 = (-2.0, 1.5)^T$, $\boldsymbol{\mu}_2 = (2.0, -1.5)^T$, and $\mathbf{\Phi}_1 = \mathbf{\Phi}_2 = \mathbf{I}_2$; and (II) ξ_{ij} are independently drawn from $\sum_{l=0}^{7} N[3\{(2/3)^l - 1\} + 1.919, (2/3)^{2l}]/8$ for $j = 1, 2$. Hence, the true distributions of $\boldsymbol{\xi}_i$ under (I) and (II) are bimodal and skewed, respectively. Based on these settings, random samples with $n = 800$ are generated.

In this simulation study, $G = 50$ is taken in the modified truncated DP. Prior inputs for the hyperparameters in the prior distributions relating to the parameters involved in the nonparametric component (see (11.25)) are $\sigma_M = 100$, $\rho_1 = \rho_2 = 0.01$, and $\tau_1 = \tau_2 = 2.0$; while prior inputs in the prior distributions corresponding to the parameters involved in the parametric component (see (11.24)) are $\alpha_{0\epsilon j} = \alpha_{0\delta j} = 9$, $\beta_{0\epsilon j} = \beta_{0\delta j} = 8$, $\mathbf{H}_{0yj}$ and $\mathbf{H}_{0\omega j}$ are diagonal matrices with the diagonal elements 1.0, and elements in $\{\mathbf{\Lambda}_{0yj}, \mathbf{\Lambda}_{0\omega j}\}$ are equal to the true values. A few test runs revealed that the blocked Gibbs sampler converged within 2000 iterations. Here, 2000 observations were collected after 3000 burn-in iterations in computing the absolute bias (Bias) and root mean squares (RMS) of the estimates and the true values in 100 replications. Results obtained using the modified truncated DP (MTDP) with stick-breaking priors, and a parametric approach based on the assumption that $\boldsymbol{\xi}_i$ is distributed as normal, are reported in Table 11.1. It can be seen that the results obtained through the MTDP are reasonably accurate with small bias and RMS values; and that estimates of some parameters (e.g. a_7, a_8, a_9, γ_2, and ψ_δ) associated with the unordered categorical variables obtained through the parametric model are not accurate with large bias and RMS values. Plots of the estimated densities of $\{\xi_{i1}, \xi_{i2}\}$ under (I) and (II) obtained from MTDP based on 100 replications are displayed in (I1), (I2), (II1), and (II2) of Figure 11.3, respectively. Note that the estimated density of ξ_{i2} associated with the unordered categorical observed variables is

Table 11.1 Performance of the semiparametric and parametric Bayesian estimates.

	$\xi_i \stackrel{D}{=}$ MTDP				$\xi_i \stackrel{D}{=}$ Normal			
	(I)		(II)		(I)		(II)	
Parameter	Bias	RMS	Bias	RMS	Bias	RMS	Bias	RMS
$a_1 = 0.7$	0.008	0.056	−0.008	0.058	0.013	0.057	0.010	0.059
$a_2 = 0.7$	0.001	0.044	0.003	0.046	0.005	0.044	0.000	0.048
$a_3 = 0.7$	0.006	0.048	−0.005	0.049	0.010	0.049	0.002	0.051
$a_4 = 0.7$	−0.008	0.085	0.001	0.042	−0.015	0.083	0.000	0.040
$a_5 = 0.7$	−0.004	0.075	−0.002	0.038	−0.010	0.073	−0.001	0.045
$a_6 = 0.7$	−0.007	0.076	−0.003	0.041	−0.012	0.075	−0.006	0.044
$a_7 = 0.7$	−0.019	0.105	0.009	0.073	**−0.307**	**0.313**	**−0.182**	**0.186**
$a_8 = 0.7$	0.005	0.090	0.014	0.068	**−0.283**	**0.287**	**−0.205**	**0.209**
$a_9 = 0.7$	0.011	0.093	0.003	0.060	**−0.258**	**0.263**	**−0.185**	**0.190**
$\lambda_{21} = 0.8$	0.002	0.031	0.004	0.039	0.005	0.031	0.000	0.035
$\lambda_{31} = 0.8$	0.003	0.035	0.007	0.036	0.006	0.036	−0.002	0.038
$\lambda_{52} = 0.8$	0.004	0.019	0.009	0.056	0.004	0.020	0.027	0.073
$\lambda_{62} = 0.8$	0.002	0.021	0.012	0.056	0.001	0.021	0.013	0.066
$\lambda_{83} = 0.8$	0.029	0.102	0.057	0.139	0.072	0.093	0.015	0.076
$\lambda_{93} = 0.8$	0.025	0.093	0.030	0.131	0.097	0.111	0.026	0.087
$\psi_{\epsilon x1} = 1.0$	−0.003	0.069	0.000	0.072	0.003	0.071	0.002	0.076
$\psi_{\epsilon x2} = 1.0$	0.002	0.064	−0.020	0.069	0.001	0.063	−0.005	0.067
$\psi_{\epsilon x3} = 1.0$	−0.009	0.063	0.003	0.066	−0.010	0.063	−0.004	0.065
$\psi_{\epsilon x4} = 1.0$	−0.009	0.077	0.021	0.085	−0.012	0.078	0.009	0.086
$\psi_{\epsilon x5} = 1.0$	0.008	0.065	0.002	0.061	0.008	0.066	−0.016	0.078
$\psi_{\epsilon x6} = 1.0$	−0.004	0.065	0.004	0.066	−0.003	0.065	−0.006	0.069
$b_1 = 1.0$	0.001	0.054	−0.000	0.072	0.053	0.076	0.064	0.089
$\gamma_1 = 0.5$	0.070	0.090	0.015	0.059	−0.087	0.097	0.012	0.076
$\gamma_2 = 0.7$	0.051	0.119	0.044	0.141	**0.204**	**0.231**	**0.466**	**0.502**
$\psi_\delta = 1.0$	−0.068	0.128	0.001	0.090	**0.176**	**0.207**	0.045	0.129

not as close to the true density as that corresponding to ξ_{i1} associated with the continuous observed variables. The corresponding plots obtained under the parametric approach revealed that the estimated densities of ξ_{i1} and ξ_{i2} are not close to the true densities. Plots obtained from the inferior parametric approach are not provided here.

We use the following competing models to illustrate the performance of the $L_{0.5}$-measure in model selection:

M_1: the above model with measurement equation (11.28) and structural equation (11.29);
M_2: measurement equation (11.28) and $\eta_i = \gamma_1\xi_{i1} + \gamma_2\xi_{i2} + \delta_i$;
M_3: $x_{ij} = \boldsymbol{\Lambda}_j^T\boldsymbol{\omega}_i^* + \epsilon_{ij}$, $j = 1, \ldots, 6$, and $v_{ij,l} = \boldsymbol{\Lambda}_j^T\boldsymbol{\omega}_i^+ + \epsilon_{ij,l}$, $j = 7, 8, 9$, $l = 1, 2$, with the structural equation $\eta_i = \gamma_1\xi_{i1} + \gamma_2\xi_{i2} + \delta_i$.

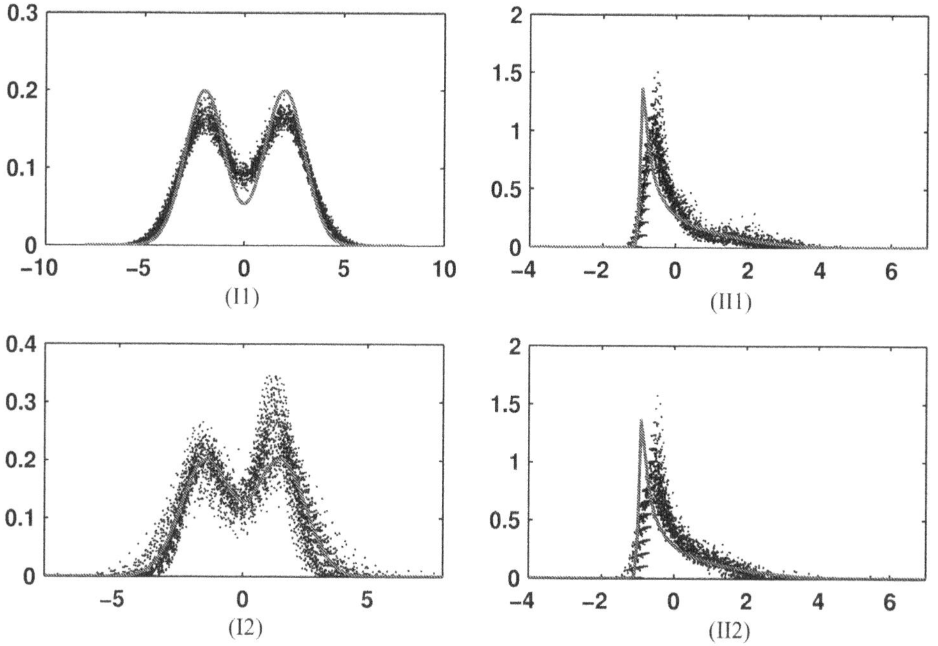

Figure 11.3 True densities (solid lines), and estimated densities via MTDP in 100 replications.

For each of the 100 replications, observations obtained through the blocked Gibbs sampler are used to compute $L_{0.5}$-measures (see equation (11.27)) for M_1, M_2, and M_3. The $L_{0.5}$-measure selects the true model if its value for M_1 is the smallest. Under (I), with a bimodal distribution of ξ_i, it correctly selected M_1 in 84 replications, and incorrectly selected M_2 and M_3 in the other 7 and 9 replications, respectively. Under (II) with a skewed distribution of ξ_i, it correctly selected M_1 in all replications. The means and standard deviations of the $L_{0.5}$-measures obtained from the 100 replications are presented in Table 11.2. Additional simulation studies with smaller sample sizes show that larger sample sizes lead to better performance.

11.3.5 Real example: Diabetic nephropathy study

We illustrate the methodology with an application to a study of diabetic kidney disease (see Section 11.2.2). In this application, several observed phenotype and genotype variables were

Table 11.2 Mean and standard deviation (SD) of $L_{0.5}$-measures in 100 replications.

	Model	Mean	SD		Model	Mean	SD
	M_1	10 930	229		M_1	9470	183
(I)	M_2	11 570	311	(II)	M_2	9490	197
	M_3	11 500	341		M_3	9810	175

selected. Two observed continuous phenotype variables, log urinary albumin creatinine ratio (lnACR) and log plasma creatinine (lnPCr), were used to form the outcome latent variable for diabetic kidney disease. Based on a preliminary data analysis, and motivated by medical findings, phenotype and genotype observed variables were selected to form the explanatory latent variables that are expected to have substantial effects on diabetic kidney disease. In particular, the following explanatory latent variables are considered: (i) 'lipid control' via the continuous phenotype observed variables non-high-density lipoprotein cholesterol (non-HDL-C), lower-density lipoprotein cholesterol (LDL-C), and log plasma triglyceride (lnTG); (ii) 'glycemic control' via the continuous phenotype observed variables fasting plasma glucose (FPG) and glycated hemoglobin (HbA1c); (iii) 'β adrenergic receptor' via the genotype variables beta-2 adrenergic receptor SNP1 (ADRβ21), beta-2 adrenergic receptor SNP2 (ADRβ22), and beta-3 adrenergic receptor (ADRβ3); and (iv) 'plasminogen activator inhibitor' via the genotype variables tumor necrosis factor beta (LTA2), plasminogen activator inhibitor1 SNP1 (PAI11), and plasminogen activator inhibitor1 SNP2 (PAI12). Note that the genotype variables are unordered categorical. These phenotype and genotype observed variables are grouped into their corresponding latent variables through the measurement equation. Then the outcome latent variable of diabetic kidney disease is regressed on the explanatory latent variables through the structural equation. As the distributions of some observed variables are nonnormal, we apply the Bayesian semiparametric SEM to analyze this data set.

The sample size of the data set is 353. There are some missing data which were treated as missing at random. To roughly unify the scale, the continuous variables were standardized using the fully observed data points. The genotype variables LTA2, PAI11, PAI12, ADRβ21, ADRβ22, and ADRβ3 are coded with $\{$AA, Aa, aa$\}$; their frequencies are equal to $\{78, 177, 96\}$, $\{61, 178, 112\}$, $\{72, 173, 106\}$, $\{127, 164, 48\}$, $\{266, 79, 0\}$, and $\{307, 43, 0\}$, respectively.

Let $\mathbf{y} =$ (lnACR, lnPCr, HbA1c, FPG, non-HDL-C, LDL-C, lnTG, LTA2, PAI11, PAI12, ADRβ21, ADRβ22, ADRβ3$)^T$ be the vector of the observed variables. The following loading matrix $\mathbf{\Lambda}$ in the measurement equation with $\boldsymbol{\omega}_i = (\eta_i, \xi_{i1}, \xi_{i2}, \xi_{i3}, \xi_{i4})^T$ is considered:

$$\mathbf{\Lambda}^T = \begin{bmatrix} 1 & \lambda_{21} & 0 & 0 & 0 & 0 & 0 & 0 & 0 & 0 & 0 & 0 & 0 \\ 0 & 0 & 1 & \lambda_{42} & 0 & 0 & 0 & 0 & 0 & 0 & 0 & 0 & 0 \\ 0 & 0 & 0 & 0 & 1 & \lambda_{63} & \lambda_{73} & 0 & 0 & 0 & 0 & 0 & 0 \\ 0 & 0 & 0 & 0 & 0 & 0 & 0 & 1 & \lambda_{94} & \lambda_{10,4} & 0 & 0 & 0 \\ 0 & 0 & 0 & 0 & 0 & 0 & 0 & 0 & 0 & 0 & 1 & \lambda_{12,5} & \lambda_{13,5} \end{bmatrix},$$

where the 1s and 0s are treated as fixed parameters. Although other $\mathbf{\Lambda}$ structures could be used, we consider the above non-overlapping structure for the sake of clear interpretation of the latent variables.

To illustrate the L_ν-measure in model selection, we consider the following competing models with different fixed covariates:

M_1: $y^*_{ik} = a_{k1}c_{i1} + a_{k2}c_{i2} + \mathbf{\Lambda}_k^T\boldsymbol{\omega}_i + \epsilon_{ik}, \quad \eta_i = b_1 d_{i1} + b_2 d_{i2} + \gamma_1\xi_{i1} + \gamma_2\xi_{i2} + \gamma_3\xi_{i3} + \gamma_4\xi_{i4} + \delta_i$,

M_2: $y^*_{ik} = a_{k1}c_{i1} + \mathbf{\Lambda}_k^T\boldsymbol{\omega}_i + \epsilon_{ik}, \eta_i = b_1 d_{i1} + b_2 d_{i2} + \gamma_1\xi_{i1} + \gamma_2\xi_{i2} + \gamma_3\xi_{i3} + \gamma_4\xi_{i4} + \delta_i$,

M_3: $y^*_{ik} = a_{k2}c_{i2} + \mathbf{\Lambda}_k^T\boldsymbol{\omega}_i + \epsilon_{ik}, \eta_i = b_1 d_{i1} + b_2 d_{i2} + \gamma_1\xi_{i1} + \gamma_2\xi_{i2} + \gamma_3\xi_{i3} + \gamma_4\xi_{i4} + \delta_i$,

M_4: $y^*_{ik} = a_{k1}c_{i1} + a_{k2}c_{i2} + \mathbf{\Lambda}_k^T\boldsymbol{\omega}_i + \epsilon_{ik}, \eta_i = \gamma_1\xi_{i1} + \gamma_2\xi_{i2} + \gamma_3\xi_{i3} + \gamma_4\xi_{i4} + \delta_i$,

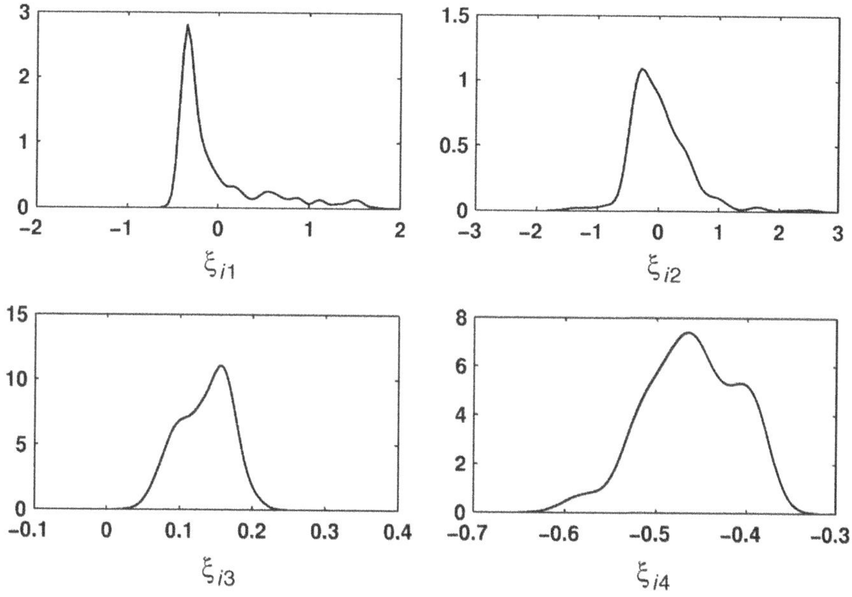

Figure 11.4 Estimated densities of ξ_{i1}, ξ_{i2}, ξ_{i3}, and ξ_{i4}.

where c_{i1} and c_{i2} are continuous fixed covariates related to age at onset and duration of disease, and d_{i1} and d_{i2} are binary variables related to smoking and alcohol. The Bayesian semiparametric approach with $G = 50$ in the MTDP (see (11.19)) was applied to obtain the parameter estimates. The following prior inputs for the hyperparameters in the conjugate prior distributions (see (11.24) and (11.25)) were used: $\alpha_{0\epsilon j} = 15$, $\beta_{0\epsilon j} = (\alpha_{0\epsilon j} - 1)\tilde{\psi}_{\epsilon xj}$, $\mathbf{\Lambda}_{0yj} = \tilde{\mathbf{\Lambda}}_{yj}$, $\mathbf{H}_{0yj} = \mathbf{I}_7$, $\alpha_{0\delta j} = 15$, $\beta_{0\delta j} = (\alpha_{0\delta j} - 1)\tilde{\psi}_{\delta j}$, $\mathbf{\Lambda}_{0\omega j} = \tilde{\mathbf{\Lambda}}_{\omega j}$, $\mathbf{H}_{0\omega j} = \mathbf{I}_6$, $\rho_1 = \rho_2 = 0.01$, $\tau_1 = \tau_2 = 2.0$, $\sigma_M = 10\,000$, and $\tilde{\boldsymbol{\theta}}$ denotes the Bayesian estimates of $\boldsymbol{\theta}$ obtained from the analysis of a 'control group' sample of diabetes patients. Results were obtained with 10 000 observations sampled by the blocked Gibbs sampler after 10 000 burn-in iterations.

The $L_{0.5}$-measures for M_1, M_2, M_3, and M_4 are 59 270, 58 822, 59 206, and 59 245, respectively. Hence, M_2 is selected. The estimated densities based on 10 000 simulated observations of $\xi_{i1}, \ldots, \xi_{i4}$ are presented in Figure 11.4. These plots indicate that the distributions of $\xi_{i1}, \ldots, \xi_{i4}$ are not normal. A path diagram illustrating the relationships among observed and latent variables is presented in Figure 11.5. Parameter estimates, together with 5% and 95% quantiles, are reported in Table 11.3. We note that most of the [5%, 95%] quantile ranges are reasonably short. The estimates of the coefficients $\hat{a}_{kj}$ corresponding to the fixed covariate 'age at onset', and the factor loading estimates $\hat{\lambda}_{kj}$ in the measurement equation can be interpreted according to a standard confirmatory factor analysis model. The estimated structural equation is

$$\eta_i = -0.023d_{i1} + 0.031d_{i2} - 0.122\xi_{i1} + 0.533\xi_{i2} + 0.726\xi_{i3} + 0.563\xi_{i4}.$$

This structural equation can be interpreted according to a standard regression model. It seems that the effects of 'smoking' and 'alcohol' are minor, but the other phenotype and genotype

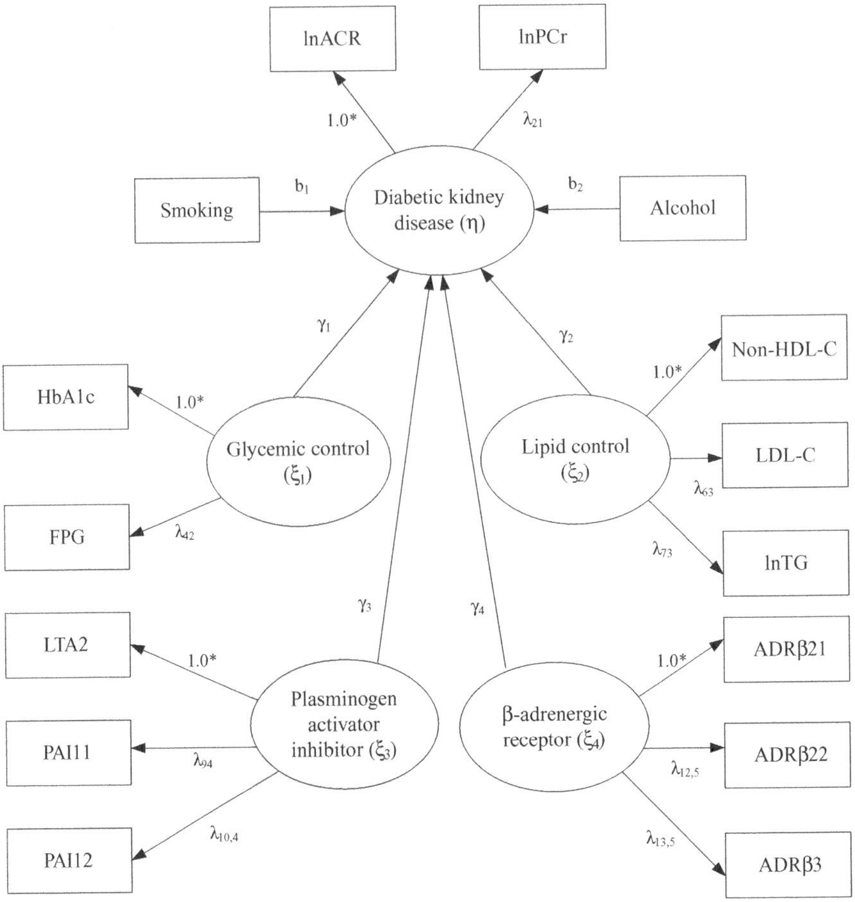

Figure 11.5 Path diagram of the selected model for analyzing the real data set.

latent variables have substantial effects on diabetic kidney disease. Other straightforward interpretations are not discussed here.

To assess the sensitivity of the results to the prior inputs of the hyperparameters in prior distributions corresponding to the parametric component, the data set was reanalyzed with some perturbations of the above *ad hoc* prior inputs, for example, $\mathbf{H}_{0yj} = 10\mathbf{I}_7$ and $\mathbf{H}_{0\omega j} = 10\mathbf{I}_6$. We obtained close Bayesian estimates and very similar estimated densities of the latent variables compared to those given above.

To examine the difference between the semiparametric and parametric approaches, the data set was reanalyzed using a parametric approach under the assumption that $\boldsymbol{\xi}_i$ is distributed as $N(\mathbf{0}, \boldsymbol{\Phi})$. The prior distribution of $\boldsymbol{\Phi}$ is taken as $\text{IW}(\tilde{\boldsymbol{\Phi}}, 20)$, where $\tilde{\boldsymbol{\Phi}}$ is the Bayesian estimate of $\boldsymbol{\Phi}$ obtained from the analysis of a 'control group' sample of diabetes patients. The prior distributions of other parameters are the same as before. For comparison, the estimates obtained are also presented in Table 11.3. We observe that some of the parameter estimates, in particular those associated with unordered categorical variables, such as $\hat{\lambda}_{94}$, $\hat{\lambda}_{12,5}$, $\hat{\gamma}_3$, and $\hat{\gamma}_4$, are quite different from the estimates obtained using the semiparametric approach. Given

Table 11.3 Estimation and standard error estimate for kidney disease data under M_2.

	$\xi_i \stackrel{D}{=}$ MTDP			$\xi_i \stackrel{D}{=}$ Normal	
Para.	EST	[5%, 95%] Quantiles	Para.	EST	[5%, 95%] Quantiles
a_{11}	0.005	[−0.139, 0.105]	a_{11}	0.007	[−0.143, 0.110]
a_{21}	0.163	[0.026, 0.260]	a_{21}	0.165	[0.027, 0.263]
a_{31}	−0.078	[−0.193, 0.014]	a_{31}	−0.071	[−0.224, 0.021]
a_{41}	−0.024	[−0.134, 0.067]	a_{41}	−0.016	[−0.170, 0.077]
a_{51}	−0.124	[−0.245, −0.030]	a_{51}	−0.117	[−0.264, −0.023]
a_{61}	−0.044	[−0.148, 0.047]	a_{61}	−0.033	[−0.181, 0.066]
a_{71}	0.004	[−0.120, 0.114]	a_{71}	0.024	[−0.143, 0.136]
a_{81}	−0.037	[−0.176, 0.051]	a_{81}	−0.046	[−0.206, 0.057]
a_{91}	−0.021	[−0.172, 0.077]	a_{91}	−0.020	[−0.158, 0.075]
$a_{10,1}$	0.034	[−0.100, 0.129]	$a_{10,1}$	0.034	[−0.110, 0.130]
$a_{11,1}$	−0.024	[−0.149, 0.059]	$a_{11,1}$	−0.026	[−0.178, 0.072]
$a_{12,1}$	−0.011	[−0.166, 0.073]	$a_{12,1}$	−0.019	[−0.173, 0.086]
$a_{13,1}$	−0.024	[−0.228, 0.058]	$a_{13,1}$	−0.048	[−0.312, 0.115]
λ_{21}	0.745	[0.428, 0.972]	λ_{21}	0.723	[0.415, 0.953]
λ_{42}	1.275	[0.856, 1.342]	λ_{42}	0.976	[0.753, 1.136]
λ_{63}	1.856	[1.444, 2.047]	λ_{63}	1.651	[1.379, 1.882]
λ_{73}	2.224	[1.710, 2.469]	λ_{73}	1.861	[1.539, 2.142]
λ_{94}	0.054	[−0.073, 0.106]	λ_{94}	−0.159	[−0.685, 0.254]
$\lambda_{10,4}$	0.432	[0.249, 0.681]	$\lambda_{10,4}$	0.489	[−0.151, 1.087]
$\lambda_{12,5}$	2.242	[1.963, 2.504]	$\lambda_{12,5}$	1.030	[0.565, 1.455]
$\lambda_{13,5}$	3.087	[2.845, 3.272]	$\lambda_{13,5}$	2.752	[1.775, 3.665]
$\psi_{\epsilon 1}$	0.712	[0.540, 0.837]	$\psi_{\epsilon 1}$	0.699	[0.540, 0.837]
$\psi_{\epsilon 2}$	0.849	[0.665, 0.984]	$\psi_{\epsilon 2}$	0.845	[0.662, 0.981]
$\psi_{\epsilon 3}$	0.667	[0.470, 0.710]	$\psi_{\epsilon 3}$	0.562	[0.434, 0.658]
$\psi_{\epsilon 4}$	0.518	[0.391, 0.621]	$\psi_{\epsilon 4}$	0.594	[0.461, 0.700]
$\psi_{\epsilon 5}$	0.768	[0.623, 0.866]	$\psi_{\epsilon 5}$	0.759	[0.621, 0.861]
$\psi_{\epsilon 6}$	0.249	[0.193, 0.287]	$\psi_{\epsilon 6}$	0.242	[0.187, 0.279]
$\psi_{\epsilon 7}$	0.323	[0.252, 0.383]	$\psi_{\epsilon 7}$	0.323	[0.248, 0.379]
b_1	−0.023	[−0.173, 0.069]	b_1	−0.027	[−0.175, 0.069]
b_2	0.031	[−0.111, 0.126]	b_2	0.036	[−0.107, 0.133]
γ_1	−0.122	[−0.346, 0.028]	γ_1	−0.188	[−0.418, −0.044]
γ_2	0.533	[0.240, 0.708]	γ_2	0.521	[0.217, 0.730]
γ_3	0.726	[0.431, 1.574]	γ_3	−0.106	[−0.685, 0.301]
γ_4	0.563	[0.330, 0.811]	γ_4	0.103	[−0.197, 0.309]
ψ_δ	0.315	[0.205, 0.416]	ψ_δ	0.383	[0.227, 0.511]

the fact that the distributions of $\xi_{i1}, \ldots, \xi_{i4}$ are not normal (see Figure 11.4), and the results obtained from the simulation study reported in Section 11.3.4, we expect the semiparametric solution to be better.

The computer program for analyzing this data set is written in C, and the code is available from:

`www.wiley.com/go/medical_behavioral_sciences`

Appendix 11.1 Full conditional distributions

The full conditional distribution in step (a) of the Gibbs sampler is:

$$p(\mathbf{X}_{\text{mis}}|\mathbf{X}_{\text{obs}}, \mathbf{U}_{\text{obs}}, \mathbf{V}_{\text{obs}}, \mathbf{V}_{\text{mis}}, \boldsymbol{\Omega}, \boldsymbol{\theta}) = \prod_{i=1}^{n} p(\mathbf{x}_{i,\text{mis}}|\boldsymbol{\omega}_i, \boldsymbol{\theta}),$$

$$[\mathbf{x}_{i,\text{mis}}|\boldsymbol{\omega}_i, \boldsymbol{\theta}] \stackrel{D}{=} N[\boldsymbol{\mu}_{i,\text{mis}} + \boldsymbol{\Lambda}_{i,\text{mis}}\boldsymbol{\omega}_i, \boldsymbol{\Psi}_{\epsilon xi}], \tag{11.A1}$$

where $\boldsymbol{\mu}_{i,\text{mis}}$ is an $r_i \times 1$ subvector of $\boldsymbol{\mu}$ with rows corresponding to $\mathbf{x}_{i,\text{mis}}$, $\boldsymbol{\Lambda}_{i,\text{mis}}$ is an $r_i \times q$ submatrix of $\boldsymbol{\Lambda}$ with rows corresponding to $\mathbf{x}_{i,\text{mis}}$, and $\boldsymbol{\Psi}_{\epsilon xi}$ is the submatrix of $\boldsymbol{\Psi}_{\epsilon x}$ corresponding to $\mathbf{x}_{i,\text{mis}}$.

The full conditional distribution in step (b) of the Gibbs sampler is

$$p(\mathbf{V}_{\text{obs}}|\mathbf{X}_{\text{obs}}, \mathbf{U}_{\text{obs}}, \mathbf{X}_{\text{mis}}, \mathbf{V}_{\text{mis}}, \boldsymbol{\Omega}, \boldsymbol{\theta}) = \prod_{i=1}^{n}\prod_{j=r+1}^{p} p(\mathbf{v}_{ij,\text{obs}}|u_{ij,\text{obs}}, \boldsymbol{\omega}_i, \boldsymbol{\theta}),$$

$$\big[\mathbf{v}_{ij,\text{obs}}|u_{ij,\text{obs}}, \boldsymbol{\omega}_i, \boldsymbol{\theta}\big] \stackrel{D}{=} N\big[\mathbf{1}_{K_j-1}\mu_j + \mathbf{1}_{K_j-1}\boldsymbol{\Lambda}_j^T\boldsymbol{\omega}_i, \mathbf{I}_{K_j-1}\big]I(\mathfrak{R}_{ij,\text{obs}}), \tag{11.A2}$$

where

$$\mathfrak{R}_{ij,\text{obs}} = \begin{cases} \{\mathbf{v}_{ij,\text{obs}} : v_{ij,k,\text{obs}} > \max(\mathbf{v}_{ij,-k,\text{obs}}, 0)\}, & \text{if } u_{ij,\text{obs}} = k \neq 0, \\ \{\mathbf{v}_{ij,\text{obs}} : \max(v_{ij,\text{obs}}) < 0\}, & \text{if } u_{ij,\text{obs}} = 0, \end{cases}$$

where $\mathbf{v}_{ij,-k,\text{obs}}$ is $\mathbf{v}_{ij,\text{obs}}$ with $v_{ij,k,\text{obs}}$ deleted. The distribution of $[\mathbf{v}_{ij,\text{obs}}|u_{ij,\text{obs}}, \boldsymbol{\omega}_i, \boldsymbol{\theta}]$ in (11.A2) is a truncated multivariate normal distribution truncated over the appropriate cone $\mathfrak{R}_{ij,\text{obs}}$ in R^{K_j-1}. To sample $\mathbf{v}_{ij,\text{obs}}$, we use the following partitioning of the variables to successively simulate observations in $\{v_{ij,1,\text{obs}}, \ldots, v_{ij,K_j-1,\text{obs}}\}$ via the Gibbs sampler (see Geweke, 1991). This approach replaces the difficult draw from $[\mathbf{v}_{ij,\text{obs}}|u_{ij,\text{obs}}, \boldsymbol{\omega}_i, \boldsymbol{\theta}]$ with simpler univariate draws. The distribution of the utility differential $v_{ij,k,\text{obs}}$, given $\mathbf{v}_{ij,-k,\text{obs}}$, $u_{ij,\text{obs}}$, $\boldsymbol{\omega}_i$, and $\boldsymbol{\theta}$, is a univariate truncated normal distribution with the truncation point depending on whether $u_{ij,\text{obs}} = k$ or not. That is,

$$[v_{ij,k,\text{obs}}|\mathbf{v}_{ij,-k,\text{obs}}, u_{ij,\text{obs}}, \boldsymbol{\omega}_i, \boldsymbol{\theta}] \stackrel{D}{=} N\big[\mu_j + \boldsymbol{\Lambda}_j^T\boldsymbol{\omega}_i, 1\big]\Big[I_{\{u_{ij,\text{obs}}=k\}}I_{[\max(\mathbf{v}_{ij,-k,\text{obs}},0),\infty)}(v_{ij,k,\text{obs}})$$
$$+ I_{\{u_{ij,\text{obs}}\neq k\}}I_{\{u_{ij,\text{obs}}\neq 0\}}I_{(-\infty,\max(\mathbf{v}_{ij,-k,\text{obs}},0)]}(v_{ij,k,\text{obs}}) + I_{\{u_{ij,\text{obs}}\neq k\}}I_{\{u_{ij,\text{obs}}=0\}}I_{(-\infty,0)}(v_{ij,k,\text{obs}})\Big].$$

The full conditional distribution in step (c) of the Gibbs sampler is

$$p(\mathbf{V}_{\text{mis}}|\mathbf{X}_{\text{obs}}, \mathbf{U}_{\text{obs}}, \mathbf{X}_{\text{mis}}, \mathbf{V}_{\text{obs}}, \boldsymbol{\Omega}, \boldsymbol{\theta}) = p(\mathbf{V}_{\text{mis}}|\boldsymbol{\Omega}, \boldsymbol{\theta}) = \prod_{i=1}^{n}\prod_{j=r+1}^{p} p(\mathbf{v}_{ij,\text{mis}}|\boldsymbol{\omega}_i, \boldsymbol{\theta})$$

$$\big[v_{ij,k,\text{mis}}|\boldsymbol{\omega}_i, \boldsymbol{\theta}\big] \stackrel{D}{=} N\big[\mu_j + \boldsymbol{\Lambda}_j^T\boldsymbol{\omega}_i, 1\big], \quad \text{for } k = 1, \ldots, K_j - 1, \tag{11.A3}$$

where $v_{ij,k,\text{mis}}$ is the kth component of $\mathbf{v}_{ij,\text{mis}}$.

The full conditional distribution in step (d) of the Gibbs sampler is $\prod_{i=1}^n p(\boldsymbol{\omega}_i|\ \mathbf{y}_i^*, \boldsymbol{\theta})$, where $\mathbf{y}_i^* = \{\mathbf{x}_{i,\text{obs}}, \mathbf{x}_{i,\text{mis}}, \mathbf{V}_{i,\text{obs}}, \mathbf{V}_{i,\text{mis}}\}$ and

$$p(\boldsymbol{\omega}_i|\mathbf{y}_i^*, \boldsymbol{\theta}) \propto \exp\left\{ -\frac{1}{2}\boldsymbol{\xi}_i^T\boldsymbol{\Phi}^{-1}\boldsymbol{\xi}_i - \frac{1}{2}\sum_{j=1}^{r}\left(x_{ij} - \mu_j - \boldsymbol{\Lambda}_j^T\boldsymbol{\omega}_i\right)^T\psi_{\epsilon xj}^{-1}\left(x_{ij} - \mu_j - \boldsymbol{\Lambda}_j^T\boldsymbol{\omega}_i\right)\right.$$
$$-\frac{1}{2}\sum_{j=r+1}^{p}\sum_{k=1}^{K_j-1}\left(v_{ij,k} - \mu_j - \boldsymbol{\Lambda}_j^T\boldsymbol{\omega}_i\right)^T\left(v_{ij,k} - \mu_j - \boldsymbol{\Lambda}_j^T\boldsymbol{\omega}_i\right)$$
$$\left. -\frac{1}{2}[\boldsymbol{\eta}_i - \boldsymbol{\Lambda}_\omega\mathbf{G}(\boldsymbol{\omega}_i)]^T\boldsymbol{\Psi}_\delta^{-1}[\boldsymbol{\eta}_i - \boldsymbol{\Lambda}_\omega\mathbf{G}(\boldsymbol{\omega}_i)]\right\}. \tag{11.A4}$$

As the parameter vector $\boldsymbol{\theta}$ contains the unknown parameters in $\boldsymbol{\mu}$, $\boldsymbol{\Lambda}$, $\boldsymbol{\Phi}$, $\boldsymbol{\Lambda}_\omega$, $\boldsymbol{\Psi}_{\epsilon x}$, and $\boldsymbol{\Psi}_\delta$, the full conditional distribution in step (e) of the Gibbs sampler consists of several components that depend on the respective prior distributions. Based on the rationale given in the previous chapters, the following independent conjugate prior distributions are used:

$$\boldsymbol{\mu} \stackrel{D}{=} N[\boldsymbol{\mu}_0, \boldsymbol{\Sigma}_0],\ [\boldsymbol{\Lambda}_j|\psi_{\epsilon xj}] \stackrel{D}{=} N[\boldsymbol{\Lambda}_{0j}, \psi_{\epsilon xj}\mathbf{H}_{0j}],\ \psi_{\epsilon xj}^{-1} \stackrel{D}{=} \text{Gamma}[\alpha_{0j}, \beta_{0j}], \quad j = 1, \ldots, r,$$
$$\boldsymbol{\Lambda}_j \stackrel{D}{=} N[\boldsymbol{\Lambda}_{0j}, \mathbf{H}_{0j}],\ j = r+1, \ldots, p, \quad \boldsymbol{\Phi}^{-1} \stackrel{D}{=} W_{q_2}[\mathbf{R}_0, \rho_0],$$
$$[\boldsymbol{\Lambda}_{\omega j}|\psi_{\delta j}] \stackrel{D}{=} N[\boldsymbol{\Lambda}_{0\omega j}, \psi_{\delta j}\mathbf{H}_{0\omega j}],\ \psi_{\delta j}^{-1} \stackrel{D}{=} \text{Gamma}[\alpha_{0\delta j}, \beta_{0\delta j}], \quad j = 1, \ldots, q_1, \tag{11.A5}$$

where $\boldsymbol{\Lambda}_{\omega j}^T$ is jth row of $\boldsymbol{\Lambda}_\omega$, $\psi_{\epsilon xj}$ and $\psi_{\delta j}$ are the jth diagonal elements of $\boldsymbol{\Psi}_{\epsilon x}$ and $\boldsymbol{\Psi}_\delta$, respectively; and $\boldsymbol{\mu}_0$, $\boldsymbol{\Lambda}_{0j}$, $\boldsymbol{\Lambda}_{0\omega j}$, α_{0j}, β_{0j}, $\alpha_{0\delta j}$, $\beta_{0\delta j}$, ρ_0, and positive definite matrices $\boldsymbol{\Sigma}_0$, $\mathbf{H}_{0j}$, $\mathbf{H}_{0\omega j}$, and $\mathbf{R}_0$ are hyperparameters whose values are assumed to be given by the prior information.

Let $\mathbf{Y}^* = (\mathbf{y}_1^* - \mathbf{E}\boldsymbol{\mu}, \ldots, \mathbf{y}_n^* - \mathbf{E}\boldsymbol{\mu})$, $\tilde{\mathbf{Y}}^* = (\mathbf{y}_1^*, \ldots, \mathbf{y}_n^*)$, $\boldsymbol{\Omega}_1 = (\boldsymbol{\eta}_1, \ldots, \boldsymbol{\eta}_n)$, $\boldsymbol{\Omega}_2 = (\boldsymbol{\xi}_1, \ldots, \boldsymbol{\xi}_n)$, and $\mathbf{G} = (\mathbf{G}(\boldsymbol{\omega}_1), \ldots, \mathbf{G}(\boldsymbol{\omega}_n))$; and let $\mathbf{Y}_j^{*T}$ and $\boldsymbol{\Omega}_{1j}^T$ be the jth rows of $\mathbf{Y}^*$ and $\boldsymbol{\Omega}_1$, respectively. Under these prior distributions, the conditional distributions of the components of $\boldsymbol{\theta}$ are as follows:

$$[\boldsymbol{\mu}|\tilde{\mathbf{Y}}^*, \boldsymbol{\Omega}, \boldsymbol{\Lambda}, \boldsymbol{\Psi}_{\epsilon x}] \stackrel{D}{=} N\left[\boldsymbol{\Sigma}_\mu\left\{\mathbf{E}^T\boldsymbol{\Psi}_\epsilon^{-1}\sum_{i=1}^{n}(\mathbf{y}_i^* - \mathbf{E}\boldsymbol{\Lambda}\boldsymbol{\omega}_i) + \boldsymbol{\Sigma}_0^{-1}\boldsymbol{\mu}_0\right\}, \boldsymbol{\Sigma}_\mu\right], \tag{11.A6}$$

$$[\boldsymbol{\Lambda}_j|\mathbf{Y}^*, \boldsymbol{\Omega}, \psi_{\epsilon xj}] \stackrel{D}{=} N[\mathbf{m}_j, \psi_{\epsilon xj}\boldsymbol{\Sigma}_j],\ [\psi_{\epsilon xj}^{-1}|\mathbf{Y}^*, \boldsymbol{\Omega}] \stackrel{D}{=} \text{Gamma}[n/2 + \alpha_{0j}, \beta_j], \quad j = 1, \ldots, r,$$
$$[\boldsymbol{\Lambda}_j|\mathbf{Y}^*, \boldsymbol{\Omega}] \stackrel{D}{=} N[\mathbf{m}_j, \boldsymbol{\Sigma}_j],\ j = r+1, \ldots, p, \quad [\boldsymbol{\Phi}|\boldsymbol{\Omega}_2] \stackrel{D}{=} \text{IW}_{q_2}\left[\left(\boldsymbol{\Omega}_2\boldsymbol{\Omega}_2^T + \mathbf{R}_0^{-1}\right), n + \rho_0\right],$$
$$[\boldsymbol{\Lambda}_{\omega j}|\boldsymbol{\Omega}, \psi_{\delta j}] \stackrel{D}{=} N[\mathbf{m}_{\omega j}, \psi_{\delta j}\boldsymbol{\Sigma}_{\omega j}],\ [\psi_{\delta j}^{-1}|\boldsymbol{\Omega}] \stackrel{D}{=} \text{Gamma}[n/2 + \alpha_{0\delta j}, \beta_{\delta j}], \quad j = 1\ldots, q_1,$$

where

$$\boldsymbol{\Sigma}_\mu = \left(n\mathbf{E}^T\boldsymbol{\Psi}_\epsilon^{-1}\mathbf{E} + \boldsymbol{\Sigma}_0^{-1}\right)^{-1}, \quad \boldsymbol{\Psi}_\epsilon = \begin{bmatrix} \boldsymbol{\Psi}_{\epsilon x} & \mathbf{0} & \cdots & \mathbf{0} \\ \mathbf{0} & \mathbf{I}_{K_{r+1}-1} & \cdots & \mathbf{0} \\ \vdots & \vdots & \ddots & \vdots \\ \mathbf{0} & \mathbf{0} & \cdots & \mathbf{I}_{K_p-1} \end{bmatrix},$$

$\mathbf{m}_j = \boldsymbol{\Sigma}_j(\mathbf{H}_{0j}^{-1}\boldsymbol{\Lambda}_{0j} + \boldsymbol{\Omega}\mathbf{Y}_j^*)$, $\boldsymbol{\Sigma}_j = (\mathbf{H}_{0j}^{-1} + \boldsymbol{\Omega}\boldsymbol{\Omega}^T)^{-1}$, $\beta_j = \beta_{0j} + [\mathbf{Y}_j^{*T}\mathbf{Y}_j^* - \mathbf{m}_j^T\boldsymbol{\Sigma}_j^{-1}\mathbf{m}_j + \boldsymbol{\Lambda}_{0j}^T\mathbf{H}_{0j}^{-1}\boldsymbol{\Lambda}_{0j}]/2$, $\mathbf{m}_{\omega j} = \boldsymbol{\Sigma}_{\omega j}(\mathbf{H}_{0\omega j}^{-1}\boldsymbol{\Lambda}_{0\omega j} + \mathbf{G}\boldsymbol{\Omega}_{1j})$, $\boldsymbol{\Sigma}_{\omega j} = (\mathbf{H}_{0\omega j}^{-1} + \mathbf{G}\mathbf{G}^T)^{-1}$, and $\beta_{\delta j} = \beta_{0\delta j} + [\boldsymbol{\Omega}_{1j}^T\boldsymbol{\Omega}_{1j} - \mathbf{m}_{\omega j}^T\boldsymbol{\Sigma}_{\omega j}^{-1}\mathbf{m}_{\omega j} + \boldsymbol{\Lambda}_{0\omega j}^T\mathbf{H}_{0\omega j}^{-1}\boldsymbol{\Lambda}_{0\omega j}]/2$.

Simulating observations from the distributions involved in steps (a), (c), and (e) is straightforward. However, the conditional distributions of $\mathbf{V}_{\text{obs}}$ in step (b) and $\boldsymbol{\Omega}$ in step (d) are nonstandard. The approach developed in Geweke (1991) and the MH algorithm (Metropolis *et al.*, 1953; Hastings, 1970) will be applied to simulate observations from these distributions.

Appendix 11.2 Path sampling

Utilizing data augmentation, the difficulty of MCMC sampling is alleviated by augmenting $(\mathbf{X}_{\text{obs}}, \mathbf{U}_{\text{obs}})$ with $(\mathbf{X}_{\text{mis}}, \mathbf{V}_{\text{obs}}, \mathbf{V}_{\text{mis}}, \boldsymbol{\Omega})$ as in the estimation. Let t be a continuous parameter in [0, 1] to link the competing models M_0 and M_1, $p(\mathbf{X}_{\text{obs}}, \mathbf{U}_{\text{obs}}, \mathbf{X}_{\text{mis}}, \mathbf{V}_{\text{obs}}, \mathbf{V}_{\text{mis}}, \boldsymbol{\Omega}; \boldsymbol{\theta}, t)$ be the complete-data likelihood, and $U(\mathbf{X}_{\text{obs}}, \mathbf{U}_{\text{obs}}, \mathbf{X}_{\text{mis}}, \mathbf{V}_{\text{obs}}, \mathbf{V}_{\text{mis}}, \boldsymbol{\Omega}, \boldsymbol{\theta}, t) = d \log p(\mathbf{X}_{\text{obs}}, \mathbf{U}_{\text{obs}}, \mathbf{X}_{\text{mis}}, \mathbf{V}_{\text{obs}}, \mathbf{V}_{\text{mis}}, \boldsymbol{\Omega}|\boldsymbol{\theta}, t)/dt$. It can be shown by the similar reasoning to that in Gelman and Meng (1998) that

$$\log B_{10} = \int_0^1 E_{\mathbf{X}_{\text{mis}}, \mathbf{V}_{\text{obs}}, \mathbf{V}_{\text{mis}}, \boldsymbol{\Omega}, \boldsymbol{\theta}}[U(\mathbf{X}_{\text{obs}}, \mathbf{U}_{\text{obs}}, \mathbf{X}_{\text{mis}}, \mathbf{V}_{\text{obs}}, \mathbf{V}_{\text{mis}}, \boldsymbol{\Omega}, \boldsymbol{\theta}, t)]dt, \qquad (11.\text{A}7)$$

where $E_{\mathbf{X}_{\text{mis}}, \mathbf{V}_{\text{obs}}, \mathbf{V}_{\text{mis}}, \boldsymbol{\Omega}, \boldsymbol{\theta}}$ is the expectation with respect to the distribution $p(\mathbf{X}_{\text{mis}}, \mathbf{V}_{\text{obs}}, \mathbf{V}_{\text{mis}}, \boldsymbol{\Omega}, \boldsymbol{\theta}|\mathbf{X}_{\text{obs}}, \mathbf{U}_{\text{obs}}, t)$. This integral can be numerically evaluated via the trapezoidal rule. Specifically, let S different fixed grids $\{t_{(s)}\}_{s=1}^S$ be ordered as $0 = t_{(0)} < t_{(1)} < t_{(2)} < \ldots < t_{(S)} < t_{(S+1)} = 1$. Then, $\log B_{10}$ can be computed as

$$\widehat{\log B_{10}} = \frac{1}{2}\sum_{s=0}^{S}(t_{(s+1)} - t_{(s)})(\bar{U}_{(s+1)} + \bar{U}_{(s)}), \qquad (11.\text{A}8)$$

where $\bar{U}_{(s)}$ is the average of the $U(\mathbf{X}_{\text{obs}}, \mathbf{U}_{\text{obs}}, \mathbf{X}_{\text{mis}}, \mathbf{V}_{\text{obs}}, \mathbf{V}_{\text{mis}}, \boldsymbol{\Omega}, \boldsymbol{\theta}, t)$ on the basis of all simulation draws for which $t = t_{(s)}$, that is,

$$\bar{U}_{(s)} = L^{-1}\sum_{l=1}^{L} U\big(\mathbf{X}_{\text{obs}}, \mathbf{U}_{\text{obs}}, \mathbf{X}_{\text{mis}}^{(l)}, \mathbf{V}_{\text{obs}}^{(l)}, \mathbf{V}_{\text{mis}}^{(l)}, \boldsymbol{\Omega}^{(l)}, \boldsymbol{\theta}^{(l)}, t_{(s)}\big), \qquad (11.\text{A}9)$$

in which $\{(\mathbf{X}_{\text{mis}}^{(l)}, \mathbf{V}_{\text{obs}}^{(l)}, \mathbf{V}_{\text{mis}}^{(l)}, \boldsymbol{\Omega}^{(l)}, \boldsymbol{\theta}^{(l)}), l = 1, \ldots, L\}$ are simulated observations drawn from $p(\mathbf{X}_{\text{mis}}, \mathbf{V}_{\text{obs}}, \mathbf{V}_{\text{mis}}, \boldsymbol{\Omega}, \boldsymbol{\theta}|\mathbf{X}_{\text{obs}}, \mathbf{U}_{\text{obs}}, t_{(s)})$.

Appendix 11.3 A modified truncated DP related to equation (11.19)

To construct an appropriate random probability measure, we consider a finite nonnull measure ν on the space of real numbers R and the set containing all the subsets of $\mathcal{B}$, where R is a real-valued space, and $\mathcal{B}$ is a Borel σ-field on R. Further, we assume that the median of ν is zero, that is, $\nu(-\infty, 0) = \nu(0, \infty)$. We denote by $\mathcal{D}_\nu$ the Dirichlet process over all the distributions defined on $(R, \mathcal{B})$ with the parameter ν. Let $\nu_+(B) = \nu\{B \cap (0, \infty)\} + 0.5\nu\{B \cap \{0\}\}$ and $\nu_-(B) = \nu\{B \cap (-\infty, 0)\} + 0.5\nu\{B \cap \{0\}\}$, for $B \in \mathcal{B}$. We consider

$$P = \frac{1}{2}P_+ + \frac{1}{2}P_-, \tag{11.A10}$$

where P_+ and P_- are taken independently from $\mathcal{D}_{\nu_+}$ and $\mathcal{D}_{\nu_-}$, respectively. Thus, the median of P is zero. This defines a random probability measure $\mathcal{D}_\nu^*$ on the set of all distribution functions P on R with median zero. A similar random probability measure has been used in Bayesian semiparametric estimation of the median in a distribution (Doss, 1985), and median regression modeling (Kottas and Gelfand, 2001). It can be shown by reasoning similar to that in Sethurman (1994) that $\mathcal{D}_{\nu_+}$ generates $P_+ = \sum_{k=1}^{\infty} \pi_k \delta_{z_k}(\cdot)$ with $\pi_k = \prod_{j=1}^{k-1}(1 - v_j^+)v_k^+$, where $v_k^+ \overset{D}{=} \text{Beta}(1, \nu_+(R))$, and $z_k \overset{D}{=} \nu_+/\nu_+(R)$. Similarly, $\mathcal{D}_{\nu_-}$ generates $P_- = \sum_{k=1}^{\infty} p_k \delta_{w_k}(\cdot)$ with $p_k = \prod_{j=1}^{k-1}(1 - v_j^-)v_k^-$, where $v_k^- \overset{D}{=} \text{Beta}(1, \nu_-(R))$, and $w_k \overset{D}{=} \nu_-/\nu_-(R)$. Note that $\{z_k\}_{k=1}^{\infty}$, $\{w_k\}_{k=1}^{\infty}$, $\{\pi_k\}_{k=1}^{\infty}$, and $\{p_k\}_{k=1}^{\infty}$ are independent. For $\nu(\cdot) = \alpha H_\theta(\cdot)(\alpha > 0)$ with some distribution $H_\theta(\cdot)$, we have $v_k^- \overset{D}{=} \text{Beta}(1, \alpha M^-)$ with $M^- = H_\theta((-\infty, 0])$, and $w_k \overset{D}{=} H_\theta^-$, where H_θ^- is a truncated distribution function at $(-\infty, 0)$. We also have similar results for v_k^+, and π_k. Consequently, $\mathcal{D}_\nu^*$ generates

$$P = \frac{1}{2}P_+ + \frac{1}{2}P_- = \frac{1}{2}\sum_{k=1}^{\infty} \pi_k \delta_{z_k}(\cdot) + \frac{1}{2}\sum_{k=1}^{\infty} p_k \delta_{w_k}(\cdot). \tag{11.A11}$$

This gives (11.19), the MTDP for modeling ξ_i.

Appendix 11.4 Conditional distributions and the MH algorithm for the Bayesian semiparametric model

The full conditional distribution $p(\mathbf{X}_{\text{mis}}|\mathbf{V}_{\text{obs}}, \mathbf{V}_{\text{mis}}, \boldsymbol{\Omega}_1, \boldsymbol{\theta}, \boldsymbol{\pi}, \mathbf{Z}, \mathbf{L}, \boldsymbol{\beta}, \mathbf{X}_{\text{obs}}, \mathbf{U}_{\text{obs}})$ is

$$p(\mathbf{X}_{\text{mis}}|\mathbf{V}_{\text{obs}}, \mathbf{V}_{\text{mis}}, \boldsymbol{\Omega}_1, \boldsymbol{\theta}, \boldsymbol{\pi}, \mathbf{Z}, \mathbf{L}, \boldsymbol{\beta}, \mathbf{X}_{\text{obs}}, \mathbf{U}_{\text{obs}}) = \prod_{i=1}^{n} p(\mathbf{x}_{i,\text{mis}}|\boldsymbol{\omega}_i, \boldsymbol{\theta}),$$

$$[\mathbf{x}_{i,\text{mis}}|\boldsymbol{\omega}_i, \boldsymbol{\theta}] \stackrel{D}{=} N[\mathbf{A}_{i,\text{mis}}\mathbf{c}_i + \boldsymbol{\Lambda}_{i,\text{mis}}\boldsymbol{\omega}_i, \boldsymbol{\Psi}_{\epsilon xi}]$$

where $\mathbf{A}_{i,\text{mis}}$ is an $r_i \times t$ subvector of $\mathbf{A}$ with rows corresponding to $\mathbf{x}_{i,\text{mis}}$, $\mathbf{c}_i$ is a $t \times 1$ vector of covariates, $\boldsymbol{\Lambda}_{i,\text{mis}}$ is an $r_i \times q$ submatrix of $\boldsymbol{\Lambda}$ with rows corresponding to $\mathbf{x}_{i,\text{mis}}$, and $\boldsymbol{\Psi}_{\epsilon xi}$ is the submatrix of $\boldsymbol{\Psi}_{\epsilon x}$ corresponding to $\mathbf{x}_{i,\text{mis}}$.

The full conditional distribution $p(\mathbf{V}_{\text{obs}}|\mathbf{X}_{\text{mis}}, \mathbf{V}_{\text{mis}}, \boldsymbol{\Omega}_1, \boldsymbol{\theta}, \boldsymbol{\pi}, \mathbf{Z}, \mathbf{L}, \boldsymbol{\beta}, \mathbf{X}_{\text{obs}}, \mathbf{U}_{\text{obs}})$ is given by

$$p(\mathbf{V}_{\text{obs}}|\mathbf{X}_{\text{mis}}, \mathbf{V}_{\text{mis}}, \boldsymbol{\Omega}_1, \boldsymbol{\theta}, \boldsymbol{\pi}, \mathbf{Z}, \mathbf{L}, \boldsymbol{\beta}, \mathbf{X}_{\text{obs}}, \mathbf{U}_{\text{obs}}) = \prod_{i=1}^{n}\prod_{j=r+1}^{p} p(\mathbf{v}_{ij}|u_{ij}, \boldsymbol{\omega}_i, \boldsymbol{\theta}),$$

$$p(\mathbf{v}_{ij}|u_{ij}, \boldsymbol{\omega}_i, \boldsymbol{\theta}) \propto N\big[\mathbf{1}_{K_j-1}\mathbf{A}_j^T\mathbf{c}_i + \mathbf{1}_{K_j-1}\boldsymbol{\Lambda}_j^T\boldsymbol{\omega}_i^+, \mathbf{I}_{K_j-1}\big]I(\mathfrak{R}_{i,u_{ij}}).$$

It can be shown that if $u_{ij} = 0$,

$$p(\mathbf{v}_{ij}|u_{ij}, \boldsymbol{\omega}_i, \boldsymbol{\theta}) = \prod_{l=1}^{K_j-1} p(v_{ij,l}|u_{ij}, \boldsymbol{\omega}_i, \boldsymbol{\theta}) \propto \prod_{l=1}^{K_j-1} N\big[\mathbf{A}_j^T\mathbf{c}_i + \boldsymbol{\Lambda}_j^T\boldsymbol{\omega}_i^+, 1\big]I_{(-\infty,\, 0)},$$

and if $u_{ij} = k \neq 0$,

$$p(v_{ij,l}|u_{ij}, v_{ij,t}, t \neq l, \boldsymbol{\omega}_i, \boldsymbol{\theta}) \propto \begin{cases} N\big[\mathbf{A}_j^T\mathbf{c}_i + \boldsymbol{\Lambda}_j^T\boldsymbol{\omega}_i^+, 1\big]I_{(-\infty,\, v_{ij,k}\vee 0]} & \text{if } l \neq k, \\ N\big[\mathbf{A}_j^T\mathbf{c}_i + \boldsymbol{\Lambda}_j^T\boldsymbol{\omega}_i^+, 1\big]I_{(\max_{t\neq k} v_{ij,t}\vee 0,\, +\infty)} & \text{if } l = k, \end{cases}$$

where $a \vee b$ means the maximum of a and b.

The full conditional distribution $p(\mathbf{V}_{\text{mis}}|\mathbf{X}_{\text{mis}}, \mathbf{V}_{\text{obs}}, \boldsymbol{\Omega}_1, \boldsymbol{\theta}, \boldsymbol{\pi}, \mathbf{Z}, \mathbf{L}, \boldsymbol{\beta}, \mathbf{X}_{\text{obs}}, \mathbf{U}_{\text{obs}})$ is given by

$$p(\mathbf{V}_{\text{mis}}|\mathbf{X}_{\text{mis}}, \mathbf{V}_{\text{obs}}, \boldsymbol{\Omega}_1, \boldsymbol{\theta}, \boldsymbol{\pi}, \mathbf{Z}, \mathbf{L}, \boldsymbol{\beta}, \mathbf{X}_{\text{obs}}, \mathbf{U}_{\text{obs}}) = \prod_{i=1}^{n}\prod_{j=r+1}^{p} p(\mathbf{v}_{ij,\text{mis}}|\boldsymbol{\omega}_i, \boldsymbol{\theta}),$$

$$[\mathbf{v}_{ij,\text{mis}}|\boldsymbol{\omega}_i, \boldsymbol{\theta}] \stackrel{D}{=} N\big[\mathbf{1}_{K_j-1}\big(\mathbf{A}_j^T\mathbf{c}_i + \boldsymbol{\Lambda}_j^T\boldsymbol{\omega}_i^+\big), \mathbf{I}_{K_j-1}\big].$$

The full conditional distribution $p(\boldsymbol{\Omega}_1|\mathbf{X}_{\text{mis}}, \mathbf{V}_{\text{obs}}, \mathbf{V}_{\text{mis}}, \boldsymbol{\theta}, \boldsymbol{\pi}, \mathbf{Z}, \mathbf{L}, \boldsymbol{\beta}, \mathbf{X}_{\text{obs}}, \mathbf{U}_{\text{obs}})$ is given by

$$p(\boldsymbol{\Omega}_1|\mathbf{X}_{\text{mis}}, \mathbf{V}_{\text{obs}}, \mathbf{V}_{\text{mis}}, \boldsymbol{\theta}, \boldsymbol{\pi}, \mathbf{Z}, \mathbf{L}, \boldsymbol{\beta}, \mathbf{X}_{\text{obs}}, \mathbf{U}_{\text{obs}}) = \prod_{i=1}^{n} p(\boldsymbol{\eta}_i|\boldsymbol{\xi}_i, \mathbf{y}_i^*, \boldsymbol{\theta}),$$

$$[\boldsymbol{\eta}_i|\boldsymbol{\xi}_i, \mathbf{y}_i^*, \boldsymbol{\theta}] \stackrel{D}{=} N[\boldsymbol{\mu}_{\eta_i}, \boldsymbol{\Sigma}_\eta], \quad i = 1, \ldots, n,$$

where $\mathbf{\Sigma}_\eta = (\mathbf{\Lambda}_\eta^T \mathbf{\Psi}_M^{-1} \mathbf{\Lambda}_\eta + \mathbf{\Pi}_0^T \mathbf{\Psi}_\delta^{-1} \mathbf{\Pi}_0)^{-1}$, $\boldsymbol{\mu}_{\eta_i} = \mathbf{\Sigma}_\eta \{ \mathbf{\Lambda}_\eta^T \mathbf{\Psi}_M^{-1} (\bar{\mathbf{y}}_{i\cdot}^* - \mathbf{A}\mathbf{c}_i - \mathbf{\Lambda}_\xi \boldsymbol{\xi}_i) + \mathbf{\Pi}_0^T \mathbf{\Psi}_\delta^{-1} (\mathbf{B}\mathbf{d}_i + \mathbf{\Gamma}\boldsymbol{\xi}_i) \}$, $\bar{\mathbf{y}}_{i\cdot}^* = (\mathbf{x}_i^T, \bar{v}_{i(r+1)\cdot}, \ldots, \bar{v}_{ip\cdot})^T$ with $\bar{v}_{ij\cdot} = \sum_{k=1}^{K_j - 1} v_{ij,k}/(K_j - 1)$, $j = r+1, \ldots, p$, and

$$\mathbf{\Psi}_M^{-1} = \begin{bmatrix} \mathbf{\Psi}_{\epsilon x}^{-1} & \mathbf{0} & \cdots & \mathbf{0} \\ \mathbf{0} & K_{r+1} - 1 & \cdots & 0 \\ \vdots & \vdots & \ddots & \vdots \\ \mathbf{0} & 0 & \cdots & K_p - 1 \end{bmatrix}.$$

The full conditional distribution $p(\boldsymbol{\theta}|\mathbf{X}_{\text{mis}}, \mathbf{V}_{\text{obs}}, \mathbf{V}_{\text{mis}}, \mathbf{\Omega}_1, \boldsymbol{\pi}, \mathbf{Z}, \mathbf{L}, \boldsymbol{\beta}, \mathbf{X}_{\text{obs}}, \mathbf{U}_{\text{obs}})$ is further partitioned into the following parts. Let $\mathbf{w}_i = (\mathbf{c}_i^T, \boldsymbol{\omega}_i^T)^T$, $\mathbf{g}_i = (\mathbf{d}_i^T, \boldsymbol{\omega}_i^T)^T$, $\mathbf{W} = (\mathbf{w}_1, \ldots, \mathbf{w}_n)$, $\mathbf{G} = (\mathbf{g}_1, \ldots, \mathbf{g}_n)$, $\mathbf{X} = (\mathbf{x}_1, \ldots, \mathbf{x}_n)$, and $\mathbf{Y}^* = (\mathbf{y}_1^*, \ldots, \mathbf{y}_n^*)$; and let $\mathbf{X}_j^T$ and $\mathbf{\Omega}_{1j}^T$ be the jth rows of $\mathbf{X}$ and $\mathbf{\Omega}_1$, respectively. Under the prior (11.24), the full conditional distributions are given as follows:

$$[\mathbf{\Lambda}_{yj}|\mathbf{Y}^*, \mathbf{\Omega}, \psi_{\epsilon xj}] \stackrel{D}{=} N[\mathbf{m}_{xj}, \psi_{\epsilon xj}\mathbf{\Sigma}_{xj}],\ [\psi_{\epsilon xj}^{-1}|\mathbf{Y}^*, \mathbf{\Omega}] \stackrel{D}{=} \text{Gamma}[n/2 + \alpha_{0\epsilon j}, \beta_{\epsilon xj}],$$
$$j = 1, \ldots, r,$$

$$[\mathbf{\Lambda}_{yj}|\mathbf{Y}^*, \mathbf{\Omega}] \stackrel{D}{=} N[\mathbf{m}_{vj}, \mathbf{\Sigma}_{vj}], \quad j = r+1, \ldots, p,$$

$$[\mathbf{\Lambda}_{\omega j}|\mathbf{\Omega}, \psi_{\delta j}] \stackrel{D}{=} N[\mathbf{m}_{\omega j}, \psi_{\delta j}\mathbf{\Sigma}_{\omega j}],\ [\psi_{\delta j}^{-1}|\mathbf{\Omega}] \stackrel{D}{=} \text{Gamma}[n/2 + \alpha_{0\delta j}, \beta_{\delta j}], \quad j = 1, \ldots, q_1,$$

where

$$\mathbf{m}_{xj} = \mathbf{\Sigma}_{xj}[\mathbf{H}_{0yj}^{-1}\mathbf{\Lambda}_{0yj} + \mathbf{W}\mathbf{X}_j], \quad \mathbf{\Sigma}_{xj} = (\mathbf{H}_{0yj}^{-1} + \mathbf{W}\mathbf{W}^T)^{-1},$$

$$\beta_{\epsilon xj} = \beta_{0\epsilon j} + [\mathbf{X}_j^T\mathbf{X}_j - \mathbf{m}_{xj}^T\mathbf{\Sigma}_{xj}^{-1}\mathbf{m}_{xj} + \mathbf{\Lambda}_{0yj}^T\mathbf{H}_{0yj}^{-1}\mathbf{\Lambda}_{0yj}]/2,$$

$$\mathbf{m}_{vj} = \mathbf{\Sigma}_{vj}[\mathbf{H}_{0yj}^{-1}\mathbf{\Lambda}_{0yj} + (K_j - 1)\mathbf{W}\bar{\mathbf{v}}_{(k)}], \quad \mathbf{\Sigma}_{vj} = [\mathbf{H}_{0yj}^{-1} + (K_j - 1)\mathbf{W}\mathbf{W}^T]^{-1},$$

$$\mathbf{m}_{\omega j} = \mathbf{\Sigma}_{\omega j}[\mathbf{H}_{0\omega j}^{-1}\mathbf{\Lambda}_{0\omega j} + \mathbf{G}\mathbf{\Omega}_{1j}], \quad \mathbf{\Sigma}_{\omega j} = (\mathbf{H}_{0\omega j}^{-1} + \mathbf{G}\mathbf{G}^T)^{-1},$$

$$\beta_{\delta j} = \beta_{0\delta j} + [\mathbf{\Omega}_{1j}^T\mathbf{\Omega}_{1j} - \mathbf{m}_{\omega j}^T\mathbf{\Sigma}_{\omega j}^{-1}\mathbf{m}_{\omega j} + \mathbf{\Lambda}_{0\omega j}^T\mathbf{H}_{0\omega j}^{-1}\mathbf{\Lambda}_{0\omega j}]/2,$$

with $\bar{\mathbf{v}}_{(k)} = (\bar{v}_{1k\cdot}, \ldots, \bar{v}_{nk\cdot})^T$.

To simulate $(\boldsymbol{\pi}, \mathbf{Z})$ from $p(\boldsymbol{\pi}, \mathbf{Z}|\mathbf{X}_{\text{mis}}, \mathbf{V}_{\text{obs}}, \mathbf{V}_{\text{mis}}, \mathbf{\Omega}_1, \boldsymbol{\theta}, \mathbf{L}, \boldsymbol{\beta}, \mathbf{X}_{\text{obs}}, \mathbf{U}_{\text{obs}})$, we draw $(\boldsymbol{\pi}_l, \mathbf{Z}_l)$ from $p(\boldsymbol{\pi}_l, \mathbf{Z}_l|\mathbf{X}_{\text{mis}}, \mathbf{V}_{\text{obs}}, \mathbf{V}_{\text{mis}}, \mathbf{\Omega}_1, \boldsymbol{\theta}, \mathbf{L}, \boldsymbol{\beta}, \mathbf{X}_{\text{obs}}, \mathbf{U}_{\text{obs}})$, for $l = 1, \ldots, q_2$. To simulate $(\boldsymbol{\pi}_l, \mathbf{Z}_l)$ from $p(\boldsymbol{\pi}_l, \mathbf{Z}_l|\mathbf{X}_{\text{mis}}, \mathbf{V}_{\text{obs}}, \mathbf{V}_{\text{mis}}, \mathbf{\Omega}_1, \boldsymbol{\theta}, \mathbf{L}, \boldsymbol{\beta}, \mathbf{X}_{\text{obs}}, \mathbf{U}_{\text{obs}})$, let $\mathbf{Z}_{-l} = \{\mathbf{Z}_1, \ldots, \mathbf{Z}_{l-1}, \mathbf{Z}_{l+1}, \ldots, \mathbf{Z}_{q_2}\}$, $\boldsymbol{\pi}_{-l} = \{\boldsymbol{\pi}_1, \ldots, \boldsymbol{\pi}_{l-1}, \boldsymbol{\pi}_{l+1}, \ldots, \boldsymbol{\pi}_{q_2}\}$, and $\mathbf{L}_{-l} = \{\mathbf{L}^1, \ldots, \mathbf{L}^{l-1}, \mathbf{L}^{l+1}, \ldots, \mathbf{L}^{q_2}\}$. Let $\{L_j^{l*}, j = 1, \ldots, n_l\}$ be the unique set of L_i^l values in $\mathbf{L}^l$, and $n_{jl} = \#\{i : L_i^l = L_j^{l*}\}$, the number of L_i^l equal to L_j^{l*}. Then

$$p(\boldsymbol{\pi}_l, \mathbf{Z}_l|\mathbf{X}_{\text{mis}}, \mathbf{V}_{\text{obs}}, \mathbf{V}_{\text{mis}}, \mathbf{\Omega}_1, \boldsymbol{\theta}, \mathbf{L}, \boldsymbol{\beta}, \mathbf{X}_{\text{obs}}, \mathbf{U}_{\text{obs}})$$
$$\propto \prod_{j=1}^{n_l} \left\{ p(Z_{L_j^{l*},l}|\mu_{zl}, \sigma_{zl}) \times \prod_{\{i:L_i^l = L_j^{l*}\}} p(\mathbf{y}_i^*|\boldsymbol{\eta}_i, \boldsymbol{\theta}, Z_{L_j^{l*},l}, \mathbf{L}_{-l}, \mathbf{Z}_{-l}) p(\boldsymbol{\eta}_i|\boldsymbol{\theta}, Z_{L_j^{l*},l}, \mathbf{L}_{-l}, \mathbf{Z}_{-l}) \right\}$$
$$\times\, p(\mathbf{Z}_{(-L^l),l}|\mu_{zl}, \sigma_{zl}) p(\mathbf{L}^l|\boldsymbol{\pi}_l) p(\boldsymbol{\pi}_l),$$

where $\mathbf{Z}_{(-L^l),l}$ corresponds to those values in $\mathbf{Z}_l$ excluding $\mathbf{Z}_{L^l,l} = \{Z_{L_1^{l*},l}, \ldots, Z_{L_{n_l}^{l*},l}\}$.

It can be shown that, for $j = 1, \ldots, n_l$,

$$Z_{L_j^{l*},l} \stackrel{D}{=} \begin{cases} N[\mu_{wjl}, \sigma_{wjl}]I\{(-\infty,\ 0]\}, & \text{if } L_j^{l*} \leq G, \\ N[\mu_{wjl}, \sigma_{wjl}]I\{(0,\ \infty)\}, & \text{if } L_j^{l*} > G, \end{cases}$$

where $\sigma_{wjl} = [\sigma_{zl}^{-1} + n_{jl}(\boldsymbol{\Lambda}_{\xi l}^T \boldsymbol{\Psi}_M^{-1} \boldsymbol{\Lambda}_{\xi l} + \boldsymbol{\Gamma}_l^T \boldsymbol{\Psi}_\delta^{-1} \boldsymbol{\Gamma}_l)]^{-1}$ and

$$\mu_{wjl} = \sigma_{wjl} \left\{ \boldsymbol{\Lambda}_{\xi l}^T \boldsymbol{\Psi}_M^{-1} \sum_{\{i: L_i^l = L_j^{l*}\}} \left(\bar{\mathbf{y}}_{i\cdot}^* - \mathbf{A}\mathbf{c}_i - \boldsymbol{\Lambda}_\eta \boldsymbol{\eta}_i - \sum_{\{l'=1:\ l' \neq l\}}^{q_2} \boldsymbol{\Lambda}_{\xi l'} \xi_{il'} \right) \right.$$

$$\left. + \boldsymbol{\Gamma}_l^T \boldsymbol{\Psi}_\delta^{-1} \sum_{\{i: L_i^l = L_j^{l*}\}} \left(\boldsymbol{\Pi}_0 \boldsymbol{\eta}_i - \mathbf{B}\mathbf{d}_i - \sum_{\{l'=1:\ l' \neq l\}}^{q_2} \boldsymbol{\Gamma}_{l'} \xi_{il'} \right) + \sigma_{zl}^{-1} \mu_{zl} \right\},$$

where $\boldsymbol{\Lambda}_{\xi l}$ and $\boldsymbol{\Gamma}_l$ are the lth columns of $\boldsymbol{\Lambda}_\xi$ and $\boldsymbol{\Gamma}$, respectively.

The components of $(\mathbf{Z}_{(-L^l),l} | \boldsymbol{\mu}_z, \boldsymbol{\Sigma}_z)$ are i.i.d. with the following distribution:

$$Z_{L_i^l,l} \stackrel{D}{=} \begin{cases} N[\mu_{zl}, \sigma_{zl}]I\{(-\infty,\ 0]\}, & L_i^l \leq G \text{ and } L_i^l \neq L_j^{l*},\ j = 1,\ \ldots, n_l, \\ N[\mu_{zl}, \sigma_{zl}]I\{(0,\ \infty)\}, & L_i^l > G \text{ and } L_i^l \neq L_j^{l*},\ j = 1,\ \ldots, n_l. \end{cases}$$

Let $n_{kl}^- = \#\{i : L_i^l = k, k \leq G\}$, $n_{kl}^+ = \#\{i : L_i^l = G + k, k \leq G\}$, $a_{kl}^- = 1 + n_{kl}^-$, $b_{kl}^- = M_l^- \alpha_l + \sum_{j=k+1}^G n_{jl}^-$, $a_{kl}^+ = 1 + n_{kl}^+$, and $b_{kl}^+ = M_l^+ \alpha_l + \sum_{j=k+1}^G n_{jl}^+$. The conditional distribution of $p(\boldsymbol{\pi}|\mathbf{L}, \boldsymbol{\alpha})$ can be obtained as follows:

$$\pi_{1l}^* = V_{1l}^*,$$

$$\pi_{kl}^* = (1 - V_{1l}^*) \ldots (1 - V_{k-1,l}^*) V_{kl}^*, \quad k = 2, \ldots, G - 1,$$

$$\pi_{Gl}^* = (1 - V_{1l}^*) \ldots (1 - V_{G-1,l}^*),$$

$$\pi_{G+1,l}^* = U_{1l}^*, \quad \pi_{G+k,l}^* = (1 - U_{1l}^*) \ldots (1 - U_{k-1,l}^*) U_{kl}^*, \quad k = 2, \ldots, G - 1,$$

$$\pi_{2G,l}^* = (1 - U_{1l}^*) \ldots (1 - U_{G-1,l}^*),$$

where $V_{kl}^* \stackrel{D}{=} \text{Beta}[a_{kl}^-, b_{kl}^-]$ and $U_{kl}^* \stackrel{D}{=} \text{Beta}[a_{kl}^+, b_{kl}^+]$.

To simulate $\mathbf{L}$ from $p(\mathbf{L}|\mathbf{X}_{\text{mis}}, \mathbf{V}_{\text{obs}}, \mathbf{V}_{\text{mis}}, \boldsymbol{\Omega}_1, \boldsymbol{\theta}, \boldsymbol{\pi}, \mathbf{Z}, \boldsymbol{\beta}, \mathbf{X}_{\text{obs}}, \mathbf{U}_{\text{obs}})$, we draw $\mathbf{L}^l = (L_1^l, \ldots, L_n^l)^T$ from $p(\mathbf{L}^l|\mathbf{X}_{\text{mis}}, \mathbf{V}_{\text{obs}}, \mathbf{V}_{\text{mis}}, \boldsymbol{\Omega}_1, \boldsymbol{\theta}, \boldsymbol{\pi}, \mathbf{Z}, \mathbf{L}_{-l}, \boldsymbol{\beta}, \mathbf{X}_{\text{obs}}, \mathbf{U}_{\text{obs}})$, $l = 1, \ldots, q_2$. It can be shown that the conditional distribution of $\mathbf{L}_i^l$ is given by

$$[\mathbf{L}_i^l|\mathbf{X}_{\text{mis}}, \mathbf{V}_{\text{obs}}, \mathbf{V}_{\text{mis}}, \boldsymbol{\Omega}_1, \boldsymbol{\theta}, \boldsymbol{\pi}, \mathbf{Z}, \mathbf{L}_{-l}, \boldsymbol{\beta}, \mathbf{X}_{\text{obs}}, \mathbf{U}_{\text{obs}}] \stackrel{D}{=} \sum_{k=1}^{2G} \tilde{\pi}_{kl}^* \delta_k(\cdot),$$

where $\tilde{\pi}_{kl}^* \propto \frac{1}{2}\pi_{kl} p(\mathbf{y}_i^*|\boldsymbol{\eta}_i, \boldsymbol{\theta}, Z_{kl}, \mathbf{Z}_{-l}) p(\boldsymbol{\eta}_i|\boldsymbol{\theta}, Z_{kl}, \mathbf{Z}_{-l})$, $k = 1, \ldots, 2G$, satisfying $\sum_{k=1}^{2G} \tilde{\pi}_{kl}^* = 1.0$.

Note that the conditional distribution $p(\boldsymbol{\beta}|\mathbf{X}_{\text{mis}}, \mathbf{V}_{\text{obs}}, \mathbf{V}_{\text{mis}}, \boldsymbol{\Omega}_1, \boldsymbol{\theta}, \boldsymbol{\pi}, \mathbf{Z}, \mathbf{L}, \mathbf{X}_{\text{obs}}, \mathbf{U}_{\text{obs}})$ only depends on $\boldsymbol{\pi}$ and $\mathbf{Z}$. To simulate $\boldsymbol{\beta}$, we draw $p(\boldsymbol{\alpha}|\boldsymbol{\mu}_z, \boldsymbol{\Sigma}_z, \boldsymbol{\pi}, \mathbf{Z})$ and $p(\boldsymbol{\mu}_z, \boldsymbol{\Sigma}_z|\boldsymbol{\alpha}, \boldsymbol{\pi}, \mathbf{Z})$. Moreover, $p(\boldsymbol{\alpha}|\boldsymbol{\mu}_z, \boldsymbol{\Sigma}_z, \boldsymbol{\pi}, \mathbf{Z}) = \prod_{l=1}^{q_2} p(\alpha_l|\boldsymbol{\mu}_z, \boldsymbol{\Sigma}_z, \boldsymbol{\pi})$, and

$$[\alpha_l|\boldsymbol{\mu}_z, \boldsymbol{\Sigma}_z, \boldsymbol{\pi}] \stackrel{D}{=} \text{Gamma}\left[2G - 2 + \tau_1, \tau_2 - M_l^- \sum_{k=1}^{G-1} \log\left(1 - V_{kl}^*\right) - M_l^+ \sum_{k=1}^{G-1} \log\left(1 - U_{kl}^*\right)\right].$$

It follows from (11.23) that $p(\boldsymbol{\mu}_z, \boldsymbol{\Sigma}_z|\boldsymbol{\alpha}, \mathbf{Z}, \boldsymbol{\pi})$ can be obtained as a product of the following $p(\mu_{zl}, \sigma_{zl}|\boldsymbol{\alpha}, \mathbf{Z}, \boldsymbol{\pi})$:

$$p(\mu_{zl}, \sigma_{zl}|\boldsymbol{\alpha}, \mathbf{Z}, \boldsymbol{\pi}) \propto \left(\prod_{i=1}^{2G} p(Z_{il}|\mu_{zl}, \sigma_{zl})p(\mu_{zl})p(\sigma_{zl})\right)\left(\prod_{i=1}^{G-1} p(V_{il}|\mu_{zl}, \sigma_{zl})p(U_{il}|\mu_{zl}, \sigma_{zl})\right). \tag{11.A12}$$

The MH algorithm can be used to draw observations from this target distribution. Under $\boldsymbol{\mu}_z = \mathbf{0}$ with $M_l^- = M_l^+ = 0.5$, (11.A12) does not involve $\boldsymbol{\pi}$, and the conditional distribution of σ_{zl} is given by

$$[\sigma_{zl}^{-1}|\mathbf{Z}] \overset{D}{=} \text{Gamma}\left[G + \rho_1, \rho_2 + \frac{1}{2}\sum_{i=1}^{2G} Z_{il}^2\right].$$

Finally, in the derivation of the full conditional distributions relating to $\boldsymbol{\mu}_z, \boldsymbol{\Sigma}_z$, it can be shown that

$$\begin{aligned}\log p(\mu_{zl}|\sigma_{zl}, \boldsymbol{\alpha}, \mathbf{Z}, \boldsymbol{\pi}) &\propto (G-1)[\log M_l^- + \log M_l^+] + \alpha_l[M_l^- \log \pi_{Gl} + M_l^+ \log \pi_{2G,l}] \\ &\quad \times \log p(\mu_{zl}|\sigma_M) + \sum_{i=1}^{2G} \log p(Z_{il}|\mu_{zl}, \sigma_{zl}), \\ \log p(\sigma_{zl}^{-1}|\mu_{zl}, \boldsymbol{\alpha}, \mathbf{Z}, \boldsymbol{\pi}) &\propto (G-1)[\log M_l^- + \log M_l^+] + \alpha_l[M_l^- \log \pi_{Gl} + M_l^+ \log \pi_{2G,l}] \\ &\quad \times \log p(\sigma_{zl}^{-1}|\rho_1, \rho_2) + \sum_{i=1}^{2G} \log p(Z_{il}|\mu_{zl}, \sigma_{zl}), \\ -\frac{d^2 \log p(\mu_{zl}|\sigma_{zl}, \mathbf{Z}, \boldsymbol{\pi})}{d\mu_{zl}^2}\bigg|_{\mu_{zl}=0} &= \sigma_{zl}^{-1}[2G + 4(G-1)/\pi] + \sigma_M^{-1}.\end{aligned}$$

In the implementation of the algorithm, we draw a candidate μ_{zl}^* from the proposal distribution $N(\cdot|\mu_{zl}, r\sigma_{zl})$ at the current values μ_{zl}, where r is a constant for adjusting the acceptance rate, accepting μ_{zl}^* with probability

$$\min\left\{1, \frac{p(\mu_{zl}^*|\sigma_{zl}, \boldsymbol{\alpha}, \mathbf{Z}, \boldsymbol{\pi})}{p(\mu_{zl}|\sigma_{zl}, \boldsymbol{\alpha}, \mathbf{Z}, \boldsymbol{\pi})}\right\}.$$

An independent sampler is used to sample σ_{zl}^{-1}. Specifically, draw σ_{zl}^{-1*} from $q(\cdot|\mu_{zl}, \mathbf{Z})$ with

$$q(\cdot|\mu_{zl}, \mathbf{Z}) \overset{D}{=} \text{Gamma}\left[G + \rho_1, \rho_2 + \frac{1}{2}\sum_{i=1}^{2G}(Z_{il} - \mu_{zl})^2\right],$$

accepting σ_{zl}^{-1*} with probability

$$\min\left\{1, \frac{p(\sigma_{zl}^{-1*}|\mu_{zl}, \boldsymbol{\alpha}, \mathbf{Z}, \boldsymbol{\pi})q(\sigma_{zl}^{-1}|\mu_{zl}, \mathbf{Z})}{p(\sigma_{zl}^{-1}|\mu_{zl}, \boldsymbol{\alpha}, \mathbf{Z}, \boldsymbol{\pi})q(\sigma_{zl}^{-1*}|\mu_{zl}, \mathbf{Z})}\right\}.$$

References

Albert, J. H. and Chib, S. (1993) Bayesian analysis of binary and polychotomous response data. *Journal of the American Statistical Association*, **88**, 669–679.

Chen, C. C., Lu, R. B., Chan, Y. C., Wang, M. F. Chang, Y. C., Li, Y. K. and Yin, S. J. (1999) Interaction between the functional polymorphisms of the alcohol-metabolism genes in protection against alcoholism. *American Journal of Human Genetics*, **65**, 795–807.

Cheng, S., Grow, M. A., Pallaud, C., Klitz, W., Erlich, H. A., Visvikis, S., Chen, J. J., Pullinger, C. R., Malloy, M. J., Siest, G. and Kane, J. P. (1999) A multilocus genotyping assay for candidate markers of cardiovascular disease risk. *Genome Research*, **9**, 936–949.

Dunson, D. B. (2000) Bayesian latent variable models for clustered mixed outcomes. *Journal of the Royal Statistical Society, Series B*, **62**, 355–366.

Doss H. (1985) Bayesian nonparametric estimation of the median, I: Computation of the estimates. *Annals of Statistics*, **13**, 1432–1444.

Gelman, A. and Meng, X. L. (1998) Simulating normalizing constants: From importance sampling to bridge sampling to path sampling. *Statistical Science*, **13**, 163–185.

Gelman, A., Meng, X. L. and Stern, H. (1996) Posterior predictive assessment of model fitness via realized discrepancies. *Statistica Sinica*, **6**, 733–807.

Geman, S. and Geman, D. (1984) Stochastic relaxation, Gibbs distributions, and the Bayesian restoration of images. *IEEE Transactions on Pattern Analysis and Machine Intelligence*, **6**, 721–741.

Geweke, J. (1991) Efficient simulation from the multivariate normal and Student-*t* distributions subject to linear constraints and the evaluation of constraint probabilities. In E. M. Keramidas and S. M. Kaufman (eds), *Computer Science and Statistics: Proceedings of the 23rd Symposium on the Interface*, pp. 571–578. Fairfax Station, VA: Interface Foundation.

Hastings, W. K. (1970) Monte Carlo sampling methods using Markov chains and their applications. *Biometrika*, **57**, 97–109.

Ibrahim, J. G., Chen, M. H. and Sinha, D. (2001) Criterion-based methods for Bayesian model assessment. *Statistica Sinica*, **11**, 419–443.

Imai, K. and van Dyk, D. A. (2005) A Bayesian analysis of the multinomial probit model using marginal data augmentation. *Journal of Econometrics*, **124**, 311–334.

Ishwaran, H. and James, L. F. (2001) Gibbs sampling methods for stick-breaking priors. *Journal of the American Statistical Association*, **96**, 161–173.

Kass, R. E. and Raftery, A. E. (1995) Bayes factors. *Journal of the American Statistical Association*, **90**, 773–795.

Kleinman, K. P. and Ibrahim, J. G. (1998) A semiparametric Bayesian approach to the random effects model. *Biometrics*, **54**, 921–938.

Kottas, A. and Gelfand, A. E. (2001) Bayesian semiparametric median regression modeling. *Journal of the American Statistical Association*, **96**, 1458–1468.

Lee, S. Y. (2007) *Structural Equation Modeling: A Bayesian Approach*. Chichester: John Wiley & Sons, Ltd.

Lee, S. Y. and Song, X. Y. (2003) Bayesian analysis of structural equation models with dichotomous variables. *Statistics in Medicine*, **22**, 3073–3088.

Lee, S. Y. and Song, X. Y. (2004) Maximum likelihood analysis of a general latent variable model with hierarchically mixed data. *Biometrics*, **60**, 624–636.

Lee, S. Y., Lu, B. and Song, X. Y. (2008) Semiparametric Bayesian analysis of structural equation models with fixed covariates. *Statistics in Medicine*, **27**, 2341–2360.

Little, R. J. A. and Rubin, D. B. (2002) *Statistical Analysis with Missing Data* (2nd edn). Hoboken, NJ: Wiley.

McCulloch, R. and Rossi, P. E. (1994) An exact likelihood analysis of the multinomial probit model. *Journal of Econometrics*, **64**, 207–240.

Meng, X. L. and Schilling, S. (1996) Fitting full-information item factor models and an empirical investigation of bridge sampling. *Journal of the American Statistical Association*, **91**, 1254–1267.

Metropolis, N., Rosenbluth, A. W., Rosenbluth, M. N., Teller, A. H. and Teller, E. (1953) Equations of state calculations by fast computing machines. *Journal of Chemical Physics*, **21**, 1087–1092.

Müller, P. and Rosner, G. (1997) A Bayesian population model with hierarchical mixture priors applied to blood count data. *Journal of the American Statistical Association*, **92**, 1279–1292.

Seaquist, E. R., Goetz, F. C., Rich, S. and Barbosa, J. (1989) Familial clustering of diabetic kidney disease: evidence for genetic susceptibility to diabetic nephropathy. *New England Journal of Medicine*, **320**, 1161–1165.

Sethuraman, J. (1994) A constructive definition of the Dirichlet priors. *Statistica Sinica*, **4**, 639–650.

Shi, J. Q. and Lee, S. Y. (2000) Latent variable models with mixed continuous and polytomous data. *Journal of the Royal Statistical Society, Series B*, **62**, 77–87.

Song, X. Y., Lee, S. Y., Ng, M. C. Y., So, W. Y. and Chan, J. C. N. (2007) Bayesian analysis of structural equation models with multinomial variable and an application to type 2 diabetic nephropathy. *Statistics in Medicine*, **26**, 2348–2369.

Song, X. Y., Xia, Y. M. and Lee, S. Y. (2009) Bayesian semiparametric analysis of structural equation models with mixed continuous and unordered categorical variables. *Statistics in Medicine*, **28**, 2253–2276.

12

Structural equation models with nonparametric structural equations

12.1 Introduction

In Chapters 10 and 11, we presented semiparametric SEMs in which the distributions of explanatory latent variables are assumed unknown, and the Bayesian approach with the stick-breaking prior and the blocked Gibbs sampler is used to model the unknown distributions of latent variables. Unlike the semiparametric modeling described in the previous chapter, this chapter presents another kind of SEM in which a nonparametric structural equation is used to model the functional relationships among latent variables and covariates. The Bayesian approach, together with a Bayesian analogue of P-splines, is used to estimate the nonparametric functions and unknown parameters in the model.

Nonparametric modeling with various smoothing techniques has been extensively developed in the statistics literature. Approaches to nonparametric modeling include – but are not limited to – smoothing splines (Green and Silverman, 1994), kernel methods with local polynomials (Fan and Gijbels, 1996; Fan and Zhang, 1999), and penalized splines (Ruppert *et al.*, 2003). More recently, due to some nice features of the Bayesian approach and its related powerful sampling-based tools, such as the Markov chain Monte Carlo (MCMC) techniques, the development of Bayesian methodology for the estimation of smooth functions has become both extensive and fruitful; see, for example, DiMatteo *et al.* (2001), Biller and Fahrmeir (2001), Behseta *et al.* (2005), and Panagiotelis and Smith (2008). In particular, Bayesian P-splines (Berry *et al.*, 2002; Lang and Brezger, 2004), which are basically a Bayesian approach to penalized splines, are appealing because they can flexibly fit an unknown smooth function using a large number of basis functions with a simple penalty on differences between

Basic and Advanced Bayesian Structural Equation Modeling: With Applications in the Medical and Behavioral Sciences,
First Edition. Xin-Yuan Song and Sik-Yum Lee.

coefficients of adjacent basis functions, and simultaneously estimate smooth functions and smoothing parameters. Fahrmeir and Raach (2007) applied the Bayesian P-splines approach to analyze a specific latent variable model, in which the structural equation includes observed covariates and spatial effects, but does not include any explanatory latent variable. As their focus was on observed covariates and spatial effects, relationships between latent variables were not involved in their model, and nonparametric smooth functions of the important latent variables were not accommodated in their structural equation. Hence, existing nonparametric methods cannot be applied to analyze functional relationships among latent variables.

To extend the applicability of SEMs, we introduce a nonparametric SEM, in which the important structural equation is formulated via unspecified smooth functions of latent variables, along with covariates if applicable. The nonparametric structural equation in the model can be regarded as a generalization of the ordinary nonparametric regression model with the new inclusion of unknown smooth functions of latent variables. The Bayesian P-splines approach, together with a MCMC algorithm will be introduced to estimate smooth functions, unknown parameters, and latent variables in the model.

12.2 Nonparametric SEMs with Bayesian P-splines

12.2.1 Model description

Let $\mathbf{y}_i = (y_{i1}, \ldots, y_{ip})^T$ be a random vector of observed variables and $\boldsymbol{\omega}_i = (\omega_{i1}, \ldots, \omega_{iq})^T$ be a random vector of latent variables for n observations, $p > q$. The relationship between $\mathbf{y}_i$ and $\boldsymbol{\omega}_i$ is given by the measurement equation

$$\mathbf{y}_i = \mathbf{A}\mathbf{c}_i + \boldsymbol{\Lambda}\boldsymbol{\omega}_i + \boldsymbol{\epsilon}_i, \tag{12.1}$$

where $\mathbf{c}_i$ is a vector of fixed covariates, $\mathbf{A}$ is a matrix of coefficients, $\boldsymbol{\Lambda}$ is the factor loading matrix, and $\boldsymbol{\epsilon}_i$ is a residual random vector which is independent of $\boldsymbol{\omega}_i$ and has a distribution $N[\mathbf{0}, \boldsymbol{\Psi}]$, in which $\boldsymbol{\Psi}$ is a diagonal matrix.

Based on the objective of the substantive study, the latent variables in $\boldsymbol{\omega}_i$ are distinguished into outcome and explanatory latent variables, then the functional effects of explanatory latent variables on the outcome latent variables are assessed by a nonparametric structural equation. For this purpose, $\boldsymbol{\omega}_i$ is partitioned as $(\boldsymbol{\eta}_i^T, \boldsymbol{\xi}_i^T)^T$, where $\boldsymbol{\eta}_i$ $(q_1 \times 1)$ and $\boldsymbol{\xi}_i$ $(q_2 \times 1)$ are outcome and explanatory latent vectors, respectively. It is assumed that the distribution of $\boldsymbol{\xi}_i$ is $N[\mathbf{0}, \boldsymbol{\Phi}]$, with a nondiagonal covariance matrix $\boldsymbol{\Phi}$. To assess the functional effects of $\boldsymbol{\xi}_i = (\xi_{i1}, \ldots, \xi_{iq_2})^T$ on $\boldsymbol{\eta}_i = (\eta_{i1}, \ldots, \eta_{iq_1})^T$, the following nonparametric structural equation (see Song and Lu, 2010) is used: for an arbitrary element η_{ih} in $\boldsymbol{\eta}_i$, $i = 1, \ldots, n$ and $h = 1, \ldots, q_1$,

$$\eta_{ih} = g_{h1}(x_{i1}) + \ldots + g_{hm}(x_{im}) + f_{h1}(\xi_{i1}) + \ldots + f_{hq_2}(\xi_{iq_2}) + \delta_{ih}, \tag{12.2}$$

where $x_{i1}, \ldots, x_{im}$ are fixed covariates that can be directly observed such as age and weight, $g_{h1}, \ldots, g_{hm}, f_{h1}, \ldots, f_{hq_2}$ are unspecified smooth functions with continuous second-order derivatives, and δ_{ih} is the residual error with a distribution $N[0, \psi_{\delta h}]$ and is independent of $\boldsymbol{\xi}_i$ and δ_{ij} for $j \neq h$. For notational simplicity, we suppress the subscript h in equation (12.2) by assuming $q_1 = 1$ in the subsequent sections. An extension to the case with $q_1 > 1$ is straightforward.

Fahrmeir and Raach (2007) developed an SEM which has a measurement equation similar to equation (12.1) but a different structural equation as follows:

$$\omega_{ih} = g_{h1}(x_{i1}) + \ldots + g_{hm}(x_{im}) + g_{h,\text{spat}}(e_i) + \boldsymbol{\Gamma}_h^T\mathbf{u}_i + \delta_{ih}, \tag{12.3}$$

where ω_{ih} is the hth component of $\boldsymbol{\omega}_i$, $g_{h1}, \ldots, g_{hm}$ are nonparametric smooth functions of fixed covariates $x_{i1}, \ldots, x_{im}$, $g_{h,\text{spat}}$ is a spatial effect of the location e_i, $\mathbf{u}_i$ is another vector of fixed covariates, $\boldsymbol{\Gamma}_h$ is the vector of regression coefficients, and δ_{ih} is the random error with variance 1.0 and is independent of δ_{ij} for $j \neq h$. The current model with structural equation (12.2) is different from that of Fahrmeir and Raach (2007) with structural equation (12.3) in various respects. First, their model focused on the effects of fixed covariates and a spatial effect of a given location, involved no partition of $\boldsymbol{\omega}_i$ into outcome latent vector $\boldsymbol{\eta}_i$ and explanatory latent vector $\boldsymbol{\xi}_i$, and their structural equation did not involve explanatory latent variables $\xi_{i1}, \ldots, \xi_{iq_2}$. As a result, neither parametric nor nonparametric effects related to latent variables can be assessed by their approach. Second, the covariance matrix of their latent vector $\boldsymbol{\omega}_i$ was assumed to be an identity matrix. In our model, the covariance matrices of $\boldsymbol{\xi}_i$ and $\boldsymbol{\omega}_i$ can be nondiagonal. As latent variables in practical applications are usually correlated, it is important to be able to accommodate nondiagonal covariance matrices. Third, due to the presence of explanatory latent variables in the nonparametric structural equation (12.2), some extra computational difficulties are encountered in estimating unknown smooth functions of latent variables. In Section 12.2.3 some methodologies for solving these difficulties are illustrated; see also Song and Lu (2010).

12.2.2 General formulation of the Bayesian P-splines

In the analysis of the nonparametric SEM defined by equations (12.1) and (12.2), modeling smooth nonparametric functions is an important issue. Because of the nice features of Bayesian P-splines (see Lang and Brezger, 2004) and the advantages of the Bayesian approach in analyzing SEMs (see Dunson, 2000; Lee, 2007), we use the Bayesian P-splines approach. To present the basic ideas, we first consider the simple case of

$$\eta_i = f(\xi_i) + \delta_i, \tag{12.4}$$

and then extend it to the more general case as defined by equation (12.2). We make the common assumption that $f(\xi_i)$ has a continuous second-order derivative and can be modeled by a sum of B-splines (De Boor, 1978) basis with a series of knots in the domain of ξ_i as follows:

$$f(\xi_i) = \sum_{k=1}^{K} \beta_k B_k(\xi_i), \tag{12.5}$$

where K is the number of splines determined by the number of knots, β_k is an unknown parameter, and $B_k(\cdot)$ is a B-spline of appropriate order. A common choice is the cubic B-spline. In practice, a choice of K in the range of 10 to 30 provides flexibility of fitting. To prevent overfitting due to the use of a relatively large number of knots, Eilers and Marx (1996) proposed using a difference penalty on coefficients of adjacent B-splines. More specifically, the following expression is minimized:

$$\sum_{i=1}^{n} \left(\eta_i - \sum_{k=1}^{K} \beta_k B_k(\xi_i) \right)^2 + \lambda \sum_{k=m+1}^{K} (\Delta^m \beta_k)^2, \tag{12.6}$$

where λ is a smoothing parameter to control the penalty, and $\Delta^m \beta_k$ is the difference penalty defined in a recursive manner by $\Delta^m \beta_k = \Delta^{m-1} \beta_k - \Delta^{m-1} \beta_{k-1}$ (e.g. $\Delta \beta_k = \beta_k - \beta_{k-1}$, $\Delta^2 \beta_k = \Delta \beta_k - \Delta \beta_{k-1} = \beta_k - 2\beta_{k-1} + \beta_{k-2}$). It can be shown that (12.6) can be expressed as

$$\sum_{i=1}^{n}\left(\eta_i - \sum_{k=1}^{K} \beta_k B_k(\xi_i)\right)^2 + \lambda \boldsymbol{\beta}^T \mathbf{M} \boldsymbol{\beta}, \tag{12.7}$$

where $\boldsymbol{\beta} = (\beta_1, \ldots, \beta_K)^T$, and $\mathbf{M}$ is the penalty matrix that is obtained with the specified difference penalty.

In the Bayesian framework (Lang and Brezger, 2004), coefficients β_k are treated as random and the difference penalty in (12.7) is replaced by its stochastic analogue, $\beta_k = \beta_{k-1} + u_k$, where u_k is i.i.d. $N[0, \tau_\beta]$. With this model framework, the amount of smoothness is controlled by the additional variance parameter τ_β, which corresponds to the inverse of smoothing parameter λ in (12.7). Consequently, τ_β can be regarded as a new smoothing parameter. Let $K^* = \text{rank}(\mathbf{M})$; the complete-data log-likelihood based on (12.5) is

$$-\frac{1}{2}\left[\frac{1}{\psi_\delta}\sum_{i=1}^{n}\left\{\eta_i - \sum_{k=1}^{K}\beta_k B_k(\xi_i)\right\}^2 + \frac{1}{\tau_\beta}\boldsymbol{\beta}^T\mathbf{M}\boldsymbol{\beta}\right] - \frac{n}{2}\log(\psi_\delta) - \frac{K^*}{2}\log(\tau_\beta) + \text{constant}. \tag{12.8}$$

The above approach can be applied to the more general situation defined by (12.2). By using the sum of B-splines basis in (12.5) to model each of the smooth nonparametric functions, the structural equation (12.2) is reformulated as

$$\eta_i = \sum_{j=1}^{m}\sum_{k=1}^{K_{bj}} b_{jk}B_{jk}^x(x_{ij}) + \sum_{j=1}^{q_2}\sum_{k=1}^{K_j}\beta_{jk}B_{jk}(\xi_{ij}) + \delta_i, \tag{12.9}$$

and the corresponding complete-data log-likelihood is

$$-\frac{1}{2}\left[\frac{1}{\psi_\delta}\sum_{i=1}^{n}\left\{\eta_i - \sum_{j=1}^{m}\sum_{k=1}^{K_{bj}} b_{jk}B_{jk}^x(x_{ij}) - \sum_{j=1}^{q_2}\sum_{k=1}^{K_j}\beta_{jk}B_{jk}(\xi_{ij})\right\}^2 + \sum_{j=1}^{m}\frac{1}{\tau_{bj}}\mathbf{b}_j^T\mathbf{M}_{bj}\mathbf{b}_j\right.$$

$$\left. + \sum_{j=1}^{q_2}\frac{1}{\tau_{\beta j}}\boldsymbol{\beta}_j^T\mathbf{M}_{\beta j}\boldsymbol{\beta}_j\right] - \frac{n}{2}\log(\psi_\delta) - \sum_{j=1}^{m}\frac{K_{bj}^*}{2}\log(\tau_{bj}) - \sum_{j=1}^{q_2}\frac{K_j^*}{2}\log(\tau_{\beta j}) + \text{constant}, \tag{12.10}$$

where $\{b_{jk}, B_{jk}^x, \mathbf{b}_j, \mathbf{M}_{bj}, K_{bj}^*, \tau_{bj}\}$ and $\{\beta_{jk}, B_{jk}, \mathbf{M}_{\beta j}, K_j, \tau_{\beta j}\}$ are defined similarly to $\{\beta_k, B_k, \mathbf{M}, K^*, \tau_\beta\}$ in (12.8).

12.2.3 Modeling nonparametric functions of latent variables

The modeling of nonparametric functions of latent variables is a major challenge. Compared with the existing literature, some additional difficulties will be encountered in the current analysis involving nonparametric smooth functions of latent variables.

First, traditional B-splines are defined in finite intervals. This induces some difficulties since observations of the latent variables obtained in MCMC iterations may be outside these intervals. To tackle this problem, we consider the B-spline basis for natural cubic splines: $N_{jk}(\xi_{ij})$, $1 \leq k \leq K_j$, $1 \leq j \leq q_2$. Suppose $(\kappa_{j1}, \kappa_{j2}, \ldots, \kappa_{j,K_j-1}, \kappa_{jK_j})$ are the knots and $(\kappa_{j1}, \kappa_{jK_j})$ are the boundary knots. Each $N_{jk}(\xi_{ij})$ is a piecewise cubic spline which smoothly joins at knots. This property is similar to B-splines inside the boundaries. Moreover, in $(-\infty, \kappa_{j1})$ and (κ_{jK_j}, ∞), $N_{jk}(\xi_{ij})$ is linear and smoothly joins at κ_{j1} and κ_{jK_j} with the part inside the boundaries. Hence, $\sum_{k=1}^{K_j} \beta_{jk} N_{jk}(\xi_{ij})$ is used to model the unknown smooth function $f_j(\xi_{ij})$. Even if some ξ_{ij} generated in a MCMC iteration exceed the boundaries, $\sum_{j=1}^{q_2} \sum_{k=1}^{K_j} \beta_{jk} N_{jk}(\xi_{ij})$ is still well defined. Thus, the formulation in (12.9) is modified as

$$\eta_i = \sum_{j=1}^{m} \sum_{k=1}^{K_{bj}} b_{jk} B_{jk}^x(x_{ij}) + \sum_{j=1}^{q_2} \sum_{k=1}^{K_j} \beta_{jk} N_{jk}(\xi_{ij}) + \delta_i. \tag{12.11}$$

The second difficulty is caused by the unknown scales of latent variables, which makes it impossible to determine the range of a latent variable and the positions of the knots beforehand. To solve this problem, for each ξ_{ij} we choose the product of a free scale parameter s_j and fixed quantiles of $N[0, 1]$ as knots. For example, if the quantiles are $(\kappa_1, \kappa_2, \ldots, \kappa_{K_j})$, then the knots for constructing $\{N_{jk}(\xi_{ij})\}_{1 \le k \le K_j}$ are $(s_j\kappa_1, s_j\kappa_2, \ldots, s_j\kappa_{K_j})$. Now, as the $\{N_{jk}(\xi_{ij})\}_{1 \le k \le K_j}$ depend on the scale parameter s_j, the formulation in (12.11) should be further modified as

$$\eta_i = \sum_{j=1}^{m} \sum_{k=1}^{K_{bj}} b_{jk} B_{jk}^x(x_{ij}) + \sum_{j=1}^{q_2} \sum_{k=1}^{K_j} \beta_{jk} N_{jk}(\xi_{ij}|s_j) + \delta_i. \tag{12.12}$$

The third difficulty is related to the fact that each function $f_j(\xi_{ij})$, $j = 1, \ldots, q_2$, is not identified up to a constant. Inspired by Panagiotelis and Smith (2008) in a simpler nonparametric regression context, we solve this problem by imposing a constraint on $\boldsymbol{\beta}_j$. Denote $\mathbf{F}_j = (f_j(\xi_{1j}), f_j(\xi_{2j}), \ldots, f_j(\xi_{nj}))^T$ and $\mathbf{1}_n$ be an $n \times 1$ vector of 1s. In each MCMC iteration, we let $\mathbf{1}_n^T \mathbf{F}_j = 0$. It can be shown that this is equivalent to $\mathbf{1}_n^T \mathbf{N}_j \boldsymbol{\beta}_j = 0$, where $\mathbf{N}_j = [N_{jk}(\xi_{ij}|s_j)]_{n \times K_j}$ is a matrix in which the elements are the B-spline basis of natural cubic splines. Let $\mathbf{Q}_j = \mathbf{1}_n^T \mathbf{N}_j$; then the above constraint can be written as $\mathbf{Q}_j \boldsymbol{\beta}_j = 0$. A similar constraint will also be imposed on $\mathbf{b}_j$ to identify nonparametric functions $g_j(x_{ij})$, $j = 1, \ldots, m$. Let $\mathbf{B}_{bj} = [B_{jk}^x(x_{ij})]_{n \times K_{bj}}$ and $\mathbf{Q}_{bj} = \mathbf{1}_n^T \mathbf{B}_{bj}$; then the constraint on $\mathbf{b}_j$ can be written as $\mathbf{Q}_{bj} \mathbf{b}_j = 0$.

12.2.4 Prior distributions

First, we hope to control the scale parameter s_j such that it is not too small or too large. If s_j is too small, many generated samples of ξ_{ij} may fall outside the boundary knots $(s_j\kappa_1, s_j\kappa_{K_j})$. As discussed in Section 12.2.3, natural cubic splines are defined with linear functions outside the boundary knots. As a result, the nonlinear function of ξ_{ij}, $f_j(\xi_{ij})$, would be estimated by a linear function over a large range of ξ_{ij}, leading to a poor estimation of $f_j(\xi_{ij})$. If s_j is too large, the generated sample of ξ_{ij} would vary within a small part of a large range, leading to many spline knots being wasted. Consequently, the remaining knots may not be enough to accurately estimate the unknown function of ξ_{ij}. For this purpose, inspired by the form of normal distribution in (12.14) and (12.17) below, we propose the prior distribution of $\mathbf{S} = (s_1, \ldots, s_{q_2})^T$ as follows:

$$p(\mathbf{S}|\tau_{s1}, \ldots, \tau_{sq_2}) = \prod_{j=1}^{q_2} \frac{1}{(2\pi\tau_{sj})^{K_j/2}} \exp\left[-\frac{1}{2\tau_{sj}} \sum_{k=1}^{K_j} \{\log(|s_j\kappa_k|)\}^2 \right], \tag{12.13}$$

where κ_k is the kth quantile of $N[0, 1]$. The prior distribution in (12.13) is equivalent to penalizing $\{s_1, \ldots, s_{q_2}\}$ with the penalty $\sum_{j=1}^{q_2} \sum_{k=1}^{K_j} [\log(|s_j\kappa_k|)]^2/(2\tau_{sj})$. Based on (12.13), we have

$$\log p(\mathbf{S}|\cdot) = -\frac{1}{2\psi_\delta}\left[\sum_{i=1}^{n}\left\{\eta_i - \sum_{j=1}^{m}\sum_{k=1}^{K_{bj}} b_{jk}B_{jk}^x(x_{ij}) - \sum_{j=1}^{q_2}\sum_{k=1}^{K_j}\beta_{jk}N_{jk}(\xi_{ij}|s_j)\right\}^2\right]$$
$$-\frac{1}{2}\sum_{j=1}^{q_2}\sum_{k=1}^{K_j}\frac{\{\log(|s_j\kappa_k|)\}^2}{\tau_{sj}} + \text{constant},$$

which consists of a quadratic term and a penalty term. A too small or too large s_j results in a large penalty and a small $\log p(\mathbf{S}|\cdot)$. Hence, for a given τ_{sj}, it is less likely to draw a too small or too large scale parameter s_j under prior distribution (12.13). Here, τ_{sj} is an unknown parameter for determining the amount of penalty put on s_j, and it plays a similar role to $\tau_{\beta j}$ and τ_{bj} in the prior distributions specified in (12.14) and (12.17) below. As we never know the true scales of latent variables, this unknown parameter can help to capture the information from the data and thus automatically updates the amount of penalty on s_j in the MCMC iterations.

Second, to identify the unspecified smooth function $f_j(\xi_{ij})$, the identifiability constraint $\mathbf{Q}_j\boldsymbol{\beta}_j = 0$ should be imposed on $\boldsymbol{\beta}_j$. Under this constraint, the prior distribution of the unknown parameter $\boldsymbol{\beta}_j$ is assigned as

$$p(\boldsymbol{\beta}_j|\tau_{\beta j}) \propto \exp\left\{-\frac{1}{2\tau_{\beta j}}\boldsymbol{\beta}_j^T\mathbf{M}_{\beta j}\boldsymbol{\beta}_j\right\} I(\mathbf{Q}_j\boldsymbol{\beta}_j = 0), \tag{12.14}$$

with appropriate penalty matrix $\mathbf{M}_{\beta j}$, which is a linearly constrained Gaussian density. The prior distribution given in (12.14) is a conjugate type because the posterior distribution of $\boldsymbol{\beta}_j$ given others is still linearly constrained Gaussian with the density

$$N[\boldsymbol{\beta}_j^*, \boldsymbol{\Sigma}_j^*]I(\mathbf{Q}_j\boldsymbol{\beta}_j = 0), \tag{12.15}$$

where $\boldsymbol{\Sigma}_j^* = (\mathbf{N}_j^T\mathbf{N}_j/\psi_\delta + \mathbf{M}_{\beta j}/\tau_{\beta j})^{-1}$, $\boldsymbol{\beta}_j^* = \boldsymbol{\Sigma}_j^*\mathbf{N}_j^T\boldsymbol{\eta}^*/\psi_\delta$, and $\boldsymbol{\eta}^* = (\eta_1^*, \ldots, \eta_n^*)^T$, in which

$$\eta_i^* = \eta_i - \sum_{j=1}^{m}\sum_{k=1}^{K_{bj}} b_{jk}B_{jk}^x(x_{ij}) - \sum_{l\neq j}\sum_{k=1}^{K_l}\beta_{lk}N_{lk}(\xi_{il}|s_l).$$

According to Panagiotelis and Smith (2008), sampling an observation $\boldsymbol{\beta}_j$ from (12.15) is equivalent to sampling an observation $\boldsymbol{\beta}_j^{(\text{new})}$ from $N[\boldsymbol{\beta}_j^*, \boldsymbol{\Sigma}_j^*]$; then $\boldsymbol{\beta}_j^{(\text{new})}$ is transformed to $\boldsymbol{\beta}_j$ by

$$\boldsymbol{\beta}_j = \boldsymbol{\beta}_j^{(\text{new})} - \boldsymbol{\Sigma}_j^*\mathbf{Q}_j^T\left(\mathbf{Q}_j\boldsymbol{\Sigma}_j^*\mathbf{Q}_j^T\right)^{-1}\mathbf{Q}_j\boldsymbol{\beta}_j^{(\text{new})}. \tag{12.16}$$

Similarly, under the identifiability constraint $\mathbf{Q}_{bj}\mathbf{b}_j = 0$, the prior distribution of the unknown parameter $\mathbf{b}_j$ is assigned as

$$p(\mathbf{b}_j|\tau_{bj}) \propto \exp\left\{-\frac{1}{2\tau_{bj}}\mathbf{b}_j^T\mathbf{M}_{bj}\mathbf{b}_j\right\} I(\mathbf{Q}_{bj}\mathbf{b}_j = 0), \tag{12.17}$$

and the posterior distribution of $\mathbf{b}_j$ given others is

$$N[\mathbf{b}_j^*, \boldsymbol{\Sigma}_{bj}^*]I(\mathbf{Q}_{bj}\mathbf{b}_j = 0), \tag{12.18}$$

where $\boldsymbol{\Sigma}^*_{bj} = (\mathbf{B}^T_{bj}\mathbf{B}_{bj}/\psi_\delta + \mathbf{M}_{bj}/\tau_{bj})^{-1}$, $\mathbf{b}^*_j = \boldsymbol{\Sigma}^*_{bj}\mathbf{B}^T_{bj}\boldsymbol{\eta}^*_x/\psi_\delta$, and $\boldsymbol{\eta}^*_x = (\eta^*_{x1}, \ldots, \eta^*_{xn})^T$, in which

$$\eta^*_{xi} = \eta_i - \sum_{l \neq j}\sum_{k=1}^{K_{bl}} b_{lk}B^x_{lk}(x_{il}) - \sum_{j=1}^{q_2}\sum_{k=1}^{K_j} \beta_{jk}N_{jk}(\xi_{ij}|s_j).$$

Moreover, in a full Bayesian analysis, the inverse smooth parameters τ_{bj}, $\tau_{\beta j}$, and τ_{sj} are also treated as random and estimated simultaneously with the unknown $\mathbf{b}_j$, $\boldsymbol{\beta}_j$, and s_j. According to common practice in the literature (see, for example, Lang and Brezger, 2004; Fahrmeir and Raach, 2007; and references therein), highly dispersed (but proper) inverted gamma priors are assigned to these parameters:

$$\begin{aligned} &\tau_{bj}^{-1} \stackrel{D}{=} \text{Gamma}[\alpha_{0b}, \beta_{0b}], \quad j = 1, \ldots, m, \\ &\tau_{\beta j}^{-1} \stackrel{D}{=} \text{Gamma}[\alpha_{0\beta}, \beta_{0\beta}], \ \tau_{sj}^{-1} \stackrel{D}{=} \text{Gamma}[\alpha_{0\tau}, \beta_{0\tau}], \quad j = 1, \ldots, q_2, \end{aligned} \tag{12.19}$$

where α_{0b}, β_{0b}, $\alpha_{0\beta}$, $\beta_{0\beta}$, $\alpha_{0\tau}$, and $\beta_{0\tau}$ are hyperparameters whose values are preassigned. The common choices for these hyperparameters are $\alpha_{0b} = \alpha_{0\beta} = \alpha_{0\tau} = 1$, and β_{0b}, $\beta_{0\beta}$, and $\beta_{0\tau}$ are small. Throughout this chapter we set $\alpha_{0b} = \alpha_{0\beta} = \alpha_{0\tau} = 1$ and $\beta_{0b} = \beta_{0\beta} = \beta_{0\tau} = 0.005$.

Finally, for structural parameters such as $\mathbf{A}$, $\boldsymbol{\Lambda}$, $\boldsymbol{\Psi}$, ψ_δ, and $\boldsymbol{\Phi}$, the following conjugate prior distributions are assigned according to common practice in SEMs: for $j = 1, \ldots, p$,

$$\begin{aligned} &[\boldsymbol{\Lambda}_j|\psi_j] \stackrel{D}{=} N[\boldsymbol{\Lambda}_{0j}, \psi_j\boldsymbol{\Sigma}_{0j}], \quad \psi_j^{-1} \stackrel{D}{=} \text{Gamma}[\alpha_{0j}, \beta_{0j}], \\ &\mathbf{A}_j \stackrel{D}{=} N[\mathbf{A}_{0j}, \boldsymbol{\Sigma}_{0aj}], \quad \psi_\delta^{-1} \stackrel{D}{=} \text{Gamma}[\alpha_{0\delta}, \beta_{0\delta}], \quad \boldsymbol{\Phi}^{-1} \stackrel{D}{=} W[\mathbf{R}_0, \rho_0], \end{aligned} \tag{12.20}$$

where $\mathbf{A}^T_j$ and $\boldsymbol{\Lambda}^T_j$ are the jth row of $\mathbf{A}$ and $\boldsymbol{\Lambda}$ respectively, ψ_j is the jth diagonal element of $\boldsymbol{\Psi}$, and $\mathbf{A}_{0j}$, $\boldsymbol{\Lambda}_{0j}$, α_{0j}, β_{0j}, $\alpha_{0\delta}$, $\beta_{0\delta}$, ρ_0, and positive definite matrices $\boldsymbol{\Sigma}_{0aj}$, $\boldsymbol{\Sigma}_{0j}$, and $\mathbf{R}_0$ are hyperparameters whose values are assumed to be given by the prior information.

12.2.5 Posterior inference via Markov chain Monte Carlo sampling

Let $\mathbf{Y} = (\mathbf{y}_1, \ldots, \mathbf{y}_n)$, $\boldsymbol{\Omega} = (\boldsymbol{\omega}_1, \ldots, \boldsymbol{\omega}_n)$, $\boldsymbol{\Omega}_1 = (\eta_1, \ldots, \eta_n)$, $\boldsymbol{\Omega}_2 = (\boldsymbol{\xi}_1, \ldots, \boldsymbol{\xi}_n)$, $\mathbf{b} = (\mathbf{b}_1, \ldots, \mathbf{b}_m)$, $\boldsymbol{\beta} = (\boldsymbol{\beta}_1, \ldots, \boldsymbol{\beta}_{q_2})$, $\mathbf{S} = (s_1, \ldots, s_{q_2})$, $\boldsymbol{\tau}_b = (\tau_{b1}, \ldots, \tau_{bm})$, $\boldsymbol{\tau}_\beta = (\tau_{\beta 1}, \ldots, \tau_{\beta q_2})$, $\boldsymbol{\tau}_s = (\tau_{s1}, \ldots, \tau_{sq_2})$, and $\boldsymbol{\theta} = \{\mathbf{A}, \boldsymbol{\Lambda}, \boldsymbol{\Psi}, \psi_\delta, \boldsymbol{\Phi}, \boldsymbol{\tau}_b, \boldsymbol{\tau}_\beta, \boldsymbol{\tau}_s, \mathbf{b}, \boldsymbol{\beta}, \mathbf{S}\}$. The Bayesian estimate of $\boldsymbol{\theta}$ is obtained using observations drawn from $p(\boldsymbol{\Omega}, \boldsymbol{\theta}|\mathbf{Y})$ with MCMC tools such as the Gibbs sampler (Geman and Geman, 1984) and the Metropolis–Hastings algorithm (Metropolis *et al.*, 1953; Hastings, 1970). The computing algorithm in our method is implemented as follows. At the $(t+1)$th iteration with current values $\{\boldsymbol{\Omega}^{(t)}, \boldsymbol{\theta}^{(t)}\}$:

(a) Draw $\boldsymbol{\Omega}^{(t+1)}$ from $[\boldsymbol{\Omega}|\mathbf{Y}, \mathbf{A}^{(t)}, \boldsymbol{\Lambda}^{(t)}, \boldsymbol{\Psi}^{(t)}, \psi_\delta^{(t)}, \boldsymbol{\Phi}^{(t)}, \mathbf{b}^{(t)}, \boldsymbol{\beta}^{(t)}, \mathbf{S}^{(t)}]$.

(b) Draw $\boldsymbol{\theta}^{(t+1)}$ from $[\boldsymbol{\theta}|\mathbf{Y}, \boldsymbol{\Omega}^{(t+1)}]$. Due to its complexity, step (b) is further decomposed into the following substeps:

(b1) Draw $\mathbf{A}^{(t+1)}$ from $[\mathbf{A}|\mathbf{Y}, \boldsymbol{\Omega}^{(t+1)}, \boldsymbol{\Lambda}^{(t)}, \boldsymbol{\Psi}^{(t)}]$.

(b2) Draw $(\boldsymbol{\Lambda}^{(t+1)}, \boldsymbol{\Psi}^{(t+1)})$ from $[\boldsymbol{\Lambda}, \boldsymbol{\Psi}|\mathbf{Y}, \boldsymbol{\Omega}^{(t+1)}, \mathbf{A}^{(t+1)}]$.

(b3) Draw $\psi_\delta^{(t+1)}$ from $[\psi_\delta|\boldsymbol{\Omega}^{(t+1)}, \mathbf{b}^{(t)}, \boldsymbol{\beta}^{(t)}, \mathbf{S}^{(t)}]$.

(b4) Draw $\boldsymbol{\Phi}^{(t+1)}$ from $[\boldsymbol{\Phi}|\boldsymbol{\Omega}_2^{(t+1)}]$.

(b5) Draw $\boldsymbol{\tau}_b^{(t+1)}$ from $[\boldsymbol{\tau}_b|\mathbf{b}^{(t)}]$, $\boldsymbol{\tau}_\beta^{(t+1)}$ from $[\boldsymbol{\tau}_\beta|\boldsymbol{\beta}^{(t)}]$, and $\boldsymbol{\tau}_s^{(t+1)}$ from $[\boldsymbol{\tau}_s|\mathbf{S}^{(t)}]$.

(b6) Draw $\mathbf{b}^{(t+1)}$ from $[\mathbf{b}|\boldsymbol{\Omega}^{(t+1)}, \psi_\delta^{(t+1)}, \boldsymbol{\tau}_b^{(t+1)}, \boldsymbol{\beta}^{(t)}, \mathbf{S}^{(t)}]$.

(b7) Draw $(\boldsymbol{\beta}^{(t+1)}, \mathbf{S}^{(t+1)})$ from $[\boldsymbol{\beta}, \mathbf{S}|\boldsymbol{\Omega}^{(t+1)}, \psi_\delta^{(t+1)}, \boldsymbol{\tau}_\beta^{(t+1)}, \boldsymbol{\tau}_s^{(t+1)}, \mathbf{b}^{(t+1)}]$.

The conditional distributions involved in steps (b1)–(b6) are normal, truncated normal, inverted gamma, and inverted Wishart, respectively. Simulating observations from them is standard (see Lee, 2007). However, the conditional distributions involved in steps (a) and (b7) are nonstandard and need to be derived. The MH algorithm is used to simulate observations from these nonstandard distributions. All the full conditional distributions and the implementation of the MH algorithm are given in Appendix 12.1.

12.2.6 Simulation study

The main purpose of this simulation study is to illustrate the empirical performance of the approach presented. The data set is obtained on the basis of the model defined by (12.1) and (12.2) with $p = 12$, $q = 4$, $q_1 = 1$, $q_2 = 3$, and $m = 1$. For $i = 1, \ldots, 300$, the covariate c_i is fixed at 1.0 such that $\mathbf{A}^T = (a_1, \ldots, a_{12})$ is a vector of intercepts, the covariate x_i is independently drawn from $N[0, 1]$, and the latent vector $\boldsymbol{\xi}_i = (\xi_{i1}, \xi_{i2}, \xi_{i3})^T$ is drawn from $N[\mathbf{0}, \boldsymbol{\Phi}]$. The structure of the loading matrix is

$$\boldsymbol{\Lambda}^T = \begin{bmatrix} 1 & \lambda_{21} & \lambda_{31} & 0 & 0 & 0 & 0 & 0 & 0 & 0 & 0 & 0 \\ 0 & 0 & 0 & 1 & \lambda_{52} & \lambda_{62} & 0 & 0 & 0 & 0 & 0 & 0 \\ 0 & 0 & 0 & 0 & 0 & 0 & 1 & \lambda_{83} & \lambda_{93} & 0 & 0 & 0 \\ 0 & 0 & 0 & 0 & 0 & 0 & 0 & 0 & 0 & 1 & \lambda_{11,4} & \lambda_{12,4} \end{bmatrix},$$

where the 1s and 0s are fixed parameters to give an identified model, and the λ_{kj} are unknown parameters. The nonparametric structural equation is

$$\eta_i = g(x_i) + f_1(\xi_{i1}) + f_2(\xi_{i2}) + f_3(\xi_{i3}) + \delta_i, \qquad (12.21)$$

with $g(x_i) = (x_i/2)^3$, $f_1(\xi_{i1}) = \sin(1.5\xi_{i1}) - \xi_{i1}$, $f_2(\xi_{i2}) = 1.65 - \exp(\xi_{i2})$, and $f_3(\xi_{i3}) = -0.5 + \exp(2\xi_{i3})/[1 + \exp(2\xi_{i3})]$. The true population values are taken as $a_j = 0.5$, $\psi_j = \psi_\delta = 0.3$, $j = 1, \ldots, 12$, $\lambda_{21} = \lambda_{31} = \lambda_{52} = \lambda_{62} = \lambda_{83} = \lambda_{93} = \lambda_{11,4} = \lambda_{12,4} = 0.8$, and $\{\phi_{11}, \phi_{12}, \phi_{13}, \phi_{22}, \phi_{23}, \phi_{33}\}$ in $\boldsymbol{\Phi}$ are $\{1.0, 0.2, 0.2, 1.0, 0.2, 1.0\}$.

In the simulation study, the conjugate priors specified in Section 12.2.4 with the following hyperparameters were used. The elements in $\mathbf{A}_{0j}$ and $\boldsymbol{\Lambda}_{0j}$ were taken as zeros, and $\boldsymbol{\Sigma}_{0aj}$ and $\boldsymbol{\Sigma}_{0j}$ were taken as identity matrices with appropriate dimensions. $\alpha_{0j} = \alpha_{0\delta} = 9$, $\beta_{0j} = \beta_{0\delta} = 4$, $\rho_0 = 7$, $\mathbf{R}_0^{-1} = 3\mathbf{I}_3$, $\alpha_{0b} = \alpha_{0\beta} = \alpha_{0\tau} = 1$, and $\beta_{0b} = \beta_{0\beta} = \beta_{0\tau} = 0.005$.

A total of 20 equidistant knots were used to construct cubic P-splines of covariate x_i. A further 20 knots based on quantiles of $N[0, 1]$ multiplied by the scale parameter s_j were used to construct a B-spline basis for natural cubic splines of the latent variables ξ_{i1}, ξ_{i2}, and ξ_{i3}. Second-order random walk penalties were used for the Bayesian P-splines to estimate the unknown smooth functions. On the basis of 100 replications, the bias (Bias) and the root mean squares (RMS) between the Bayesian estimates and the true population values of the parameters were computed. The main results are presented in the 'Nonpara SEM' column in Table 12.1; some less important parameters (a_j and ψ_j, $j = 1, \ldots, 12$) are omitted. We observe that the 'Bias' and 'RMS' are small, which indicates that the Bayesian estimates of unknown

Table 12.1 Comparison of parameter estimates under three models in the simulation study ($n = 300$, number of replications = 100).

		Nonpara SEM		Linear SEM		Nonlinear SEM	
Par.	True	Bias	RMS	Bias	RMS	Bias	RMS
λ_{21}	0.80	−0.001	0.018	0.005	0.021	0.001	0.019
λ_{31}	0.80	−0.001	0.019	0.003	0.020	−0.001	0.019
λ_{52}	0.80	0.022	0.044	0.022	0.054	0.013	0.049
λ_{62}	0.80	0.021	0.048	0.021	0.045	0.009	0.037
λ_{83}	0.80	0.022	0.050	0.015	0.049	0.012	0.046
λ_{93}	0.80	0.023	0.048	0.008	0.053	0.007	0.051
$\lambda_{11,4}$	0.80	0.007	0.049	0.016	0.049	0.014	0.048
$\lambda_{12,4}$	0.80	0.016	0.046	0.017	0.047	0.014	0.046
ϕ_{11}	1.00	−0.057	0.110	−0.069	0.126	−0.049	0.111
ϕ_{12}	0.20	−0.022	0.070	−0.003	0.054	−0.004	0.054
ϕ_{13}	0.20	−0.010	0.064	−0.019	0.068	−0.017	0.067
ϕ_{22}	1.00	−0.037	0.113	−0.037	0.122	−0.029	0.117
ϕ_{23}	0.20	0.003	0.058	−0.006	0.073	−0.003	0.074
ϕ_{33}	1.00	−0.025	0.116	−0.043	0.111	−0.040	0.111
ψ_δ	0.30	0.020	0.040	**2.080**	**2.814**	0.036	0.056
b_1	1.00	0.003	0.151	**−0.708**	**0.720**	−0.019	0.130
γ_1	1.00	0.022	0.128	**−1.511**	**1.523**	0.027	0.121
γ_2	1.00	0.030	0.088	**0.695**	**0.736**	0.041	0.103
γ_3	1.00	0.023	0.186	**−0.719**	**0.731**	−0.029	0.163

Reproduced by permission of the American Statistical Association from Song, X. Y. and Lu, Z. H. (2010). Semiparametric latent variable models with Bayesian P-splines. *Journal of Computational and Graphical Statistics*, **19**, 590–608.

parameters are accurate. Based on 100 replications, the average of the pointwise posterior means of nonparametric functions, together with the 5% and 95% pointwise quantiles, are presented in Figure 12.1. Compared with their true functions (represented by solid curves), the estimated curves correctly capture the true functional relationships among latent and observed variables.

In order to compare the empirical performance of the nonparametric SEM with some parametric SEMs, the data sets in the 100 replications were reanalyzed on the basis of M_1, a simple linear SEM with structural equation $\eta_i = b_1 x_i + \gamma_1\xi_{i1} + \gamma_2\xi_{i2} + \gamma_3\xi_{i3} + \delta_i$; and M_2, a nonlinear parametric SEM with structural equation $\eta_i = b_1 g(x_i) + \gamma_1 f_1(\xi_{i1}) + \gamma_2 f_2(\xi_{i2}) + \gamma_3 f_3(\xi_{i3}) + \delta_i$, where the exact forms of functions g, f_1, f_2, and f_3 are known. The estimates of unknown parameters and unknown smooth functions are respectively presented in Table 12.1 (columns 'Linear SEM' and 'Nonlinear SEM') and Figure 12.2. These show that the results obtained from the nonparametric SEM are close to those obtained under M_2. Note that the b_1, γ_1, γ_2, and γ_3 in the current approach were estimated by fitting true parametric functions to $\hat{g}(x_i)$ and $\hat{f}_j(\xi_{ij})$. They also show that, as the misspecification in M_1 only focuses on the structural equation, the performance of parameter estimates associated with the measurement

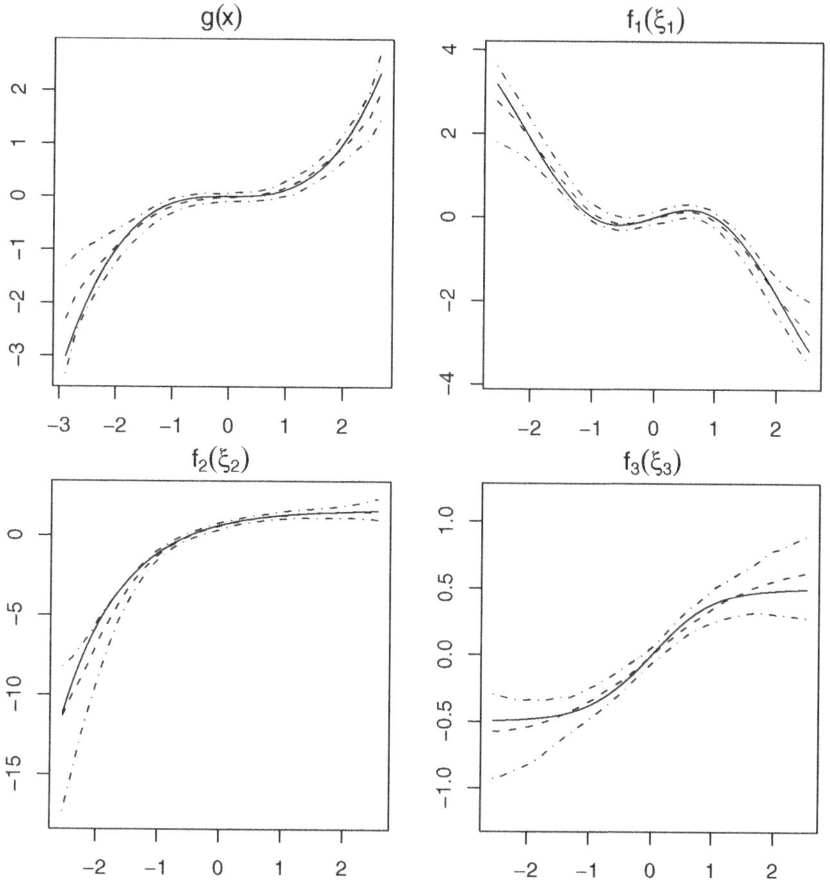

Figure 12.1 Estimates of the unknown smooth functions in the simulation study. The solid curves represent the true curves, the dashed and dot-dashed curves respectively represent the average and the 5% and 95% pointwise quantiles of the posterior means based on 100 replications. Reproduced by permission of the American Statistical Association from Song, X. Y. and Lu, Z. H. (2010). Semiparametric latent variable models with Bayesian P-splines. *Journal of Computational and Graphical Statistics*, **19**, 590–608.

equation in M_1 is similar to that in M_2 and the current approach. However, the results associated with the structural equation in M_1 are very misleading (see Figure 12.2 and the bold-faced parameter estimates in Table 12.1). In particular, the large estimated variance of the residual in the structural equation, $\hat{\psi}_\delta$, reveals the inadequacy of a linear SEM in capturing unknown functional relationships between latent variables and covariates.

The above analysis was repeated for two different choices of (1, 0.05) and (0.001, 0.001) for $\alpha_{0b} = \alpha_{0\beta} = \alpha_{0\tau}$ and $\beta_{0b} = \beta_{0\beta} = \beta_{0\tau}$, and some perturbations of the hyperparamters in the prior distributions of structural parameters. The sensitivity analysis reveals that the Bayesian results are robust to different choices of $\{(\alpha_{0b}, \beta_{0b}), (\alpha_{0\beta}, \beta_{0\beta}), (\alpha_{0\tau}, \beta_{0\tau})\}$ and the hyperparameters related to structural parameters.

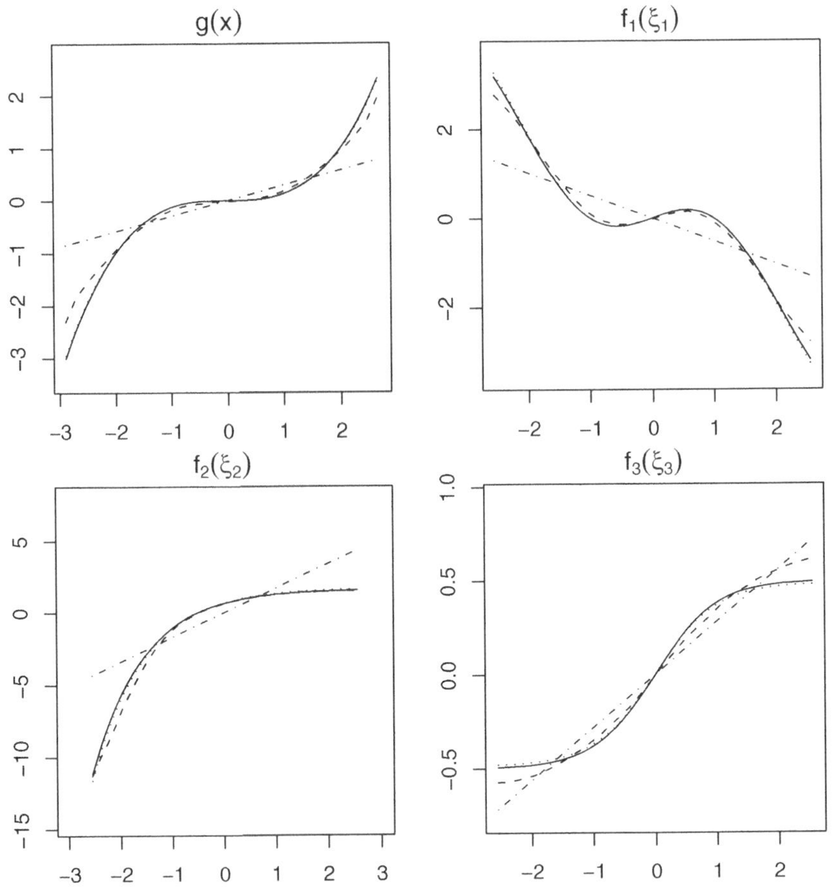

Figure 12.2 Estimates of the unknown smooth functions in the simulation study. The dashed curves are estimated with the nonparametric SEM. The dot-dashed curves are estimated with a linear SEM. The dotted curves are estimated with a nonlinear parametric SEM when the exact forms of g, f_1, f_2, and f_3 are known. The solid curves are true curves. All the estimated curves are obtained on the basis of 100 replications. Reproduced by permission of the American Statistical Association from Song, X. Y. and Lu, Z. H. (2010). Semiparametric latent variable models with Bayesian P-splines. *Journal of Computational and Graphical Statistics*, **19**, 590–608.

12.2.7 A study on osteoporosis prevention and control

The methodology was applied to a partial study on osteoporosis prevention and control. This study concerns the influence of serum concentration of sex hormones, and their precursors and metabolites on bone mineral density in older men. It was part of a multicenter prospective cohort study of risk factors of osteoporotic fractures in older people. A total of 1446 Chinese men aged 65 years and above were recruited using a combination of private solicitation and public advertising from community centers and public housing estates. The main objective of this analysis is to investigate the functional influences of serum concentration of sex hormones, and their precursors and metabolites on bone mineral density (BMD) in older men. The following observed variables were selected in establishing a model to achieve the objective: spine BMD, hip BMD, estrone (E1), estrone sulfate (E1-S), estradiol (E2), testosterone (TESTO), 5-androstenediol (5-DIOL), dihydrotestosterone (DHT), androstenedione (4-DIONE), dehydroepiandrosterone (DHEA), DHEA sulfate (DHEA-S), androsterone (ADT), ADT glucuronide (ADT-G), 3a-diol-3G (3G), and 3d-diol-17G (17G). Moreover, weight and age were also included as covariates. All the above continuous measurements were standardized.

Based on the medical meaning of the observed variables, we identified five latent variables through the measurement equation (12.1). More specifically, spine BMD and hip BMD were grouped into a latent variable 'BMD'; similarly, {E1, E1-S, E2}, {TESTO, 5-DIOL, DHT}, {4-DIONE, DHEA, DHEA-S}, and {ADT, ADT-G, 3G, 17G} were respectively grouped into four latent variables which could be interpreted as 'estrogen', 'androgen', 'precursors', and 'metabolites', respectively. Hence, we considered a measurement equation with $\mathbf{A} = \mathbf{0}$, a 5×1 random vector $\boldsymbol{\omega}$ containing the above latent variables, and the non-overlapping factor loading matrix

$$\boldsymbol{\Lambda}^T = \begin{bmatrix} 1 & \lambda_{21} & 0 & 0 & 0 & 0 & 0 & 0 & 0 & 0 & 0 & 0 & 0 & 0 & 0 \\ 0 & 0 & 1 & \lambda_{42} & \lambda_{52} & 0 & 0 & 0 & 0 & 0 & 0 & 0 & 0 & 0 & 0 \\ 0 & 0 & 0 & 0 & 0 & 1 & \lambda_{73} & \lambda_{83} & 0 & 0 & 0 & 0 & 0 & 0 & 0 \\ 0 & 0 & 0 & 0 & 0 & 0 & 0 & 0 & 1 & \lambda_{10,4} & \lambda_{11,4} & 0 & 0 & 0 & 0 \\ 0 & 0 & 0 & 0 & 0 & 0 & 0 & 0 & 0 & 0 & 0 & 1 & \lambda_{13,5} & \lambda_{14,5} & \lambda_{15,5} \end{bmatrix}, \tag{12.22}$$

where the 1s and 0s are fixed parameters to identify the model in accordance with common practice in SEMs; see Lee (2007). The λ_{kj} represent unknown factor loadings and reflect the associations between latent variables and the corresponding observed variables. According to the main objective of this study, the investigation of the functional effects of 'estrogen', 'androgen', 'precursors', and 'metabolites' on 'BMD', the outcome latent variable is defined as $\eta =$ BMD, and the vector of explanatory latent variables $\boldsymbol{\xi}$ is defined as $(\xi_1, \xi_2, \xi_3, \xi_4)^T =$ (estrogen, androgen, precursors, metabolites)^T. Finally, to take also the effects of fixed covariates, weight and age, into account, the nonparametric structural equation was defined by

$$\eta_i = g_1(x_{i1}) + g_2(x_{i2}) + f_1(\xi_{i1}) + f_2(\xi_{i2}) + f_3(\xi_{i3}) + f_4(\xi_{i4}) + \delta_i. \tag{12.23}$$

The weight and age effects were modeled by cubic P-splines, and the effects of the explanatory latent variables on BMD were modeled by natural cubic P-splines. A first-order random walk penalty and 20 knots were used in the analysis. As specified in Section 12.2.4, the conjugate priors were used as the prior distributions for most of the unknown parameters. The diffuse hyperparameters $\alpha_{0b} = \alpha_{0\beta} = \alpha_{0\tau} = 1$ and $\beta_{0b} = \beta_{0\beta} = \beta_{0\tau} = 0.005$ were used for the inverse smoothing parameters in $\boldsymbol{\tau}_b$, $\boldsymbol{\tau}_\beta$, and $\boldsymbol{\tau}_s$. To obtain some prior knowledge of the structural parameters, a preliminary analysis of the current data set was performed using a traditional SEM, which was defined by measurement equation (12.1) and a linear structural equation $\eta_i = b_1 x_{i1} + b_2 x_{i2} + \gamma_1\xi_{i1} + \gamma_2\xi_{i2} + \gamma_3\xi_{i3} + \gamma_4\xi_{i4} + \delta_i$. The standard package LISREL 8 (Jöreskog and Sörbom, 1996) produced the maximum likelihood (ML) estimates of unknown parameters for the parametric SEM. The hyperparameters in the prior distributions of structural parameters were taken as $\boldsymbol{\Lambda}_{0j} = \hat{\boldsymbol{\Lambda}}_j$, $\alpha_{0j} = \alpha_{0\delta} = 9$, $\beta_{0j} = (\alpha_{0j} - 1)\hat{\psi}_j$,

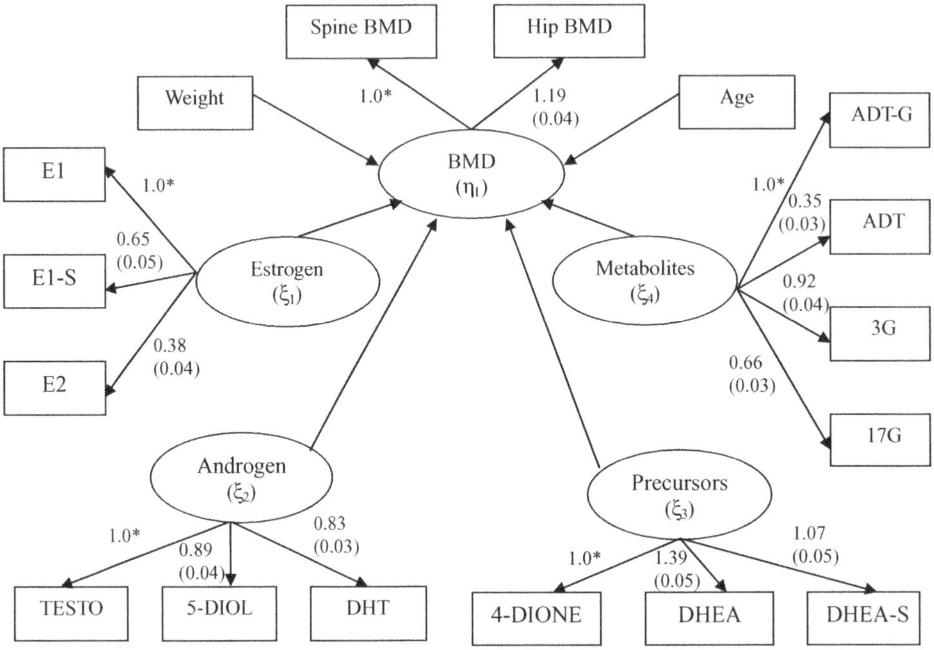

Figure 12.3 Path diagram, together with the estimated factor loadings and their standard error estimates (in parentheses), of the nonparametric SEM in the analysis of the BMD data. Reproduced by permission of the American Statistical Association from Song, X. Y. and Lu, Z. H. (2010). Semiparametric latent variable models with Bayesian P-splines. *Journal of Computational and Graphical Statistics*, **19**, 590–608.

$\beta_{0\delta} = (\alpha_{0\delta} - 1)\hat{\psi}_\delta$, $\rho_0 = 8$, and $\mathbf{R}_0^{-1} = (\rho_0 - q_2 - 1)\hat{\mathbf{\Phi}}$, where $\hat{\mathbf{\Lambda}}_j$, $\hat{\psi}_j$, $\hat{\psi}_\delta$, and $\hat{\mathbf{\Phi}}$ were the ML estimates obtained via the parametric SEM.

The MCMC algorithm was found to converge within 10 000 iterations. After discarding 10 000 burn-in iterations, 20 000 observations generated by the MCMC algorithm were used to obtain the Bayesian results. The estimates of factor loadings and their standard error estimates are reported in Figure 12.3. For clarity, the less important structural parameters in $\mathbf{\Psi}$, ψ_δ, and $\mathbf{\Phi}$ are omitted. The pointwise posterior means of unknown smooth functions, together with the 10% and 90% pointwise quantiles, are depicted in Figure 12.4. We observe that most of the fitted curves are neither linear nor quadratic. This fact provides verification that traditional parametric SEMs with linear and/or quadratic terms of latent variables may not correctly reflect the true functional relationships between latent and observed variables, and would give misleading conclusions if the data were analyzed via a parametric approach.

The specific interpretation of the functional relationships is as follows. (i) Weight had a positive effect on BMD. Roughly speaking, this effect rose linearly. The rate of increase slowed down when subjects were overweight, say with weights exceeding 80 kg. (ii) The effect of age on BMD was basically negative. This negative effect was less significant for men aged 65–75 years, but became increasingly significant when the subjects were over 75 years old. (iii) The influence of estrogen on BMD rose with estrogen score, indicating that the subjects with a higher level of estrogen would have had a higher level of BMD and thus a lower

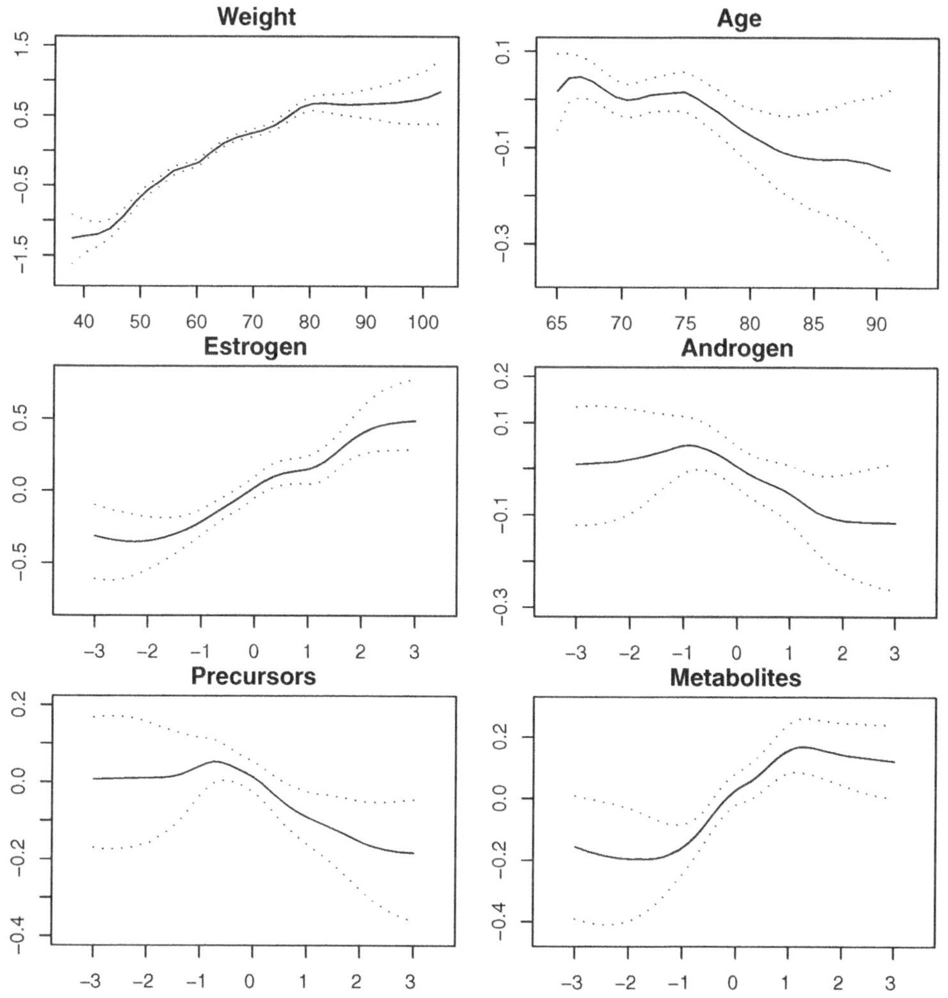

Figure 12.4 Estimates of the unknown smooth functions in the BMD study. The solid curves represent the pointwise posterior mean curves, while the dotted curves represent the 10% and 90% pointwise quantiles. Reproduced by permission of the American Statistical Association from Song, X. Y. and Lu, Z. H. (2010). Semiparametric latent variable models with Bayesian P-splines. *Journal of Computational and Graphical Statistics*, **19**, 590–608.

risk of osteoporotic fractures. (iv) The influence of androgen on BMD exhibited a nonlinear pattern. It changed direction from positive to negative, indicating a positive effect for subjects with low androgen scores and a negative effect for those with moderate or high androgen scores. Therefore, some insight into the influence of androgen on BMD might be gained: increasing androgen might have had a positive impact on BMD for those with a low level of androgen, but, for most subjects, controlling androgen level could have helped improve BMD and thus prevent the development of osteoporotic fractures. (v) The influence of precursors on BMD was hardly significant when the level of precursors was low, and it became more and more significant as the level of precursors increased. Since precursors played an important role in producing sex hormones, for older men with a relatively high level of precursors, controlling precursors might have helped control androgen and thus improve BMD. (vi) The influence of metabolites on BMD presented a composite effect of an increasing trend and a sinusoidal shape, which resulted in an overall increasing trend but with significant changes in both tails of the curve. If we partitioned the subjects into three types with respectively low, middle, and high levels of metabolites, the estimated curve revealed that the effect of metabolites on BMD was clearly nonlinear and had completely different patterns for each type of subjects. Therefore, different treatments should be given to improve BMD and thus prevent the development of osteoporotic fractures in older men with low, middle, and high levels of metabolites. The above insights obtained from nonlinear curves cannot be gained using parametric SEMs.

To assess the sensitivity of the Bayesian results to inputs of hyperparameters in the prior distributions, the above analysis was repeated with some *ad hoc* perturbations of the current prior inputs. In particular, two different choices of $\alpha_{0b} = \alpha_{0\beta} = \alpha_{0\tau} = 1$, $\beta_{0b} = \beta_{0\beta} = \beta_{0\tau} = 0.05$ and $\alpha_{0b} = \alpha_{0\beta} = \alpha_{0\tau} = 0.001$, $\beta_{0b} = \beta_{0\beta} = \beta_{0\tau} = 0.001$ were used. As close Bayesian estimates of unknown parameters and similar estimated curves of unknown smooth functions were obtained, the Bayesian results are not very sensitive to different prior inputs. The program is written in R, and the code is available from the following website:

`www.wiley.com/go/medical_behavioral_sciences`

12.3 Generalized nonparametric structural equation models

As mixed data types – continuous, count, ordered, and unordered categorical – are increasingly used and collected in practical studies, the inclusion of mixed-mode data has consistently attracted a high level of interest in the development of SEMs (see, for example, Arminger and Küsters, 1988; Moustaki, 1996, 2003; Bartholomew and Knott, 1999; Shi and Lee, 2000; Jöreskog and Moustaki, 2001; Skrondal and Rabe-Hesketh, 2004; Sánchez *et al.*, 2005; Song and Lee, 2007; Song *et al.*, 2007; Huber *et al.*, 2009). In this section, the nonparametric SEM discussed in the previous section is extended to include various types of discrete data. The generalized nonparametric SEM discussed can simultaneously handle mixed data types, including continuous, ordered and unordered categorical, and count data, as well as allowing users to visually examine and interpret the functional relationship between latent variables of interest. In addition to visual inspection, in this section we introduce strategies to statistically assess whether the nonparametric approach is necessary and whether it offers meaningful benefits over its simpler parametric counterparts, and to compare the performance – in terms of goodness of fit – between different nonparametric models as well as between these models and their parametric counterparts.

12.3.1 Model description

We consider a $p \times 1$ random vector composed of ordered categorical, continuous, count, and unordered categorical variables. Without loss of generality, for $i = 1, \ldots, n$, let $\mathbf{d}_i = (d_{i1}, \ldots, d_{ip})^T = (z_{i1}, \ldots, z_{ir_1}, y_{i,r_1+1}, \ldots, y_{ir_2}, v_{i,r_2+1}, \ldots, v_{ir_3}, u_{i,r_3+1}, \ldots, u_{ir_4})^T$, where z_{ij}, y_{ij}, v_{ij}, and u_{ij} denote ordered categorical, continuous, count, and unordered categorical variables, respectively. To provide a unified framework for modeling different types of data, let $\mathbf{d}_i^* = (z_{i1}^*, \ldots, z_{ir_1}^*, y_{i,r_1+1}^*, \ldots, y_{ir_2}^*, v_{i,r_2+1}^*, \ldots, v_{ir_3}^*, \mathbf{w}_{i,r_3+1}^T, \ldots, \mathbf{w}_{ir_4}^T)^T$ be the underlying vector, which is linked to the vector $\mathbf{d}_i$ as follows (Song *et al.*, 2011):

$$\begin{cases} z_{ij} = h_j(z_{ij}^*), & j = 1, \ldots, r_1, \\ y_{ij} = h_j(y_{ij}^*), & j = r_1 + 1, \ldots, r_2, \\ \kappa_{ij} = h_j(v_{ij}^*), & j = r_2 + 1, \ldots, r_3, \\ u_{ij} = h_j(\mathbf{w}_{ij}), & j = r_3 + 1, \ldots, r_4, \end{cases} \tag{12.24}$$

where $\kappa_{ij} = E(v_{ij})$, and the $h_j(\cdot)$ are threshold, identity, exponential, and multinomial probit link functions, respectively, as defined below.

For ordered categorical variables z_{ij} that take integer values in $\{0, 1, \ldots, H_j\}$, a threshold link function $h_j(\cdot)$ is used as follows (Muthén, 1984; Lee, 2007):

$$z_{ij} = h_j\left(z_{ij}^*\right) = \sum_{l=0}^{H_j} l \cdot I\left(\alpha_{j,l} \le z_{ij}^* < \alpha_{j,l+1}\right), \tag{12.25}$$

where $I(\cdot)$ is an indicator function, which takes the value 1 if $\alpha_{j,l} \le z_{ij}^* < \alpha_{j,l+1}$ and 0 otherwise. Here, $\{-\infty = \alpha_{j,0} < \alpha_{j,1} < \ldots < \alpha_{j,H_j} < \alpha_{j,H_j+1} = +\infty\}$ is a set of thresholds defining the $H_j + 1$ categories.

For continuous variables y_{ij}, $h_j(\cdot)$ is the identity link; that is,

$$y_{ij} = h_j(y_{ij}^*) = y_{ij}^*. \tag{12.26}$$

For count variables v_{ij}, we assume $v_{ij} \stackrel{D}{=} \text{Pois}(\kappa_{ij})$, where $\text{Pois}(\cdot)$ denotes the Poisson distribution. Under the generalized linear model framework (McCullagh and Nelder, 1989), the log link $h_j^{-1}(\cdot)$ or exponential link $h_j(\cdot)$ is given by

$$\log \kappa_{ij} = h_j^{-1}\left(E(v_{ij})\right) = v_{ij}^* \quad \text{or} \quad \kappa_{ij} = E(v_{ij}) = h_j\left(v_{ij}^*\right) = \exp\left(v_{ij}^*\right). \tag{12.27}$$

For unordered categorical variables u_{ij} with L_j categories, we assume that the u_{ij} take values in $\{0, 1, \ldots, L_j - 1\}$. For simplicity, we assume that $L_j = L$ for all j. This assumption can be relaxed without difficulty. Following Imai and van Dyk (2005) and Song *et al.* (2007), u_{ij} is modeled in terms of an underlying vector $\mathbf{w}_{ij} = (w_{ij,1}, \ldots, w_{ij,L-1})^T$ with a multinomial probit link function $h_j(\cdot)$ defined as follows:

$$u_{ij} = h_j(\mathbf{w}_{ij}) = \begin{cases} 0, & \text{if } \max(\mathbf{w}_{ij}) < 0, \\ l, & \text{if } \max(\mathbf{w}_{ij}) = w_{ij,l} > 0. \end{cases} \tag{12.28}$$

For example, for an unordered categorical variable u_{ij} with three categories, we have $\mathbf{w}_{ij} = (w_{ij,1}, w_{ij,2})^T$, $u_{ij} = 0$ if both $w_{ij,1}$ and $w_{ij,2}$ are less than zero, $u_{ij} = 1$ if $w_{ij,1} > w_{ij,2}$ and $w_{ij,1} > 0$, and $u_{ij} = 2$ if $w_{ij,2} > w_{ij,1}$ and $w_{ij,2} > 0$.

The measurement equations for $\mathbf{d}_i$ are defined through equations (12.24) and (12.29)–(12.32) below. For z_{ij}, y_{ij}, and v_{ij}, the measurement equations are given by

$$z_{ij}^* = \mu_j + \boldsymbol{\Lambda}_j^T \boldsymbol{\omega}_i + \epsilon_{ij}, \tag{12.29}$$

$$y_{ij}^* = \mu_j + \boldsymbol{\Lambda}_j^T \boldsymbol{\omega}_i + \epsilon_{ij}, \tag{12.30}$$

$$v_{ij}^* = \mu_j + \boldsymbol{\Lambda}_j^T \boldsymbol{\omega}_i, \tag{12.31}$$

where μ_j is an intercept, $\mathbf{\Lambda}_j(q \times 1)$ is a vector of factor loadings, $\boldsymbol{\omega}_i(q \times 1)$ is a vector of latent variables, and ϵ_{ij} is a random error following $N[0, \psi_j]$ that is independent of $\boldsymbol{\omega}_i$. For u_{ij}, the measurement equation is given by

$$\mathbf{w}_{ij} = \boldsymbol{\mu}_j + \mathbf{1}_{L-1}\mathbf{\Lambda}_j^T\boldsymbol{\omega}_i + \boldsymbol{\epsilon}_{ij}, \tag{12.32}$$

where $\boldsymbol{\mu}_j = (\mu_{j,1}, \ldots, \mu_{j,L-1})^T$ is the intercept vector, $\mathbf{1}_{L-1}$ is an $(L-1) \times 1$ vector of 1s, $\mathbf{\Lambda}_j$ is the factor loading vector defined previously, and $\boldsymbol{\epsilon}_{ij}$ is a random error vector distributed as $N[\mathbf{0}, \mathbf{\Psi}_{wj}]$ and independent of $\boldsymbol{\omega}_i$. The probability mass function of u_{ij} is

$$p(u_{ij} = l|\boldsymbol{\omega}_i, \boldsymbol{\mu}_j, \mathbf{\Lambda}_j, \mathbf{\Psi}_{wj}) = \int_{\mathfrak{R}_l} \phi_{L-1}\big(\mathbf{w}_{ij};\ \boldsymbol{\mu}_j + \mathbf{1}_{L-1}\mathbf{\Lambda}_j^T\boldsymbol{\omega}_i, \mathbf{\Psi}_{wj}\big)d\mathbf{w}_{ij}, \tag{12.33}$$

where $\phi_{L-1}(\cdot\ ; \boldsymbol{\mu}, \mathbf{\Sigma})$ is the density function of the $(L-1)$-variate normal distribution with mean $\boldsymbol{\mu}$ and covariance matrix $\mathbf{\Sigma}$, and

$$\mathfrak{R}_l = \begin{cases} \{\mathbf{w}_{ij} : \max(\mathbf{w}_{ij}) < 0\}, & l = 0, \\ \{\mathbf{w}_{ij} : \max(\mathbf{w}_{ij}) = w_{ij,l} > 0\}, & 0 < l \le L-1. \end{cases}$$

Hence, $p(\mathbf{w}_{ij}|u_{ij} = l, \boldsymbol{\omega}_i, \boldsymbol{\mu}_j, \mathbf{\Lambda}_j, \mathbf{\Psi}_{wj})$ is proportional to the truncated multivariate normal distribution with density function $\phi_{L-1}(\mathbf{w}_{ij};\ \boldsymbol{\mu}_j + \mathbf{1}_{L-1}\mathbf{\Lambda}_j^T\boldsymbol{\omega}_i, \mathbf{\Psi}_{wj})I(\mathbf{w}_{ij} \in \mathfrak{R}_l)$, where $I(\mathbf{w}_{ij} \in \mathfrak{R}_l)$ is an indicator function which takes value 1 if $\mathbf{w}_{ij} \in \mathfrak{R}_l$ and 0 otherwise.

The measurement equations defined in equations (12.29)–(12.32) are not identified. Following common practice in SEMs (Lee, 2007), the appropriate elements in $\mathbf{\Lambda}_j$ are fixed at preassigned values to identify the scale of the latent variables. Another model indeterminacy is due to the existence of ordered and unordered variables. Ordered categorical variables can be identified by fixing $\alpha_{j,1}$ and α_{j,H_j} at preassigned values (see Shi and Lee, 2000). For dichotomous variables which can be regarded as a special case of ordered categorical variables with two categories, it is necessary to fix ψ_j at 1 in order to achieve identifiability. Unordered categorical variables are also not identified; multiplying each $w_{ij,k}$ by an arbitrary positive constant does not change the values of u_{ij} in (12.28). Following Dunson (2000) and Song *et al.* (2007), $\mathbf{\Psi}_{wj}$ is fixed at an identity matrix to identify the unordered categorical variables.

For the structural component of the nonparametric SEM, a partition of $\boldsymbol{\omega}_i = (\boldsymbol{\eta}_i^T, \boldsymbol{\xi}_i^T)^T$ is considered. Here, $\boldsymbol{\eta}_i = (\eta_{i1}, \ldots, \eta_{iq_1})^T$ is a $q_1 \times 1$ outcome latent vector, and $\boldsymbol{\xi}_i = (\xi_{i1}, \ldots, \xi_{iq_2})^T$ is a $q_2 \times 1$ explanatory latent vector assumed to follow $N[\mathbf{0}, \mathbf{\Phi}]$, where $\mathbf{\Phi}$ is a covariance matrix. In order to examine the functional effects of explanatory latent variables in $\boldsymbol{\xi}_i$ and covariates in $\mathbf{x}_i$ on outcome latent variables in $\boldsymbol{\eta}_i$, we use the following nonparametric structural equation: for an arbitrary element η_{ih} in $\boldsymbol{\eta}_i$, and $h = 1, \ldots, q_1$,

$$\eta_{ih} = g_{h1}(x_{i1}) + \ldots + g_{hm}(x_{im}) + f_{h1}(\xi_{i1}) + \ldots + f_{hq_2}(\xi_{iq_2}) + \delta_{ih}, \tag{12.34}$$

where $g_{h1}(\cdot), \ldots, g_{hm}(\cdot), f_{h1}(\cdot), \ldots, f_{hq_2}(\cdot)$ are unspecified smooth functions with continuous second-order derivatives, and δ_{ih} is a random residual distributed as $N[0, \psi_{\delta h}]$ and independent of $\boldsymbol{\xi}_i$ and δ_{ij} for $j \neq h$. For notational simplicity, we suppress the subscript h in (12.34) by assuming $q_1 = 1$ throughout Section 12.3.2.

12.3.2 Bayesian P-splines

The smooth functions $g(\cdot)$ and $f(\cdot)$ in (12.34) can be modeled by a sum of B-splines (De Boor, 1978) based on a large number of knots in the x or ξ domain. Here, $f(\xi_i)$ is approximated by $f(\xi_i) = \sum_{k=1}^{K} \beta_k B_k(\xi_i)$, where K is the number of splines determined by the number of knots, the β_k are the unknown parameters, and the functions $B_k(\cdot)$ are B-splines of appropriate order. As discussed in Section 12.2.3, some difficulties will be encountered in the use of the traditional B-spline basis functions $B_k(\cdot)$ in this approximation. First, traditional B-splines are defined in a predetermined finite interval, but the observations of the latent variables generated in the MCMC iterations may lie outside the fixed interval. Second, the unknown scales of latent variables make it impossible to determine in advance the ranges of the latent variables and positions of the knots. Two solutions are presented in Section 12.2.3 to address these difficulties. One is to use natural cubic splines in place of the B-splines functions (see also Song and Lu, 2010). With the use of natural cubic splines, the sum $\sum_{k=1}^{K} \beta_k B_k(\xi_i)$ would always be well defined even if the observations of ξ_i at certain MCMC iterations exceeded the boundaries of the predetermined interval. The other solution is to introduce an additional scale parameter to construct flexible knots for latent variables with unknown scales. Useful as this solution may be, it requires both careful specification of the prior distribution of the scale parameter and nontrivial posterior simulation from the associated complex conditional distribution. Here, we consider a simpler method to solve the aforementioned difficulties through 'probit transformation' applied to explanatory latent variables. Specifically, instead of using $B_k(\xi_i)$ in a B-splines approximation directly, we model $f(\xi_i)$ as follows:

$$f(\xi_i) = \sum_{k=1}^{K} \beta_k B_k\big(\Phi^*(\xi_i)\big), \tag{12.35}$$

where $\Phi^*(\cdot)$ is the cumulative distribution of $N[0, 1]$. Equation (12.35) transforms the original scale of ξ_i to the scale of the cumulative probability $p(\xi \leq \xi_i)$. The modeling method in (12.35) has the following advantages. First, it forces $\Phi^*(\xi_i)$ to fall into a fixed interval [0, 1], regardless of original ranges of ξ_i. Second, it is easy to determine the positions of knots in the domain of ξ_i *a priori*. For example, the knots can be chosen as equally spaced grids. Third, it renders the additional parameters for handling latent variables with unknown scales in Section 12.2.3 unnecessary. This procedure therefore saves substantial effort with regard to prior specification and posterior simulation. In other words, this computational algorithm for estimating the unknown function $f(\xi_i)$ is simpler, more efficient, and easier to use (Song *et al.*, 2011).

Using (12.35), the structural equation (12.34) is reformulated as

$$\eta_i = \sum_{j=1}^{m} \sum_{k=1}^{K_{bj}} b_{jk} B_{jk}^x(x_{ij}) + \sum_{j=1}^{q_2} \sum_{k=1}^{K_j} \beta_{jk} B_{jk}(\Phi^*(\xi_{ij})) + \delta_i, \tag{12.36}$$

where b_{jk}, $B_{jk}^x(\cdot)$, β_{jk}, $B_{jk}(\cdot)$, K_{bj}, and K_j are defined as in equation (12.9). The stochastic analogues to the difference penalty are equivalent to assigning the coefficients of B-splines the following prior distributions:

$$[\mathbf{b}_j|\tau_{bj}] \stackrel{D}{=} \left(\frac{1}{2\pi\tau_{bj}}\right)^{(K_{bj}^*/2)} \exp\left\{-\frac{1}{2\tau_{bj}}\mathbf{b}_j^T \mathbf{M}_{bj} \mathbf{b}_j\right\}, \quad j = 1, \ldots, m, \tag{12.37}$$

$$[\boldsymbol{\beta}_j|\tau_{\beta j}] \stackrel{D}{=} \left(\frac{1}{2\pi\tau_{\beta j}}\right)^{(K_j^*/2)} \exp\left\{-\frac{1}{2\tau_{\beta j}}\boldsymbol{\beta}_j^T \mathbf{M}_{\beta j} \boldsymbol{\beta}_j\right\}, \quad j = 1, \ldots, q_2, \tag{12.38}$$

where $\mathbf{b}_j$, τ_{bj}, $\mathbf{M}_{bj}$, $\boldsymbol{\beta}_j$, $\tau_{\beta j}$, and $\mathbf{M}_{\beta j}$, are defined as previously described, and $K_{bj}^* = \text{rank}(\mathbf{M}_{bj})$, $K_j^* = \text{rank}(\mathbf{M}_{\beta j})$.

Note that each function $f_j(\xi_{ij})$, $j = 1, \ldots, q_2$, defined in (12.34) is not identified up to a constant. As before, we solve this identification problem by first imposing a constraint on $\boldsymbol{\beta}_j$. For every j, let $\mathbf{F}_j = (f_j(\xi_{1j}), \ldots, f_j(\xi_{nj}))^T$, and $\mathbf{1}_n$ be an $n \times 1$ vector of 1s; at each MCMC iteration, impose the restriction $\mathbf{1}_n^T \mathbf{F}_j = 0$. This constraint is equivalent to $\mathbf{1}_n^T \mathbf{B}_j \boldsymbol{\beta}_j = 0$, where $\mathbf{B}_j$ is an $n \times K_j$ matrix with the element in the ith row and kth column being $B_{jk}\big(\Phi^*(\xi_{ij})\big)$. Additionally, a similar constraint, $\mathbf{1}_n^T \mathbf{B}_j^x \mathbf{b}_j = 0$, is imposed on $\mathbf{b}_j$, where $\mathbf{B}_j^x$ is an $n \times K_{bj}$ matrix with the element in the ith row and kth column being $B_{jk}^x(x_{ij})$.

12.3.3 Prior distributions

Let $\boldsymbol{\mu} = \{\mu_1, \ldots, \mu_{r_3}, \boldsymbol{\mu}_{r_3+1}, \ldots, \boldsymbol{\mu}_{r_4}\}$, $\boldsymbol{\Lambda} = \{\boldsymbol{\Lambda}_1, \ldots, \boldsymbol{\Lambda}_p\}$, $\boldsymbol{\Psi} = \{\psi_1, \ldots, \psi_{r_2}\}$, and $\boldsymbol{\theta}_s$ denote the collection of unknown structural parameters in the model; that is, $\boldsymbol{\theta}_s = \{\boldsymbol{\mu}, \boldsymbol{\Lambda}, \boldsymbol{\Psi}, \psi_\delta, \boldsymbol{\Phi}\}$. Furthermore, let $\mathbf{b} = \{\mathbf{b}_1, \ldots, \mathbf{b}_m\}$, $\boldsymbol{\beta} = \{\boldsymbol{\beta}_1, \ldots, \boldsymbol{\beta}_{q_2}\}$, $\boldsymbol{\tau}_b = \{\tau_{b1}, \ldots, \tau_{bm}\}$, $\boldsymbol{\tau}_\beta = \{\tau_{\beta 1}, \ldots, \tau_{\beta q_2}\}$, and $\boldsymbol{\theta}_f$ denote the collection of parameters that are associated with the P-splines approximation; that is, $\boldsymbol{\theta}_f = \{\mathbf{b}, \boldsymbol{\beta}, \boldsymbol{\tau}_b, \boldsymbol{\tau}_\beta\}$. Finally, let $\boldsymbol{\alpha} = \{\boldsymbol{\alpha}_1, \ldots, \boldsymbol{\alpha}_{r_1}\}$ be a set of unknown thresholds, where $\boldsymbol{\alpha}_j = (\alpha_{j,2}, \ldots, \alpha_{j,H_j-1})$. In a full Bayesian analysis, an important issue is the specification of appropriate prior distributions for the unknown parameters. First, we consider the prior distributions for $\mathbf{b}$ and $\boldsymbol{\beta}$. As mentioned previously, the identifiability constraints $\mathbf{1}_n^T \mathbf{B}_j^x \mathbf{b}_j = 0$ and $\mathbf{1}_n^T \mathbf{B}_j \boldsymbol{\beta}_j = 0$ should be respectively imposed on $\mathbf{b}_j$ and $\boldsymbol{\beta}_j$ to identify the smooth functions $g(\cdot)$ and $f(\cdot)$. With these constraints, the following truncated Gaussian priors for $\mathbf{b}_j$ and $\boldsymbol{\beta}_j$ are specified:

$$p(\mathbf{b}_j|\tau_{bj}) \propto \exp\left\{-\frac{1}{2\tau_{bj}}\mathbf{b}_j^T \mathbf{M}_{bj} \mathbf{b}_j\right\} I\big(\mathbf{1}_n^T \mathbf{B}_j^x \mathbf{b}_j = 0\big), \quad j = 1, \ldots, m, \tag{12.39}$$

$$p(\boldsymbol{\beta}_j|\tau_{\beta j}) \propto \exp\left\{-\frac{1}{2\tau_{\beta j}}\boldsymbol{\beta}_j^T \mathbf{M}_{\beta j} \boldsymbol{\beta}_j\right\} I\big(\mathbf{1}_n^T \mathbf{B}_j \boldsymbol{\beta}_j = 0\big), \quad j = 1, \ldots, q_2. \tag{12.40}$$

Second, following the existing literature (Lang and Brezger, 2004; Song and Lu, 2010), highly dispersed (but proper) inverted gamma priors are assigned for the smoothing parameters τ_{bj} and $\tau_{\beta j}$:

$$\begin{aligned} \tau_{bj}^{-1} &\stackrel{D}{=} \text{Gamma}[\alpha_{0b}, \beta_{0b}], \quad j = 1, \ldots, m, \\ \tau_{\beta j}^{-1} &\stackrel{D}{=} \text{Gamma}[\alpha_{0\beta}, \beta_{0\beta}], \quad j = 1, \ldots, q_2, \end{aligned} \tag{12.41}$$

where α_{0b}, β_{0b}, $\alpha_{0\beta}$, and $\beta_{0\beta}$ are hyperparameters with preassigned values. To obtain highly dispersed priors, common choices for these hyperparameters are $\alpha_{0b} = \alpha_{0\beta} = 1$; β_{0b} and $\beta_{0\beta}$ are small. In Section 12.3.5, $\alpha_{0b} = \alpha_{0\beta} = 1$ and $\beta_{0b} = \beta_{0\beta} = 0.005$ are used in the numerical anlaysis.

Third, for the structural parameters that are involved in the measurement equations (12.29)–(12.32) and the structural equation (12.36), the following conjugate priors are considered:

$$
\begin{aligned}
&\mu_j \stackrel{D}{=} N[\mu_{0j}, \sigma_{0j}^2], \quad \text{for } j = 1, \ldots, r_3, \\
&\boldsymbol{\mu}_j \stackrel{D}{=} N[\boldsymbol{\mu}_{0j}, \mathbf{H}_{0\mu j}], \quad \text{for } j = r_3 + 1, \ldots, r_4, \\
&[\boldsymbol{\Lambda}_j | \psi_j] \stackrel{D}{=} N[\boldsymbol{\Lambda}_{0j}, \psi_j \mathbf{H}_{0j}], \ \psi_j^{-1} \stackrel{D}{=} \text{Gamma}[\alpha_{0j}, \beta_{0j}], \quad \text{for } j = 1, \ldots, r_2 \qquad (12.42) \\
&\boldsymbol{\Lambda}_j \stackrel{D}{=} N[\boldsymbol{\Lambda}_{0j}, \mathbf{H}_{0j}], \quad \text{for } j = r_2 + 1, \ldots, r_4, \\
&\psi_\delta^{-1} \stackrel{D}{=} \text{Gamma}[\alpha_{0\delta}, \beta_{0\delta}], \quad \text{and} \quad \boldsymbol{\Phi}^{-1} \stackrel{D}{=} W[\mathbf{R}_0, \rho_0],
\end{aligned}
$$

where μ_{0j}, σ_{0j}^2, $\boldsymbol{\mu}_{0j}$, $\mathbf{H}_{0\mu j}$, $\boldsymbol{\Lambda}_{0j}$, $\mathbf{H}_{0j}$, α_{0j}, β_{0j}, $\alpha_{0\delta}$, $\beta_{0\delta}$, $\mathbf{R}_0$, and ρ_0 are hyperparameters with preassigned values.

Finally, for the thresholds that define ordered categorical variables, the following noninformative prior distribution is used to reflect the fact that very little information is available for these parameters. Thus, for $\alpha_{j,2} < \ldots < \alpha_{j,H_j-1}$,

$$p(\boldsymbol{\alpha}_j) = p(\alpha_{j,2}, \ldots, \alpha_{j,H_j-1}) \propto \text{constant}, \quad j = 1, \ldots, r_1.$$

12.3.4 Bayesian estimation and model comparison

Let $\mathbf{D} = \{\mathbf{d}_1, \ldots, \mathbf{d}_n\}$ with $\mathbf{d}_i = \{\mathbf{z}_i, \mathbf{y}_i, \mathbf{v}_i, \mathbf{u}_i\}$, where $\mathbf{z}_i$, $\mathbf{y}_i$, $\mathbf{v}_i$, and $\mathbf{u}_i$ are the vectors of ordered categorical, continuous, count, and unordered categorical variables, respectively. Let $\boldsymbol{\theta}_* = \{\boldsymbol{\theta}_s, \boldsymbol{\theta}_f, \boldsymbol{\alpha}\}$. The Bayesian estimate of $\boldsymbol{\theta}_*$ can then be obtained through the sample mean of a sufficiently large number of observations drawn from the posterior distribution $p(\boldsymbol{\theta}_*|\mathbf{D})$. However, this posterior distribution is intractable due to the existence of latent variables and discrete data. Let $\mathbf{z}_i^* = (z_{i1}^*, \ldots, z_{i,r_1}^*)^T$, $\mathbf{w}_i = \{\mathbf{w}_{i,r_3+1}, \ldots, \mathbf{w}_{i,r_4}\}$, $\mathbf{Z}^* = \{\mathbf{z}_1^*, \ldots, \mathbf{z}_n^*\}$, $\mathbf{W} = \{\mathbf{w}_1, \ldots, \mathbf{w}_n\}$, and $\boldsymbol{\Omega} = \{\boldsymbol{\omega}_1, \ldots, \boldsymbol{\omega}_n\}$. To solve the problem, we again utilize the data augmentation procedure, which is implemented by augmenting the observed data $\mathbf{D}$ with the latent quantities $\mathbf{F} = \{\mathbf{Z}^*, \mathbf{W}, \boldsymbol{\Omega}\}$ in the posterior analysis. A sequence of random observations is drawn from the joint posterior distribution $p(\boldsymbol{\theta}_*, \mathbf{F}|\mathbf{D})$ using MCMC methods such as the Gibbs sampler (Geman and Geman, 1984) and the MH algorithm (Metropolis *et al.*, 1953; Hastings, 1970). More specifically, $(\boldsymbol{\alpha}, \mathbf{Z}^*)$, $\mathbf{W}$, $\boldsymbol{\Omega}$, $\boldsymbol{\theta}_s$, and $\boldsymbol{\theta}_f$ are generated iteratively from the corresponding full conditional distributions. These full conditional distributions are derived in Appendix 12.2. Note that sampling from some of these full conditional distributions is not straightforward. For example, the full conditional distribution of $\mathbf{w}_{ij}$ is a multivariate truncated normal distribution, and the parameter spaces of $\mathbf{b}_j$ and $\boldsymbol{\beta}_j$ are constrained and degenerate. Hence, additional effort is required to simulate observations from such nonstandard distributions (see Appendix 12.2).

A specific question regarding model selection is whether or not an advanced (more complex) model is actually 'better' than an elementary (simple) one. The issue is particularly relevant here: if it can be shown that a parametric SEM using simple linear equations can provide a better fit to the observed data, then the case for using a nonparametric model would be difficult to establish. The Bayes factor (Kass and Raftery, 1995) is a common Bayesian model comparison statistic designed for this purpose. Song *et al.* (2007) demonstrated that the path sampling procedure proposed by Gelman and Meng (1998) is useful for computing the Bayes factor. However, defining a link model between the nonparametric SEM and conventional parametric SEMs within the path sampling procedure is nontrivial. Moreover, as pointed out by Song *et al.* (2007), the path sampling procedure for calculating the Bayes factor is computationally very intensive. Apparently, the computational cost for the current complex model is even higher. Here, we use an index based on the DIC (Spiegelhalter *et al.*, 2002) to conduct model comparison. The DIC is designed to seek an appropriate model by finding a balance between goodness of fit to the data and model complexity. The model with a smallest DIC-based index is selected in a model comparison procedure. Celeux *et al.* (2006) explored several versions of the DIC and pointed out that the complete DIC based on the complete-data log-likelihood function is the best of all the versions when latent variables or missing data are included. The complete DIC is defined as follows:

$$\text{DIC} = -4\text{E}_{\boldsymbol{\theta}_*,\mathbf{F}}\{\log p(\mathbf{D},\mathbf{F}|\boldsymbol{\theta}_*)|\mathbf{D}\} + 2\text{E}_{\mathbf{F}}\{\log p(\mathbf{D},\mathbf{F}|\text{E}_{\boldsymbol{\theta}_*}[\boldsymbol{\theta}_*|\mathbf{D},\mathbf{F}])|\mathbf{D}\}, \qquad (12.43)$$

where $\log p(\mathbf{D},\mathbf{F}|\boldsymbol{\theta}_*)$ is the complete-data log-likelihood function. For generalized nonparametric SEMs, $\log p(\mathbf{D},\mathbf{F}|\boldsymbol{\theta}_*)$ can be written as

$$\log p(\mathbf{D},\mathbf{F}|\boldsymbol{\theta}_*) = \sum_{i=1}^{n} \log p\big(\mathbf{d}_i, \mathbf{z}_i^*, \mathbf{w}_i, \boldsymbol{\omega}_i|\boldsymbol{\theta}_*\big),$$

where

$$\begin{aligned}
&\log p\big(\mathbf{d}_i, \mathbf{z}_i^*, \mathbf{w}_i, \boldsymbol{\omega}_i|\boldsymbol{\theta}_*\big) \\
&= \log p\big(\mathbf{d}_i, \mathbf{z}_i^*, \mathbf{w}_i|\boldsymbol{\omega}_i, \boldsymbol{\theta}_*\big) + \log p(\boldsymbol{\eta}_i|\boldsymbol{\xi}_i,\boldsymbol{\theta}_*) + \log p(\boldsymbol{\xi}_i|\boldsymbol{\theta}_*) \\
&= -\frac{1}{2}\left[\sum_{j=1}^{r_2}\log(\psi_j) + \sum_{j=1}^{r_1}\big(z_{ij}^* - \mu_j - \boldsymbol{\Lambda}_j^T\boldsymbol{\omega}_i\big)^2/\psi_j + \sum_{j=r_1+1}^{r_2}\big(y_{ij} - \mu_j - \boldsymbol{\Lambda}_j^T\boldsymbol{\omega}_i\big)^2/\psi_j\right] \\
&\quad + \sum_{j=r_2+1}^{r_3}\left[v_{ij}\big(\mu_j + \boldsymbol{\Lambda}_j^T\boldsymbol{\omega}_i\big) - \exp\big(\mu_j + \boldsymbol{\Lambda}_j^T\boldsymbol{\omega}_i\big) - \log(v_{ij}!)\right] \\
&\quad - \frac{1}{2}\sum_{j=r_3+1}^{r_4}\big(\mathbf{w}_{ij} - \boldsymbol{\mu}_j - \mathbf{1}_{L-1}\boldsymbol{\Lambda}_j^T\boldsymbol{\omega}_i\big)^T\big(\mathbf{w}_{ij} - \boldsymbol{\mu}_j - \mathbf{1}_{L-1}\boldsymbol{\Lambda}_j^T\boldsymbol{\omega}_i\big) \qquad (12.44) \\
&\quad - \frac{1}{2\psi_\delta}\left[\eta_i - \sum_{j=1}^{m}\sum_{k=1}^{K_{bj}} b_{jk}B_{jk}^x(x_{ij}) - \sum_{j=1}^{q_2}\sum_{k=1}^{K_j}\beta_{jk}B_{jk}(\Phi^*(\xi_{ij}))\right]^2 - \frac{1}{2}\log(\psi_\delta) \\
&\quad - \frac{1}{2}\big(\log|\boldsymbol{\Phi}| + \boldsymbol{\xi}_i^T\boldsymbol{\Phi}^{-1}\boldsymbol{\xi}_i\big) + \text{constant}, \quad \text{for}\, \mathbf{z}_i^* \in \mathbf{R}_i^*,
\end{aligned}$$

and $\mathbf{R}_i^* = \prod_{j=1}^{r_1}[\alpha_{j,z_{ij}}, \alpha_{j,z_{ij}+1})$. The first expectation in (12.43) can be obtained using the following approximation with the MCMC samples $\{(\mathbf{F}^{(t)}, \boldsymbol{\theta}_*^{(t)}) : t = 1,\ldots,T\}$:

$$\text{E}_{\boldsymbol{\theta}_*,\mathbf{F}}\{\log p(\mathbf{D},\mathbf{F}|\boldsymbol{\theta}_*)|\mathbf{D}\} \approx \frac{1}{T}\sum_{t=1}^{T}\log p(\mathbf{D},\mathbf{F}^{(t)}|\boldsymbol{\theta}_*^{(t)}).$$

Furthermore, if we let $\{\boldsymbol{\theta}_*^{(m,t)} : m = 1,\ldots,M\}$ denote the observations generated from $p(\boldsymbol{\theta}_*|\mathbf{D},\mathbf{F}^{(t)})$ via the MCMC methods described above, then we have the approximation

$$\text{E}_{\boldsymbol{\theta}_*}[\boldsymbol{\theta}_*|\mathbf{D},\mathbf{F}^{(t)}] \approx \bar{\boldsymbol{\theta}}_*^{(t)} = \frac{1}{M}\sum_{m=1}^{M}\boldsymbol{\theta}_*^{(m,t)}.$$

Consequently, the second expectation in (12.43) can be approximated by

$$\mathrm{E}_{\mathbf{F}}\{\log p(\mathbf{D}, \mathbf{F}|\mathrm{E}_{\boldsymbol{\theta}_*}[\boldsymbol{\theta}_*|\mathbf{D}, \mathbf{F}])|\mathbf{D}\} \approx \frac{1}{T}\sum_{t=1}^{T} \log p\big(\mathbf{D}, \mathbf{F}^{(t)}|\bar{\boldsymbol{\theta}}_*^{(t)}\big).$$

Note that the complete DIC is computed based on MCMC samples, which are by-products in the estimation procedure. As a result, the computational burden of obtaining DIC values is light.

12.3.5 National longitudinal surveys of youth study

In this subsection, we illustrate the methodology using NLSY data (Center for Human Resource Research, 2004). The four-decade-long NLSY is one of the most comprehensive longitudinal studies of youth conducted in North America. Although the NLSY originally focused on labor force behavior, the content of the survey evolved and became considerably broader in later years. The NLSY is a nationally representative sample of youths who were 14–21 years old in 1979 and 29–36 years old in 1994. The data set derived for this analysis included 1660 observations with a few missing entries. For simplicity, the missing data in this analysis were imputed under a missing at random (MAR) assumption.

In the current study, we focus on the effects of a child's 'behavior problem', 'home environment', 'mother's alcoholic problem', and 'friendship' on his/her 'academic achievement'. Given that one can never directly measure these variables of primary interest, they were modeled as latent constructs that are measured by two or more observed variables. Following the existing literature, 'academic achievement' was measured by the Peabody Individual Achievement Tests (PIAT) with continuous scales in the following domains: math, reading comprehension, and reading recognition (Dunn and Markwardt, 1970). 'Behavior problem' was measured by the Behavior Problem Index (BPI) on an ordinal scale in the following domains: anti-social, anxious, dependent, headstrong, and hyperactive behaviors (Zill, 1985). In the BPI, higher scores represent higher levels of behavior problems. 'Home environment' was measured by two continuous variables, namely cognitive stimulation and emotional support, and one unordered categorical variable coded $\{0, 1, 2\}$ representing a child who 'lives with a biological father', 'lives with a stepfather', or 'neither'. The probabilities of the unordered categorical variable taking 0, 1, and 2 are related to the latent score of 'home environment' through equations (12.28), (12.32), and (12.33). The results in the following analysis show that the estimated factor loading of 'home environment' corresponding to this unordered categorical variable is negative, indicating that a higher probability of $u_{ij} = 0$ (lives with a biological father) is associated with a higher score on 'home environment' (better home environment). The instruments for measuring these constructs come from a short form of the Home Observation for Measurement of the Environment (HOME) Inventory (Caldwell and Bradley, 1984). 'Mother's alcoholic problem' was measured by two dichotomous variables, namely 'whether mother is a binge drinker' and 'whether mother is a heavy drinker'. Finally, 'friendship' is measured by two count variables, namely the number of boyfriends and the number of girlfriends. In a preliminary analysis with a linear SEM, we find that children's 'behavior problem', 'home environment', 'mother's alcoholic problem', and 'friendship' with others have significant effects on their 'academic achievement'. Substantive studies have demonstrated that the conventional linear or quadratic structural equation may not be adequate to capture the true relationships between latent variables (see, for example, Fahrmeir and Raach, 2007; Song and Lu, 2010). For this purpose, we use a generalized nonparametric SEM, in which the

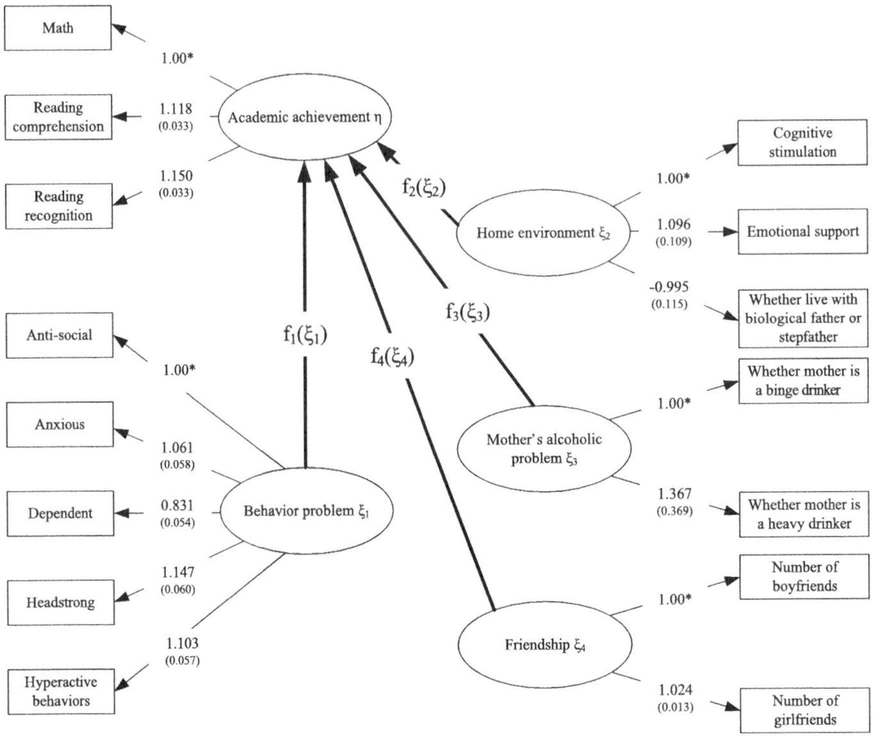

Figure 12.5 Path diagram, together with the estimated factor loadings and their standard error estimates (in parentheses), of the nonparametric SEM in the analysis of the NLSY data set.

observed variables are mixed continuous, count, and ordered and unordered categorical, and the structural equation is formulated using a series of unknown smooth functions of explanatory latent variables. The path diagram, which shows the relationships between the observed variables and their corresponding latent variables, as well as the interrelationships between latent variables, is presented in Figure 12.5. Operationally, the main goal of this analysis is to investigate how the explanatory latent variables 'behavior problem' (ξ_1), 'home environment' (ξ_2), 'mother's alcoholic problem' (ξ_3), and 'friendship' (ξ_4) influence the outcome latent variable 'academic achievement' (η). Given that the continuous variables have very different scales, they were all standardized prior to the analysis.

Based on the apparent meaning of the latent constructs, we consider the following non-overlapping structure of the loading matrix for the corresponding latent variables:

$$\boldsymbol{\Lambda}^T = \begin{bmatrix} \boldsymbol{\Lambda}_1 & \cdots & \boldsymbol{\Lambda}_{15} \end{bmatrix}$$

$$= \begin{bmatrix} 1 & \lambda_{21} & \lambda_{31} & 0 & 0 & 0 & 0 & 0 & 0 & 0 & 0 & 0 & 0 & 0 & 0 \\ 0 & 0 & 0 & 1 & \lambda_{52} & \lambda_{62} & \lambda_{72} & \lambda_{82} & 0 & 0 & 0 & 0 & 0 & 0 & 0 \\ 0 & 0 & 0 & 0 & 0 & 0 & 0 & 0 & 1 & \lambda_{10,3} & \lambda_{11,3} & 0 & 0 & 0 & 0 \\ 0 & 0 & 0 & 0 & 0 & 0 & 0 & 0 & 0 & 0 & 0 & 1 & \lambda_{13,4} & 0 & 0 \\ 0 & 0 & 0 & 0 & 0 & 0 & 0 & 0 & 0 & 0 & 0 & 0 & 0 & 1 & \lambda_{15,5} \end{bmatrix},$$

where the 1s and 0s are fixed parameters to give an identified model.

To examine the functional effects of the explanatory latent variables $\xi_{i1}, \ldots, \xi_{i4}$ on the outcome latent variable η_i, the following nonparametric structural equation is considered:

$$\eta_i = f_1(\xi_{i1}) + f_2(\xi_{i2}) + f_3(\xi_{i3}) + f_4(\xi_{i4}) + \delta_i. \tag{12.45}$$

A total of 25 equidistant knots were used to construct cubic P-splines for the ξs. The second-order random walk penalty was used for the Bayesian P-splines in estimating the unknown smooth functions. With very little information about the unknown parameters in this study, we used a relatively vague prior input in (12.42) as follows: μ_{0j}, $j = 1, \ldots, r_3$, and the elements in $\boldsymbol{\mu}_{0j}$, $j = r_3 + 1, \ldots, r_4$, and $\boldsymbol{\Lambda}_{0j}$ were zeros; $\sigma_{0j}^2 = 1$; $\mathbf{H}_{0\mu j}$, $\mathbf{H}_{0j}$, and $\mathbf{R}_0$ were identity matrices with appropriate dimensions; $\alpha_{0j} = \alpha_{0\delta} = 9$, $\beta_{0j} = \beta_{0\delta} = 4$, and $\rho_0 = 6$. Preliminary tests suggested that the MCMC algorithm converged within 10 000 iterations. Based on this information, 10 000 observations subsequent to discarding the first 10 000 burn-in iterations were collected to make the Bayesian inference. Table 12.2 and Figure 12.5 present the Bayesian estimates (Est) of the unknown structural parameters and their corresponding standard error estimates (SE). Figure 12.6 depicts the Bayesian estimates of the unknown functions, together with the 5% and 95% pointwise quantiles. From this figure, we observed that – perhaps with the

Table 12.2 Bayesian estimates of the structural parameters in the study of the NLSY data set.

Par.	Est	SE	Par.	Est	SE
μ_1	−0.003	0.025	$\lambda_{13,4}$	1.367	0.369
μ_2	−0.010	0.024	$\lambda_{15,5}$	1.024	0.013
μ_3	−0.007	0.025	ψ_1	0.457	0.020
μ_4	0.102	0.027	ψ_2	0.317	0.018
μ_5	−0.002	0.029	ψ_3	0.272	0.017
μ_6	0.003	0.030	ψ_4	0.388	0.031
μ_7	0.004	0.030	ψ_5	0.449	0.025
μ_8	0.000	0.029	ψ_6	0.646	0.042
μ_9	−0.006	0.024	ψ_7	0.373	0.023
μ_{10}	−0.008	0.025	ψ_8	0.419	0.024
$\mu_{11,1}$	−0.599	0.040	ψ_9	0.676	0.038
$\mu_{11,2}$	−0.304	0.038	ψ_{10}	0.618	0.043
μ_{12}	−1.325	0.154	ϕ_{11}	0.485	0.045
μ_{13}	−3.244	0.494	ϕ_{21}	−0.135	0.018
μ_{14}	1.874	0.025	ϕ_{22}	0.322	0.040
μ_{15}	1.919	0.026	ϕ_{31}	0.169	0.056
λ_{21}	1.118	0.033	ϕ_{32}	−0.288	0.059
λ_{31}	1.150	0.033	ϕ_{33}	3.909	0.961
λ_{52}	1.061	0.058	ϕ_{41}	0.001	0.019
λ_{62}	0.831	0.054	ϕ_{42}	−0.048	0.019
λ_{72}	1.147	0.060	ϕ_{43}	0.087	0.071
λ_{82}	1.103	0.057	ϕ_{44}	0.900	0.038
$\lambda_{10,3}$	1.096	0.109	ψ_δ	0.421	0.031
$\lambda_{11,3}$	−0.995	0.115			

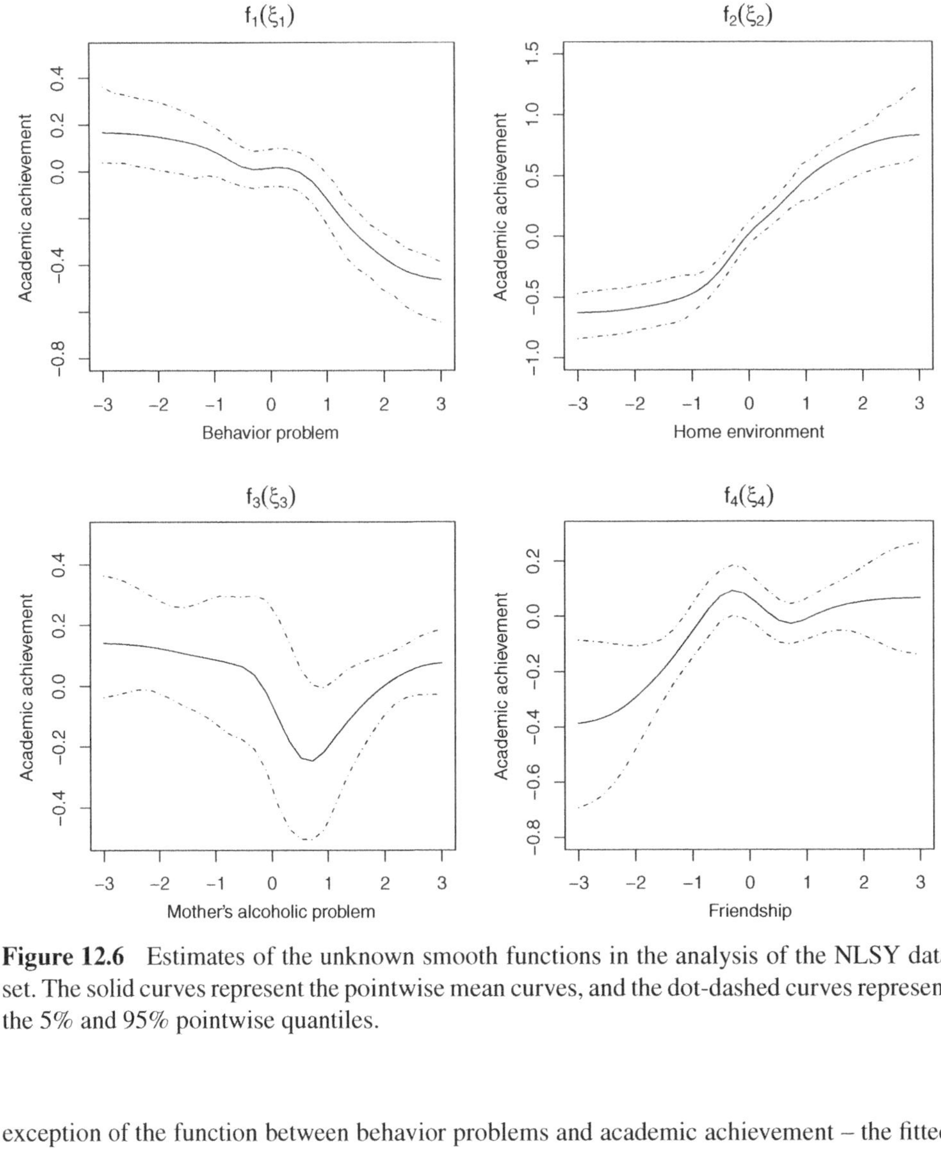

Figure 12.6 Estimates of the unknown smooth functions in the analysis of the NLSY data set. The solid curves represent the pointwise mean curves, and the dot-dashed curves represent the 5% and 95% pointwise quantiles.

exception of the function between behavior problems and academic achievement – the fitted curves were neither linear nor quadratic. This suggests that nonparametric models could be a better choice than their parametric counterparts. The performances of conventional parametric SEMs and nonparametric SEM were further compared by considering the model comparison statistics of the following competing models, which were specified by the same measurement equations (see equations (12.29)–(12.32) and Figure 12.5) but different structural equations:

M_N : nonparametric SEM, with structural equation (12.45);

M_L : linear SEM, with $\eta_i = \gamma_1\xi_{i1} + \gamma_2\xi_{i2} + \gamma_3\xi_{i3} + \gamma_4\xi_{i4} + \delta_i$; and

M_Q : quadratic SEM, with $\eta_i = \gamma_1\xi_{i1} + \gamma_2\xi_{i2} + \gamma_3\xi_{i3} + \gamma_4\xi_{i4} + \gamma_5\xi_{i1}^2 + \gamma_6\xi_{i2}^2 + \gamma_7\xi_{i3}^2 + \gamma_8\xi_{i4}^2 + \delta_i$.

The DIC values for M_N, M_L, and M_Q are 93 542, 93 613, and 94 133, respectively, suggesting that M_N is the best model.

The above results are instructive in that they demonstrate the power of the nonparametric SEM in revealing subtle patterns in the functional relationship between latent variables. They are also illustrative because they show how the nonparametric SEM can be used both as an exploratory tool for investigating functional forms and as a confirmatory tool for selecting models through statistically based criteria.

The functional effects obtained can be interpreted as follows. (i) 'Behavior problem' has an essentially negative effect on 'academic achievement'. This negative effect is mild when a child's behavior problem is not severe, but becomes significant when his/her behavior problem gets worse. (ii) 'Home environment' has a positive effect on 'academic achievement'. In general, a child with a better home environment is more likely to show higher academic achievement. This positive effect, however, appears to be neither linear nor quadratic. The functional form exhibits a logistic function-like pattern over the range of the home environment score: the rate of change of the home effect is slow, fast, and then back to slow respectively at low, medium, and high levels of the home environment score. Such a pattern reveals that at least a moderately good home environment is important for academic achievement. (iii) 'Mother's alcoholic problem' appears to have a negative impact on a child's academic achievement. This effect is especially pronounced when the consumption level increases beyond moderate. We are, however, puzzled by the upward bounce toward the end of the alcoholism scale. One plausible explanation is that the mother was no longer taking care of the home environment. Further investigation will be required to resolve this dilemma. (iv) 'Friendship' has a positive effect on 'academic achievement'. The effect is not unexpected; what is surprising is that the effect appears to be nonlinear: it increases steeply at the low level of the friendship scale, attains a maximum at around the medium level, and then remains more or less stable.

To assess the sensitivity of the Bayesian results to the prior input, the above analysis was repeated with some *ad hoc* perturbations to the current prior input. For instance, μ_{0j} and the elements in $\boldsymbol{\mu}_{0j}$ and $\boldsymbol{\Lambda}_{0j}$ were set to 1; $\mathbf{H}_{0\mu j}$, $\mathbf{H}_{0j}$, and $\mathbf{R}_0^{-1}$ were set to values 10 times the identity matrices; $\alpha_{0j} = \alpha_{0\delta} = 5$, $\beta_{0j} = \beta_{0\delta} = 6$, and $\rho_0 = 14$. Compared with the reported results, the sensitivity analysis showed that both complete DIC values and estimates of the unknown parameters and smooth functions were similar. In summary, our Bayesian results are robust to prior specification and input. The computer program is written in R with compiled C code. The code is available from the following website:

`www.wiley.com/go/medical_behavioral_sciences`

12.4 Discussion

In this chapter nonparametric SEMs with continuous and/or various types of discrete data are presented to assess the functional relationships between latent and observed variables. Unlike traditional SEMs, nonparametric SEMs formulate the structural equation nonparametrically by introducing a series of unspecified smooth functions. We use the Bayesian P-splines incorporating MCMC techniques to estimate the unknown smooth functions and parameters in the model. The DIC is used for model comparison. The adapted version of the complete DIC is used to support decision making in choosing between nonparametric SEMs and conventional parametric SEMs. Results obtained from a simulation study demonstrate the empirical performance of the methodology. The Bayesian nonparametric SEMs described in this chapter have been applied to two real-life studies; some interesting functional relationships among latent and/or observed variables have been identified.

There are several possible extensions of the current analysis. First, the model assumes normality of latent variables and random errors. This assumption may be violated in practical applications. Further research is required to develop a more robust method for handling non-normal data. Second, the interactions between explanatory latent variables are not considered in the current model. For $j \neq l$, a two-dimensional smooth function $f_{hjl}(\xi_{ij}, \xi_{il})$ can be used to model the interaction between ξ_{ij} and ξ_{il}, which leads to a nonparametric structural equation of the form

$$\eta_{ih} = g_{h1}(x_{i1}) + \ldots + g_{hm}(x_{im}) + f_{h1}(\xi_{i1}) + \ldots + f_{hq_2}(\xi_{iq_2}) + \sum_{j \neq l} f_{hjl}(\xi_{ij}, \xi_{il}) + \delta_{ih}. \tag{12.46}$$

Because equation (12.46) involves two-dimensional nonparametric functions of latent variables, substantial effort will be required to solve the technical challenges in the representation, computation, and interpretation of such models. Finally, the current method only applies to cross-sectional data. A dynamic nonparametric SEM for analyzing multi-dimensional longitudinal data would be a valuable addition to the SEM toolbox.

Appendix 12.1 Conditional distributions and the MH algorithm: Nonparametric SEMs

The conditional distributions involved in steps (a) and (b1)–(b7) (see Section 12.4.2), and the implementation of the MH algorithm are given below.

Conditional Distribution of $\boldsymbol{\Omega}$ *in Step (a)*

We have

$$p(\boldsymbol{\Omega}|\mathbf{Y},\boldsymbol{\theta}) = \prod_{i=1}^{n} p(\boldsymbol{\omega}_i|\mathbf{y}_i,\boldsymbol{\theta}) \propto \prod_{i=1}^{n} p(\mathbf{y}_i|\boldsymbol{\omega}_i,\boldsymbol{\theta})p(\eta_i|\boldsymbol{\xi}_i,\boldsymbol{\theta})p(\boldsymbol{\xi}_i|\boldsymbol{\theta})$$

$$\propto \prod_{i=1}^{n}\left[\left\{\prod_{j=1}^{p} p(y_{ij}|\boldsymbol{\omega}_i,\mathbf{A}_j,\boldsymbol{\Lambda}_j,\psi_j)\right\} p(\eta_i|\boldsymbol{\xi}_i,\psi_\delta,\mathbf{b},\boldsymbol{\beta},\mathbf{s})p(\boldsymbol{\xi}_i|\boldsymbol{\Phi})\right].$$

So

$$p(\boldsymbol{\omega}_i|\mathbf{y}_i,\boldsymbol{\theta}) \propto \exp\left\{-\sum_{j=1}^{p}\frac{1}{2\psi_j}(y_{ij}-\mathbf{A}_j^T\mathbf{c}_i-\boldsymbol{\Lambda}_j^T\boldsymbol{\omega}_i)^2\right\}\exp\left(-\frac{1}{2}\boldsymbol{\xi}_i^T\boldsymbol{\Phi}^{-1}\boldsymbol{\xi}_i\right) \quad (12.A1)$$

$$\times \exp\left[-\frac{1}{2\psi_\delta}\left\{\eta_i-\sum_{j=1}^{m}\sum_{k=1}^{K_{bj}} b_{jk}B_{jk}^x(x_{ij})-\sum_{j=1}^{q_2}\sum_{k=1}^{K_j}\beta_{jk}N_{jk}(\xi_{ij}|s_j)\right\}^2\right].$$

The conditional distribution given in (12.A1) is nonstandard and complex. Hence, the MH algorithm is used to generate observations from this conditional distribution. For the target density $p(\boldsymbol{\omega}_i|\mathbf{y}_i,\boldsymbol{\theta})$, we choose $N[\boldsymbol{\mu}_\omega,\sigma_\omega^2\boldsymbol{\Sigma}_\omega]$ as the proposal distribution, where

$$\boldsymbol{\Sigma}_\omega = \left[\begin{pmatrix} \psi_\delta^{-1} & -\psi_\delta^{-1}\boldsymbol{\beta}\boldsymbol{\Delta} \\ -\psi_\delta^{-1}(\boldsymbol{\beta}\boldsymbol{\Delta})^T & \boldsymbol{\Phi}^{-1}+\psi_\delta^{-1}\boldsymbol{\Delta}^T\boldsymbol{\beta}^T\boldsymbol{\beta}\boldsymbol{\Delta}\end{pmatrix} + \boldsymbol{\Lambda}^T\boldsymbol{\Psi}^{-1}\boldsymbol{\Lambda}\right]^{-1}$$

in which $\boldsymbol{\Delta} = (\partial\sum_{j=1}^{q_2}\sum_{k=1}^{K_j}\beta_{jk}N_{jk}(\xi_{ij}|s_j)/\partial\boldsymbol{\xi}_i)^T|_{\boldsymbol{\xi}_i=\mathbf{0}}$. Let $q(\cdot|\boldsymbol{\mu}_\omega,\sigma_\omega,\boldsymbol{\Sigma}_\omega)$ be the proposal density corresponding to $N[\boldsymbol{\mu}_\omega,\sigma_\omega^2\boldsymbol{\Sigma}_\omega]$. The MH algorithm is implemented as follows: at the $(t+1)$th iteration with a current value $\boldsymbol{\omega}_i^{(t)}$, a new candidate $\boldsymbol{\omega}_i$ is generated from $q(\cdot|\boldsymbol{\omega}_i^{(t)},\sigma_\omega,\boldsymbol{\Sigma}_\omega)$ and accepted with probability

$$\min\left\{1,\frac{p(\boldsymbol{\omega}_i|\mathbf{y}_i,\boldsymbol{\theta})}{p(\boldsymbol{\omega}_i^{(t)}|\mathbf{y}_i,\boldsymbol{\theta})}\right\}.$$

The variance σ_ω^2 can be chosen such that the average acceptance rate is approximately 0.25 or more; see Gelman *et al.* (1996) for more details.

Conditional Distributions of Structural Parameters $\mathbf{A}$, $\boldsymbol{\Lambda}$, $\boldsymbol{\Psi}$, ψ_δ, and $\boldsymbol{\Phi}$ *in Steps (b1)–(b4)*

Let $y_{ij}^* = y_{ij}-\boldsymbol{\Lambda}_j^T\boldsymbol{\omega}_i$, $\mathbf{y}_j^* = (y_{1j}^*,\ldots,y_{nj}^*)^T$, $\tilde{y}_{ij} = y_{ij}-\mathbf{A}_j^T\mathbf{c}_i$, $\tilde{\mathbf{y}}_j = (\tilde{y}_{1j},\ldots,\tilde{y}_{nj})^T$, and $\mathbf{C} = (\mathbf{c}_1,\ldots,\mathbf{c}_n)$. The full conditional distributions of $\mathbf{A}_j$, $\boldsymbol{\Lambda}_j$, ψ_j, ψ_δ, and $\boldsymbol{\Phi}$ are as follows:

$$[\mathbf{A}_j|\cdot] \stackrel{D}{=} N[\boldsymbol{\mu}_{aj},\boldsymbol{\Sigma}_{aj}],\quad [\boldsymbol{\Lambda}_j|\cdot] \stackrel{D}{=} N[\boldsymbol{\mu}_{\lambda j},\boldsymbol{\Sigma}_{\lambda j}],\quad \left[\psi_j^{-1}|\cdot\right] \stackrel{D}{=} \mathrm{Gamma}[\alpha_{0j}+n/2,\beta_{\lambda j}],$$

$$\left[\psi_\delta^{-1}|\cdot\right] \stackrel{D}{=} \mathrm{Gamma}[n/2+\alpha_{0\delta},\beta_\delta],\quad [\boldsymbol{\Phi}|\cdot] \stackrel{D}{=} \mathrm{IW}\left[\left(\boldsymbol{\Omega}_2\boldsymbol{\Omega}_2^T+\mathbf{R}_0^{-1}\right),n+\rho_0\right],$$

where $\boldsymbol{\Sigma}_{aj} = (\psi_j^{-1}\mathbf{C}\mathbf{C}^T + \boldsymbol{\Sigma}_{0aj}^{-1})^{-1}$, $\boldsymbol{\mu}_{aj} = \boldsymbol{\Sigma}_{aj}(\boldsymbol{\Sigma}_{0aj}^{-1}\mathbf{A}_{0j} + \psi_j^{-1}\mathbf{C}\mathbf{y}_j^*)$, $\boldsymbol{\Sigma}_{\lambda j} = (\boldsymbol{\Omega}\boldsymbol{\Omega}^T + \boldsymbol{\Sigma}_{0j}^{-1})^{-1}$, $\boldsymbol{\mu}_{\lambda j} = \boldsymbol{\Sigma}_{\lambda j}(\boldsymbol{\Sigma}_{0j}^{-1}\boldsymbol{\Lambda}_{0j} + \boldsymbol{\Omega}\tilde{\mathbf{y}}_j)$, $\beta_{\lambda j} = \beta_{0j} + (\tilde{\mathbf{y}}_j^T\tilde{\mathbf{y}}_j - \boldsymbol{\mu}_{\lambda j}^T\boldsymbol{\Sigma}_{\lambda j}^{-1}\boldsymbol{\mu}_{\lambda j} + \boldsymbol{\Lambda}_{0j}^T\boldsymbol{\Sigma}_{0j}^{-1}\boldsymbol{\Lambda}_{0j})/2$, $\beta_\delta = \beta_{0\delta} + \sum_{i=1}^n\{\eta_i - \sum_{j=1}^m\sum_{k=1}^{K_{bj}} b_{jk}B_{jk}^x(x_{ij}) - \sum_{j=1}^{q_2}\sum_{k=1}^{K_j}\beta_{jk}N_{jk}(\xi_{ij}|s_j)\}^2/2$.

Conditional Distributions of $\boldsymbol{\tau}_b$, $\boldsymbol{\tau}_\beta$ and $\boldsymbol{\tau}_s$ *in Step (b5)*

It can be shown that the full conditional distributions of $\boldsymbol{\tau}_b$, $\boldsymbol{\tau}_\beta$, and $\boldsymbol{\tau}_s$ are:

$$[\tau_{\beta j}^{-1}|\cdot] \stackrel{D}{=} \text{Gamma}\big[K_j^*/2 + \alpha_{0\beta}, \beta_{0\beta} + \boldsymbol{\beta}_j^T\mathbf{M}_{\beta j}\boldsymbol{\beta}_j/2\big], \quad j = 1, \ldots, q_2,$$

$$[\tau_{bj}^{-1}|\cdot] \stackrel{D}{=} \text{Gamma}\big[K_{bj}^*/2 + \alpha_{0b}, \beta_{0b} + \mathbf{b}_j^T\mathbf{M}_{bj}\mathbf{b}_j/2\big], \quad j = 1, \ldots, m,$$

$$[\tau_{sj}^{-1}|\cdot] \stackrel{D}{=} \text{Gamma}\left[K_j/2 + \alpha_{0\tau}, \beta_{0\tau} + \sum_{k=1}^{K_j}\{\log(|s_j\kappa_k|)\}^2/2\right], \quad j = 1, \ldots, q_2.$$

Distribution of $\mathbf{b}_j$ *in Step (b6).*

The distribution of $\mathbf{b}_j$ is

$$N\big[\mathbf{b}_j^*, \boldsymbol{\Sigma}_{bj}^*\big]I(\mathbf{Q}_{bj}\mathbf{b}_j = 0),$$

where $\boldsymbol{\Sigma}_{bj}^* = (\mathbf{B}_{bj}^T\mathbf{B}_{bj}/\psi_\delta + \mathbf{M}_{bj}/\tau_{bj})^{-1}$, $\mathbf{b}_j^* = \boldsymbol{\Sigma}_{bj}^*\mathbf{B}_{bj}^T\boldsymbol{\eta}_x^*/\psi_\delta$, and $\boldsymbol{\eta}_x^* = (\eta_{x1}^*, \ldots, \eta_{xn}^*)^T$ with

$$\eta_{xi}^* = \eta_i - \sum_{l\neq j}\sum_{k=1}^{K_{bl}} b_{lk}B_{lk}^x(x_{il}) - \sum_{j=1}^{q_2}\sum_{k=1}^{K_j}\beta_{jk}N_{jk}(\xi_{ij}|s_j).$$

From the discussion in Section 12.2.4, sampling an observation $\mathbf{b}_j$ from $N[\mathbf{b}_j^*, \boldsymbol{\Sigma}_{bj}^*]I(\mathbf{Q}_{bj}\mathbf{b}_j = 0)$ is equivalent to sampling an observation $\mathbf{b}_j^{(\text{new})}$ from $N[\mathbf{b}_j^*, \boldsymbol{\Sigma}_{bj}^*]$, then transforming $\mathbf{b}_j^{(\text{new})}$ to $\mathbf{b}_j$ by letting

$$\mathbf{b}_j = \mathbf{b}_j^{(\text{new})} - \boldsymbol{\Sigma}_{bj}^*\mathbf{Q}_{bj}^T\big(\mathbf{Q}_{bj}\boldsymbol{\Sigma}_{bj}^*\mathbf{Q}_{bj}^T\big)^{-1}\mathbf{Q}_{bj}\mathbf{b}_j^{(\text{new})}.$$

Conditional Distribution of $(\boldsymbol{\beta}_j, s_j)$ *in Step (b7)*

For $j = 1, \ldots, q_2$, let $\boldsymbol{\beta}_{-j}$ and $\mathbf{s}_{-j}$ denote subvectors of $\boldsymbol{\beta}$ and $\mathbf{s}$ that exclude $\boldsymbol{\beta}_j$ and s_j, respectively. The conditional distribution of $(\boldsymbol{\beta}_j, s_j)$ is

$$p(\boldsymbol{\beta}_j, s_j|\boldsymbol{\Omega}, \psi_\delta, \tau_{\beta j}, \tau_{sj}, \mathbf{b}, \boldsymbol{\beta}_{-j}, \mathbf{s}_{-j}) \propto p(\boldsymbol{\beta}_j|\boldsymbol{\Omega}, \psi_\delta, \tau_{\beta j}, \mathbf{b}, \boldsymbol{\beta}_{-j}, \mathbf{s})p(s_j|\tau_{sj}) \tag{12.A2}$$

$$\propto \exp\left[-\frac{1}{2\psi_\delta}\sum_{i=1}^n\left\{\eta_i^* - \sum_{k=1}^{K_j}\beta_{jk}N_{jk}(\xi_{ij}|s_j)\right\}^2 - \frac{1}{2\tau_{\beta j}}\boldsymbol{\beta}_j^T\mathbf{M}_{\beta j}\boldsymbol{\beta}_j - \frac{1}{2\tau_{sj}}\sum_{k=1}^{K_j}\{\log(|s_j\kappa_k|)\}^2\right].$$

The reason for updating $(\boldsymbol{\beta}_j, s_j)$ in a block is given below. It is noticed from $f_j(\xi_{ij}) = \sum_{k=1}^{K_j}\beta_{jk}N_{jk}(\xi_{ij}|s_j)$ that the highly correlated $\boldsymbol{\beta}_j$ and s_j are used to model the unknown smooth function f_j together. Updating them within a block will accelerate MCMC convergence.

As the conditional distribution in (12.A2) is nonstandard, the MH algorithm is used to simulate observations from it. Inspired by Rue and Held (2005), given the current $s_j^{(t-1)}$, we first generate a new $s_j^{(t)}$ using the random walk defined by $s_j^{(t)} = f\cdot s_j^{(t-1)}$, with $p(f) \propto 1 + 1/f$, $f \in [1/C, C]$ $(C > 1)$, in which C is a tuning parameter. It can be shown that

$$q\left(s_j^{(t)}|s_j^{(t-1)}\right) \propto \frac{1}{s_j^{(t)}} + \frac{1}{s_j^{(t-1)}}. \tag{12.A3}$$

The random walk defined in (12.A3) is symmetric in that $q(s_j^{(t)}|s_j^{(t-1)}) = q(s_j^{(t-1)}|s_j^{(t)})$. With this proposal density, a new sample $\{\boldsymbol{\beta}_j^{(t)}, s_j^{(t)}\}$ is accepted with probability $\min\{1, R_j\}$, where

$$R_j = \frac{p\left(s_j^{(t)}|\cdot\right)}{p\left(s_j^{(t-1)}|\cdot\right)},$$

in which $p(s_j^{(t)}|\cdot)$ is the marginal distribution of full conditional distribution $p(\boldsymbol{\beta}_j^{(t)}, s_j^{(t)}|\cdot)$, which can be derived analytically as follows:

$$\begin{aligned} p(s_j|\cdot) &\propto \exp\left\{-\frac{1}{2\tau_{sj}}\sum_{k=1}^{K_j}\{\log(|s_j\kappa_k|)\}^2\right\} \\ &\quad\times \int \exp\left[-\frac{1}{2}\left\{\boldsymbol{\beta}_j^T\left(\frac{1}{\psi_\delta}\mathbf{N}_j^T\mathbf{N}_j + \frac{1}{\tau_{\beta j}}\mathbf{M}_{\beta j}\right)\boldsymbol{\beta}_j - 2\boldsymbol{\beta}_j^T\left(\frac{\mathbf{N}_j^T\boldsymbol{\eta}^*}{\psi_\delta}\right)\right\}\right]d\boldsymbol{\beta}_j \\ &\propto \left|\boldsymbol{\Sigma}_j^*\right|^{1/2}\exp\left\{\frac{1}{2}\boldsymbol{\beta}_j^{*T}\boldsymbol{\Sigma}_j^{*-1}\boldsymbol{\beta}_j^* - \frac{1}{2\tau_{sj}}\sum_{k=1}^{K_j}\{\log(|s_j\kappa_k|)\}^2\right\}. \end{aligned}$$

Since R_j depends only on $s_j^{(t)}$ and $s_j^{(t-1)}$ and not on $\boldsymbol{\beta}_j$, a new observation of $\boldsymbol{\beta}_j$ is generated from $N[\boldsymbol{\beta}_j^*, \boldsymbol{\Sigma}_j^*]I(\mathbf{Q}_j\boldsymbol{\beta}_j = 0)$ when $s_j^{(t)}$ is accepted. As discussed in Section 12.4.1, sampling an observation $\boldsymbol{\beta}_j$ from $N[\boldsymbol{\beta}_j^*, \boldsymbol{\Sigma}_j^*]I(\mathbf{Q}_j\boldsymbol{\beta}_j = 0)$ is equivalent to sampling an observation $\boldsymbol{\beta}_j^{(\text{new})}$ from $N[\boldsymbol{\beta}_j^*, \boldsymbol{\Sigma}_j^*]$, then transforming $\boldsymbol{\beta}_j^{(\text{new})}$ to $\boldsymbol{\beta}_j$ by letting

$$\boldsymbol{\beta}_j = \boldsymbol{\beta}_j^{(\text{new})} - \boldsymbol{\Sigma}_j^*\mathbf{Q}_j^T\left(\mathbf{Q}_j\boldsymbol{\Sigma}_j^*\mathbf{Q}_j^T\right)^{-1}\mathbf{Q}_j\boldsymbol{\beta}_j^{(\text{new})}.$$

Appendix 12.2 Conditional distributions in generalized nonparametric SEMs

The conditional distribution of $\boldsymbol{\Omega}$ is given by

$$p(\boldsymbol{\Omega}|\mathbf{D}, \mathbf{Z}^*, \mathbf{W}, \boldsymbol{\theta}_*) = \prod_{i=1}^{n} p(\boldsymbol{\omega}_i|\mathbf{d}_i, \mathbf{z}_i^*, \mathbf{w}_i, \boldsymbol{\theta}_*)$$

and

$$p(\boldsymbol{\omega}_i|\mathbf{d}_i, \mathbf{z}_i^*, \mathbf{w}_i, \boldsymbol{\theta}_*) \propto p(\mathbf{d}_i, \mathbf{z}_i^*, \mathbf{w}_i|\boldsymbol{\omega}_i, \boldsymbol{\theta}_*)p(\eta_i|\boldsymbol{\xi}_i, \boldsymbol{\theta}_*)p(\boldsymbol{\xi}_i|\boldsymbol{\theta}_*)$$

$$\propto \exp\left\{-\frac{1}{2}\left[\sum_{j=1}^{r_1}\left(z_{ij}^* - \mu_j - \boldsymbol{\Lambda}_j^T\boldsymbol{\omega}_i\right)^2/\psi_j + \sum_{j=r_1+1}^{r_2}\left(y_{ij} - \mu_j - \boldsymbol{\Lambda}_j^T\boldsymbol{\omega}_i\right)^2/\psi_j\right]\right.$$

$$+ \sum_{j=r_2+1}^{r_3}\left[v_{ij}\left(\mu_j + \boldsymbol{\Lambda}_j^T\boldsymbol{\omega}_i\right) - \exp\left(\mu_j + \boldsymbol{\Lambda}_j^T\boldsymbol{\omega}_i\right)\right]$$

$$-\frac{1}{2}\sum_{j=r_3+1}^{r_4}\left(\mathbf{w}_{ij} - \boldsymbol{\mu}_j - \mathbf{1}_{L-1}\boldsymbol{\Lambda}_j^T\boldsymbol{\omega}_i\right)^T\left(\mathbf{w}_{ij} - \boldsymbol{\mu}_j - \mathbf{1}_{L-1}\boldsymbol{\Lambda}_j^T\boldsymbol{\omega}_i\right)$$

$$\left.-\frac{1}{2\psi_\delta}\left[\eta_i - \sum_{j=1}^{m}\sum_{k=1}^{K_{bj}} b_{jk}B_{jk}^x(x_{ij}) - \sum_{j=1}^{q_2}\sum_{k=1}^{K_j}\beta_{jk}B_{jk}\left(\Phi^*(\xi_{ij})\right)\right]^2 - \frac{1}{2}\boldsymbol{\xi}_i^T\boldsymbol{\Phi}^{-1}\boldsymbol{\xi}_i\right\}.$$

The conditional distribution of $\mathbf{W}$ is given by

$$p(\mathbf{W}|\mathbf{D}, \mathbf{Z}^*, \boldsymbol{\Omega}, \boldsymbol{\theta}_*) = \prod_{i=1}^{n}\prod_{j=r_3+1}^{r_4} p(\mathbf{w}_{ij}|u_{ij}, \boldsymbol{\omega}_i, \boldsymbol{\theta}_*)$$

and

$$[\mathbf{w}_{ij}|u_{ij} = l, \boldsymbol{\omega}_i, \boldsymbol{\theta}_*] \stackrel{D}{=} N\left[\boldsymbol{\mu}_j + \mathbf{1}_{L-1}\boldsymbol{\Lambda}_j^T\boldsymbol{\omega}_i, \mathbf{I}_{L-1}\right]I(\mathbf{w}_{ij} \in \mathfrak{R}_l),$$

where $\mathbf{I}_{L-1}$ is an identity matrix with order $L-1$, and

$$\mathfrak{R}_l = \begin{cases}\{\mathbf{w}_{ij} : \max(\mathbf{w}_{ij}) \leq 0\}, & \text{if} \quad l = 0,\\ \left\{\mathbf{w}_{ij} : \max(\mathbf{w}_{ij}) = w_{ij,l} > 0\right\}, & \text{if} \quad 0 < l \leq L-1.\end{cases}$$

The distribution of $p(\mathbf{w}_{ij}|u_{ij}, \boldsymbol{\omega}_i, \boldsymbol{\theta}_*)$ is a truncated multivariate normal distribution. Following Song *et al.* (2007), we use the following partitioning of variables to simulate observations $\{w_{ij,1}, \ldots, w_{ij,L-1}\}$ via the Gibbs sampler. Let $\mathbf{w}_{ij,-l}$ be $\mathbf{w}_{ij}$ with $w_{ij,l}$ deleted. The distribution of $w_{ij,l}$ given u_{ij}, $\mathbf{w}_{ij,-l}$, $\boldsymbol{\omega}_i$, and $\boldsymbol{\theta}_*$ is a univariate truncated normal distribution as follows:

$$[w_{ij,l}|u_{ij}, \mathbf{w}_{ij,-l}, \boldsymbol{\omega}_i, \boldsymbol{\theta}_*] \stackrel{D}{=} \begin{cases}N\left[\mu_{jl} + \boldsymbol{\Lambda}_j^T\boldsymbol{\omega}_i, 1\right]I(w_{ij,l} > \max\{\mathbf{w}_{ij,-l}, 0\}), & \text{if} \quad u_{ij} = l,\\ N\left[\mu_{jl} + \boldsymbol{\Lambda}_j^T\boldsymbol{\omega}_i, 1\right]I(w_{ij,l} \leq \max\{\mathbf{w}_{ij,-l}, 0\}), & \text{if} \quad u_{ij} \neq l.\end{cases}$$

The conditional distribution of $\mathbf{b}_j$ is

$$[\mathbf{b}_j|\cdot] \stackrel{D}{=} N\left[\mathbf{b}_j^*, \boldsymbol{\Sigma}_{bj}^*\right]I\left(\mathbf{1}_n^T\mathbf{B}_j^x\mathbf{b}_j = 0\right), \quad j = 1, \ldots, m,$$

where $\boldsymbol{\Sigma}_{bj}^* = (\mathbf{B}_j^{xT}\mathbf{B}_j^x/\psi_\delta + \mathbf{M}_{bj}/\tau_{bj})^{-1}$, $\mathbf{b}_j^* = \boldsymbol{\Sigma}_{bj}^*\mathbf{B}_j^{xT}\boldsymbol{\eta}_x^*/\psi_\delta$, and $\boldsymbol{\eta}_x^* = (\eta_{x1}^*, \ldots, \eta_{xn}^*)^T$ with

$$\eta_{xi}^* = \eta_i - \sum_{l \neq j}\sum_{k=1}^{K_{bl}} b_{lk}B_{lk}^x(x_{il}) - \sum_{j=1}^{q_2}\sum_{k=1}^{K_j} \beta_{jk}B_{jk}(\Phi^*(\xi_{ij})).$$

To sample an observation $\mathbf{b}_j$ from its full conditional distribution with the constraint, we can sample an observation $\mathbf{b}_j^{(\text{new})}$ from $N[\mathbf{b}_j^*, \boldsymbol{\Sigma}_{bj}^*]$, then transform $\mathbf{b}_j^{(\text{new})}$ to $\mathbf{b}_j$ as follows:

$$\mathbf{b}_j = \mathbf{b}_j^{(\text{new})} - \boldsymbol{\Sigma}_{bj}^*\mathbf{B}_j^{xT}\mathbf{1}_n\left(\mathbf{1}_n^T\mathbf{B}_j^x\boldsymbol{\Sigma}_{bj}^*\mathbf{B}_j^{xT}\mathbf{1}_n\right)^{-1}\mathbf{1}_n^T\mathbf{B}_j^x\mathbf{b}_j^{(\text{new})}.$$

The conditional distribution of $\boldsymbol{\beta}_j$ is

$$[\boldsymbol{\beta}_j|\cdot] \stackrel{D}{=} N\left[\boldsymbol{\beta}_j^*, \boldsymbol{\Sigma}_{\beta j}^*\right]I\left(\mathbf{1}_n^T\mathbf{B}_j\boldsymbol{\beta}_j = 0\right), \quad j = 1, \ldots, q_2,$$

where $\boldsymbol{\Sigma}_{\beta j}^* = (\mathbf{B}_j^T\mathbf{B}_j/\psi_\delta + \mathbf{M}_{\beta j}/\tau_{\beta j})^{-1}$, $\boldsymbol{\beta}_j^* = \boldsymbol{\Sigma}_{\beta j}^*\mathbf{B}_j^T\boldsymbol{\eta}^*/\psi_\delta$, and $\boldsymbol{\eta}^* = (\eta_1^*, \ldots, \eta_n^*)^T$ with

$$\eta_i^* = \eta_i - \sum_{j=1}^{m}\sum_{k=1}^{K_{bj}} b_{jk}B_{jk}^x(x_{ij}) - \sum_{l \neq j}\sum_{k=1}^{K_l} \beta_{lk}B_{lk}(\Phi^*(\xi_{il})).$$

Similar to $\mathbf{b}_j$, we can sample an observation $\boldsymbol{\beta}_j^{(\text{new})}$ from $N[\boldsymbol{\beta}_j^*, \boldsymbol{\Sigma}_{\beta j}^*]$, then transform $\boldsymbol{\beta}_j^{(\text{new})}$ to $\boldsymbol{\beta}_j$ as follows:

$$\boldsymbol{\beta}_j = \boldsymbol{\beta}_j^{(\text{new})} - \boldsymbol{\Sigma}_{\beta j}^*\mathbf{B}_j^T\mathbf{1}_n\left(\mathbf{1}_n^T\mathbf{B}_j\boldsymbol{\Sigma}_{\beta j}^*\mathbf{B}_j^T\mathbf{1}_n\right)^{-1}\mathbf{1}_n^T\mathbf{B}_j\boldsymbol{\beta}_j^{(\text{new})}.$$

The conditional distributions of $\boldsymbol{\tau}_b$ and $\boldsymbol{\tau}_\beta$ are as follows:

$$\left[\tau_{bj}^{-1}|\cdot\right] \stackrel{D}{=} \text{Gamma}\left[\alpha_{0b} + K_{bj}^*/2, \beta_{0b} + \mathbf{b}_j^T\mathbf{M}_{bj}\mathbf{b}_j/2\right], \quad j = 1, \ldots, m,$$

$$\left[\tau_{\beta j}^{-1}|\cdot\right] \stackrel{D}{=} \text{Gamma}\left[\alpha_{0\beta} + K_j^*/2, \beta_{0\beta} + \boldsymbol{\beta}_j^T\mathbf{M}_{\beta j}\boldsymbol{\beta}_j/2\right], \quad j = 1, \ldots, q_2.$$

The conditional distribution of $\boldsymbol{\mu}$ is as follows:

$$[\mu_j|\cdot] \stackrel{D}{=} N\left[\mu_j^*, \sigma_j^{*^2}\right], \quad j = 1, \ldots, r_1,$$

$$[\mu_j|\cdot] \stackrel{D}{=} N\left[\mu_j^{**}, \sigma_j^{*^2}\right], \quad j = r_1 + 1, \ldots, r_2,$$

$$p(\mu_j|\cdot) \propto \exp\left\{\sum_{i=1}^{n}\left[v_{ij}(\mu_j + \boldsymbol{\Lambda}_j^T\boldsymbol{\omega}_i) - \exp\left(\mu_j + \boldsymbol{\Lambda}_j^T\boldsymbol{\omega}_i\right)\right] - \frac{(\mu_j - \mu_{0j})^2}{2\sigma_{0j}^2}\right\},$$

$$j = r_2 + 1, \ldots, r_3,$$

$$[\boldsymbol{\mu}_j|\cdot] \stackrel{D}{=} N[\tilde{\boldsymbol{\mu}}_j, \boldsymbol{\Sigma}_{\mu j}], \quad j = r_3 + 1, \ldots, r_4,$$

where $\sigma_j^{*^2} = (\sigma_{0j}^{-2} + n\psi_j^{-1})^{-1}$, $\mu_j^* = \sigma_j^{*^2}(n\bar{z}_j^*/\psi_j + \mu_{0j}/\sigma_{0j}^2)$ with $\bar{z}_j^* = n^{-1}\sum_{i=1}^n(z_{ij}^* - \boldsymbol{\Lambda}_j^T\boldsymbol{\omega}_i)$, $\mu_j^{**} = \sigma_j^{*^2}(n\bar{y}_j/\psi_j + \mu_{0j}/\sigma_{0j}^2)$ with $\bar{y}_j = n^{-1}\sum_{i=1}^n(y_{ij} - \boldsymbol{\Lambda}_j^T\boldsymbol{\omega}_i)$, $\boldsymbol{\Sigma}_{\mu j} = (n\mathbf{I}_{L-1} + \mathbf{H}_{0\mu j}^{-1})^{-1}$, and $\tilde{\boldsymbol{\mu}}_j = \boldsymbol{\Sigma}_{\mu j}(n\bar{\mathbf{w}}_j + \mathbf{H}_{0\mu j}^{-1}\boldsymbol{\mu}_{0j})$ with $\bar{\mathbf{w}}_j = n^{-1}\sum_{i=1}^n(\mathbf{w}_{ij} - \mathbf{1}_{L-1}\boldsymbol{\Lambda}_j^T\boldsymbol{\omega}_i)$.

The conditional distributions of $\mathbf{\Lambda}$ and $\mathbf{\Psi}$ are as follows:

$$[\mathbf{\Lambda}_j|\cdot] \stackrel{D}{=} N\left[\mathbf{\Lambda}_j^*, \psi_j\mathbf{H}_j^*\right], \ \left[\psi_j^{-1}|\cdot\right] \stackrel{D}{=} \text{Gamma}\left[n/2+\alpha_{0j}, \beta_j^*\right] \quad j=1,\ldots,r_1,$$

$$[\mathbf{\Lambda}_j|\cdot] \stackrel{D}{=} N\left[\mathbf{\Lambda}_j^{**}, \psi_j\mathbf{H}_j^*\right], \ \left[\psi_j^{-1}|\cdot\right] \stackrel{D}{=} \text{Gamma}\left[n/2+\alpha_{0j}, \beta_j^{**}\right], \quad j=r_1+1,\ldots,r_2,$$

$$p(\mathbf{\Lambda}_j|\cdot) \propto \exp\left\{\sum_{i=1}^n \left[v_{ij}(\mu_j+\mathbf{\Lambda}_j^T\boldsymbol{\omega}_i) - \exp\left(\mu_j+\mathbf{\Lambda}_j^T\boldsymbol{\omega}_i\right)\right] -\frac{1}{2}(\mathbf{\Lambda}_j-\mathbf{\Lambda}_{0j})^T\mathbf{H}_{0j}^{-1}(\mathbf{\Lambda}_j-\mathbf{\Lambda}_{0j})\right\}, \quad j=r_2+1,\ldots,r_3,$$

$$[\mathbf{\Lambda}_j|\cdot] \stackrel{D}{=} N\left[\mathbf{\Lambda}_j^{***}, \mathbf{H}_j^{**}\right], \quad j=r_3+1,\ldots,r_4,$$

where $\mathbf{H}_j^* = (\mathbf{H}_{0j}^{-1}+\mathbf{\Omega}\mathbf{\Omega}^T)^{-1}$, $\mathbf{\Lambda}_j^* = \mathbf{H}_j^*[\mathbf{H}_{0j}^{-1}\mathbf{\Lambda}_{0j}+\mathbf{\Omega}\widetilde{\mathbf{Z}}_j^*]$, $\mathbf{\Lambda}_j^{**} = \mathbf{H}_j^*[\mathbf{H}_{0j}^{-1}\mathbf{\Lambda}_{0j}+\mathbf{\Omega}\widetilde{\mathbf{Y}}_j]$, $\beta_j^* = \beta_{0j}+[\widetilde{\mathbf{Z}}_j^{*T}\widetilde{\mathbf{Z}}_j^* - \mathbf{\Lambda}_j^{*T}\mathbf{H}_j^{*-1}\mathbf{\Lambda}_j^* + \mathbf{\Lambda}_{0j}^T\mathbf{H}_{0j}^{-1}\mathbf{\Lambda}_{0j}]/2$, $\beta_j^{**} = \beta_{0j}+[\widetilde{\mathbf{Y}}_j^T\widetilde{\mathbf{Y}}_j - \mathbf{\Lambda}_j^{**T}\mathbf{H}_j^{*-1}\mathbf{\Lambda}_j^{**} + \mathbf{\Lambda}_{0j}^T\mathbf{H}_{0j}^{-1}\mathbf{\Lambda}_{0j}]/2$, with $\widetilde{\mathbf{Z}}_j^* = (z_{1j}^*-\mu_j,\ldots,z_{nj}^*-\mu_j)^T$ and $\widetilde{\mathbf{Y}}_j = (y_{1j}-\mu_j,\ldots,y_{nj}-\mu_j)^T$. Finally, $\mathbf{H}_j^{**} = (\mathbf{H}_{0j}^{-1}+(L-1)\mathbf{\Omega}\mathbf{\Omega}^T)^{-1}$ and $\mathbf{\Lambda}_j^{***} = \mathbf{H}_j^{**}[\mathbf{H}_{0j}^{-1}\mathbf{\Lambda}_{0j}+\mathbf{\Omega}\widetilde{\mathbf{W}}_j]$ with $\widetilde{\mathbf{W}}_j = \left(\mathbf{1}_{L-1}^T(\mathbf{w}_{1j}-\boldsymbol{\mu}_j),\ldots,\mathbf{1}_{L-1}^T(\mathbf{w}_{nj}-\boldsymbol{\mu}_j)\right)^T$.

The conditional distributions of ψ_δ and $\mathbf{\Phi}$ are as follows:

$$\left[\psi_\delta^{-1}|\cdot\right] \stackrel{D}{=} \text{Gamma}\left[n/2+\alpha_{0\delta}, \beta_\delta^*\right], \quad [\mathbf{\Phi}|\cdot] \stackrel{D}{=} \text{IW}\left[\left(\sum_{i=1}^n \boldsymbol{\xi}_i\boldsymbol{\xi}_i^T+\mathbf{R}_0^{-1}\right), n+\rho_0\right],$$

where $\beta_\delta^* = \beta_{0\delta}+\sum_{i=1}^n\left[\eta_i - \sum_{j=1}^m\sum_{k=1}^{K_{bj}} b_{jk}B_{jk}^x(x_{ij}) - \sum_{j=1}^{q_2}\sum_{k=1}^{K_j}\beta_{jk}B_{jk}(\Phi^*(\xi_{ij}))\right]^2/2$.

The conditional distributions of $\boldsymbol{\alpha}$ and $\mathbf{Z}^*$ are as follows. For $j=1,\ldots,r_1$, let $\mathbf{Z}_j^* = (z_{1j}^*,\ldots,z_{nj}^*)^T$, $\mathbf{Z}_j = (z_{1j},\ldots,z_{nj})^T$. We have $p(\boldsymbol{\alpha},\mathbf{Z}^*|\mathbf{D},\mathbf{W},\mathbf{\Omega},\boldsymbol{\theta}_s) = \prod_{j=1}^{r_1} p(\boldsymbol{\alpha}_j,\mathbf{Z}_j^*|\mathbf{Z}_j,\mathbf{\Omega},\boldsymbol{\theta}_s)$ and $p(\boldsymbol{\alpha}_j,\mathbf{Z}_j^*|\mathbf{Z}_j,\mathbf{\Omega},\boldsymbol{\theta}_s) = p(\boldsymbol{\alpha}_j|\mathbf{Z}_j,\mathbf{\Omega},\boldsymbol{\theta}_s)p(\mathbf{Z}_j^*|\boldsymbol{\alpha}_j,\mathbf{Z}_j,\mathbf{\Omega},\boldsymbol{\theta}_s)$, with

$$p(\boldsymbol{\alpha}_j|\mathbf{Z}_j,\mathbf{\Omega},\boldsymbol{\theta}_s) \propto \prod_{i=1}^n\left\{\Phi^*\left[\psi_j^{-1/2}\left(\alpha_{j,z_{ij}+1}-\mu_j-\mathbf{\Lambda}_j^T\boldsymbol{\omega}_i\right)\right] - \Phi^*\left[\psi_j^{-1/2}\left(\alpha_{j,z_{ij}}-\mu_j-\mathbf{\Lambda}_j^T\boldsymbol{\omega}_i\right)\right]\right\}.$$

Finally, $p(\mathbf{Z}_j^*|\boldsymbol{\alpha}_j,\mathbf{Z}_j,\mathbf{\Omega},\boldsymbol{\theta}_*) = \prod_{i=1}^n p(z_{ij}^*|\boldsymbol{\alpha}_j,z_{ij},\boldsymbol{\omega}_i,\boldsymbol{\theta}_*)$, and

$$p\left(z_{ij}^*|\boldsymbol{\alpha}_j,z_{ij},\boldsymbol{\omega}_i,\boldsymbol{\theta}_*\right) \stackrel{D}{=} N\left[\mu_j+\mathbf{\Lambda}_j^T\boldsymbol{\omega}_i,\psi_j\right]I_{[\alpha_{j,z_{ij}},\alpha_{j,z_{ij}+1})}\left(z_{ij}^*\right).$$

References

Arminger, G. and Küsters, U. (1988) Latent trait models with indicators of mixed measurement level. In R. Langeheine and J. Rost (eds), *Latent Trait and Latent Class Models*, pp. 51–73. New York: Plenum.

Bartholomew, D. J. and Knott, M. (1999) *Latent Variable Models and Factor Analysis*, Vol. 7 of Kendall's Library of Statistics (2nd edn). London: Arnold.

Behseta, S., Kass, R. E. and Wallstrom, G. L. (2005) Hierarchical models for assessing variability among functions. *Biometrika*, **92**, 419–434.

Berry, S. M., Carroll, R. J. and Ruppert, D. (2002) Bayesian smoothing and regression splines for measurement error problems. *Journal of the American Statistical Association*, **97**, 160–169.

Biller, C. and Fahrmeir, L. (2001) Bayesian varying-coefficient models using adaptive regression splines. *Statistical Modelling*, **1**, 195–211.

Caldwell, B. M. and Bradley, R. H. (1984) *Home Observation for Measurement of the Environment*. Little Rock: University of Arkansas at Little Rock, Center for Child Development and Education.

Celeux, G., Forbes, F., Robert, C. P. and Titterington, D. M. (2006) Deviance information criteria for missing data models. *Bayesian Analysis*, **1**, 651–674.

Center for Human Resource Research. (2004) *The National Longitudinal Surveys NLSY User's Guide, 1979–2004*. US Department of Labor, Bureau of Labor Statistics. Columbus, OH: Center for Human Resource Research, Ohio State University.

De Boor, C. (1978) *A Practical Guide to Splines*. New York: Springer-Verlag.

DiMatteo, I., Genovese, C. R. and Kass, R. E. (2001) Bayesian curve-fitting with free-knot splines. *Biometrika*, **88**, 1055–1071.

Dunn, L. M. and Markwardt, F. C. (1970) *Peabody Individual Achievement Test Manual*. Circle Pines, MN: American Guidance Services.

Dunson, D. B. (2000) Bayesian latent variable models for clustered mixed outcomes. *Journal of the Royal Statistical Society, Series B*, **62**, 355–366.

Eilers, P. H. C. and Marx, B. D. (1996) Flexible smoothing with B-splines and penalties. *Statistical Science*, **11**, 89–121.

Fahrmeir, L. and Raach, A. (2007) A Bayesian semiparametric latent variable model for mixed responses. *Psychometrika*, **72**, 327–346.

Fan, J. and Gijbels, I. (1996) *Local Polynomial Modelling and Its Applications*. London: Chapman & Hall.

Fan, J. and Zhang, W. (1999) Statistical estimation in varying coefficient models. *Annals of Statistics*, **27**, 1491–1518.

Gelman, A. and Meng, X. L. (1998) Simulating normalizing constants: From importance sampling to bridge sampling to path sampling. *Statistical Science*, **13**, 163–185.

Gelman, A., Roberts, G. O. and Gilks, W. R. (1996) Efficient Metropolis jumping rules. In J. M. Bernardo, J. O. Berger, A. P. Dawid and A. F. M. Smith (eds), *Bayesian Statistics 5*, pp. 599–607. Oxford: Oxford University Press.

Geman, S. and Geman, D. (1984) Stochastic relaxation, Gibbs distributions, and the Bayesian restoration of images. *IEEE Transactions on Pattern Analysis and Machine Intelligence*, **6**, 721–741.

Green, P. J. and Silverman, B. W. (1994) *Nonparametric Regression and Generalized Linear Models: A Roughness Penalty Approach*. London: Chapman & Hall.

Hastings, W. K. (1970) Monte Carlo sampling methods using Markov chains and their applications. *Biometrika*, **57**, 97–109.

Huber, P., Scaillet, O. and Victoria-Feser, M. P. (2009) Assessing multivariate predictors of financial market movements: A latent factor framework for ordinal data. *Annals of Applied Statistics*, **3**, 249–271.

Imai, K. and van Dyk, D. A. (2005) A Bayesian analysis of the multinomial probit model using marginal data augmentation. *Journal of Econometrics*, **124**, 311–334.

Jöreskog, K. G. and Moustaki, I. (2001) Factor analysis for ordinal variables: a comparison of three approaches. *Multivariate Behavioral Research*, **36**, 347–387.

Jöreskog, K. G. and Sörbom, D. (1996) *LISREL 8: Structural Equation Modeling with the SIMPLIS Command Language*. Hove: Scientific Software International.

Kass, R. E. and Raftery, A. E. (1995) Bayes factors. *Journal of the American Statistical Association*, **90**, 773–795.

Lang, S. and Brezger, A. (2004) Bayesian P-splines. *Journal of Computational and Graphical Statistics*, **13**, 183–212.

Lee, S. Y. (2007) *Structural Equation Modeling: A Bayesian Approach*. Chichester: John Wiley & Sons, Ltd.

Metropolis, N., Rosenbluth, A. W., Rosenbluth, M. N., Teller, A. H. and Teller, E. (1953) Equation of state calculations by fast computing machines. *Journal of Chemical Physics*, **21**, 1087–1092.

McCullagh, P. and Nelder, J. A. (1989) *Generalized Linear Models* (2nd edn). London: Chapman & Hall.

Moustaki, I. (1996) A latent trait and a latent class model for mixed observed variables. *British Journal of Mathematical and Statistical Psychology*, **49**, 313–334.

Moustaki, I. (2003) A general class of latent variable models for ordinal manifest variables with covariate effects on the manifest and latent variables. *British Journal of Mathematical and Statistical Psychology*, **56**, 337–357.

Muthén, B. (1984) A general structural equation model with dichotomous, ordered categorical, and continuous latent variable indicators. *Psychometrika*, **49**, 115–132.

Panagiotelis, A. and Smith, M. (2008) Bayesian identification, selection and estimation of semiparametric functions in high-dimensional additive models. *Journal of Econometrics*, **143**, 291–316.

Rue, H. and Held, L. (2005) *Gaussian Markov Random Fields: Theory and Applications*. Boca Raton, FL: Chapman & Hall/CRC.

Ruppert, D., Wand, M. P. and Carroll, R. J. (2003) *Semiparametric Regression*. Cambridge: Cambridge University Press.

Sánchez, B. N., Budtz-Jorgensen, E., Ryan, L. M. and Hu, H. (2005) Structural equation models: A review with applications to environmental epidemiology. *Journal of the American Statistical Association*, **100**, 1443–1455.

Shi, J. Q. and Lee, S. Y. (2000) Latent variable models with mixed continuous and polytomous data. *Journal of the Royal Statistical Society, Series B*, **62**, 77–87.

Skrondal, A. and Rabe-Hesketh, S. (2004) *Generalized Latent Variable Modeling: Multilevel, Longitudinal, and Structural Equation Models*. Boca Raton, FL: Chapman & Hall/CRC.

Song, X. Y. and Lee, S. Y. (2007) Bayesian analysis of latent variable models with non-ignorable missing outcomes from exponential family. *Statistics in Medicine*, **26**, 681–693.

Song, X. Y. and Lu, Z. H. (2010) Semiparametric latent variable models with Bayesian P-splines. *Journal of Computational and Graphical Statistics*, **19**, 590–608.

Song, X. Y., Lee, S. Y., Ng, M. C. Y., So, W. Y. and Chan, J. C. N. (2007) Bayesian analysis of structural equation models with multinomial variables and an application to type 2 diabetic nephropathy. *Statistics in Medicine*, **26**, 2348–2369.

Song, X. Y., Lu, Z. H., Cai, J. H. and Ip, H. S. (2012) A Bayesian analysis of generalized semiparametric structural equation models. *Psychometrika*, under revision.

Spiegelhalter, D. J., Best, N. G., Carlin, B. P. and van der Linde, A. (2002) Bayesian measures of model complexity and fit (with discussion). *Journal of the Royal Statistical Society, Series B*, **64**, 583–639.

Zill, N. (1985) *Behavior problem scales developed from the 1981 child health supplement to the national health interview survey*. Washington, DC: Child Trends, Inc.

13

Transformation structural equation models

13.1 Introduction

Analysis of SEMs with nonnormal data has received a great deal of attention in the field. Many parametric and nonparametric/semiparametric methods have been proposed. Parametric methods include, but are not limited to, the asymptotically distribution-free (ADF) approach (Bentler, 1983; Browne, 1984), robust methods (Shapiro and Browne, 1987; Kano *et al.*, 1993; Yuan *et al.*, 2000), and finite mixture modeling (Jedidi *et al.*, 1997; Yung, 1997; Dolan and van der Maas, 1998; Arminger *et al.*, 1999). While these methods are useful for analyzing certain kinds of nonnormal data, they have limitations. For instance, the ADF approach requires a huge sample size to achieve accurate results (Hu *et al.*, 1992; Bentler and Dudgeon, 1996). Robust methods based on the t-distribution are effective in handling symmetrically heavy-tailed nonnormal data but less efficient for skewed and other nonsymmetric data. Finite mixture SEMs with a fixed number of components are useful for heterogeneous data, but not effective for highly skewed and/or heavy-tailed data. Recently, some semiparametric SEMs have been developed to analyze nonnormal data. These models assume the distributions of latent variables or random errors are unknown, and formulate these unknown distributions through a truncated or centered Dirichlet process with stick-breaking priors (see Lee *et al.*, 2008; Yang and Dunson, 2010; Chow *et al.*, 2011; Chapters 10 and 11 above). However, these semiparametric methods still encounter problems when analyzing extremely nonnormal data. For instance, in the polydrug use example in Section 13.7, the distributions of most variables are extremely nonnormal, and the Bayesian semiparametric SEM approach cannot produce meaningful results.

Another research direction lies in transforming response variables so that the resulting model can justify the model assumptions. Box and Cox (1964) proposed a family of power

Basic and Advanced Bayesian Structural Equation Modeling: With Applications in the Medical and Behavioral Sciences, First Edition. Xin-Yuan Song and Sik-Yum Lee.

transformations, the so-called Box–Cox transformations, to tackle the nonnormality of data. Since then, various extensions and other parametric transformation families have been developed under both the maximum likelihood and Bayesian frameworks (see, for example, John and Draper, 1980; Bickel and Doksum, 1981; Pericchi, 1981; David, 1993; Hoeting *et al.*, 2002; Mallick and Walker, 2003; Yin and Ibrahim, 2006). As parametric transformation families may not be flexible enough to capture the different shapes of nonnormal distributions, the more comprehensive nonparametric transformation modeling has received much attention (see, for example, Carroll and Ruppert, 1988; Ramsay, 1988, 1998; Nychka and Ruppert, 1995; He and Shen, 1997; Ruppert, 2001). Although there has been rather rapid development of parametric/nonparametric transformation modeling in the statistical literature, only a few works are directly relevant to transformation SEMs and Bayesian nonparametric transformation modeling. Mallick and Walker (2003) developed a Bayesian semiparametric transformation regression model without latent variables based on mixture modeling with unknown weights. Van Montfort *et al.* (2009) applied the Box–Cox transformation to analyze SEM with nonnormal variables. Song and Lu (2012) proposed transformation random effect models with Bayesian P-splines.

In this chapter we present a transformation SEM for handling various kinds of highly nonnormal data and stabilizing error variances simultaneously. The model has the following features: (i) nonparametric transformations are applied to response variables so that the resulting model can justify the model assumptions in SEMs; and (ii) fixed covariates are incorporated into both the measurement and structural equations to help establish a better model. Inspired by recently developed efficient Bayesian methods for analyzing general nonparametric functions, such as DiMatteo *et al.* (2001), Biller and Fahrmeir (2001), Lang and Brezger (2004), Brezger and Steiner (2008), and Song and Lu (2010, 2012), an MCMC algorithm with Bayesian P-splines is used to estimate the transformation functions, unknown parameters, and latent variables in the transformation SEM.

13.2 Model description

Let $\mathbf{y}_i = (y_{i1}, \ldots, y_{ip})^T$ be a random vector of observed variables and $\boldsymbol{\omega}_i = (\omega_{i1}, \ldots, \omega_{iq})^T$ be a random vector of latent variables for n observations, and $p \geq q$. A transformation SEM is defined by

$$\mathbf{f}(\mathbf{y}_i) = \mathbf{A}\mathbf{x}_i + \boldsymbol{\Lambda}\boldsymbol{\omega}_i + \boldsymbol{\epsilon}_i, \tag{13.1}$$

where $\mathbf{f}(\mathbf{y}_i) = (f_1(y_{i1}), \ldots, f_p(y_{ip}))^T$, the $f_j(\cdot)$ are unspecified smooth transformation functions, $\mathbf{x}_i$ is a vector of covariates, $\mathbf{A}$ is a matrix of coefficients, $\boldsymbol{\Lambda}$ is a factor loading matrix, and $\boldsymbol{\epsilon}_i$ is a residual random vector that is independent of $\boldsymbol{\omega}_i$ and distributed as $N(\mathbf{0}, \boldsymbol{\Psi})$, in which $\boldsymbol{\Psi}$ is diagonal. The unknown functions $f_j(\cdot)$, $j = 1, \ldots, p$, are assumed to be strictly monotonically increasing.

To investigate the interrelationships between latent variables, $\boldsymbol{\omega}_i$ is partitioned into $(\boldsymbol{\eta}_i^T, \boldsymbol{\xi}_i^T)^T$, where $\boldsymbol{\eta}_i$ $(q_1 \times 1)$ and $\boldsymbol{\xi}_i$ $(q_2 \times 1)$ are outcome and explanatory latent vectors, respectively. The structural equation is defined as

$$\boldsymbol{\eta}_i = \mathbf{C}\mathbf{z}_i + \boldsymbol{\Pi}\boldsymbol{\eta}_i + \boldsymbol{\Gamma}\boldsymbol{\xi}_i + \boldsymbol{\delta}_i, \tag{13.2}$$

where $\mathbf{z}_i$ is a vector of covariates, $\mathbf{C}$, $\boldsymbol{\Pi}$, and $\boldsymbol{\Gamma}$ are matrices of unknown coefficients, and $\boldsymbol{\delta}_i$ is a residual random vector that is independent of $\boldsymbol{\xi}_i$ and distributed as $N[\mathbf{0}, \boldsymbol{\Psi}_\delta]$, in which $\boldsymbol{\Psi}_\delta$ is diagonal. Moreover, we assume that $\mathbf{I} - \mathbf{\Pi}$ is nonsingular, its determinant is independent of $\mathbf{\Pi}$, and $\boldsymbol{\xi}_i$ is distributed as $N[\mathbf{0}, \mathbf{\Phi}]$. Let $\mathbf{\Lambda}_\omega = (\mathbf{\Pi}, \mathbf{\Gamma})$; model (13.2) can then be rewritten as

$$\boldsymbol{\eta}_i = \mathbf{C}\mathbf{z}_i + \mathbf{\Lambda}_\omega \boldsymbol{\omega}_i + \boldsymbol{\delta}_i. \tag{13.3}$$

The transformation SEM defined in equations (13.1) and (13.2) is an important extension of the traditional SEMs. As pointed out by Ruppert (2001), the transformations $f_j(\cdot)$ in equation (13.1) can play one or more roles, including: (i) inducing a normal distribution or removing extreme skewness or irregularity so that the data are more appropriate for modeling; (ii) inducing a simple systematic relationship between responses and latent/observed variables in the measurement equation; and (iii) stabilizing variances so that residuals have constant variances. As each transformation $f_j(\cdot)$ is strictly monotonically increasing, the transformed measurement equation will not change the directions and rankings of the associations between observed and latent variables. Hence, the interrelationships among latent variables in the structural equation will not be distorted in transformation SEMs.

13.3 Modeling nonparametric transformations

The transformations $f_j(\cdot)$ introduced in equation (13.1) are strictly monotonically increasing smooth functions, which are unspecified and need to be determined by data. Bayesian P-splines (Lang and Brezger, 2004), which are the Bayesian analogue of the P-splines method proposed by Eilers and Marx (1996), have been found very useful in modeling unspecified smooth functions. The idea of P-splines is that the unknown smooth function $f_j(\cdot)$ is approximated by $\sum_{k=1}^{K} \beta_k B_k(\cdot)$ (De Boor, 1978), where K is the number of splines determined by the number of knots, the β_k are unknown coefficients, and the $B_k(\cdot)$ are B-splines of appropriate order. A common choice of $B_k(\cdot)$ is the cubic B-spline. In practice, a choice of K in the range of 10 to 30 provides sufficient flexibility of fitting. Note that we suppress the subscript j in the summation throughout this chapter to simplify the notation. The extension to the general case where $\sum_{k=1}^{K_j} \beta_{jk} B_{jk}(\cdot)$ approximates $f_j(\cdot)$ is straightforward. Approximating $f_j(\cdot)$ with the P-splines, equation (13.1) can be rewritten as

$$\sum_{k=1}^{K} \beta_k B_k(y_{ij}) = \mathbf{A}_j^T \mathbf{x}_i + \mathbf{\Lambda}_j^T \boldsymbol{\omega}_i + \epsilon_{ij}, \tag{13.4}$$

where $\mathbf{A}_j^T$ and $\mathbf{\Lambda}_j^T$ are the jth rows of $\mathbf{A}$ and $\mathbf{\Lambda}$, respectively. The smoothness of $f_j(\cdot)$ is controlled by penalizing very large differences between coefficients of adjacent B-splines. In a Bayesian framework, this penalization is conveniently incorporated by introducing a random walk prior to β_k. The first- and second-order random walks are defined as

$$\beta_k = \beta_{k-1} + u_k \quad \text{and} \quad \beta_k = 2\beta_{k-1} - \beta_{k-2} + u_k, \tag{13.5}$$

with $u_k \overset{D}{=} N(0, \sigma^2)$, a diffuse prior $\beta_1 \propto$ constant for the first-order random walk, and $\beta_1 \propto$ constant and $\beta_2 \propto$ constant for the second-order random walk. The variance σ^2 can be viewed as an inverse smoothing parameter, which determines the smoothness of the resulting function $f_j(\cdot)$. In practice, this global smoothness prior may not be adequate when the 'true' curve is highly oscillating, which leads to large fluctuation of the differences between β_k. To consider this situation, a local smoothness prior $u_k \overset{D}{=} N(0, \sigma^2/\tau_k)$ is used, and the additional independent weights τ_k can be viewed as local smoothing parameters which help control the local smoothness of a highly oscillating curve.

There are two kinds of approaches to determining K in the literature. One is to fix K, and the other is to treat K as random and use the reversible jump MCMC algorithm or birth-and-death method (Stephens, 2000; Biller and Fahrmeir, 2001). Lang and Brezger (2004) compared them and found that the approach that fixes K performed better for functions with moderate curvature, while the approach that treats K as random performed better for highly oscillating functions. As the transformation functions defined in (13.1) are monotonic, they are more likely to be functions with moderate curvature. Hence, we fix K in (13.4) to simplify the MCMC procedure and achieve better efficiency.

13.4 Identifiability constraints and prior distributions

The transformation SEM defined by equations (13.1)–(13.4) is not identified without identifiability constraints. We consider the model identification in the following aspects. First, we fix the diagonal elements in $\boldsymbol{\Psi}$ at 1.0 and $\sum_{i=1}^{n}\sum_{k=1}^{K}\beta_k B_k(y_{ij})=0$ to solve the indeterminacies in the scale and location of the unknown functions. Let $\boldsymbol{\beta}=(\beta_1,\ldots,\beta_K)^T$, $\mathbf{B}=[B_k(y_{ij})]_{n\times K}$, $\mathbf{1}=(1,\ldots,1)^T$, and $\mathbf{Q}=\mathbf{1}^T\mathbf{B}$; the constraint on the summation can then be rewritten as $\mathbf{Q}\boldsymbol{\beta}=0$. Second, to ensure the approximation is strictly monotonically increasing, the constraint $\beta_1<\ldots<\beta_K$ is needed. Finally, to identify the scale of the latent variables, some elements in $\boldsymbol{\Lambda}$ should be fixed at preassigned values that are chosen on a problem-by-problem basis. Incorporating these identifiability constraints, we consider the following local smoothing prior distribution of $\boldsymbol{\beta}$:

$$\left(\frac{1}{\sqrt{2\pi}\sigma}\right)^{K-d}\exp\left\{-\frac{1}{2\sigma^2}\boldsymbol{\beta}^T\mathbf{M}(\boldsymbol{\tau})\boldsymbol{\beta}\right\}I(\beta_1<\ldots<\beta_K,\mathbf{Q}\boldsymbol{\beta}=0), \tag{13.6}$$

where d is the order of the random walk, $\mathbf{M}(\boldsymbol{\tau})=(D_{d-1}\times\ldots\times D_0)^T\mathrm{diag}(\boldsymbol{\tau})(D_{d-1}\times\ldots\times D_0)$, $\boldsymbol{\tau}=(\tau_{d+1},\ldots,\tau_K)$, D_l is a $(K-l-1)\times(K-l)$ penalty matrix that can be derived from the random walk penalty specified in (13.5) and is given by

$$D_l=\begin{pmatrix}-1 & 1 & 0 & \cdots & 0\\ 0 & \ddots & \ddots & \ddots & \vdots\\ \vdots & \ddots & \ddots & \ddots & 0\\ 0 & \ldots & 0 & -1 & 1\end{pmatrix},\quad l=0,\cdots,d-1,$$

and $I(\cdot)$ is an indicator function.

In a full Bayesian analysis, the inverse smoothing parameters σ^2 and τ_k are also treated as random. According to common practice, for $k=d+1,\ldots,K$,

$$\sigma^{-2}\stackrel{D}{=}\mathrm{Gamma}[\alpha_1,\alpha_2],\quad \tau_k\stackrel{D}{=}\mathrm{Gamma}[\nu/2,\nu/2], \tag{13.7}$$

where α_1, α_2, and ν are specified hyperparameters. We use $\alpha_1=1$ and $\alpha_2=0.005$ to obtain a highly dispersed (but proper) gamma prior for σ^{-2} and use $\nu=1$ to obtain a Cauchy distribution for u_k in (13.5).

For the structural parameters involved in equations (13.1) and (13.3), the common conjugate prior distributions are assigned: for $k = 1, \ldots, p$ and $j = 1, \ldots, q_1$,

$$\begin{aligned} &\mathbf{A}_k \stackrel{D}{=} N[\mathbf{A}_{0k}, \boldsymbol{\Sigma}_{0ak}], \quad \boldsymbol{\Lambda}_k \stackrel{D}{=} N[\boldsymbol{\Lambda}_{0k}, \boldsymbol{\Sigma}_{0\lambda k}], \qquad \boldsymbol{\Phi}^{-1} \stackrel{D}{=} W[\boldsymbol{\Phi}_0, r_0], \\ &\mathbf{C}_j \stackrel{D}{=} N[\mathbf{C}_{0j}, \boldsymbol{\Sigma}_{0cj}], \quad \boldsymbol{\Lambda}_{\omega j} \stackrel{D}{=} N[\boldsymbol{\Lambda}_{0\omega j}, \boldsymbol{\Sigma}_{0\omega j}], \quad \psi_{\delta j}^{-1} \stackrel{D}{=} \text{Gamma}[c_{j1}, c_{j2}], \end{aligned} \tag{13.8}$$

where $\mathbf{A}_k^T$ and $\boldsymbol{\Lambda}_k^T$ are the kth rows of $\mathbf{A}$ and $\boldsymbol{\Lambda}$, respectively, $\mathbf{C}_j^T$ and $\boldsymbol{\Lambda}_{\omega j}^T$ are the jth rows of $\mathbf{C}$ and $\boldsymbol{\Lambda}_\omega$, respectively, $\psi_{\delta j}$ is the jth diagonal element of $\boldsymbol{\Psi}_\delta$, and $\mathbf{A}_{0k}$, $\boldsymbol{\Lambda}_{0k}$, $\mathbf{C}_{0j}$, $\boldsymbol{\Lambda}_{0\omega j}$, r_0, c_{j1}, c_{j2}, and positive definite matrices $\boldsymbol{\Sigma}_{0ak}$, $\boldsymbol{\Sigma}_{0\lambda k}$, $\boldsymbol{\Sigma}_{0cj}$, $\boldsymbol{\Sigma}_{0\omega j}$, $\boldsymbol{\Phi}_0$ are hyperparameters whose values are assumed to be given by the prior information.

13.5 Posterior inference with MCMC algorithms

Let $\mathbf{Y} = \{\mathbf{y}_i, i = 1, \ldots, n\}$, $\boldsymbol{\Omega} = \{\boldsymbol{\omega}_i, i = 1, \ldots, n\}$, and $\boldsymbol{\theta}$ be a vector of all unknown parameters in the transformation SEM defined by (13.1)–(13.4). To obtain the Bayesian estimate of $\boldsymbol{\theta}$ and $\boldsymbol{\Omega}$, the main task is to draw observations from the joint posterior distribution $p(\boldsymbol{\theta}, \boldsymbol{\Omega}|\mathbf{Y})$. Due to the complexity of the model, this posterior distribution involves high-dimensional integrals and does not have a closed form. Markov chain Monte Carlo methods, including the Gibbs sampler (Geman and Geman, 1984) and other sampling techniques, are used to draw observations from $p(\boldsymbol{\theta}, \boldsymbol{\Omega}|\mathbf{Y})$. The related conditional distributions corresponding to the components of $(\boldsymbol{\theta}, \boldsymbol{\Omega})$ to implement the Gibbs sampler are presented next.

13.5.1 Conditional distributions

(a) *Conditional distribution of* $\boldsymbol{\beta}$

The full conditional distribution of $\boldsymbol{\beta}$ is given by

$$\begin{aligned} p(\boldsymbol{\beta}|\mathbf{Y}, \boldsymbol{\Omega}, \boldsymbol{\theta}_{-\boldsymbol{\beta}}) \propto \prod_{i=1}^{n}\prod_{j=1}^{p}\left[\exp\left\{-\frac{1}{2}\left(\sum_{k=1}^{K}\beta_k B_k(y_{ij}) - \mathbf{A}_j^T\mathbf{x}_i - \boldsymbol{\Lambda}_j^T\boldsymbol{\omega}_i\right)^2\right\}\sum_{k=1}^{K}\beta_k B_k'(y_{ij})\right] \\ \times \exp\left\{-\frac{1}{2\sigma^2}\boldsymbol{\beta}^T\mathbf{M}(\boldsymbol{\tau})\boldsymbol{\beta}\right\} I(\beta_1 < \ldots < \beta_K, \mathbf{Q}\boldsymbol{\beta} = 0), \end{aligned} \tag{13.9}$$

where $\boldsymbol{\theta}_{-\boldsymbol{\beta}}$ is the subvector of $\boldsymbol{\theta}$ excluding $\boldsymbol{\beta}$, $\sum_{k=1}^{K}\beta_k B_k'(y_{ij})$ is the Jacobian of the transformation, and $B_k'(y_{ij})$ is the first derivative of $B_k(y_{ij})$. This full conditional distribution is irregular, and the constrained parameter space $S = \{\boldsymbol{\beta} = (\beta_1, \ldots, \beta_K); \beta_1 < \ldots < \beta_K, \mathbf{Q}\boldsymbol{\beta} = 0\}$ is truncated and degenerate. The conventional Metropolis–Hastings algorithm (Metropolis *et al.*, 1953; Hastings, 1970) cannot be applied to sample $\boldsymbol{\beta}$ in S. The algorithm used to draw samples from this distribution is given in Sections 13.5.2 and 13.5.3.

(b) *Conditional distributions of smoothing parameters* σ^2 and τ_k

Based on the prior distributions given in (13.7), for $k = d + 1, \ldots, K$ and $j = 1, \ldots, p$,

$$[\sigma^{-2}|\boldsymbol{\beta}, \boldsymbol{\tau}] \stackrel{D}{=} \text{Gamma}\left[\alpha_1 + \frac{K-d}{2}, \alpha_2 + \frac{1}{2}\boldsymbol{\beta}^T\mathbf{M}(\boldsymbol{\tau})\boldsymbol{\beta}\right], \tag{13.10}$$

$$[\tau_k|\boldsymbol{\beta}, \sigma^2] \stackrel{D}{=} \text{Gamma}\left[\frac{\nu+1}{2}, \frac{1}{2}\left(\nu + \frac{u_k^2}{\sigma^2}\right)\right], \tag{13.11}$$

where u_k is equal to $\beta_k - \beta_{k-1}$ and $\beta_k - 2\beta_{k-1} + \beta_{k-2}$ for the first- and second-order random walks, respectively.

(c) *Conditional distributions of* $\mathbf{\Omega}$, $\mathbf{A}$, $\mathbf{\Lambda}$, $\mathbf{C}$, $\mathbf{\Lambda}_\omega$, $\mathbf{\Phi}$, and $\mathbf{\Psi}_\delta$

Given $\mathbf{Y}$ and $\boldsymbol{\beta}$ or equivalently $f(y_{ij}) = \sum_{k=1}^{K} \beta_k B_k(y_{ij})$, the conditional distributions of $\mathbf{\Omega}$, $\mathbf{A}$, $\mathbf{\Lambda}$, $\mathbf{C}$, $\mathbf{\Lambda}_\omega$, $\mathbf{\Phi}$, and $\mathbf{\Psi}_\delta$ given others are standard distributions, such as normal, inverted gamma, and inverted Wishart distributions (see Appendix 5.1). The MCMC sampling scheme can be implemented similarly to models without transformation.

13.5.2 The random-ray algorithm

When implementing the Gibbs sampler for Bayesian estimation, simulating $\boldsymbol{\beta}$ from (13.9) is challenging because the corresponding conditional distribution is nonstandard, and the parameter space is truncated and denerate. It is difficult to apply the conventional MH algorithm with a multivariate normal proposal distribution in sampling $\boldsymbol{\beta}$ in S because it is difficult to generate a candidate in a truncated and degenerate space. Moreover, the normalizing constants of the proposal distributions involved in the conventional MH algorithm depend on the current state of $\boldsymbol{\beta}$, which can be neither canceled out in the acceptance ratio nor calculated analytically. Chen and Schmeiser (1993) proposed the Hit-and-Run (HR) algorithm, which is suitable for sampling observations in a constrained parameter space. Based on a current state $\boldsymbol{\beta}^{(t)}$, the HR algorithm randomly generates a direction vector $\mathbf{e}$ and a scalar r, providing a candidate $\boldsymbol{\beta}^{(t)} + r\mathbf{e}$. Consequently, sampling in a multivariate constrained space is converted to sampling in a univariate truncated space of r. Liu *et al.* (2000) proposed a Random-Ray (RR) algorithm that combines the ideas of the HR algorithm and the Multiple-Try Metropolis (MTM) algorithm. The MTM algorithm can increase the acceptance rate without narrowing the Metropolis jumps, but at the expense of generating multiple candidates from the proposal distribution at each iteration.

The RR algorithm for generating $\boldsymbol{\beta}$ from the full conditional distribution $p(\boldsymbol{\beta}|\cdot)$ in (13.9) at the current state $\boldsymbol{\beta}^{(t)}$ is as follows:

(a) Randomly generate a directional unit vector $\mathbf{e}$ (see Section 13.5.3).

(b) Draw $\mathbf{w}_1, \ldots, \mathbf{w}_m$ along the direction $\mathbf{e}$ by generating a scalar r_{1k} from a univariate proposal distribution $T_e(\mathbf{w}, \boldsymbol{\beta}^{(t)})$, and calculate $\mathbf{w}_k = \boldsymbol{\beta}^{(t)} + r_{1k}\mathbf{e}$, $k = 1, \ldots, m$.

(c) Choose $\mathbf{w}^*$ from candidates $\mathbf{w}_1, \ldots, \mathbf{w}_m$ with the following probabilities:

$$p(\mathbf{w}^* = \mathbf{w}_k) \propto p(\mathbf{w}_k|\cdot)T_e\big(\mathbf{w}_k, \boldsymbol{\beta}^{(t)}\big), \quad k = 1, \ldots, m.$$

(d) Draw $\mathbf{v}_1, \ldots, \mathbf{v}_{m-1}$ along the direction $\mathbf{e}$ by generating r_{2k} from $T_e(\mathbf{w}^*, \mathbf{v})$, and calculate $\mathbf{v}_k = \mathbf{w}^* + r_{2k}\mathbf{e}$. Let $\mathbf{v}_m = \boldsymbol{\beta}^{(t)}$, and let r_{2m} be the scalar such that $\boldsymbol{\beta}^{(t)} = \mathbf{w}^* + r_{2m}\mathbf{e}$. Compute the generalized Metropolis ratio:

$$R^{(t)} = \min\left\{1, \frac{\sum_{k=1}^{m} p(\mathbf{w}_k|\cdot)T_e\big(\mathbf{w}_k, \boldsymbol{\beta}^{(t)}\big)}{\sum_{k=1}^{m} p(\mathbf{v}_k|\cdot)T_e(\mathbf{w}^*, \mathbf{v}_k)}\right\}, \tag{13.12}$$

where $p(\cdot|\cdot)$ is the target density of $\boldsymbol{\beta}$ defined in (13.9).

(e) Generate v_1 from Uniform[0, 1], and let $\boldsymbol{\beta}^{(t+1)} = \mathbf{w}^*$ if $v_1 \leq R^{(t)}$, or $\boldsymbol{\beta}^{(t+1)} = \boldsymbol{\beta}^{(t)}$ if $v_1 > R^{(t)}$.

Here, m is the number of multiple candidates. For $l = 1, 2$ and $k = 1, \ldots, m$, the truncated normal distribution $N[0, \sigma_r^2]I(l_{lk}^{(t)}, u_{lk}^{(t)})$ is used as the proposal distribution of r_{lk}, where the truncation range $(l_{lk}^{(t)}, u_{lk}^{(t)})$ is determined by $\mathbf{e}$ (see Section 13.5.3). Therefore, all $(l_{lk}^{(t)}, u_{lk}^{(t)})$ have to be updated at each MCMC iteration. In most situations here, σ_r^2 ranging from 4 to 8 and m ranging from 5 to 10 produce acceptance rates between 0.4 and 0.6. In the nonparametric transformation model with Bayesian P-splines, generating $\mathbf{e}$ is crucial because it affects the efficiency of the sampling scheme. Hence, some modifications are introduced to achieve better efficiency of the RR algorithm.

13.5.3 Modifications of the random-ray algorithm

For $r \neq 0$, let $\boldsymbol{\beta} + r\mathbf{e}$ be a candidate sample generated along the direction $\mathbf{e} = (e_1, \ldots, e_K)$ based on the current state $\boldsymbol{\beta}$. To ensure that all new samples generated by the RR algorithm are in the constrained parameter space S, the following two conditions should be satisfied:

(1) $\mathbf{Qe} = 0$. Since $\mathbf{Q}\boldsymbol{\beta} = 0$, we have $\mathbf{Qe} = 0$ if and only if $\mathbf{Q}(\boldsymbol{\beta} + r\mathbf{e}) = 0$.

(2) $\beta_{k+1} + re_{k+1} > \beta_k + re_k$, for $k = 1, \ldots, K - 1$. We can determine the range of r as follows. For $k = 1, \ldots, K - 1$,

$$r \in \begin{cases} [-(\beta_{k+1} - \beta_k)/(e_{k+1} - e_k), \infty], & e_{k+1} > e_k, \\ [-\infty, -(\beta_{k+1} - \beta_k)/(e_{k+1} - e_k)], & e_{k+1} < e_k. \end{cases}$$

Let $I_l = \{k | e_{k+1} > e_k\}$ and $I_u = \{k | e_{k+1} < e_k\}$. The domain of r is the intersection of these $K - 1$ intervals:

$$\left[\max\left\{-\infty, \max_{k \in I_l}\left(-\frac{\beta_{k+1} - \beta_k}{e_{k+1} - e_k}\right)\right\}, \min\left\{\min_{k \in I_u}\left(-\frac{\beta_{k+1} - \beta_k}{e_{k+1} - e_k}\right), \infty\right\}\right]. \tag{13.13}$$

The directional vector $\mathbf{e}$ affects the range of r, thus it also affects the efficiency of the algorithm. One approach (Chen and Schmeiser, 1993; Liu *et al.*, 2000) is to generate $\tilde{e}_k$ from Uniform$[-1, 1]$, $k = 1, \ldots, K$, and $e_k = \tilde{e}_k / \sqrt{\sum_k \tilde{e}_k^2}$. However, this sampling scheme ignores the characteristic of $p(\boldsymbol{\beta}|\cdot)$, leading to inefficient exploration in the parameter space S. Hence, we aim to modify the conventional sampling of $\mathbf{e}$ by drawing $\mathbf{e}$ from $N(\mathbf{0}, \boldsymbol{\Sigma}(\boldsymbol{\beta}))I(\mathbf{Qe} = 0)$ with $\boldsymbol{\Sigma}(\boldsymbol{\beta}) = \partial^2\{-\log p(\boldsymbol{\beta}|\cdot)\}/\partial\boldsymbol{\beta}\partial\boldsymbol{\beta}^T = \mathbf{B}^T\mathbf{B} + \mathbf{M}(\boldsymbol{\tau})/\sigma^2 + (\mathbf{B}')^T\mathbf{D}(\boldsymbol{\beta})\mathbf{B}'$, in which $\mathbf{B}' = (\mathbf{B}_1', \ldots, \mathbf{B}_n')^T$, $\mathbf{B}_i' = (B_1'(y_i), \ldots, B_K'(y_i))^T$, and $\mathbf{D}(\boldsymbol{\beta}) = \text{diag}(1/(\boldsymbol{\beta}^T\mathbf{B}_1')^2, \ldots, 1/(\boldsymbol{\beta}^T\mathbf{B}_n')^2)$. However, (13.12) is valid only when step (a) in the RR algorithm is independent of the current state of $\boldsymbol{\beta}$. Otherwise, it should include the conditional distributions of $\mathbf{e}$ given $\mathbf{w}_k$ and $\mathbf{v}_k$, which requires the factorization of $2m$ covariance matrices at each iteration and leads to considerable computation. To simplify the generalized Metropolis ratio, we modify step (a) in the RR algorithm by using the following two phases:

(a1) In the burn-in phase, take $\boldsymbol{\Sigma} = \mathbf{B}^T\mathbf{B} + \mathbf{M}(\boldsymbol{\tau})/\sigma^2$ as a rough approximation of $\boldsymbol{\Sigma}(\boldsymbol{\beta})$ in generating $\mathbf{e}$.

(a2) After the burn-in phase, take $\boldsymbol{\Sigma}(\boldsymbol{\beta}_0)$ as an approximation of $\boldsymbol{\Sigma}(\boldsymbol{\beta})$ in generating $\mathbf{e}$, where $\boldsymbol{\beta}_0$ is the mean of samples of $\boldsymbol{\beta}$ obtained with the burn-in samples.

Phases (a1) and (a2) consider the characteristic of $p(\boldsymbol{\beta}|\cdot)$ and simultaneously simplify the calculation of the generalized Metropolis ratio. According to our numerical experience, this modification leads to better efficiency in exploring the constrained parameter space of $\boldsymbol{\beta}$. Moreover, generating the directional vector $\mathbf{e}$ from $N[\mathbf{0}, \boldsymbol{\Sigma}]I(\mathbf{Qe} = 0)$ in (a1) and from $N(\mathbf{0}, \boldsymbol{\Sigma}(\boldsymbol{\beta}_0))I(\mathbf{Qe} = 0)$ in (a2) is efficient through the algorithm in Rue and Held (2005) because the covariance matrices are band matrices.

13.6 Simulation study

In this section, we present a simulation study to examine the empirical performance of the transformation SEM. The model is defined by equations (13.1) and (13.2) with $p = 9$, $\boldsymbol{\Pi} = \mathbf{0}$, $\boldsymbol{\omega}_i = (\eta_i, \xi_{i1}, \xi_{i2})^T$ as follows: for $i = 1, \ldots, 500$, $j = 1, \ldots, 9$,

$$f_j(y_{ij}) = a_j x_i + \boldsymbol{\Lambda}_j^T \boldsymbol{\omega}_i + \epsilon_{ij}, \quad \eta_i = c_1 z_{i1} + c_2 z_{i2} + \gamma_1 \xi_{i1} + \gamma_2 \xi_{i2} + \delta_i.$$

Although a general case where $f_j(\cdot)$ has different forms for different j can be considered, in this simulation we use the same $f(y) = 5\,\mathrm{logit}[(y + 10)/20] + 15$ to produce highly skewed y_{ij}. Here, x_i, z_{i1}, and z_{i2} are independently simulated from the exponential distribution Exp(0.2), $\boldsymbol{\Lambda}_j^T = (\lambda_{j1}, 0, 0)$, $j = 1, 2, 3$, $\boldsymbol{\Lambda}_j^T = (0, \lambda_{j2}, 0)$, $j = 4, 5, 6$, $\boldsymbol{\Lambda}_j^T = (0, 0, \lambda_{j3})$, $j = 7, 8, 9$, $\boldsymbol{\Phi} = (\phi_{ij})_{2\times 2}$, and $\boldsymbol{\Psi}_\delta = \psi_\delta$, in which λ_{11}, λ_{42}, and λ_{73} are fixed at 1 to identify the transformation SEM.

In this simulation study, P-splines with $K = 15$ were used to approximate the transformation function $f(\cdot)$. The prior inputs in (13.8) were taken as: $\mathbf{A}_0 = \mathbf{0}$, $\boldsymbol{\Lambda}_0 = \mathbf{0}$, $\mathbf{C}_0 = \mathbf{0}$, $\boldsymbol{\Lambda}_{0\omega} = \mathbf{0}$, $\boldsymbol{\Sigma}_{0a}$, $\boldsymbol{\Sigma}_{0\lambda}$, $\boldsymbol{\Sigma}_{0c}$, $\boldsymbol{\Sigma}_{0\omega}$ were taken as $10^{-4}\mathbf{I}$, $c_{j1} = 9$, $c_{j2} = 4$, $r_0 = 5$, and $\boldsymbol{\Phi}_0 = \boldsymbol{\Phi}$. The EPSR convergence diagnostic statistic (Gelman and Rubin, 1992) showed that the algorithm converged within 5000 iterations. The estimates of the unknown transformation function and unknown parameters were obtained using the Bayesian P-splines approach based on 100 replications. In each replication, 5000 burn-in iterations were discarded, and 10 000 samples were acquired as posterior samples. The bias (Bias) and root mean square (RMS) between the true values of the parameters and their estimates are reported in Tables 13.1 and 13.2, showing that the nonparametric transformation SEM performs well for the response variables with a highly nonnormal distribution.

To study the sensitivity of the Bayesian results to prior inputs, the simulated data sets were reanalyzed using two different prior settings: (I) $\mathbf{A}_0 = 2\mathbf{A}$, $\boldsymbol{\Lambda}_0 = 2\boldsymbol{\Lambda}$, $\mathbf{C}_0 = 2\mathbf{C}$, $\boldsymbol{\Lambda}_{0\omega} = 2\boldsymbol{\Lambda}_\omega$, $\boldsymbol{\Sigma}_{0a}$, $\boldsymbol{\Sigma}_{0\lambda}$, $\boldsymbol{\Sigma}_{0c}$, $\boldsymbol{\Sigma}_{0\omega}$ are taken as the identity matrix, $c_{j1} = 15$, $c_{j2} = 5$, $r_0 = 5$, $\boldsymbol{\Phi}_0 = 2\boldsymbol{\Phi}$, $\alpha_1 = 1$, and $\alpha_2 = 0.05$; and (II) $\mathbf{A}_0 = 0.5\mathbf{A}$, $\boldsymbol{\Lambda}_0 = 0.5\boldsymbol{\Lambda}$, $\mathbf{C}_0 = 0.5\mathbf{C}$, $\boldsymbol{\Lambda}_{0\omega} = 0.5\boldsymbol{\Lambda}_\omega$, $\boldsymbol{\Sigma}_{0a}$, $\boldsymbol{\Sigma}_{0\lambda}$, $\boldsymbol{\Sigma}_{0c}$, $\boldsymbol{\Sigma}_{0\omega}$ are taken as the identity matrix, $c_{j1} = 6$, $c_{j2} = 3$, $r_0 = 5$, $\boldsymbol{\Phi}_0 = 0.5\boldsymbol{\Phi}$, $\alpha_1 = 0.001$, and $\alpha_2 = 0.001$, in which $\mathbf{A}$, $\boldsymbol{\Lambda}$, $\mathbf{C}$, $\boldsymbol{\Lambda}_\omega$, and $\boldsymbol{\Phi}$ denote true population values. Note that ν is taken as 1 throughout this chapter because $\nu = 1$ means assigning the Cauchy distribution as the prior of β_j, which gives the model the most flexibility to capture local fluctuation compared to other possible choices of ν. The estimated unknown parameters are close to those reported in Tables 13.1 and 13.2, indicating that the Bayesian results are not very sensitive to prior inputs under the given sample sizes and model settings.

To study the sensitivity of the Bayesian estimation to the choice of K, a sensitivity analysis regarding the choice of K under the same simulation setting was carried out. The same data sets were reanalyzed with $K = 10$, 15, and 30. The estimation is not as good when $K = 10$, but is robust to the choice of K when K is larger than 15. The following guidelines on making this choice in practice are given. If the distribution of a variable does not include many outliers, it is safe to use K in the range 20–40. Otherwise, a larger K, in the range 40–60 say, should be taken.

Table 13.1 Bayesian estimates of unknown parameters in the measurement equation.

Parameter		Our method	Threshold method	Box–Cox transformation $\rho = 1$	$\rho = 0.5$	$\rho = 0$	$\rho = -0.5$	$\rho = -1$
	Bias	−0.04	−0.54	−0.32	−0.33	−0.61	−0.91	−1.04
$a_1 = 1.2$	RMS	0.07	0.54	0.32	0.34	0.61	0.92	1.05
	Bias	0.01	−0.45	0.02	−0.14	−0.55	−0.04	−1.05
$a_2 = 1.2$	RMS	0.06	0.45	0.09	0.15	0.55	0.94	1.06
	Bias	0.01	−0.47	−0.01	−0.17	−0.54	−0.91	−1.03
$a_3 = 1.2$	RMS	0.06	0.47	0.07	0.17	0.54	0.91	1.03
	Bias	−0.04	−0.30	0.23	−0.08	−0.55	−0.95	−1.11
$a_4 = 1.2$	RMS	0.08	0.31	0.26	0.09	0.55	0.95	1.11
	Bias	0.01	−0.26	0.26	−0.06	−0.55	−0.94	−1.07
$a_5 = 1.2$	RMS	0.06	0.26	0.28	0.07	0.55	0.95	1.08
	Bias	−0.00	−0.26	0.32	−0.05	−0.53	−0.93	−0.88
$a_6 = 1.2$	RMS	0.05	0.26	0.34	0.05	0.53	0.93	0.90
	Bias	−0.03	−0.30	0.19	−0.10	−0.56	−0.94	−1.06
$a_7 = 1.2$	RMS	0.08	0.30	0.21	0.11	0.56	0.94	1.07
	Bias	0.01	−0.29	0.27	−0.05	−0.53	−0.92	−1.05
$a_8 = 1.2$	RMS	0.07	0.29	0.28	0.06	0.54	0.92	1.07
	Bias	0.01	−0.27	0.30	−0.05	−0.54	−0.95	−1.05
$a_9 = 1.2$	RMS	0.06	0.28	0.31	0.06	0.54	0.95	1.06
	Bias	0.04	0.06	0.30	0.18	0.12	0.05	2.83
$\lambda_{21} = 0.8$	RMS	0.07	0.07	0.32	0.19	0.13	0.34	8.76
	Bias	0.04	0.05	0.28	0.15	0.14	0.16	1.70
$\lambda_{31} = 1.0$	RMS	0.08	0.07	0.30	0.16	0.14	0.33	3.44
	Bias	0.07	0.09	0.20	0.12	0.20	0.58	−5.21
$\lambda_{52} = 1.0$	RMS	0.14	0.13	0.21	0.14	0.26	1.15	32.68
	Bias	0.08	0.10	0.26	0.16	0.26	0.68	23.30
$\lambda_{62} = 1.0$	RMS	0.15	0.13	0.27	0.18	0.28	1.20	32.85
	Bias	0.09	0.03	0.26	0.16	0.16	0.23	2.02
$\lambda_{83} = 1.0$	RMS	0.16	0.09	0.28	0.17	0.17	0.37	6.03
	Bias	0.08	0.02	0.29	0.14	0.15	0.10	10.47
$\lambda_{93} = 1.0$	RMS	0.16	0.09	0.32	0.16	0.17	0.35	27.61

To compare our method with other existing methods, the simulated data were reanalyzed using the following conventional transformations. The first is the Box–Cox transformation, which is the most popular parametric transformation method. We considered Box–Cox transformations with index parameter ρ in $\{-1, -0.5, 0, 0.5, 1\}$, which are commonly used and associated with the reciprocal, reciprocal of square root, logarithm, square root, and identity transformation, respectively. The identity transformation with $\rho = 1$ is equivalent to ignoring the nonnormality and simply fitting the data to the model. The second is to discretize the nonnormal response variable y_{ij} into a categorical variable with five categories with probabilities

Table 13.2 Bayesian estimates of unknown parameters in the structural equation.

Parameter		Our method	Threshold method	Box–Cox transformation $\rho = 1$	$\rho = 0.5$	$\rho = 0$	$\rho = -0.5$	$\rho = -1$
	Bias	−0.04	−0.48	5.07	−0.01	0.38	0.11	3.98
$\phi_{11} = 1.0$	RMS	0.23	0.49	5.18	0.17	0.48	0.82	15.23
	Bias	0.03	−0.07	5.16	0.35	0.79	0.49	−0.13
$\phi_{21} = 1.0$	RMS	0.13	0.08	5.22	0.39	0.83	0.53	0.17
	Bias	−0.04	−0.43	4.71	0.04	0.58	0.80	12.39
$\phi_{22} = 1.0$	RMS	0.25	0.44	4.81	0.23	0.70	1.67	28.01
	Bias	−0.03	−0.42	−0.28	−0.26	−0.49	−0.75	−0.87
$c_1 = 1.0$	RMS	0.18	0.42	0.29	0.27	0.49	0.75	0.87
	Bias	−0.03	−0.42	−0.28	−0.27	−0.48	−0.75	−0.86
$c_2 = 1.0$	RMS	0.18	0.42	0.29	0.27	0.49	0.75	0.87
	Bias	0.02	−0.22	−0.44	−0.15	−0.12	−0.30	1.94
$\gamma_1 = 0.6$	RMS	0.09	0.24	0.45	0.18	0.16	0.51	15.06
	Bias	0.02	−0.24	−0.37	−0.16	−0.08	0.09	1.31
$\gamma_2 = 0.6$	RMS	0.09	0.25	0.38	0.18	0.12	0.48	5.37
	Bias	0.07	0.46	3.55	1.35	2.23	4.74	18.00
$\psi_\delta = 0.3$	RMS	0.15	0.46	3.57	1.43	2.30	5.82	34.30

$(0.1, 0.2, 0.4, 0.2, 0.1)$. The estimated unknown parameters produced by the conventional transformation methods are also presented in Tables 13.1 and 13.2 for comparison. The performance of the current method with the Bayesian P-splines is much better than with the Box–Cox transformation and the discretization method.

13.7 A study on the intervention treatment of polydrug use

The transformation SEM with Bayesian P-splines is applied to reanalyze the data set previously analyzed using a modified mixture SEM in Section 7.3.4. The entire data set was obtained based on self-reported and administrative questionnaire items on drug treatment dropouts, drug-related crime histories, and drug use histories; and services and tests received were collected from the participants at intake, 3-month, and 12-month follow-up interviews. We used a latent variable model in this analysis to investigate how drug use severity and convicted crime histories affect retention in the drug treatment and how this retention will affect future drug use. For a description of the variables included in the analysis, see Appendix 1.1. The first three observed variables ((Drgplm30, Drgday30, DrgN30) $= (y_1, y_2, y_3)$) reveal the characteristics of drug severity. These variables were grouped into a latent factor, 'drug severity' (ξ_1). The next three observed variables ((Incar, ArrN, Agefirstarrest) $= (y_4, y_5, y_6)$), which reflect crime history, were grouped into a latent factor, 'crime history' (ξ_2). A confirmatory factor analysis (CFA) model was used to group the observed variables into latent factors. Three observed variables, including Servicem (x_1), DrugtestTX (x_2), and DrugtestCJ (x_3), were considered as covariates because they were expected to affect Retent (y_7) according

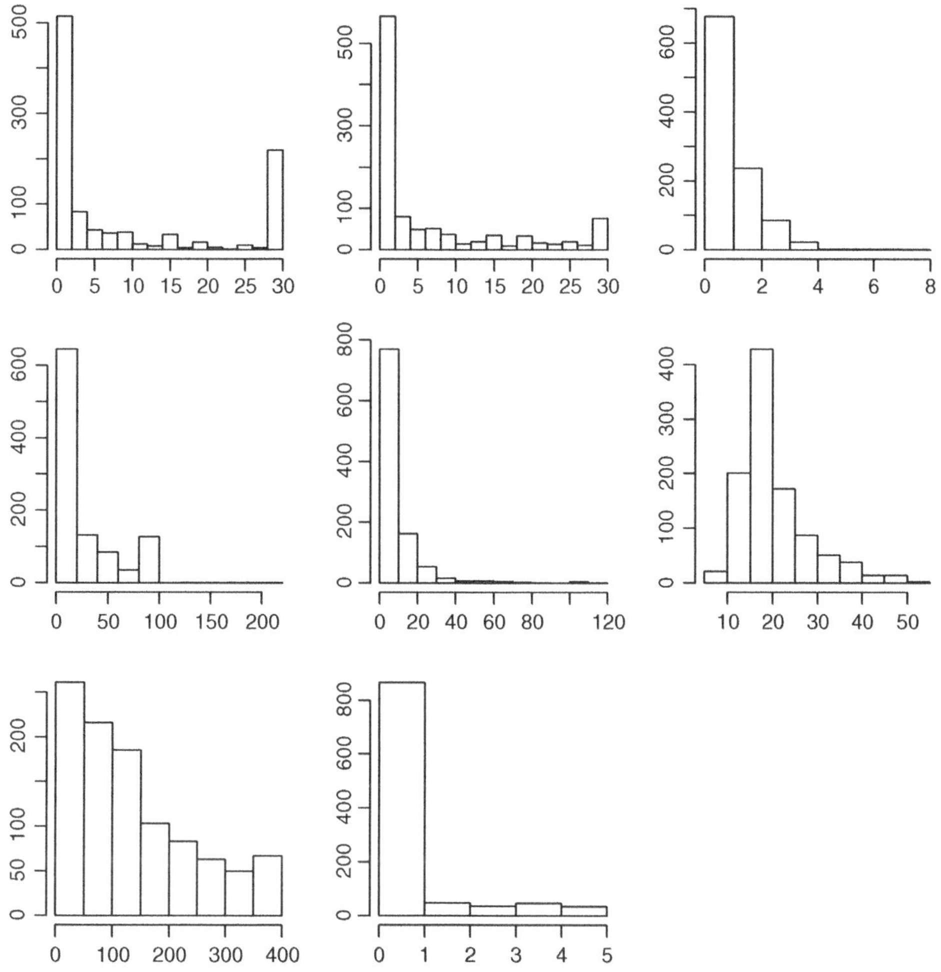

Figure 13.1 Histograms of response variables in polydrug real data example. First row from left to right: y_1, y_2, y_3. Second row from left to right: y_4, y_5, y_6. Third row from left to right: y_7, y_8. Reproduced from Song, X. Y. and Lu, Z. H. Semiparametric transformation models with Bayesian P-splines. *Statistics and Computing* (to appear), with kind permission from Springer Science and Business Media.

to prior medical knowledge. The sample size of the data set was 1028, and all variables were treated as continuous. The histograms of the variables (see Figure 13.1) showed that most distributions were nonnormal. Specifically, y_1 and y_2 were nonsymmetrically U-shaped, y_4 and y_7 were bimodal, and the rest were highly skewed to the right. For these highly nonnormal variables, the conventional parametric and discretizing transformations were not expected to work well. Therefore, we applied the nonparametric transformation in the analysis of the data set.

In formulating an appropriate model to analyze the data, y_7 plays a special role because covariates (x_1, x_2, x_3) and latent factors (ξ_1, ξ_2) influence it, and it further influences M12Drg30 (y_8). Therefore, y_7 is not only in the sets of response variables but also in the sets of covariates

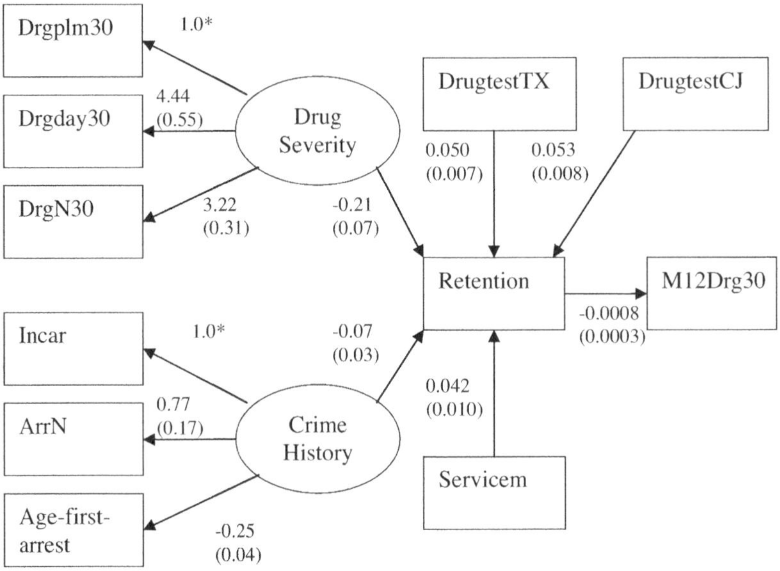

Figure 13.2 Path diagram, together with the estimated regression coefficients and their standard error estimates (in parentheses), for the polydrug data example. Reproduced from Song, X. Y. and Lu, Z. H. Semiparametric transformation models with Bayesian P-splines. *Statistics and Computing* (to appear), with kind permission from Springer Science and Business Media.

in the model. For $i = 1, \ldots, 1028$,

$$\mathbf{f}(\mathbf{y}_i) = \mathbf{A}\mathbf{x}_i + \mathbf{\Lambda}\boldsymbol{\xi}_i + \boldsymbol{\epsilon}_i, \tag{13.14}$$

where $\mathbf{f}(\mathbf{y}_i) = (f_1(y_{i1}), \ldots, f_8(y_{i8}))^T$, $\mathbf{x}_i = (x_{i1}, x_{i2}, x_{i3}, y_{i7})^T$, $\boldsymbol{\xi}_i = (\xi_{i1}, \xi_{i2})^T \stackrel{D}{=} N(\mathbf{0}, \mathbf{\Phi})$, $\boldsymbol{\epsilon}_i = (\epsilon_{i1}, \ldots, \epsilon_{i8})^T \stackrel{D}{=} N(\mathbf{0}, \mathbf{I})$, and $\mathbf{I}$ is an identity matrix to identify the model. As the patterns of nonnormality and the meaning of the variables are different for y_{ij} at distinct j, component-specific K_j and $f_j(\cdot)$ are applied to y_{ij} for each j. Based on prior knowledge of experts (Evans *et al.*, 2009) in formulating the relationships between response variables and latent factors (see the path diagram in Figure 13.2), the structures of $\mathbf{A}$ and $\mathbf{\Lambda}$ in equation (13.14) are specified as follows:

$$\mathbf{A} = \begin{bmatrix} \mathbf{0} & \mathbf{0} & \mathbf{0} & \mathbf{0} \\ a_1 & a_2 & a_3 & 0 \\ 0 & 0 & 0 & a_4 \end{bmatrix}, \quad \mathbf{\Lambda} = \begin{bmatrix} 1 & \lambda_1 & \lambda_2 & 0 & 0 & 0 & \lambda_5 & 0 \\ 0 & 0 & 0 & 1 & \lambda_3 & \lambda_4 & \lambda_6 & 0 \end{bmatrix}^T,$$

where the $\mathbf{0}$s in $\mathbf{A}$ indicate 6×1 vectors of 0s. All the 0s and 1s in $\mathbf{A}$ and $\mathbf{\Lambda}$ were fixed to define an identified CFA model (see Shi and Lee, 2000), as given in Figure 13.2. Hence, the unknown parameters are $\mathbf{a} = (a_1, a_2, a_3, a_4)^T$, $\boldsymbol{\lambda} = (\lambda_1, \ldots, \lambda_6)^T$, and $\boldsymbol{\varphi} = \{\phi_{11}, \phi_{12}, \phi_{22}\}$ in $\mathbf{\Phi}$. We encounter a problem in applying the nonparametric transformation to each y_{ij}. Although the y_{ij} vary within a wide range, most of them take integer values (e.g. number of days or number of arrests), resulting in ties. As the transformations are one to one, it is impossible to transform variables with ties to normal. To solve this problem, small random noises generated from $N[0, 0.01]$ were added to break the ties, which still maintained the orders of the patients for every variable. In this analysis, $K_4 = 40$, $K_5 = 60$, and $K_j = 30$ for the rest of the j were taken as the number of splines to approximate the unknown transformation functions $f_j(\cdot)$. The prior distributions of $\mathbf{A}$, $\mathbf{\Lambda}$, and $\mathbf{\Phi}$ were taken as those in (13.8) with the hyperparameter inputs $\mathbf{A}_0 = \hat{\mathbf{A}}$, $\mathbf{\Sigma}_{0a} = \mathbf{I}$, $\mathbf{\Lambda}_0 = \hat{\mathbf{\Lambda}}$, $\mathbf{\Sigma}_{0\lambda} = \mathbf{I}$, $r_0 = 6$, and $\mathbf{\Phi}_0 = (r_0 - q - 1)\hat{\mathbf{\Phi}}$, where $\mathbf{I}$ is the identity matrix with an appropriate dimension, q is the dimension of $\boldsymbol{\xi}_i$, and $\hat{\mathbf{A}}$, $\hat{\mathbf{\Lambda}}$, and $\hat{\mathbf{\Phi}}$ are the ML estimates obtained via the discretization method.

After checking the convergence, the MCMC algorithm was found to converge within 30 000 iterations. To be conservative, 50 000 generated samples were used to obtain the Bayesian results after discarding 50 000 burn-in iterations. Estimates of the factor loadings, regression coefficients, and their standard error estimates are reported in Figure 13.2. The pointwise posterior means of the unknown transformation functions, together with the 5% and 95% pointwise quantiles, are depicted in Figure 13.3. For most curves, the estimated credible intervals formed by the pointwise quantiles are narrow, indicating good estimates of the unknown transformation functions with the Bayesian P-splines approach.

To investigate the sensitivity of the Bayesian results to prior inputs, the analysis was repeated with some disturbances in the current prior input. In particular, one vague prior input with little information, that is, $\mathbf{A}_0 = \mathbf{0}$, $\mathbf{\Lambda}_0 = \mathbf{0}$, $\mathbf{\Sigma}_{0a} = 10^2\mathbf{I}$, $\mathbf{\Sigma}_{0\lambda} = 10^2\mathbf{I}$, $r_0 = 4$, and $\mathbf{\Phi}_0 = \mathbf{I}_2$, and two different choices of $\alpha_1 = 1$, $\alpha_2 = 0.05$ and $\alpha_1 = 0.001$, $\alpha_2 = 0.001$ were used. The Bayesian estimates of unknown parameters under different prior inputs are presented in Table 13.3, which presents the parameter estimates under the above vague prior, and those under the prior with ML estimates of parameters as hyperparameters. The Bayesian estimates of unknown parameters under these two prior inputs are similar. In addition, similar estimated curves of unknown smooth functions under the vague prior input (not presented here) were obtained.

The results are interpreted as follows. First, all factor loadings are significant, indicating strong associations between latent factors and the corresponding observed variables. The loading on 'age of first arrest' is negative, indicating that patients involved in crime earlier in their lives tend to have a history of serious crime, which may be reflected in large numbers of incarcerations and arrests. Second, 'drug severity' and 'crime history' have negative impacts on 'retention', indicating that patients with more serious 'drug severity' and worse 'crime history' tend to have lower treatment retention. Therefore, some enforcement action might be necessary for these patients. For example, more attention should be given to patients who were young criminals or serious drug users. Third, the covariates that measure services and tests at the 3-month interview give a significant indication of retention measurement. x_1 is the mean value of a questionnaire about the treatment with 42 questions at the 3-month interview, which reflects the attitude of the patients toward the treatment after the first 3 months. x_2 and x_3 are numbers of tests the patients received in the first 3 months, which reflect how much attention is given to monitoring the treatment process. Patients who received more attention were likely to stay longer in treatment. Furthermore, the results from the 3-month interview can serve as an indicator to monitor and improve the treatment process. To decrease the number of dropouts from the treatment, special attention should be given to the patients who have less positive attitude toward the treatment and received few drug tests. Finally, 'retention' has negative impact on drug use in the 12-month follow-up interview, which indicates that longer treatment retention leads to less drug use at 12 months. This finding indicates a positive effect of the Proposition 36 treatment program in reducing drug abuse.

The program was written in R. The code is available from the website:
`www.wiley.com/go/medical_behavioral_sciences`

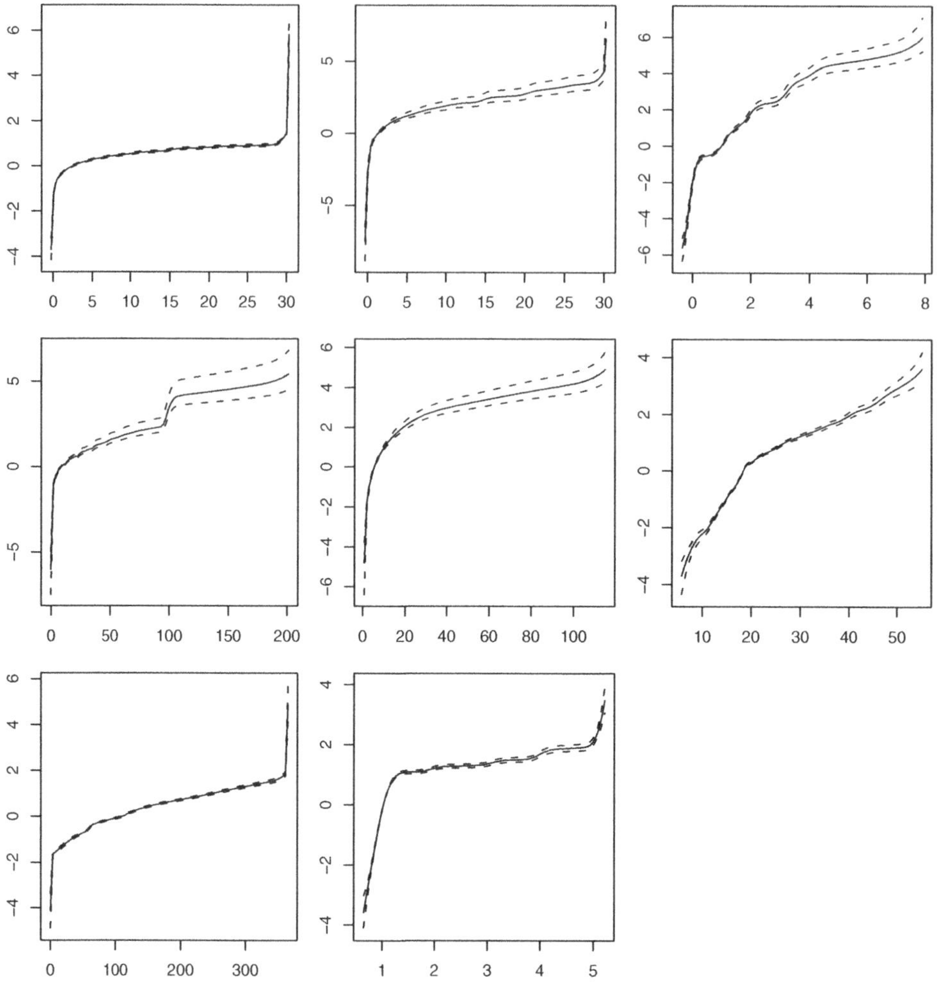

Figure 13.3 Estimates of the unknown transformation functions in the polydrug data example. The solid curves represent the pointwise posterior mean curves, while the dashed curves represent the 5% and 95% pointwise quantiles. Reproduced from Song, X. Y. and Lu, Z. H. Semiparametric transformation models with Bayesian P-splines. *Statistics and Computing* (to appear), with kind permission from Springer Science and Business Media.

13.8 Discussion

In this chapter a nonparametric transformation model was applied to analyze a data set involving highly nonnormal variables. Unlike traditional transformation methods such as the Box–Cox transformation, the current model formulates the unknown transformation function through Bayesian P-splines. To solve the difficulties encountered in the analysis, a modified constrained Bayesian P-splines approach incorporating powerful MCMC techniques was employed. A simulation study demonstrated that the transformation SEM and the methodology

Table 13.3 Bayesian estimates of parameters in the polydrug use data.

Par		Prior		Par		Prior	
		Vague	ML			Vague	ML
	Est	0.042	0.042		Est	3.08	3.22
a_1	SE	0.010	0.010	λ_2	SE	0.31	0.31
	Est	0.050	0.050		Est	0.84	0.77
a_2	SE	0.007	0.007	λ_3	SE	0.07	0.17
	Est	0.053	0.053		Est	−0.27	−0.25
a_3	SE	0.008	0.008	λ_4	SE	0.03	0.04
	Est	−0.008	−0.0008		Est	−0.21	−0.21
a_4	SE	0.0003	0.0003	λ_5	SE	0.07	0.07
	Est	4.99	4.44		Est	−0.08	−0.07
λ_1	SE	0.97	0.55	λ_6	SE	0.03	0.03

introduced perform satisfactorily in a commonly encountered highly skewed distribution. The methodology was applied to analyze a data set related to polydrug use intervention, in which observed variables were extremely nonnormal, such as U-shaped and highly skewed. Interesting findings were obtained.

There are some possible extensions of the current analysis. First, we only apply the Bayesian P-splines approach to estimate nonparametric transformation functions of the response variables. The methodology can be further extended to transform both sides of the model, as proposed by Carroll and Ruppert (1988). Second, more complicated distributions of residual errors can be considered to attain higher flexibility of modeling. Finally, when the observed nonnormal data are longitudinal, we can propose the following longitudinal transformation SEM:

$$\begin{aligned}\mathbf{f}_t(\mathbf{y}_{it}) &= \mathbf{A}_t\mathbf{x}_{it} + \boldsymbol{\Lambda}_t\boldsymbol{\omega}_{it} + \boldsymbol{\epsilon}_{it},\\ \boldsymbol{\eta}_{it} &= \boldsymbol{\Gamma}_t\mathbf{H}_t(\boldsymbol{\eta}_{i1}, \ldots, \boldsymbol{\eta}_{i,t-1}, \boldsymbol{\xi}_{i1}, \ldots, \boldsymbol{\xi}_{it}, \mathbf{z}_{i1}, \ldots, \mathbf{z}_{it}) + \boldsymbol{\delta}_{it},\end{aligned}$$

where $\boldsymbol{\omega}_{it} = (\boldsymbol{\eta}_{it}^T, \boldsymbol{\xi}_{it}^T)^T$ and the other terms are similarly defined as Chapter 9. This model is useful for analyzing the time-dependent interrelationships among longitudinal latent variables that are repeatedly measured via highly nonnormal observed variables over time.

References

Arminger, G., Stein, P. and Wittenberg, J. (1999) Mixtures of conditional mean- and covariance-structure models. *Psychometrika*, **64**, 475–494.

Bentler, P. M. (1983) Some contributions to efficient statistics in structural models: Specification and estimation of moment structures. *Psychometrika*, **48**, 493–517.

Bentler, P. M. and Dudgeon, P. (1996) Covariance structure analysis: Statistical practice, theory, and directions. *Annual Review of Psychology*, **47**, 563–592.

Bickel, P. J. and Doksum, K. A. (1981) An analysis of transformations revisited. *Journal of the American Statistical Association*, **76**, 296–311.

Biller, C. and Fahrmeir, L. (2001) Bayesian varying-coefficient models using adaptive regression splines. *Statistical Modelling*, **1**, 195–211.

Box, G. E. P. and Cox, D. R. (1964) An analysis of transformations. *Journal of the Royal Statistical Society, Series B*, **26**, 211–252.

Brezger, A. and Steiner, W. J. (2008) Monotonic regression based on Bayesian P-splines: An application to estimating price response functions from store-level scanner data. *Journal of Business & Economic Statistics*, **26**, 90–104.

Browne, M. W. (1984) Asymptotically distribution-free methods for the analysis of covariance structures. *British Journal of Mathematical and Statistical Psychology*, **37**, 62–83.

Carroll, R. J. and Ruppert, D. (1988) *Transformation and Weighting in Regression*. New York: Chapman & Hall.

Chen, M. H. and Schmeiser, B. (1993) Performance of the Gibbs, Hit-and-Run, and Metropolis samplers. *Journal of Computational and Graphical Statistics*, **2**, 251–272.

Chow, S. M., Tang, N. S., Yuan, Y., Song, X. Y. and Zhu, H. T. (2011) Bayesian estimation of semiparametric nonlinear dynamic factor analysis models using the Dirichlet process prior. *British Journal of Mathematical and Statistical Psychology*, **64**, 69–106.

David, M. R. (1993) On the beta transformation family. *Technometrics*, **35**, 72–81.

De Boor, C. (1978) *A Practical Guide to Splines*. New York: Springer-Verlag.

DiMatteo, I., Genovese, C. R. and Kass, R. E. (2001) Bayesian curve-fitting with free-knot splines. *Biometrika*, **88**, 1055–1071.

Dolan, C. V. and van der Maas, H. L. J. (1998) Fitting multivariage normal finite mixtures subject to structural equation modeling. *Psychometrika*, **63**, 227–253.

Eilers, P. H. C. and Marx, B. D. (1996) Flexible smoothing with B-splines and penalties. *Statistical Science*, **11**, 89–121.

Evans, E., Li, L. and Hser, Y. I. (2009) Client and program factors associated with dropout from court mandated drug treatment. *Evaluation and Program Planning*, **32**, 204–212.

Gelman, A. and Rubin, D. B. (1992) Inference from iterative simulation using multiple sequences. *Statistical Science*, **7**, 457–472.

Geman, S. and Geman, D. (1984) Stochastic relaxation, Gibbs distributions, and the Bayesian restoration of images. *IEEE Transactions on Pattern Analysis and Machine Intelligence*, **6**, 721–741.

Hastings, W. K. (1970) Monte Carlo sampling methods using Markov chains and their applications. *Biometrika*, **57**, 97–109.

He, X. and Shen, L. (1997) Linear regression after spline transformation. *Biometrika*, **84**, 474–481.

Hoeting, J. A., Raftery, A. E. and Madigan, D. (2002) Bayesian variable and transformation selection in linear regression. *Journal of Computational and Graphical Statistics*, **11**, 485–507.

Hu, L., Bentler, P. M. and Kano, Y. (1992) Can test statistics in covariance structure analysis be trusted? *Psychological Bulletin*, **112**, 351–362.

Jedidi, K., Jagpal, H. S. and DeSarbo, W. S. (1997) STEMM: A general finite mixture structural equation model. *Journal of Classification*, **14**, 23–50.

John, J. A. and Draper, N. R. (1980) An alternative family of transformations. *Applied Statistics*, **29**, 190–197.

Kano, Y., Bentler, P. M. and Mooijaart, A. (1993) Additional information and precision of estimators in multivariate structural models. In K. Matusita, M. L. Puri and T. Hayakawa (eds), *Statistical Sciences and Data Analysis*, pp. 187–196. Zeist: VSP International Science Publishers.

Lang, S. and Brezger, A. (2004) Bayesian P-splines. *Journal of Computational and Graphical Statistics*, **13**, 183–212.

Lee, S. Y., Lu, B. and Song, X. Y. (2008) Semiparametric Bayesian analysis of structural equation models with fixed covariates. *Statistics in Medicine*, **27**, 2341–2360.

Liu, J. S., Liang, F. and Wong, W. H. (2000) The Multiple-Try method and local optimization in Metropolis sampling. *Journal of the American Statistical Association*, **95**, 121–134.

Mallick, B. K. and Walker, S. (2003) A Bayesian semiparametric transformation model incorporating frailties. *Journal of Statistical Planning and Inference*, **112**, 159–174.

Metropolis, N., Rosenbluth, A. W., Rosenbluth, M. N., Teller, A. H. and Teller, E. (1953) Equation of state calculations by fast computing machines. *Journal of Chemical Physics*, **21**, 1087–1092.

Nychka, D. and Ruppert, D. (1995) Nonparametric transformations for both sides of a regression model. *Journal of the Royal Statistical Society, Series B*, **57**, 519–532.

Pericchi, L. R. (1981) A Bayesian approach to transformations to normality. *Biometrika*, **68**, 35–43.

Ramsay, J. O. (1988) Monotone regression splines in action. *Statistical Science*, **3**, 425–461.

Ramsay, J. O. (1998) Estimating smooth monotone functions. *Journal of the Royal Statistical Society, Series B*, **60**, 365–375.

Rue, H. and Held, L. (2005) *Gaussian Markov Random Fields: Theory and Applications*. Boca Raton, FL: Chapman & Hall/CRC.

Ruppert, D. (2001) Transformations of data. *International Encyclopedia of Social and Behavioral Sciences*. Amsterdam: Elsevier.

Shapiro, A. and Browne, M. W. (1987) Analysis of covariance structures under elliptical distributions. *Journal of the American Statistical Association*, **82**, 1092–1097.

Shi, J. Q. and Lee, S. Y. (2000) Latent variable models with mixed continuous and polytomous data. *Journal of the Royal Statistical Society, Series B*, **62**, 77–87.

Song, X. Y. and Lu, Z. H. (2010) Semiparametric latent variable models with Bayesian P-splines. *Journal of Computational and Graphical Statistics*, **19**, 590–608.

Song, X. Y. and Lu, Z. H. (2012) Semiparametric transformation models with Bayesian P-splines. *Statistics and Computing*, to appear.

Stephens, M. (2000) Bayesian analysis of mixture models with an unknown number of components – an alternative to reversible jump methods. *Annals of Statistics*, **28**, 40–74.

Van Montfort, K., Mooijaart, A. and Meijerink, F. (2009) Estimating structural equation models with non-normal variables by using transformations. *Statistica Neerlandica*, **63**, 213–226.

Yang, M. and Dunson, D. B. (2010) Bayesian semiparametric structural equation models with latent variables. *Psychometrika*, **75**, 675–693.

Yin, G. and Ibrahim, J. G. (2006) Bayesian transformation hazard models. In J. Rojo (ed.), *Optimality: The Second Erich L. Lehmann Symposium*, IMS Lecture Notes-Monograph Series Volume 49, pp. 170–182 Beachwood, OH: Institute of Mathematical Statistics.

Yuan, K. H., Chan, W. and Bentler, P. M. (2000) Robust transformation with applications to structural equation modelling. *British Journal of Mathematical and Statistical Psychology*, **53**, 31–50.

Yung, Y. F. (1997). Finite mixtures in confirmatory factor-analysis models. *Psychometrika*, **62**, 297–330.

14

Conclusion

In this book, we have introduced the Bayesian approach to analyze various types of structural equation models. Our choice is based on several of its advantages. As we have shown throughout this book, these advantages include the following. First, it can incorporate genuine prior information and/or knowledge in the analysis so that better results can be achieved. Second, as it does not depend on the asymptotic theory, it can provide more reliable results with moderate sample sizes. Third, it produces better estimates of latent variables than the classical methods. Fourth, the model comparison statistics, such as the Bayes factor and deviance information criterion, provide more reasonable and flexible tools than the classical likelihood ratio test in the maximum likelihood approach. Fifth, and finally, when coupled with data augmentation and MCMC methods, it can be efficiently and effectively applied to handle almost all complex models and/or data structures in substantive research in many fields.

As we have recognized, this book covers many comparatively well-known SEMs that are useful in practical research. These include nonlinear SEMs, SEMs with ignorable and/or nonignorable missing data, multisample SEMs, mixture SEMs, multilevel SEMs, and SEMs with variables from an exponential family. In addition, we have introduced a number of advanced SEMs that have recently been developed and have not been covered in any textbooks or reference books in the field. More specifically, a general latent curve model with second-order longitudinal variables, and a dynamic two-level SEM with a nonlinear auto-regressive structure equation are presented for analyzing various types of longitudinal data. A Bayesian semiparametric SEM, in which the explanatory latent variables in $\boldsymbol{\xi}_i$ are modeled with a general distribution through a truncated Dirichlet process with stick-breaking priors, is introduced to capture the true distribution of $\boldsymbol{\xi}_i$ and to handle some nonnormal data. We also present SEMs with unordered categorical variables for analyzing genotype variables which are frequently encountered in formulating models in many medical studies.

Basically, SEMs are regression models with latent variables. The measurement equation is a confirmatory factor analysis model which is used to identify the latent variables based on some prior knowledge of the observed variables. Clearly, this measurement equation can be

Basic and Advanced Bayesian Structural Equation Modeling: With Applications in the Medical and Behavioral Sciences,
First Edition. Xin-Yuan Song and Sik-Yum Lee.

regarded as a confirmatory tool. The interrelationships of latent variables are studied through the structural equation. In most SEM applications, the structural equation is used to assess the main hypotheses of the substantive study, and hence it is the most important component of the model. Parametric SEMs are formulated with a prespecified parametric structural equation. Hence, the structural equation is also confirmatory, as is the whole model. In many substantive studies, researchers may have no idea about the functional relationships among latent variables, so that they are unable to preassign a specific parametric form for the structural equation. Hence, it is important to develop SEMs with a general nonparametric structural equation. For nonparametric SEMs of this kind, the measurement equation is confirmatory while the structural equation is exploratory. In Chapter 12, we formulate and analyze nonparametric SEMs through Bayesian P-splines. The latter are also useful in developing transformation SEMs in Chapter 13, in which the highly nonnormal observed random variables, if they exist, are transformed through Bayesian P-splines into random variables whose distributions are close to normal. We demonstrate that this nonparametric transformation approach is effective in handling extremely nonnormal data.

Although this book provides a comprehensive coverage of topics in SEMs, there is plenty of room for further development. First of all, it is worth considering some combinations of the models and/or data structures that have been discussed. For example, for the dynamic two-level SEMs, it is desirable to use the Bayesian semiparametric approach with the truncated Dirichlet process to relax the distributional assumption of latent variables and/or residual errors. We expect that generalizations of this sort will be useful in practical applications. Another topic that has not been covered in this book is spatial SEMs; see for example, Liu *et al.* (2005). For this kind of model, the explanatory latent variables in the matrix $\Xi = (\boldsymbol{\xi}_1, \ldots, \boldsymbol{\xi}_n)$ are correlated in a certain manner. Hence, it is necessary to define a reasonable covariance structure for Ξ, and incorporate this structure in the development of the Bayesian methodologies. Another direction for further research relates to the treatment of outliers and/or influential observations. Based on the key ideas of Cook (1986) in influence analysis, methodologies based on the maximum likelihood (ML) approach have been developed; see Zhu and Lee (2001), Zhu *et al.* (2001), Lu and Song (2006), and, in particular, Song and Lee (2004a, 2004b) and Lee *et al.* (2006) in the field of SEMs. Recently, Zhu *et al.* (2011) developed a general Bayesian influence analysis for assessing various perturbation schemes for the data, the prior and the sampling distributions simultaneously. They have demonstrated some advantages of the Bayesian influence analysis over the traditional ML-based influence analysis approaches. On the other hand, Lee and Xia (2008), and Xia *et al.* (2009) have proposed robust Bayesian approaches for analyzing SEMs with outliers. They used the normal/independent distributions with random weights to model the covariance matrices of latent variables and error measurements for reducing the impacts of the outliers and distribution deviations. Naturally, their approach can be adopted to analyze some of the models considered in this book. Moreover, it is useful to develop efficient Bayesian methods with longitudinal SEMs for situations where the number of time points is large (e.g. real studies with functional data). Theoretically, the dynamic two-level SEM presented in Chapter 9 can be considered. However, as the number of parameters will increase dramatically with the number of time points, more efficient methods are needed. Finally, and perhaps most importantly, it is necessary to develop user-friendly software for applied researchers. WinBUGS (Spiegelhalter *et al.*, 2003) can be applied to analyze some of the SEMs discussed in this book. We also believe that some commercial software in the field is beginning to provide Bayesian results for some models.

However, for more advanced SEMs, such as the nonparametric SEMs and the transformation SEMs, user-friendly tailor-made software is still needed.

References

Cook, R. D. (1986). Assessment of local influence (with discussion). *Journal of the Royal Statistical Society, Series B*, **48**, 133–169.

Lee, S. Y. and Xia, Y. M. (2008) A robust Bayesian approach for structural equation models with missing data. *Psychometrika*, **73**, 343–364.

Lee, S. Y., Lu, B. and Song, X. Y. (2006) Assessing local influence for nonlinear structural equation models with ignorable missing data. *Computational Statistics and Data Analysis*, **50**, 1356–1377.

Liu, X., Wall, M. M. and Hodges J. S. (2005) Generalized spatial structural equation models. *Biostatistics*, **6**, 539–557.

Lu, B. and Song, X. Y. (2006) Local influence analysis of multivariate probit latent variable models. *Journal of Multivariate Analysis*, **97**, 1783–1798.

Song, X. Y. and Lee, S. Y. (2004a) Local influence of two-level latent variable models with continuous and polytomous data. *Statistica Sinica*, **14**, 317–332.

Song, X, Y. and Lee, S. Y. (2004b) Local influence analysis for mixture of structural equation models. *Journal of Classification*, **21**, 111–137.

Spiegelhalter, D. J., Thomas, A., Best, N. G. and Lunn, D. (2003) *WinBUGS User Manual. Version 1.4*. Cambridge: MRC Biostatistics Unit.

Xia, Y. M., Song, X. Y. and Lee, S. Y. (2009) Robustifying model fitting for the nonlinear structural equation model under normal theory. *British Journal of Mathematical and Statistical Psychology*, **62**, 529-568.

Zhu, H. T. and Lee, S. Y. (2001) Local influence for incomplete data models. *Journal of the Royal Statistical Society, Series B*, **63**, 111–126.

Zhu, H. T., Lee, S. Y., Wei, B. C. and Zhou, J. (2001) Case-deletion measures for models with incomplete data. *Biometrika*, **88**, 727–737.

Zhu, H. T., Ibrahim, J. G. and Tang, N. S. (2011) Bayesian influence analysis: A geometric approach. *Biometrika*, **98**, 307–323.

Index

Basic and Advanced Bayesian Structural Equation Modeling: With Applications in the Medical and Behavioral Sciences,
First Edition. Xin-Yuan Song and Sik-Yum Lee.

WILEY SERIES IN PROBABILITY AND STATISTICS
ESTABLISHED BY WALTER A. SHEWHART AND SAMUEL S. WILKS

The ***Wiley Series in Probability and Statistics*** is well established and authoritative. It covers many topics of current research interest in both pure and applied statistics and probability theory. Written by leading statisticians and institutions, the titles span both state-of-the-art developments in the field and classical methods.

Reflecting the wide range of current research in statistics, the series encompasses applied, methodological and theoretical statistics, ranging from applications and new techniques made possible by advances in computerized practice to rigorous treatment of theoretical approaches.

This series provides essential and invaluable reading for all statisticians, whether in academia, industry, government, or research.

† ABRAHAM and LEDOLTER • Statistical Methods for Forecasting
AGRESTI • Analysis of Ordinal Categorical Data, *Second Edition*
AGRESTI • An Introduction to Categorical Data Analysis, *Second Edition*
AGRESTI • Categorical Data Analysis, *Second Edition*
ALTMAN, GILL, and McDONALD • Numerical Issues in Statistical Computing for the Social Scientist
AMARATUNGA and CABRERA • Exploration and Analysis of DNA Microarray and Protein Array Data
ANDĚL • Mathematics of Chance
ANDERSON • An Introduction to Multivariate Statistical Analysis, *Third Edition*
* ANDERSON • The Statistical Analysis of Time Series
ANDERSON, AUQUIER, HAUCK, OAKES, VANDAELE, and WEISBERG • Statistical Methods for Comparative Studies
ANDERSON and LOYNES • The Teaching of Practical Statistics
ARMITAGE and DAVID (editors) • Advances in Biometry
ARNOLD, BALAKRISHNAN, and NAGARAJA • Records
* ARTHANARI and DODGE • Mathematical Programming in Statistics
* BAILEY • The Elements of Stochastic Processes with Applications to the Natural Sciences
BAJORSKI • Statistics for Imaging, Optics, and Photonics
BALAKRISHNAN and KOUTRAS • Runs and Scans with Applications
BALAKRISHNAN and NG • Precedence-Type Tests and Applications
BARNETT • Comparative Statistical Inference, *Third Edition*
BARNETT • Environmental Statistics
BARNETT and LEWIS • Outliers in Statistical Data, *Third Edition*
BARTHOLOMEW, KNOTT, and MOUSTAKI • Latent Variable Models and Factor Analysis: A Unified Approach, *Third Edition*
BARTOSZYNSKI and NIEWIADOMSKA-BUGAJ • Probability and Statistical Inference, *Second Edition*
BASILEVSKY • Statistical Factor Analysis and Related Methods: Theory and Applications
BATES and WATTS • Nonlinear Regression Analysis and Its Applications

*Now available in a lower priced paperback edition in the Wiley Classics Library.
†Now available in a lower priced paperback edition in the Wiley–Interscience Paperback Series.

BECHHOFER, SANTNER, and GOLDSMAN • Design and Analysis of Experiments for Statistical Selection, Screening, and Multiple Comparisons
BEIRLANT, GOEGEBEUR, SEGERS, TEUGELS, and DE WAAL • Statistics of Extremes: Theory and Applications
BELSLEY • Conditioning Diagnostics: Collinearity and Weak Data in Regression
† BELSLEY, KUH, and WELSCH • Regression Diagnostics: Identifying Influential Data and Sources of Collinearity
BENDAT and PIERSOL • Random Data: Analysis and Measurement Procedures, *Fourth Edition*
BERNARDO and SMITH • Bayesian Theory
BERZUINI • Causality: Statistical Perspectives and Applications
BHAT and MILLER • Elements of Applied Stochastic Processes, *Third Edition*
BHATTACHARYA and WAYMIRE • Stochastic Processes with Applications
BIEMER, GROVES, LYBERG, MATHIOWETZ, and SUDMAN • Measurement Errors in Surveys
BILLINGSLEY • Convergence of Probability Measures, *Second Edition*
BILLINGSLEY • Probability and Measure, *Anniversary Edition*
BIRKES and DODGE • Alternative Methods of Regression
BISGAARD and KULAHCI • Time Series Analysis and Forecasting by Example
BISWAS, DATTA, FINE, and SEGAL • Statistical Advances in the Biomedical Sciences: Clinical Trials, Epidemiology, Survival Analysis, and Bioinformatics
BLISCHKE AND MURTHY (editors) • Case Studies in Reliability and Maintenance
BLISCHKE AND MURTHY • Reliability: Modeling, Prediction, and Optimization
BLOOMFIELD • Fourier Analysis of Time Series: An Introduction, *Second Edition*
BOLLEN • Structural Equations with Latent Variables
BOLLEN and CURRAN • Latent Curve Models: A Structural Equation Perspective
BOROVKOV • Ergodicity and Stability of Stochastic Processes
BOSQ and BLANKE • Inference and Prediction in Large Dimensions
BOULEAU • Numerical Methods for Stochastic Processes
* BOX and TIAO • Bayesian Inference in Statistical Analysis
BOX • Improving Almost Anything, *Revised Edition*
* BOX and DRAPER • Evolutionary Operation: A Statistical Method for Process Improvement
BOX and DRAPER • Response Surfaces, Mixtures, and Ridge Analyses, *Second Edition*
BOX, HUNTER, and HUNTER • Statistics for Experimenters: Design, Innovation, and Discovery, *Second Editon*
BOX, JENKINS, and REINSEL • Time Series Analysis: Forcasting and Control, *Fourth Edition*
BOX, LUCEÑO, and PANIAGUA-QUIÑONES • Statistical Control by Monitoring and Adjustment, *Second Edition*
* BROWN and HOLLANDER • Statistics: A Biomedical Introduction
CAIROLI and DALANG • Sequential Stochastic Optimization
CASTILLO, HADI, BALAKRISHNAN, and SARABIA • Extreme Value and Related Models with Applications in Engineering and Science
CHAN • Time Series: Applications to Finance with R and S-Plus®, *Second Edition*
CHARALAMBIDES • Combinatorial Methods in Discrete Distributions
CHATTERJEE and HADI • Regression Analysis by Example, *Fourth Edition*
CHATTERJEE and HADI • Sensitivity Analysis in Linear Regression
CHERNICK • Bootstrap Methods: A Guide for Practitioners and Researchers, *Second Edition*
CHERNICK and FRIIS • Introductory Biostatistics for the Health Sciences
CHILÈS and DELFINER • Geostatistics: Modeling Spatial Uncertainty, *Second Edition*
CHOW and LIU • Design and Analysis of Clinical Trials: Concepts and Methodologies, *Second Edition*
CLARKE • Linear Models: The Theory and Application of Analysis of Variance
CLARKE and DISNEY • Probability and Random Processes: A First Course with Applications, *Second Edition*
* COCHRAN and COX • Experimental Designs, *Second Edition*

*Now available in a lower priced paperback edition in the Wiley Classics Library.
†Now available in a lower priced paperback edition in the Wiley–Interscience Paperback Series.

COLLINS and LANZA • Latent Class and Latent Transition Analysis: With Applications in the Social, Behavioral, and Health Sciences
CONGDON • Applied Bayesian Modelling
CONGDON • Bayesian Models for Categorical Data
CONGDON • Bayesian Statistical Modelling, *Second Edition*
CONOVER • Practical Nonparametric Statistics, *Third Edition*
COOK • Regression Graphics
COOK and WEISBERG • An Introduction to Regression Graphics
COOK and WEISBERG • Applied Regression Including Computing and Graphics
CORNELL • A Primer on Experiments with Mixtures
CORNELL • Experiments with Mixtures, Designs, Models, and the Analysis of Mixture Data, *Third Edition*
COX • A Handbook of Introductory Statistical Methods
CRESSIE • Statistics for Spatial Data, *Revised Edition*
CRESSIE and WIKLE • Statistics for Spatio-Temporal Data
CSÖRGŐ and HORVÁTH • Limit Theorems in Change Point Analysis
DAGPUNAR • Simulation and Monte Carlo: With Applications in Finance and MCMC
DANIEL • Applications of Statistics to Industrial Experimentation
DANIEL • Biostatistics: A Foundation for Analysis in the Health Sciences, *Eighth Edition*
* DANIEL • Fitting Equations to Data: Computer Analysis of Multifactor Data, *Second Edition*
DASU and JOHNSON • Exploratory Data Mining and Data Cleaning
DAVID and NAGARAJA • Order Statistics, *Third Edition*
DE ROCQUIGNY • Modelling Under Risk and Uncertainty: An Introduction to Statistical, Phenomenological and Computational Models
* DEGROOT, FIENBERG, and KADANE • Statistics and the Law
DEL CASTILLO • Statistical Process Adjustment for Quality Control
DEMARIS • Regression with Social Data: Modeling Continuous and Limited Response Variables
DEMIDENKO • Mixed Models: Theory and Applications
DENISON, HOLMES, MALLICK and SMITH • Bayesian Methods for Nonlinear Classification and Regression
DETTE and STUDDEN • The Theory of Canonical Moments with Applications in Statistics, Probability, and Analysis
DEY and MUKERJEE • Fractional Factorial Plans
DILLON and GOLDSTEIN • Multivariate Analysis: Methods and Applications
* DODGE and ROMIG • Sampling Inspection Tables, *Second Edition*
* DOOB • Stochastic Processes
DOWDY, WEARDEN, and CHILKO • Statistics for Research, *Third Edition*
DRAPER and SMITH • Applied Regression Analysis, *Third Edition*
DRYDEN and MARDIA • Statistical Shape Analysis
DUDEWICZ and MISHRA • Modern Mathematical Statistics
DUNN and CLARK • Basic Statistics: A Primer for the Biomedical Sciences, *Fourth Edition*
DUPUIS and ELLIS • A Weak Convergence Approach to the Theory of Large Deviations
EDLER and KITSOS • Recent Advances in Quantitative Methods in Cancer and Human Health Risk Assessment
* ELANDT-JOHNSON and JOHNSON • Survival Models and Data Analysis
ENDERS • Applied Econometric Time Series, *Third Edition*
† ETHIER and KURTZ • Markov Processes: Characterization and Convergence
EVANS, HASTINGS, and PEACOCK • Statistical Distributions, *Third Edition*
EVERITT, LANDAU, LEESE, and STAHL • Cluster Analysis, *Fifth Edition*
FEDERER and KING • Variations on Split Plot and Split Block Experiment Designs
FELLER • An Introduction to Probability Theory and Its Applications, Volume I, *Third Edition*, Revised; Volume II, *Second Edition*
FITZMAURICE, LAIRD, and WARE • Applied Longitudinal Analysis, *Second Edition*

*Now available in a lower priced paperback edition in the Wiley Classics Library.
†Now available in a lower priced paperback edition in the Wiley–Interscience Paperback Series.

* FLEISS • The Design and Analysis of Clinical Experiments
FLEISS • Statistical Methods for Rates and Proportions, *Third Edition*
† FLEMING and HARRINGTON • Counting Processes and Survival Analysis
FUJIKOSHI, ULYANOV, and SHIMIZU • Multivariate Statistics: High-Dimensional and Large-Sample Approximations
FULLER • Introduction to Statistical Time Series, *Second Edition*
† FULLER • Measurement Error Models
GALLANT • Nonlinear Statistical Models
GEISSER • Modes of Parametric Statistical Inference
GELMAN and MENG • Applied Bayesian Modeling and Causal Inference from Incomplete-Data Perspectives
GEWEKE • Contemporary Bayesian Econometrics and Statistics
GHOSH, MUKHOPADHYAY, and SEN • Sequential Estimation
GIESBRECHT and GUMPERTZ • Planning, Construction, and Statistical Analysis of Comparative Experiments
GIFI • Nonlinear Multivariate Analysis
GIVENS and HOETING • Computational Statistics
GLASSERMAN and YAO • Monotone Structure in Discrete-Event Systems
GNANADESIKAN • Methods for Statistical Data Analysis of Multivariate Observations, *Second Edition*
GOLDSTEIN • Multilevel Statistical Models, *Fourth Edition*
GOLDSTEIN and LEWIS • Assessment: Problems, Development, and Statistical Issues
GOLDSTEIN and WOOFF • Bayes Linear Statistics
GREENWOOD and NIKULIN • A Guide to Chi-Squared Testing
GROSS, SHORTLE, THOMPSON, and HARRIS • Fundamentals of Queueing Theory, *Fourth Edition*
GROSS, SHORTLE, THOMPSON, and HARRIS • Solutions Manual to Accompany Fundamentals of Queueing Theory, *Fourth Edition*
* HAHN and SHAPIRO • Statistical Models in Engineering
HAHN and MEEKER • Statistical Intervals: A Guide for Practitioners
HALD • A History of Probability and Statistics and their Applications Before 1750
† HAMPEL • Robust Statistics: The Approach Based on Influence Functions
HARTUNG, KNAPP, and SINHA • Statistical Meta-Analysis with Applications
HEIBERGER • Computation for the Analysis of Designed Experiments
HEDAYAT and SINHA • Design and Inference in Finite Population Sampling
HEDEKER and GIBBONS • Longitudinal Data Analysis
HELLER • MACSYMA for Statisticians
HERITIER, CANTONI, COPT, and VICTORIA-FESER • Robust Methods in Biostatistics
HINKELMANN and KEMPTHORNE • Design and Analysis of Experiments, Volume 1: Introduction to Experimental Design, *Second Edition*
HINKELMANN and KEMPTHORNE • Design and Analysis of Experiments, Volume 2: Advanced Experimental Design
HINKELMANN (editor) • Design and Analysis of Experiments, Volume 3: Special Designs and Applications
HOAGLIN, MOSTELLER, and TUKEY • Fundamentals of Exploratory Analysis of Variance
* HOAGLIN, MOSTELLER, and TUKEY • Exploring Data Tables, Trends and Shapes
* HOAGLIN, MOSTELLER, and TUKEY • Understanding Robust and Exploratory Data Analysis
HOCHBERG and TAMHANE • Multiple Comparison Procedures
HOCKING • Methods and Applications of Linear Models: Regression and the Analysis of Variance, *Second Edition*
HOEL • Introduction to Mathematical Statistics, *Fifth Edition*
HOGG and KLUGMAN • Loss Distributions
HOLLANDER and WOLFE • Nonparametric Statistical Methods, *Second Edition*
HOSMER and LEMESHOW • Applied Logistic Regression, *Second Edition*
HOSMER, LEMESHOW, and MAY • Applied Survival Analysis: Regression Modeling of Time-to-Event Data, *Second Edition*

*Now available in a lower priced paperback edition in the Wiley Classics Library.
†Now available in a lower priced paperback edition in the Wiley–Interscience Paperback Series.

HUBER • Data Analysis: What Can Be Learned From the Past 50 Years
HUBER • Robust Statistics
† HUBER and RONCHETTI • Robust Statistics, *Second Edition*
HUBERTY • Applied Discriminant Analysis, *Second Edition*
HUBERTY and OLEJNIK • Applied MANOVA and Discriminant Analysis, *Second Edition*
HUITEMA • The Analysis of Covariance and Alternatives: Statistical Methods for Experiments, Quasi-Experiments, and Single-Case Studies, *Second Edition*
HUNT and KENNEDY • Financial Derivatives in Theory and Practice, *Revised Edition*
HURD and MIAMEE • Periodically Correlated Random Sequences: Spectral Theory and Practice
HUSKOVA, BERAN, and DUPAC • Collected Works of Jaroslav Hajek—with Commentary
HUZURBAZAR • Flowgraph Models for Multistate Time-to-Event Data
INSUA, RUGGERI and WIPER • Bayesian Analysis of Stochastic Process Models
JACKMAN • Bayesian Analysis for the Social Sciences
† JACKSON • A User's Guide to Principle Components
JOHN • Statistical Methods in Engineering and Quality Assurance
JOHNSON • Multivariate Statistical Simulation
JOHNSON and BALAKRISHNAN • Advances in the Theory and Practice of Statistics: A Volume in Honor of Samuel Kotz
JOHNSON, KEMP, and KOTZ • Univariate Discrete Distributions, *Third Edition*
JOHNSON and KOTZ (editors) • Leading Personalities in Statistical Sciences: From the Seventeenth Century to the Present
JOHNSON, KOTZ, and BALAKRISHNAN • Continuous Univariate Distributions, Volume 1, *Second Edition*
JOHNSON, KOTZ, and BALAKRISHNAN • Continuous Univariate Distributions, Volume 2, *Second Edition*
JOHNSON, KOTZ, and BALAKRISHNAN • Discrete Multivariate Distributions
JUDGE, GRIFFITHS, HILL, LÜTKEPOHL, and LEE • The Theory and Practice of Econometrics, *Second Edition*
JUREK and MASON • Operator-Limit Distributions in Probability Theory
KADANE • Bayesian Methods and Ethics in a Clinical Trial Design
KADANE AND SCHUM • A Probabilistic Analysis of the Sacco and Vanzetti Evidence
KALBFLEISCH and PRENTICE • The Statistical Analysis of Failure Time Data, *Second Edition*
KARIYA and KURATA • Generalized Least Squares
KASS and VOS • Geometrical Foundations of Asymptotic Inference
† KAUFMAN and ROUSSEEUW • Finding Groups in Data: An Introduction to Cluster Analysis
KEDEM and FOKIANOS • Regression Models for Time Series Analysis
KENDALL, BARDEN, CARNE, and LE • Shape and Shape Theory
KHURI • Advanced Calculus with Applications in Statistics, *Second Edition*
KHURI, MATHEW, and SINHA • Statistical Tests for Mixed Linear Models
* KISH • Statistical Design for Research
KLEIBER and KOTZ • Statistical Size Distributions in Economics and Actuarial Sciences
KLEMELÄ • Smoothing of Multivariate Data: Density Estimation and Visualization
KLUGMAN, PANJER, and WILLMOT • Loss Models: From Data to Decisions, *Third Edition*
KLUGMAN, PANJER, and WILLMOT • Solutions Manual to Accompany Loss Models: From Data to Decisions, *Third Edition*
KOSKI and NOBLE • Bayesian Networks: An Introduction
KOTZ, BALAKRISHNAN, and JOHNSON • Continuous Multivariate Distributions, Volume 1, *Second Edition*
KOTZ and JOHNSON (editors) • Encyclopedia of Statistical Sciences: Volumes 1 to 9 with Index
KOTZ and JOHNSON (editors) • Encyclopedia of Statistical Sciences: Supplement Volume
KOTZ, READ, and BANKS (editors) • Encyclopedia of Statistical Sciences: Update Volume 1
KOTZ, READ, and BANKS (editors) • Encyclopedia of Statistical Sciences: Update Volume 2
KOWALSKI and TU • Modern Applied U-Statistics

*Now available in a lower priced paperback edition in the Wiley Classics Library.
†Now available in a lower priced paperback edition in the Wiley–Interscience Paperback Series.

KRISHNAMOORTHY and MATHEW • Statistical Tolerance Regions: Theory, Applications, and Computation
KROESE, TAIMRE, and BOTEV • Handbook of Monte Carlo Methods
KROONENBERG • Applied Multiway Data Analysis
KULINSKAYA, MORGENTHALER, and STAUDTE • Meta Analysis: A Guide to Calibrating and Combining Statistical Evidence
KULKARNI and HARMAN • An Elementary Introduction to Statistical Learning Theory
KUROWICKA and COOKE • Uncertainty Analysis with High Dimensional Dependence Modelling
KVAM and VIDAKOVIC • Nonparametric Statistics with Applications to Science and Engineering
LACHIN • Biostatistical Methods: The Assessment of Relative Risks, *Second Edition*
LAD • Operational Subjective Statistical Methods: A Mathematical, Philosophical, and Historical Introduction
LAMPERTI • Probability: A Survey of the Mathematical Theory, *Second Edition*
LAWLESS • Statistical Models and Methods for Lifetime Data, *Second Edition*
LAWSON • Statistical Methods in Spatial Epidemiology, *Second Edition*
LE • Applied Categorical Data Analysis, *Second Edition*
LE • Applied Survival Analysis
LEE • Structural Equation Modeling: A Bayesian Approach
LEE and WANG • Statistical Methods for Survival Data Analysis, *Third Edition*
LEPAGE and BILLARD • Exploring the Limits of Bootstrap
LESSLER and KALSBEEK • Nonsampling Errors in Surveys
LEYLAND and GOLDSTEIN (editors) • Multilevel Modelling of Health Statistics
LIAO • Statistical Group Comparison
LIN • Introductory Stochastic Analysis for Finance and Insurance
LITTLE and RUBIN • Statistical Analysis with Missing Data, *Second Edition*
LLOYD • The Statistical Analysis of Categorical Data
LOWEN and TEICH • Fractal-Based Point Processes
MAGNUS and NEUDECKER • Matrix Differential Calculus with Applications in Statistics and Econometrics, *Revised Edition*
MALLER and ZHOU • Survival Analysis with Long Term Survivors
MARCHETTE • Random Graphs for Statistical Pattern Recognition
MARDIA and JUPP • Directional Statistics
MARKOVICH • Nonparametric Analysis of Univariate Heavy-Tailed Data: Research and Practice
MARONNA, MARTIN and YOHAI • Robust Statistics: Theory and Methods
MASON, GUNST, and HESS • Statistical Design and Analysis of Experiments with Applications to Engineering and Science, *Second Edition*
McCULLOCH, SEARLE, and NEUHAUS • Generalized, Linear, and Mixed Models, *Second Edition*
McFADDEN • Management of Data in Clinical Trials, *Second Edition*
* McLACHLAN • Discriminant Analysis and Statistical Pattern Recognition
McLACHLAN, DO, and AMBROISE • Analyzing Microarray Gene Expression Data
McLACHLAN and KRISHNAN • The EM Algorithm and Extensions, *Second Edition*
McLACHLAN and PEEL • Finite Mixture Models
McNEIL • Epidemiological Research Methods
MEEKER and ESCOBAR • Statistical Methods for Reliability Data
MEERSCHAERT and SCHEFFLER • Limit Distributions for Sums of Independent Random Vectors: Heavy Tails in Theory and Practice
MENGERSEN, ROBERT, and TITTERINGTON • Mixtures: Estimation and Applications
MICKEY, DUNN, and CLARK • Applied Statistics: Analysis of Variance and Regression, *Third Edition*
* MILLER • Survival Analysis, *Second Edition*
MONTGOMERY, JENNINGS, and KULAHCI • Introduction to Time Series Analysis and Forecasting
MONTGOMERY, PECK, and VINING • Introduction to Linear Regression Analysis, *Fifth Edition*
MORGENTHALER and TUKEY • Configural Polysampling: A Route to Practical Robustness
MUIRHEAD • Aspects of Multivariate Statistical Theory

*Now available in a lower priced paperback edition in the Wiley Classics Library.
†Now available in a lower priced paperback edition in the Wiley–Interscience Paperback Series.

MULLER and STOYAN • Comparison Methods for Stochastic Models and Risks
MURTHY, XIE, and JIANG • Weibull Models
MYERS, MONTGOMERY, and ANDERSON-COOK • Response Surface Methodology: Process and Product Optimization Using Designed Experiments, *Third Edition*
MYERS, MONTGOMERY, VINING, and ROBINSON • Generalized Linear Models. With Applications in Engineering and the Sciences, *Second Edition*
NATVIG • Multistate Systems Reliability Theory With Applications
† NELSON • Accelerated Testing, Statistical Models, Test Plans, and Data Analyses
† NELSON • Applied Life Data Analysis
NEWMAN • Biostatistical Methods in Epidemiology
NG, TAIN, and TANG • Dirichlet Theory: Theory, Methods and Applications
OKABE, BOOTS, SUGIHARA, and CHIU • Spatial Tesselations: Concepts and Applications of Voronoi Diagrams, *Second Edition*
OLIVER and SMITH • Influence Diagrams, Belief Nets and Decision Analysis
PALTA • Quantitative Methods in Population Health: Extensions of Ordinary Regressions
PANJER • Operational Risk: Modeling and Analytics
PANKRATZ • Forecasting with Dynamic Regression Models
PANKRATZ • Forecasting with Univariate Box-Jenkins Models: Concepts and Cases
PARDOUX • Markov Processes and Applications: Algorithms, Networks, Genome and Finance
PARMIGIANI and INOUE • Decision Theory: Principles and Approaches
* PARZEN • Modern Probability Theory and Its Applications
PEÑA, TIAO, and TSAY • A Course in Time Series Analysis
PESARIN and SALMASO • Permutation Tests for Complex Data: Applications and Software
PIANTADOSI • Clinical Trials: A Methodologic Perspective, *Second Edition*
POURAHMADI • Foundations of Time Series Analysis and Prediction Theory
POWELL • Approximate Dynamic Programming: Solving the Curses of Dimensionality, *Second Edition*
POWELL and RYZHOV • Optimal Learning
PRESS • Subjective and Objective Bayesian Statistics, *Second Edition*
PRESS and TANUR • The Subjectivity of Scientists and the Bayesian Approach
PURI, VILAPLANA, and WERTZ • New Perspectives in Theoretical and Applied Statistics
† PUTERMAN • Markov Decision Processes: Discrete Stochastic Dynamic Programming
QIU • Image Processing and Jump Regression Analysis
* RAO • Linear Statistical Inference and Its Applications, *Second Edition*
RAO • Statistical Inference for Fractional Diffusion Processes
RAUSAND and HØYLAND • System Reliability Theory: Models, Statistical Methods, and Applications, *Second Edition*
RAYNER, THAS, and BEST • Smooth Tests of Goodnes of Fit: Using R, *Second Edition*
RENCHER • Linear Models in Statistics, *Second Edition*
RENCHER • Methods of Multivariate Analysis, *Second Edition*
RENCHER • Multivariate Statistical Inference with Applications
RIGDON and BASU • Statistical Methods for the Reliability of Repairable Systems
* RIPLEY • Spatial Statistics
* RIPLEY • Stochastic Simulation
ROHATGI and SALEH • An Introduction to Probability and Statistics, *Second Edition*
ROLSKI, SCHMIDLI, SCHMIDT, and TEUGELS • Stochastic Processes for Insurance and Finance
ROSENBERGER and LACHIN • Randomization in Clinical Trials: Theory and Practice
ROSSI, ALLENBY, and McCULLOCH • Bayesian Statistics and Marketing
† ROUSSEEUW and LEROY • Robust Regression and Outlier Detection
ROYSTON and SAUERBREI • Multivariate Model Building: A Pragmatic Approach to Regression Analysis Based on Fractional Polynomials for Modeling Continuous Variables
* RUBIN • Multiple Imputation for Nonresponse in Surveys
RUBINSTEIN and KROESE • Simulation and the Monte Carlo Method, *Second Edition*

*Now available in a lower priced paperback edition in the Wiley Classics Library.
†Now available in a lower priced paperback edition in the Wiley–Interscience Paperback Series.

RUBINSTEIN and MELAMED • Modern Simulation and Modeling
RYAN • Modern Engineering Statistics
RYAN • Modern Experimental Design
RYAN • Modern Regression Methods, *Second Edition*
RYAN • Statistical Methods for Quality Improvement, *Third Edition*
SALEH • Theory of Preliminary Test and Stein-Type Estimation with Applications
SALTELLI, CHAN, and SCOTT (editors) • Sensitivity Analysis
SCHERER • Batch Effects and Noise in Microarray Experiments: Sources and Solutions
* SCHEFFE • The Analysis of Variance
SCHIMEK • Smoothing and Regression: Approaches, Computation, and Application
SCHOTT • Matrix Analysis for Statistics, *Second Edition*
SCHOUTENS • Levy Processes in Finance: Pricing Financial Derivatives
SCOTT • Multivariate Density Estimation: Theory, Practice, and Visualization
* SEARLE • Linear Models
† SEARLE • Linear Models for Unbalanced Data
† SEARLE • Matrix Algebra Useful for Statistics
† SEARLE, CASELLA, and McCULLOCH • Variance Components
SEARLE and WILLETT • Matrix Algebra for Applied Economics
SEBER • A Matrix Handbook For Statisticians
† SEBER • Multivariate Observations
SEBER and LEE • Linear Regression Analysis, *Second Edition*
† SEBER and WILD • Nonlinear Regression
SENNOTT • Stochastic Dynamic Programming and the Control of Queueing Systems
* SERFLING • Approximation Theorems of Mathematical Statistics
SHAFER and VOVK • Probability and Finance: It's Only a Game!
SHERMAN • Spatial Statistics and Spatio-Temporal Data: Covariance Functions and Directional Properties
SILVAPULLE and SEN • Constrained Statistical Inference: Inequality, Order, and Shape Restrictions
SINGPURWALLA • Reliability and Risk: A Bayesian Perspective
SMALL and McLEISH • Hilbert Space Methods in Probability and Statistical Inference
SONG and LEE • Basic and Advanced Bayesian Structural Equation Modeling: With Applications in the Medical and Behavioral Sciences
SRIVASTAVA • Methods of Multivariate Statistics
STAPLETON • Linear Statistical Models, *Second Edition*
STAPLETON • Models for Probability and Statistical Inference: Theory and Applications
STAUDTE and SHEATHER • Robust Estimation and Testing
STOYAN • Counterexamples in Probability, *Second Edition*
STOYAN, KENDALL, and MECKE • Stochastic Geometry and Its Applications, *Second Edition*
STOYAN and STOYAN • Fractals, Random Shapes and Point Fields: Methods of Geometrical Statistics
STREET and BURGESS • The Construction of Optimal Stated Choice Experiments: Theory and Methods
STYAN • The Collected Papers of T. W. Anderson: 1943–1985
SUTTON, ABRAMS, JONES, SHELDON, and SONG • Methods for Meta-Analysis in Medical Research
TAKEZAWA • Introduction to Nonparametric Regression
TAMHANE • Statistical Analysis of Designed Experiments: Theory and Applications
TANAKA • Time Series Analysis: Nonstationary and Noninvertible Distribution Theory
THOMPSON • Empirical Model Building: Data, Models, and Reality, *Second Edition*
THOMPSON • Sampling, *Third Edition*
THOMPSON • Simulation: A Modeler's Approach
THOMPSON and SEBER • Adaptive Sampling
THOMPSON, WILLIAMS, and FINDLAY • Models for Investors in Real World Markets
TIERNEY • LISP-STAT: An Object-Oriented Environment for Statistical Computing and Dynamic Graphics
TSAY • Analysis of Financial Time Series, *Third Edition*
UPTON and FINGLETON • Spatial Data Analysis by Example, Volume II: Categorical and Directional Data

*Now available in a lower priced paperback edition in the Wiley Classics Library.
†Now available in a lower priced paperback edition in the Wiley–Interscience Paperback Series.

† VAN BELLE • Statistical Rules of Thumb, *Second Edition*
VAN BELLE, FISHER, HEAGERTY, and LUMLEY • Biostatistics: A Methodology for the Health Sciences, *Second Edition*
VESTRUP • The Theory of Measures and Integration
VIDAKOVIC • Statistical Modeling by Wavelets
VIERTL • Statistical Methods for Fuzzy Data
VINOD and REAGLE • Preparing for the Worst: Incorporating Downside Risk in Stock Market Investments
WALLER and GOTWAY • Applied Spatial Statistics for Public Health Data
WEISBERG • Applied Linear Regression, *Third Edition*
WEISBERG • Bias and Causation: Models and Judgment for Valid Comparisons
WELSH • Aspects of Statistical Inference
WESTFALL and YOUNG • Resampling-Based Multiple Testing: Examples and Methods for *p*-Value Adjustment
* WHITTAKER • Graphical Models in Applied Multivariate Statistics
WINKER • Optimization Heuristics in Economics: Applications of Threshold Accepting
WOODWORTH • Biostatistics: A Bayesian Introduction
WOOLSON and CLARKE • Statistical Methods for the Analysis of Biomedical Data, *Second Edition*
WU and HAMADA • Experiments: Planning, Analysis, and Parameter Design Optimization, *Second Edition*
WU and ZHANG • Nonparametric Regression Methods for Longitudinal Data Analysis
YIN • Clinical Trial Design: Bayesian and Frequentist Adaptive Methods
YOUNG, VALERO-MORA, and FRIENDLY • Visual Statistics: Seeing Data with Dynamic Interactive Graphics
ZACKS • Stage-Wise Adaptive Designs
* ZELLNER • An Introduction to Bayesian Inference in Econometrics
ZELTERMAN • Discrete Distributions—Applications in the Health Sciences
ZHOU, OBUCHOWSKI, and McCLISH • Statistical Methods in Diagnostic Medicine, *Second Edition*

*Now available in a lower priced paperback edition in the Wiley Classics Library.
†Now available in a lower priced paperback edition in the Wiley–Interscience Paperback Series.

Printed and bound by CPI Group (UK) Ltd, Croydon, CR0 4YY

27/10/2024

14580149-0004